# THE FALLING SICKNESS

# THE FALLING SICKNESS

A History of Epilepsy from the Greeks
to the Beginnings of Modern Neurology

OWSEI TEMKIN

Second Edition, Revised

THE JOHNS HOPKINS PRESS    BALTIMORE AND LONDON

The first edition of *The Falling Sickness* was published in 1945 as Volume IV in the Monograph Series of the Publications of the Institute of the History of Medicine, The Johns Hopkins University.

$\sqrt{c}$

Copyright © 1945, 1971 by The Johns Hopkins Press

Manufactured in the United States of America
The Johns Hopkins Press, Baltimore, Maryland 21218
The Johns Hopkins Press Ltd., London

Library of Congress Catalog Card Number 70-139522
ISBN 0-8018-1211-9

To the memory of

HENRY E. SIGERIST

# Preface to the Second Edition

More than twenty-five years have passed since this book was written. Faced with the choice between having it reprinted or revising it for a new edition, I have decided on the latter course, not only in order to correct mistakes and to consider new research but also in order to adapt the book to changing views of epilepsy. The influence of modern medical thought is inescapable even in a book that stops short of the present century. The advances made in neurosurgery, neurophysiology, and, above all, in electroencephalography, together with the use of new drugs, have introduced concepts, such as psychomotor epilepsy and temporal lobe epilepsy, which were as yet rare or non-existent at the writing of the first edition and have changed the meaning of others. If left unaltered, some parts of the book would have led to misunderstandings, and other parts would have seemed quite incomplete. In particular, the modern concern with temporal lobe epilepsy has made much of the work done in the later part of the nineteenth century appear in a new light. Here the changes and additions have been most substantial.

Yet a glimpse at the literature on the classification of the epilepsies published during the last two decades leaves little doubt that our knowledge of the disease is still very much in flux and far from offering a point of view secure enough to measure recent events with historical objectivity.

I have, therefore, decided to leave the character of the book unchanged. It has remained a history of epilepsy in Western civilization, and I have not extended it beyond the beginnings of modern neurology. There being no exact date for that beginning, the book does not end at any specific date. In general, the chronological limit has been extended into the eighties, rarely beyond 1890 except in the case of Hughlings Jackson, where it seemed advisable to avoid any arbitrary boundary.

Working on this new edition, I have again been vividly aware of the two opposing tendencies inherent in all historical works: to let the past speak for itself and to bring it near to the understanding of the modern reader. The copious quotations, even in the text, and restraint in the use of modern medical terminology are intended to allow the reader as much insight as possible into what past generations saw, thought, and expressed. For this reason, too, I have allowed a certain amount of repetitiousness in the descriptions of similar conditions (mainly of partial convulsions and psychic symptoms) at successive times. To avoid them altogether would have destroyed the picture of what was considered new or remarkable in a given period. On the other hand, by attempting to write a developmental history of the disease, I have unavoidably been guided by our modern interests, even where older opinions are contrary to our own.

A friendly critic raised the question whether this book really represented the history of a disease in the sense of the history of infectious diseases. I have tried to answer this question in the epilogue, where I have also elaborated some points I already made in the Preface to the first edition.

The appearance of *Epilepsy and Related Disorders*, by William G. and Margaret A. Lennox, has drawn my attention to much I had formerly overlooked, and I wish to acknowledge my indebtedness here beyond the citations in the footnotes. *Die Epilepsien*, by Dieter Janz, arrived too late to allow me to pay full justice to its many historical references. I wish to thank all those who have helped me by criticism or advice, particularly Erwin H. Ackerknecht, Dietrich Blumer, Gert Brieger, Harold Cherniss, Drossaart Lulofs, Franz Rosenthal, Walter Pagel, and A. Earl Walker.

My gratitude again goes to my wife, C. Lilian Temkin, for her stylistic assistance throughout this edition. I thank Mrs. Barbara Audi for her valuable secretarial work and the staffs of the Welch Medical Library and of the National Library of Medicine for their courteous help.

OWSEI TEMKIN

*The Johns Hopkins University*
*Institute of the History of Medicine*
*June, 1970*

# Preface to the
# First Edition

A history of epilepsy seems a premature, perhaps even a doubtful enterprise. There is no unanimity about the range of the concept of epilepsy, and the nature of the disease is as yet obscure. For, on the one hand, there are many organic diseases which may lead to the same syndrome as is exhibited in "genuine" epilepsy; on the other hand, it is very difficult, if not impossible, to draw a distinct borderline between epilepsy and certain cases of severe hysteria. The broader the point of view from which epilepsy is studied, the more the condition tends to lose its identity and merge into the domain of convulsive states, encompassing many "epilepsies" of different origin.

All these doubts and questions suggest that a history of epilepsy cannot be written in the manner in which, for instance, a history of tuberculosis might be approached. In the latter case we have definite and well-founded knowledge of the nature of the disease. This knowledge we can apply as a critical standard to the past and can separate the true from the false. At present such a procedure is not possible with regard to epilepsy, for we may easily decry as false what the future will prove to be true. Oliver Wendell Holmes once said: "If I wished to show a student the difficulties of getting at truth from medical experience, I would give him the history of epilepsy to read."[1] Such a history, however, if written from one arbitrary point of view, might easily be misleading rather than enlightening.

This being the case, there seems but one way left. We must above all find out what was meant by epilepsy, what symptoms were attributed to it, how it was explained and how treated. That means we must take the past seriously and try to understand it. And this implies that we must study the opinions of laymen, philosophers and theologians, as well as those of physicians. For this reason the popular name, "the falling sickness," known to every reader of Shakespeare's "Julius Caesar," seemed an appropriate title for this book.

---

[1] Oliver Wendell Holmes, *Medical Essays* (Boston and New York: Houghton, Mifflin and Co. [1891]), p. 192. This passage has been used as a motto by Von Storch for his "Essay on the History of Epilepsy."

After what has been said, it will become understandable why this book has to deal with many cultural aspects of epilepsy. Nevertheless, certain limits have been imposed upon its scope. Much has been written about the connection of epilepsy with prehistoric trephining. The existence of trephining in prehistoric times is a fact, but its connection with epilepsy rests on speculation and analogies. To start out with such speculations might easily become prejudicial to the understanding of the later course of events. I have, therefore, disregarded these problematic beginnings, just as I have left out a discussion of epilepsy in Eastern civilizations, in present folk medicine, and among primitive people. The ideas and practices of ancient India, China, and Japan have had little direct influence upon the development of our ideas regarding epilepsy, and the unclear chronology of their literatures makes the evaluation of any such influence almost impossible. Present folk medicine is largely a result of medical and popular thought of the past, modified according to local customs and traditions. As far as its older roots are concerned, they have found their place in the historical discussion, which an enumeration of local variations would only have served to divert from the main current. A more serious objection can be raised to the almost complete omission of primitive medicine. The existence of some basic beliefs current among all men may thereby have been overlooked. I have, nevertheless, taken this risk, because I believe that in the present state of anthropology a mere glimpse at some books on primitive medicine is no longer sufficient. To be of any value the subject would have to be studied carefully and in detail, a task quite beyond the scope of a *history* of epilepsy. By not confusing history and anthropology, I hope to present the historical material in a form which can more easily be compared with the findings of the anthropologist.

Thus, the book begins with the ancient Greeks who have left us the earliest Western writings on epilepsy, and it continues to the point where the historical perspective ends and the present debate begins. This point seemed to me to lie about the year 1880, when the impact of Jackson's and Charcot's work made itself felt. Hughlings Jackson outlined a neurological theory of epilepsy, while Charcot, on the other hand, separated epilepsy and hysteria more emphatically than any of his predecessors had done. Both men confined epilepsy to the realm of neurology, thereby dissolving the vague but more comprehensive concept of "the falling sickness." This separation was not the final word, but it impressed itself strongly upon the mind of a generation. For a book on "the falling sickness," this seemed the proper place to stop. Some readers will possibly be disappointed that the whole history of the last sixty years has been left out. Since I am not a neurologist, it would have been presumptuous on my part to pass judgment on the work of recent decades. Yet without a critical evaluation, the undertaking would have become a mere catalogue of thousands of names, a bar rather than a help to a better understanding of the present.

Nobody will expect a solution of strictly medical questions from a historical book. Its aim throughout is to understand the past and thereby help to understand the setting of present problems. Antiquity has been dealt with more thoroughly than any other period, because the ancient inheritance formed the backbone of knowledge far down into modern times. But I have nowhere aimed at completeness; rather I have tried to obtain a picture of the thought of the different periods. That such a procedure is not without danger I am fully aware. The material used is only a fraction of the tremendous literature written on the subject and I may easily have overlooked material which would give a quite different aspect.

There are few tasks more fascinating in medical history than to interpret medical ideas in the light of contemporary political, social, and cultural situations. As far as possible, however, I have resisted the temptation of sketching a picture of general historical events, trying to make the history of epilepsy fit into the pattern. The history of epilepsy is such a complicated network of confused and conflicting trends that oversimplification as well as unwarranted inferences had to be avoided and interpretation of the material seemed to be the main task.

Epilepsy has long attracted the interest of many able historians. Of recent authors I wish to name here Von Storch and Kanner who have investigated the subject from a medical and cultural point of view. Baumann in his *De Heilige Ziekte* and his shorter articles in *Janus* has particularly interested himself in the ancient history of the disease. In Baumann's work the reader may find a view somewhat different from mine. The history of epilepsy is so closely interwoven with the history of neurology on the one hand and with that of magic on the other, that I must mention two standard works here which otherwise I should have to quote on almost every page. These books are Soury's *Le système nerveux central* and Thorndike's *History of Magic and Experimental Science*. They give the general background; I have studied only one isolated disease.

I am grateful to Dr. W. G. Lennox of Boston who kindly lent me the manuscript of English translations from several medieval medical authors who had written on epilepsy. This enabled me to get a quick preliminary orientation in this particular period. Professor W. F. Albright kindly helped me in interpreting the Arabic passages quoted on p. 107, footnote 133. Personal conversations with Norbert Elias, in 1938, as well as his book *Über den Prozess der Zivilisation* have been stimulating and have turned my thoughts to points which I might perhaps otherwise have overlooked. My colleague Ludwig Edelstein has drawn my attention to several important passages in ancient authors.

The close intimacy of our work makes it impossible for me to remember all the instances where his suggestions were helpful to me and I wish therefore to thank him in this place for the active interest he has taken. Above all I have to thank my wife, C. Lilian Temkin, on whose stylistic help I have relied throughout this book. She has read and corrected the manuscript and has rendered in poetical form the translations from Callimachus, Orpheus, Nonnus, and Quintus Serenus.

In expressing my gratitude to the above, I need hardly add that the responsibility for the contents of this book rests on me alone.

The secretarial assistance rendered by Miss Virginia Davidson and Miss Janet Brock was particularly helpful in preparing the manuscript for the printer.

The publication of this book was made possible by the appropriation of a substantial grant from the Epilepsy Medical Research Fund of The Johns Hopkins University for which I wish to express my sincere appreciation.

OWSEI TEMKIN

*The Johns Hopkins University*
*Institute of the History of Medicine*

# Contents

# Illustrations

## BIBLIOGRAPHICAL NOTE

The numbers in parentheses following authors' names in the footnotes refer to the bibliography at the end of the book, where more complete references will be found.

The indication of title, book, chapter, etc. in footnotes citing primary historical source material is intended to facilitate the reader's orientation and (in the case of older authors) make him independent of any particular edition.

# THE FALLING SICKNESS

# PART ONE

# ANTIQUITY

# I
# Epilepsy: The Sacred Disease

## 1. THE CONCEPT OF THE SACRED DISEASE

Diseases can be considered as acts or invasions by gods, demons, or evil spirits, and treated by the invocation of supposedly supernatural powers. Or they are considered the effects of natural causes and are consequently treated by natural means. In the struggle between the magic and the scientific conception, the latter has gradually emerged victorious in the western world. The fight has been long and eventful, and in it epilepsy held one of the key positions. Showing both physical and psychic symptoms, epilepsy more than any other disease was open to interpretation both as a physiological process and as the effect of spiritual influences. And whereas purely mental afflictions, such as neuroses and certain maniac and melancholic reactions, often were, and even are, not recognized as pathological, epilepsy, on the other hand, was always considered a disease.

There is no reason to assume that epilepsy as it is known today spared prehistoric man. Whether or not he tried to cure it by trephining, i.e., by making a hole in the skull, a practice preserved into historical times and also found among many so-called primitives, remains a moot question.[1] The old age of the disease is attested by the fact that the Mesopotamian civilizations took account of the epileptic attack. An Accadian text speaks of a person whose neck turns left, whose hands and feet are tense and eyes wide open, froth flowing from the mouth and consciousness

---

[1]For literature on prehistoric and primitive trephining see Margetts (669).

being lost. This is diagnosed as *antašubbû* and related to "the hand of
Sin," the god of the moon, by the exorciser.[2] As soon as a rational
pathology was established, claiming to explain all diseases as merely
physical processes, its explanation of epilepsy became the test for the
validity and persuasive power of the whole system. Accordingly, the
history of epilepsy becomes, at the same time, an example of the history of magic beliefs and of their refutation by scientists and scientific
physicians.

The battle is first recorded in the book *On the Sacred Disease* in the
Hippocratic collection of medical writings from about the year 400 B.C.
This is not only the first monograph on epilepsy that we possess, but
also one of the most important documents extant of magic beliefs and
practices in ancient Greece and of their place in the religious
development of that civilization.[3] The book is written by a physician,
but it is addressed to an audience of laymen. It is an attack against
popular superstition and magicians, wizards, and charlatans who termed
the disease "sacred." This alleged divine character, the author says, is
only a shelter for ignorance and fraudulent practices. The assumption
of the gods being its cause reveals those people as fundamentally
impious, for the gods do not make men's bodies unclean as the magicians would have them believe. Epilepsy is not more divine than other
diseases are. Like all diseases, it is hereditary; its cause lies in the brain,
a brain overflowing with a superfluity of phlegm. When the phlegm
rushes into the blood vessels of the body it causes all the symptoms of
the attack. The releasing factors of the attack are cold, sun, and winds,
which change the consistency of the brain. These cosmic phenomena
the author considers divine, but since they influence all diseases all
diseases are divine, though human at the same time because of their
physiological substratum.[4] Epilepsy, therefore, can and must be treated
not by magic but by diet and drugs, provided that it has not yet
become chronic.

----

[2] See Labat (603), pp. 80–81, and ch. 26, pp. 188–99, where *antašubbû* is mentioned
repeatedly. Kinnier Wilson (583), p. 41 ff., and (582), pp. 201–3, also takes *antašubbû* as
meaning epilepsy. His interpretation of *bēl ūri* as "minor epileptic attack" does not seem to me
sufficiently supported. On *bennū* see below, footnotes 320 and 321. Regarding ancient Egypt,
Wilson, in Pritchard (825), p. 26 note 13, refers to the determinative of a word that means
prophetically possessed, and that "shows a human figure in violent motion or epileptic convulsion." This is not pathognomonic. For Ebbell's (305) alleged identification of epilepsy cf.
Temkin (1004), p. 128. In the Persian *Zend-Avesta* (67), p. 77, the goddess informs Zarathustra
that epileptics (*Fallsüchtige*) are forbidden to sacrifice to her; cf. Fichtner (355), p. 27. I do not
know whether the translation of "epileptics" is above suspicion.

[3] Cf. Lanata (608), who puts *On the Sacred Disease* in the center of her discussions. In this
connection see also Kudlien (598).

[4] The correlation of divine and natural in the book has recently been discussed by Nörenberg
(738). Miller (701) believes that the author follows Diogenes of Apollonia in accepting the air
as divine, because the air is the intelligent cosmic principle.

Thus, the history of epilepsy opens with the fundamental statement that the seat of the disease is in the brain. The author goes even further: the brain is the organ of all psychic processes both normal and pathological; not only epilepsy, but all mental diseases as well, can be explained by disturbances of the brain.[5] The identity of the author of this book is not known. He is one of the many anonymous physicians whose writings go under the name of Hippocrates. In the third century already, the book was included in one of the early "Hippocratic" editions.[6] Many of the ancients, like the scholars Erotianus and Soranus,[7] referred to it as Hippocratic; others, however, like Galen, seem to have been doubtful of its authenticity.[8] The Arabs listed it among the works of Hippocrates as "a book on the divine disease,"[9] though it is not quite certain whether it was ever wholly translated into their language. It is even more dubious whether the medieval doctors read it, for no medieval Latin translation has been found so far, and the references to it in the scholastic writings are too vague to allow definite conclusions.[10] When in the beginning of the sixteenth century the works of Hippocrates were edited, a note was found in some of the manuscripts stating that Galen had thought the work spurious and not congruous with the style and acumen of Hippocrates.[11] This note was reprinted in the Latin and Greek editions and, although the statement could not be found in the extant works of Galen, it certainly increased the doubts as

---

[5]The authenticity of chapters 14-17, which outline this idea, is disputed. But regardless of whether these chapters originally were or were not an integral part of the book, the manuscript tradition [see Rivier (854)] shows them integrated by late Antiquity, and the book constituted a unit from then on. Temkin (999) states reasons for considering chapters 14-17 genuine; see also Grensemann (429), pp. 25 f. and 98-101. For other opinions pro and con cf. Flashar (363), p. 30, footnote 15.

[6]According to Wellmann (1078), p. 2, it was contained in the edition prepared by Bakcheios.

[7]For Erotianus cf. Nachmanson (728), p. 326. For Soranus cf. Caelius Aurelianus (192), Morb. chron., I, 4, par. 131: "Hippocrates de epilepsia scribens communiter ait" etc. The Anonymus Parisinus (384), p. 77 apparently also refers to this writing, cf. Temkin (1000), pp. 142-43.

[8]Galen (392), In Hippocratis prognosticum comment., I, 4; p. 206, 13 ff. According to Diller (280), p. 168 and Edelstein (315), col. 1316, Galen here appears doubtful of Hippocrates' authorship. The classical references to the book are to be found in Grensemann (429), pp. 46-49, who offers the most recent edition (with German translation) of the Greek text of On the Sacred Disease.

[9]Ibn Abī Uṣaibi'ah (524), 'Uyūn al-anbā' fī ṭabāgāt al-aṭibbā', p. 33, 6: kitābun fī l-maraḍi l-'ilāhīyi. Ḥunain ibn Isḥāq, in his translation of Galen's (389), Compendium of Plato's Timaeus, p. 30, 14 (Arabic text) also speaks of al-maraḍu lladī yud'ā l-'ilāhīyu. I take this to correspond to τὸ νόσημα τὸ ἱερὸν καλούμενον in the Galenic text. I see no reason why Galen should have substituted θεῖον for the Platonic ἱερόν. See also below, pp. 45 and 151.

[10]Cf. below, IV-2.

[11]Cf. Littré in Hippocrates (491), vol. 1, p. 354 and Grensemann (429), p. 48. For the history of the book cf. also Dietz (490), pp. 78-93, and for an evaluation of its author cf. Diller (279). The authenticity of the book is still discussed. Pohlenz (816), p. 93, doubts that the author was dependent upon Alcmaeon and (p. 67) considers it a genuine work of Hippocrates. Edelstein (313), p. 133 ff., attacks any such attempts at identification.

to the authorship of Hippocrates. This question of authorship was not a
mere antiquarian problem. The author's pure religious views brought
him near to the Christian physicians of the sixteenth and following
centuries: ". . . it appears that this author was very pious and as far as
those (i.e., heathen) times allowed, held very religious views about the
gods," remarks Mercurialis in his edition of 1588.[12] Such sentiments
were especially shared by men like Weyer and Richard Mead, who considered him an ally in their fight against superstition. When, therefore,
in about 1700, Hippocrates was accused of atheism, the accusers denied
his authorship, whereas his defenders insisted emphatically upon it.[13]

To some degree then, the tradition of this book reflects the attitude
of physicians toward the claims of religion and magic. Not always were
the views of its author supported by his medical successors. But for the
physicians of his own period they apparently contained nothing revolu-
tionary and were shared by other writers of the Hippocratic corpus.
The idea of all diseases being equally divine was also advanced in the
writing On Airs, Waters, Places.[14] The magicians' practice of making
women who recovered from phobia sacrifice valuables to the goddess
Artemis was condemned as fraudulent in the short treatise On Virgins'
Diseases.[15] Wherever epilepsy is mentioned by the Hippocratics, it is
always explained and viewed naturally. Most of them must have opposed the popular concepts implied in the name of the "so-called"
sacred disease, as the author of the book termed it;[16] in his opinion the
assumption of its divine character arose from the inexperience and
amazement of people to whom it seemed quite different from all other
diseases.

This is perhaps the oldest attempt at explaining this mysterious
name, but it did not remain the only one. Plato, himself a younger
contemporary of Hippocrates, thought the name justified because the
disease disturbed the revolutions in the head, and these were the most
divine.[17] This idea, variously repeated,[18] is clearly of late philosophical
origin. For in older times, when the name arose, the diaphragm (or the
lungs) and the heart were considered the seat of the soul, rather than

[12]Mercurialis (683), Hippocratis Coi opera, t. II, p. 356: "quo in loco etiam apparet auc-
torem hunc valde pium fuisse, et prout ea tempora patiebantur de Diis religiose sensisse."

[13]Cf. Triller (1031), Hippocrates atheismo falso accusatus, pp. 103–5. For the history of
this curious dispute cf. Deichgräber (260), p. 56 ff.

[14]Hippocrates (489), ed. Jones, vol. 2, p. 131. Like some others before him, Grensemann
(429) tries to identify the author of this work with the author of On the Sacred Disease; he
offers the arguments pro and con on pp. 7–18. I do not believe that the issue can be decided
merely on the basis of similarities of style and content.

[15]Hippocrates (491), ed. Littré, vol. 8, p. 468.

[16]Cf. the opening sentence of On the Sacred Disease.

[17]Plato (802), Timaeus, 85 A–B; p. 228.

[18]Cf. Apuleius (43), Apologia, 50.—Caelius Aurelianus (192), Morb. chron., I, 4, p. 60:
"Appellatur . . . et sacra . . . sive quod in capite fiat quod multorum philosophorum iudicio
sacrum atque templum est partis animae in corpore natae."

the brain.[19] Another explanation, according to which the disease was called sacred or divine (*morbus divinus, lues deifica*)[20] on account of its greatness, "for the crowd has called great things sacred,"[21] seems not less artificial.[22] But it would at least find a certain corroboration in the probability that the Hippocratic corpus already used the name "great disease" for epilepsy,[23] a term which over the Latin "morbus maior"[24] found its way into medieval French as "grand mal"[25] and has now become a designation for the great epileptic attack.

The very variety of explanations proferred by the ancients shows that they themselves could only speculate about the true meaning of the name.[26] But their suggestions at least reveal some of the popular beliefs surrounding epilepsy. The disease might have been called sacred because a deity had sent it,[27] or because a demon had been thought to enter the patient, or because it attacked those who had sinned against Selene, the goddess of the moon.[28] Furthermore, it might have acquired its name because its cure was not human but divine.[29] At the bottom of all these alleged reasons lies the basic belief that the disease is an infliction or possession by a higher power and that its cure must be supernatural. So, in order to prevent and cure the disease, it seems necessary to the superstitious to find out the powers which might inflict it, to remember all the transgressions which might offend them, and, finally, to know all procedures and remedies which could ward them off or conquer them. In this way a whole system of superstitions developed, held together by those analogies, associations, instinctive certainties, and animistic images which are so hard to explain in purely rational terms. The medical lore of most primitive people shows examples of this magic conception; it is found in almost all civilizations and looms behind many strange beliefs of present-day folk medicine.[30]

---

[19] Cf. Temkin (999), p. 300. According to Onians (752), p. 24 ff., *phrenes* originally meant the lungs.

[20] Apuleius, *l. c.*, Caelius Aurelianus (192), *Morb. acut.*, II, 30, par. 162.

[21] Caelius Aurelianus (192), *Morb. chron.*, I, 4, par. 60: "... sive ob magnitudinem passionis. maiora enim vulgus sacra vocavit." Similarly Aretaeus (49), ed. Hude, III, 4, p. 38, 27–29.

[22] As pointed out by Haupt (463), p. 313.

[23] Cf. Temkin (999), p. 315.

[24] Celsus (212), *De medicina*, III, 23; vol. 1, p. 332.

[25] Cf. Du Cange (301), vol. 5, p. 517.

[26] Aretaeus (50), ed. Adams, p. 297, seems to have been conscious of this. After having listed several possible explanations (cf. the following footnotes) he adds: "from some one, or all these causes together, it has been called Sacred" (Adams' translation).

[27] Caelius Aurelianus (192), *Morb. chron.*, I, 4, par. 60.

[28] Aretaeus (49), ed. Hude, III, 4; p. 38, 26–31.

[29] Aretaeus, *ibid.* The suggestions of Aretaeus and Caelius Aurelianus are partly corroborated by Galen in his commentary on Plato's *Timaeus*; cf. Galen (393), *In Platonis Timaeum commentarii fragmenta*, pp. 29–30.

[30] Cf. particularly Hovorka-Kronfeld (516), vol. 2, p. 209 ff., and Kanner (571).

In the latter it is partly a native creation, but partly it is inherited from Antiquity, just as the very name "sacred disease" has still survived in "dat hillig" and "heiliges weh" in Mecklenburg and Alsace.[31]

The presence of a god or demon during the attack tended to give it a certain social significance. These gods and demons were dreaded, and the epileptic fit constituted a bad omen. The Romans called epilepsy the *morbus comitialis*, and they themselves attributed the name to the fact that an epileptic attack used to spoil the day of the *comitia*, the assembly of the people.[32] Quintus Serenus, the poet-physician of the third century A.D., begins his chapter "To drive away the *morbus comitialis*," with the following explanation of the name:

> A kind of sudden sickness 'tis, whose name has clung
> Since of the votes a true count it prevents.
> For often has this dread disease the people's council stopped,
> When members down in fatal weakness fell. And God himself
> Through changing phases of the unstable moon
> Proclaims conception of a man oft thus to be out-stretched.[33]

The epileptic himself was unclean; whoever touched him might become a prey to the demon. By spitting one tried to keep the demon away and thus escape infection. In his characterization of the superstitious, Theophrastus adds to the description: "When he sees a madman or an epileptic, he shudders and spits in his bosom,"[34] and 300 years later Pliny admits frankly: "In cases of epilepsy we spit, that is, we throw back contagion."[35] Among the Romans this custom must have been widespread, for it seems as if the mentioning of "the disease which is spit upon" in a play was a clear enough allusion to suggest epilepsy or madness to the audience.[36] Of an epileptic slave, Thallus, it is said that his fellow slaves used to spit, that "nobody dares to eat with him from the same dish or to drink from the same cup," and it is even suspected that he has been sent away "lest he contaminate the family."[37]

---

[31]Cf. Höfler (498), p. 227.

[32]Cf. Festus (354), *De verborum significatu*, p. 268, 13-22, s.v. Prohibere comitia.

[33]Quintus Serenus (916), *Liber medicinalis*, 56; p. 48. Johann Agricola as quoted by Martin (671), p. 108, attributed the name *morbus comitialis* to the tendency of epileptics to suffer attacks in crowded places: "Denn die lewtte, welche hie mit beschwerdt sind, fallen gemainiglich wo vil lewte sind, vielleicht von dem brunst vnd athem viler lewtte." Erasmus was acquainted with this explanation of the name, cf. Nicolson (733), p. 31.

[34]Theophrastus (1010), *Characters*, 16; p. 82.

[35]Pliny (806), *Naturalis historia*, 28, 35; vol. 4, p. 162.

[36]Plautus (805), *The Captives*, III, 4, 550 ff.; p. 514: "et illic isti qui insputatur morbus interdum venit." This has commonly been interpreted as meaning epilepsy. The context of the whole scene, however, suggests madness rather than epilepsy, and the alleged patient himself asks (*ibid.*): "Insanum esse me?" It should be kept in mind that according to Theophrastus the superstitious spat out before both madmen and epileptics.

[37]Apuleius (43), *Apologia*, 44, 11.

The magic conception according to which epilepsy was a contagious disease was one of the factors which made the epileptic's life miserable and gave him a social stigma. For it was a disgraceful disease. The epileptic who felt an attack coming on rushed home, or to a deserted place where as few as possible could see him fall, and covered his head. And whether he did it from shame for the disease, as the author of *On the Sacred Disease* thinks, or from fear of the deity, as the crowd believed,[38] his behavior was the same as that of the murderer who fled, his head covered.[39] Another closely related factor was the interpretation of the disease as a sign of sin: "But also it is reckoned a disgraceful form of disease; for it is supposed, that it is an infliction on persons who have sinned against the Moon."[40] Finally, the repulsive sight of the attack must have contributed to the feeling of aversion: "The sight of a paroxysm is disagreeable, and its departure disgusting with spontaneous evacuations of the urine and of the bowels."[41] All this together had the result that "if through treatment the man endures, he lives suffering shame, disgrace, and pain."[42]

To the ancients the epileptic was an object of horror and disgust and not a saint or prophet as has sometimes been contended. That the ancients, indeed, did not expect prophetic gifts of him is best illustrated by the *Apology* of the Roman author Apuleius, the contemporary of Galen. The whole book is a speech delivered by Apuleius in his own defense when accused of magical practices. His accusers had observed that a boy, the slave Thallus, had fallen down in his presence, and they had attributed this to some malevolent sorcery. Apuleius, however, points out that this boy was subject to epilepsy and that this natural explanation of his fall in itself refuted the possibility that he might have used the boy to obtain prophecies. For only pure and healthy boys, he adds, would, according to Plato, become mouthpieces of the gods. An epileptic would not be fit for such an office and would therefore have been useless as a medium for magical procedures.[43] Apuleius takes great pains to prove that Thallus really suffered from epilepsy, and his whole

---

[38] Cf. Hippocrates (491), *On the Sacred Disease*, ch. 12. On covering the head as a custom in folk medicine cf. Höfler (499).

[39] Cf. Wächter (1056), p. 70.

[40] Aretaeus (50), ed. Adams, p. 297 (Adams' translation). In view of Kudlien's (598), p. 310, warning against too facile an imputation of sin, the question must be left open just how far back in Greek history sin goes as a cause of epilepsy. Aretaeus mentions the belief in a demon having entered the epileptic. But according to Smith (932) the idea of intrusion of gods and demons, i.e., possession in the strict sense, was foreign to ancient Greek civilization. Even if Aretaeus were dated as early as the mid-first century A.D., as Kudlien (600), p. 1166, wants it, this would not exclude a reference to oriental rather than Greek beliefs.

[41] Aretaeus, *ibid.* (Adams' translation).

[42] Aretaeus (49), ed. Hude, p. 38, 14–15.

[43] Apuleius (43), *Apologia*, 43.

line of defense would have been senseless if an epileptic had *eo ipso* been regarded as an inspired person.

If we free ourselves from the conception that the epileptic was considered a holy person, we can recognize another implication in the name "sacred disease." What is seized by gods or demons may also be "sacred" in the sense of inspiring fear. It may be abhorred and fled from, just as the epileptic was. The "sacred disease" would then be an "awesome disease" and the epileptic an untouchable person, "taboo" particularly during his attack.[44]

## 2. THE MAGICIANS

The fatal powers which caused epilepsy might exert their influence indirectly through various objects, both alive and dead. Such objects, carriers, so to speak, of the magic virus, might produce epileptic fits and prevent the cure of the disease. They could, therefore, be used to unmask an epileptic but, on the other hand, had to be carefully avoided in the treatment of epilepsy. The so-called Carystian stone, which was probably some kind of asbestos, was believed to increase with the full moon and to shrink with the waning moon.[45] Among other things it was used for lamp wicks, and the odor rising from the burning wicks was considered a test for those suffering from the falling evil.[46] Jet was similarly believed to be subject to the influence of the moon. In a late poem attributed to the mythical singer and sorcerer Orpheus, dramatic expression is given to the supposed vengeance taken by Mene, the moon goddess, on epileptics through the medium of jet:

> Jet too he flees, which through ascending vapours
> All mortals makes to suffer with its pungency.
> Smoke-hued and flat, not large to look upon,
> It flames up brightly like some dried up fir,
> Yet to the nostrils brings destructive power; and men
> Will not escape the test thou settest

---

[44] My reference (in the first edition) to the sacred disease as the "execrable disease" is questionable because, as Professor H. J. Drossaart Lulofs kindly pointed out to me, ἱερός does not have the ambiguity of the Latin *sacer*. A subtle difference between the Greek concept and the Roman suggests itself here. However, the interpretation of epilepsy as an execrable disease was expressed as early as the sixteenth century. Gabucinius (388), *De comitiali morbo*, fol. 3 v., says: "Sunt qui sacrum id est execrabilem dictum putant: quod eum, qui illo laborat, veluti dira quadam peste infectum detestantur. Neque sane mirum; quando et benevalentibus tanquam scelesti, et abominabiles non solum stomacho comitiales sint, sed et timori. unde Plinius ait hunc morbum despui suetum; perinde ac si contagione ipsos esset invasurus. Hinc Plauto sacerrimus homo, scelestissimus dicitur." Similarly Ludovicus Septalius (914), p. 81, and Ponze Sanct a Cruz (886), p. 3.

[45] Cf. Apollonius (41), *Histor. mirab.*, 36; p. 52, 18–19.

[46] *Ibid.*, p. 52, 12–13: δοκιμάζει δὲ καὶ τοὺς πτωματιξομένους ἡ ὀσμὴ τοῦ ἐλλυχνίου καιομένου. If Apollonius really lived around the second century B.C., as suggested by Christ (221), p. 238, footnote 7, this passage would represent an early example of the concept of the "falling evil;" cf. below, I-3.

> To prove them sufferers from the sacred ill.
> For quickly will they bend and forwards tilt,
> As to the earth it draws them. Smeared by froth
> From their own mouths, hither and thither will they turn,
> And wallow on the ground. For filled with anger towards
>     them
> She laughs to see their woe, Mene, the horrid and swift![47]

In dreams the apparition of animals, connected with Selene, announces epilepsy. "A Cynocephalus means the same as the monkey," writes Artemidorus, the author of the most famous dream book, "but it adds disease to its effects, mostly that called sacred; for it is consecrated to Selene, and the ancients say that this disease, too, is consecrated to Selene."[48]

Much greater was the number of things of which the sick had to beware. The author of the book *On the Sacred Disease* records a whole list of such taboos. According to him the magicians forbade: I. Baths; II. Certain dishes, (a) Seafish: red mullet, blacktail, mullet, and eel; (b) Meat: goat, deer, pig, and dog; (c) Birds: cock, turtledove, and bustard; (d) Vegetables: mint, garlic, and onion; III. The use of black garments and goat skins and the crossing of feet and hands.[49]

Leaving the baths out for the present, most of the other taboos can be more or less easily connected with chthonic deities.[50] Black was the color of death[51] and of Hekate;[52] the onion symbolized death and mourning;[53] and as far as the animals are concerned, the avoidance of the goat was of special importance, since it was even forbidden to wear, or to lie down on, the skin. The goat was sacred to the moon goddess and to Hekate[54] and is repeatedly mentioned in connection with epilepsy.[55] Roman priests had to avoid any contact with it, and Plutarch suggested the fear of disease as a possible reason: "For it seems that, of all animals, the goat is most seized with epilepsy and gives it to those who eat or touch one taken by the disease."[56] The belief that the goat was especially prone to epilepsy is even expressed by the author of the

---

[47] Orpheus (757), *Lithica*, 474-84; p. 125.

[48] Artemidorus (60), *Onirocrit.*, II, 12; p. 104, 14-17

[49] I am here following the text of Grensemann (429), pp. 60, 26-62, 37. For the crossing of feet and hands cf. Lanata (608), p. 61 f.; generally speaking, her comments should be consulted to supplement my discussion of magic practice.

[50] Cf. Dölger (289), pp. 359-77.

[51] Hippocrates (491), *On the Sacred Disease*, vol. 6, p. 356, 7, and Grensemann (429), p. 62, 17.

[52] Cf. Sutphen (981), pp. 325-26.

[53] Cf. Arbesmann (45), p. 58.

[54] Cf. Dölger, *l.c.*, p. 367.

[55] Cf., e.g., Clemens Alexandrinus (227), *Stromata* VII, 6, 33; vol. 3, p. 280, 6-10.

[56] Plutarch (813), *The Roman Questions*, 290 A; vol. 4, p. 162.

book *On the Sacred Disease*.[57] Pliny, on the other hand, reports that
the quail is the only animal subject to it and gives this as one of the
reasons why eating the flesh of quails was repugnant to many.[58] In the
Aristotelian school, however, man was thought the only, or most frequent, victim of epileptic attacks.[59]

By the proscription of these contacts it was intended to isolate man
from the contaminating process. The fact that, strangely enough, baths
also fall into this category, may perhaps be explained on a similar basis.
For abstinence from baths belonged to the rites of personal purification
of the magicians and sorcerers,[60] rites by which they prepared themselves for the exercise of their art. And just as it helped them to attain
power over demons, it may also have been thought to remove the
epileptic from the sphere of demonic influence.[61]

This whole "magic hygiene," as the various taboos might be called,
was now supplemented by the more active procedures in the magic cure
of epilepsy. The magicians use "purifications and incantations. . . .
They purify those seized by the disease with blood and other such
things, as if they carried some miasma, or avenging spirits, or had been
bewitched by men or had performed some unholy deed."[62] These rites
were perhaps similar to the expiations after burial of a murdered man,
when women caught the blood of a sacrificed animal in a pot and used
it for purifying the mourners.[63]

In any event, the fifth century B.C. already saw the use of blood, and
in various modifications it remained one of the main magic remedies for
epilepsy. According to Orpheus and Archelaus, whose legendary names
prove the magic background, the mouth of the collapsed epileptic had
to be smeared with human blood.[64] And a most popular form was the
*drinking* of human blood, if possible as it flowed from the wound.
"While the crowd looks on," writes Pliny, "epileptics drink the blood
of gladiators, a thing horrible to see, even when wild beasts do it in the
arena. Yet, by Hercules, they think it most efficacious to suck it as it
foams warm from the man himself, and together with it the very soul

---

[57]Hippocrates (491), ed. Littré, vol. 6, p. 382, 7-8, and Grensemann (429), p. 78, 3.

[58]Pliny (806), *Nat. hist.*, 10, 69; vol. 2, p. 132, 24-27. Another connection between
epilepsy and the quail is suggested by the legend that Hercules, who gave the disease its ancient
eponym, was restored to life by means of a quail; cf. Baudissin (87), p. 305 f.

[59]Aristotle (55), *Problems*, 31, 26 and 27; vol. 2, p. 198.

[60]Cf. Abt (2), p. 40.

[61]Wellmann (1077), p. 31, footnote, connects the prohibition of bathing with old Pythagorean practices. Lanata (608), p. 51, rightly points out the contradiction between abstinence
from bathing, on the one hand, and the purifying power of water, on the other.

[62]Hippocrates (491), *On the Sacred Disease*, vol. 6, p. 362, 6-10; Grensemann (429), p. 66,
40. On the ἀλάστωρ see Lanata (608), p. 35.

[63]Cf. Wächter (1056), p. 51.

[64]Pliny (806), *Nat. hist.*, 28, 43; vol. 4, p. 163, 31-34.

out of the mouths of the wounds; yet it is not even human to put the mouth to the wounds of wild beasts."[65] Pliny then blames Osthanes, the Persian magician, for having invented, and the Greeks for having accepted, these and similar practices.

Another big group of superstitious remedies for epilepsy, namely, the use of human bones and of anything which has come in contact with the dead, can also be connected with the magicians. They believed in the curative power of the first vertebra, the Atlas,[66] and it is again Orpheus and Archelaus who are mentioned as having advised the flesh of a wild beast which had been slain by the same iron weapon with which a man had been killed.[67] The use of iron is not accidental. It was believed that an iron nail fixed at the spot where an epileptic had first put his head was a remedy ridding him of the evil.[68] And some people "superstitiously" thought that mistletoe, if collected from the oak at the new moon without the aid of an iron instrument, became more efficacious and cured epilepsy if it did not touch the earth.[69] Finally, amulets too belong to the magic materia medica. Osthanes advised the gathering of coral, peony, and the root of strychnos at the time of the waning moon, putting them into a piece of linen and hanging them around the neck.[70]

These procedures are but examples of a long and tedious list of remedies which we nowadays consider superstitious. Definitely connected with the names and recorded practices of magicians, they represent examples of almost every type of miraculous cure. In some way or another they are all associated with the belief in the supernatural origin of disease and the cult of the chthonic deities. If, for example, epilepsy is not only averted but also "cured" by spitting,[71] the logic is understandable, for what keeps demons away ought to drive them away too. Yet in most cases an attempt at a deeper understanding meets with the difficulty of the ambivalent character of the procedures. Metals, it has been contended, were believed to keep ghosts away,[72] and the iron nail was driven in so as to pin the evil spirit to the spot.[73] On the other hand, it is just the avoidance of an iron instrument which is supposed to

---

[65] *Ibid.* 28, 4; vol. 4, p. 156, 19-25.

[66] *Ibid.*, 28, 99; vol. 4, p. 174, 3-5: "... hunc spinae articulum sive nodum Atlantion vocant, est autem primus. in comitialium quoque remediis habent eum."

[67] *Ibid.*, 28, 34; vol. 4, p. 162, 4-8.

[68] *Ibid.*, 28, 63; vol. 4, p. 167, 16-18.

[69] *Ibid.*, 24, 12; vol. 4, p. 36, 1-3: "quidam id religione efficacius fieri putant" etc.

[70] Alexander of Tralles (21), I, 15; vol. 1, p. 567, Cf. to this passage Bidez and Cumont (111), vol. 2, p. 302.

[71] Plautus (805), *The Captives*, III, 4; p. 514: "ne verere, multos iste morbus homines macerat, quibus insputari saluti fuit atque is profuit." Cf., however, above, footnote 36.

[72] Cf., e.g., Abt (2), p. 163, footnote 5.

[73] Cf. Frazer (377), p. 68.

make mistletoe more efficacious. The touch of the dead causes epilepsy; one would, therefore, not expect them to lend power to a remedy. And while the goat, sacred to Hekate, is forbidden to epileptics by some, other magicians prescribe goat's flesh parched in a funeral pile.[74]

From the fifth century on we find ample evidence of the existence of magic healers of epilepsy. Some of them were of the "shamanistic" type, as Empedocles is supposed to have been,[75] whereas others were tricksters or practiced within a family tradition. Pseudo-Demosthenes tells of a man who associated himself with the servant of a sorceress. From her he obtained drugs and charms, and with her help he practiced magic and claimed to cure epileptics.[76] Other healers, probably of a magic type, were the "Elasioi" in Argos. These were supposed to be descended from Alexida, a mythical daughter of the god Amphiaraus, and were reputed to avert epileptic attacks.[77] There existed also a magic literature ascribed to such legendary names as Osthanes, Orpheus, Archelaus, where magic prescriptions were compiled and could be studied by all those interested.[78] Remnants of this literature are found in Pliny and in later physicians, and the same type of literature is also represented in the Greek magic papyri, but much of it is of late origin and falls into the period of transition from Antiquity to the Middle Ages.

It is, however, necessary to distinguish between the magic and the religious cure of epilepsy in Antiquity. This distinction was already drawn by the author of *On the Sacred Disease* when he accused the magicians of impiety. Religious treatment consisted above all in the invocation of the help of Asclepius. The patient slept in his temple, and the god might appear and either effect or advise a cure of the disease. We have, indeed, at least one record, dating from the second half of the fourth century B.C. It is from the sanctuary of Asclepius in Epidaurus and reads: "N. N. from Argos, epileptic. This man during his sleep in the curative chamber saw a vision: he dreamed that the god approached him and pressed his ring . . . upon his mouth, nostrils, and ears—and he

---

[74] Pliny (806), *Nat. hist.*, 28, 226; vol. 4, p. 198, 7 ff.: "comitialibus . . . dantur et carnes caprinae in rogo hominis tostae, ut volunt Magi, sebum earum" etc.

[75] Cf. Dodds (283), p. 145; cf. below, p. 154.

[76] Demosthenes (264), *Against Aristogeiton*, pp. 562–64.

[77] Cf. Plutarch (813), *The Greek Questions*, 23; vol. 4, p. 204. Cf. also Gruppe (437), p. 537, footnote 3. According to Halliday (810), p. 119, the *elasioi* and Alexida are not mentioned in classical literature except in this passage of Plutarch's.

[78] One of the main compilers of such texts was Democritus Bolus, who probably constituted an important source of information for late authors. Cf. Bidez and Cumont (111), vol. 1, p. 170 ff., who give the literature on him. Theodorus Priscianus (1006), *Physica*, p. 251, 1–7, gives the following extract concerning the magic cure of epilepsy: "in quarum curatione Democritus inquit pollutione opus esse, ut sunt caedis culpae et menstruae mulieris et sacrarum avium, vel vetitorum animalium carnes cibo datae et sanguinis potus. nam et epilempsin, quam ieran noson appellavere, sic curare praecipit, efficaciae potentiam praeferens et vetans inquiri rationem." This is an interesting example of magic background and alleged empirical efficacy of a treatment.

recovered."[79] Religious treatment of this kind was not opposed by the physicians.[80] We shall see with what deep reverence they themselves related such miraculous healing in contrast to magic, which most of them rejected. But before we turn again to the attitude of the physicians towards magic, we must first answer another question suggested by the term "sacred disease."

## 3. SACRED DISEASE AND EPILEPSY

So far we have taken it for granted that "the sacred disease" was a name for epilepsy. Now we must ask ourselves how far this assumption is justified.

We first meet with the expression "sacred disease" in the fragments of the philosopher Heraclitus[81] and in the writings of the historian Herodotus. The latter, relating the mad doings of the Persian king Cambyses, says that he was reported to have suffered from birth from "a certain great disease . . . which some people call sacred. And thus," Herodotus adds, "it would not be unlikely that if the body suffered from a great disease, the mind was not sound either."[82] The meaning of the passage in Heraclitus, "self-conceit is a sacred disease," is obscure, and the disease of Cambyses may or may not have been epilepsy. Both references are inconclusive. If Herodotus really meant to say that Cambyses suffered from epilepsy, his statement implies that he looked upon epilepsy as a somatic disease. This view would agree well with the attitude taken by the author of *On the Sacred Disease*.

At any rate, with this book we are on solid ground concerning the identification of the sacred disease with epilepsy. However, its first chapter contains a curious passage. "For every form of the affliction," it says, "they (i.e., magicians, etc.) attribute the cause to a god." In particular, the "Mother of the Gods" is responsible if the patient imitates a goat, gnashes his teeth, or has convulsions of the right side. Poseidon is blamed for more violent cries which make the patient resemble a horse, Enodia for the passing of feces, Apollo Nomios for thinner and more frequent feces as in birds, and Ares for frothing at the mouth and kicking. "But where nightly horrors, fear and derangement of mind occur, leaping out of the bed and flight from the house, these they say to be assaults of Hekate and attacks of the heroes."[83] This distinction of various forms is made by the magicians, not by the medi-

---

[79]Herzog (488), p. 33.

[80]Cf. Edelstein (313), p. 239 ff.

[81]Diels (270), Herakleitos, B 46, p. 86: . . . τὴν τε οἴησιν ἱερὰν νόσον ἔλεγε καὶ τὴν ὅρασιν ψεύδεσθαι.

[82] Herodotus (485), ed. Godley, III, 33; vol. 2, pp. 42-44: καὶ γὰρ τινὰ ἐκ γενεῆς νοῦσον μεγάλην λέγεται ἔχειν ὁ Καμβύσης, τὴν ἱρὴν ὀνομάζουσι τινές · οὔ νύν τοι ἀεικὲς οὐδὲν ἦν τοῦ σώματος νοῦσον μεγάλην νοσέοντος μηδὲ τὰς φρένας ὑγιαίνειν.

[83]Hippocrates (491), ed. Littré, vol. 6, pp. 360-62; Grensemann (429), pp. 64, 33-66, 38.

cal author of the book. Not only does he attack this popular classification, but the whole of the rest of the book and the clear description
of symptoms show that to him "the so-called sacred disease" is one
disease, viz., epilepsy. On the whole, this attitude remained constant
among the physicians throughout Antiquity. Wherever they speak of
the sacred disease, they think of epilepsy, which they differentiate from
hysterical attacks as well as from madness.

But the matter is more complicated if we consider popular beliefs as
represented in the above classification of the magicians. Can all the
symptoms described be attributed to epilepsy? This question is difficult
to answer. Some forms, particularly passage of feces, strongly indicate
epilepsy. The others may *conceivably* occur in epilepsy. But it cannot
be denied that the imitation of animal voices ("theriomimicry," to use
an expression of Gowers)[84] and the mental symptoms attributed to
Hekate and the Heroes are compatible with hysteria and possibly other
psychic disturbances. This impression is, furthermore, strengthened by
the attribution of the sacred disease to such gods and demons, particularly Hekate and the moon, as might also be responsible for other
ill-defined abnormalities. Of Hekate a late Greek commentator said:
"Formerly people thought that those who fell down suddenly had been
twisted in their mind by Pan especially, and Hekate."[85] This statement
deserves attention because it implies the notion of the "falling evil"
which we shall find fully developed in the Middle Ages. Moreover,
Hekate was sometimes identified with Artemis, "the raving, raging,
inspired and furious,"[86] or with the goddess of the moon, into whose
mouth a late poet put the words:

> Like unto Bacchus
> O'er insensate madness do I rule.
> And I am Mene, the Bacchante, not only since
> Through space I hurl the moon; but yet because
> O'er madness I hold sway and fury can arouse.[87]

There are more passages which attribute raving to Hekate[88] and mania
to the goddess of the moon,[89] and we have already seen that it was sin
against the moon which was believed to provoke epilepsy.

---

[84] Gowers (420), p. 140.

[85] *Scholia in Euripidem* (899), p. 203: τοὺς ἐξαίφνης καταπίπτοντες ᾤοντο τὸ παλαιὸν οἱ ἄνθρωποι ὑπὸ Πανὸς μάλιστα καὶ Ἑκάτης πεπλῆχθαι τὸν νοῦν.

[86] Plutarch (813), *How the Young Man Should Study Poetry*, 22 A; vol. 1, p. 112.

[87] Nonnus (739), *Dionysiaca*, 44, 226-29.

[88] Cf. particularly Euripides (335), *Hippolytus*, 141 ff., which the editor Harry connects with *On the Sacred Disease*.

[89] Cf., e.g., Scholia to Sophocles' Ajax (900), p. 212: τοὺς πολλοὺς γὰρ τῶν μαινομένων ἐκ σελήνης νοσεῖν ὑποτίθενται, διὰ τὸ νυκτερινῶν δεσπόζειν φασμάτων. For collection of passages cf. Roscher (869), p. 67 ff.

It has, therefore, to be admitted that the popular concept of "the sacred disease" may have been broader than that of the physicians. Just how broad it was we do not know. But we must beware of going too far. It is in relatively late sources that we find a clearly stated connection between epilepsy and the moon. Moreover, the fact that various diseases were attributed to the same god does not imply that the diseases were believed the same. Thus, we have no right to assume that the sacred disease implied all kinds of ecstatic conditions, neuroses, and mental illnesses. The author of *On the Sacred Disease* expressly mentions madness and various nightly attacks as examples of afflictions which are no less astonishing than epilepsy, and yet, he says, nobody thinks them sacred![90] Like most popular designations of diseases,[91] the name "the sacred disease" was probably used in a loose manner, but it nevertheless centered around the disease which the physicians were to call epilepsy.[92]

This, however, did not exclude the designation of diseases as "sacred" which were not necessarily epilepsy or even nervous disorders. The ancient Greeks easily conferred the attribute "sacred," with many shades of meaning, to a large variety of things.[93] Their literature even offered several sacred fishes,[94] and there are a few examples suggesting the existence of more than one sacred disease.

There is the curious story of the physician "Menecrates, surnamed Zeus, who prided himself greatly on being the sole cause of life to mankind through his skill in medicine. He used, at any rate, to compel those whom he cured of the so-called sacred diseases to sign a bond that they would obey him as his slaves if they were restored to health. And one man who became his attendant wore the dress and went by the name of Heracles; he was Nicostratus of Argos, who had been cured of a[95] sacred disease."[96] At least four other men, appearing as Hermes,

---

[90] Hippocrates (491), ed. Littré, vol. 6, pp. 352, 8-354, 12, Grensemann (429), p. 60, 5.

[91] Cf. Lessiak (637), p. 112.

[92] Accordingly, I do not believe that in Antiquity epilepsy was considered one of the main types of insanity, as has been contended by modern scholars; cf., e.g., Tambornino (991), p. 57. Nor do I believe that the ancients regarded the raving of the Bacchants (as described by Euripides) or the madness of Hercules and others (as described by the poets) as identical with "the sacred disease." Such views are often expressed, cf., e.g., Dieterich (277), pp. 53 and 403, and Weinreich (1072), p. 4. Plutarch (812), *Amatorius*, ch. 12, 755 E; vol. 9, pp. 344-45, compares the somatic "sacred disease" with calling love, a mental affliction, "sacred and divine."

[93] See Wülfing von Martitz (1111), Ramat (837), and Lanata (608), p. 27, where additional literature is cited.

[94] These probably were differing attempts to identify the sacred fish of Homer's *Iliad*, XVI, 407; cf. Plutarch (813), *The Cleverness of Animals*, 981 D; vol. 12, pp. 453-55, and the editor's notes *ibid.*

[95] ἱερὰν νόσον θεραπευθείς. Gulick (61) translates this by "cured of the sacred sickness."

[96] Athenaeus (61), *Deipnosophistae*, VII, 289 A- B; vol. 3, pp. 297-99. (Gulick's translation with the exception indicated in the preceding footnote.)

Apollo, Asclepius, and Helius, have been identified as belonging to the entourage of Menecrates. Among this total of five one was a military leader, one a statesmen, and the third a scholar and founder of the city of Uranopolis.[97] Had all these men been suffering from epilepsy (or a disease considered epilepsy by their contemporaries)? Had their cure been despaired of,[98] and had they then been healed by Menecrates? Their cure would have had to be lasting enough to make them submit to their theomaniac physician. We do not know who diagnosed their illnesses as "sacred." If the diagnosis was made by Menecrates or those near to him, it is conceivable that the label "sacred" was put on different diseases, somatic or mental.[99]

One of the poems of Callimachus (third century B.C.) deals with the story of a girl who is to contract a marriage of which the goddess Artemis does not approve. All preparations for the marriage are made:

> Toward evening was the maid with pallor seized
> From a disease that to wild goats we ban
> And wrongly sacred call; a grievous ill,
> Enfeebling her even to Hades' brink.
> A second time the nuptial bed was spread;
> A second time the maid in sickness lay,
> For seven months with quartan fever torn.
> And yet a third time did they turn their thoughts
> Unto the marriage, and the third time too
> A deathly chill took hold of Cydippe.[100]

It is tempting to believe that Callimachus thought of the disease, wrongly called sacred, as epilepsy.[101] It would allow us to think of the Elasioi, mentioned before, and if there existed a practice of banishing epilepsy to the wild goats, we would gain further understanding why the author of On the Sacred Disease investigated the skull of a goat. But the text does not suggest that Cydippe suffered from attacks of three different diseases. Nor do we have cogent reason to assume that Callimachus echoed the author of On the Sacred Disease by referring to epilepsy as the disease wrongly called sacred. In all three cases the girl

---

[97]The identifications were made by Weinreich (1072), pp. 10–16, whose study is fundamental for the historical understanding of the personality of Menecrates and the phenomenon of theomania in ancient and modern times.

[98]Thus according to Plutarch, Agesilaus, 21 as quoted by Weinreich, ibid., p. 4 ftn. 10, and p. 96.

[99]Another late author, Philostratus, also alludes to the differentiation of several sacred diseases. Pointing to the different treatment of diseases by physicians and gymnasts, Philostratus (793), Περὶ γυμναστικῆς, ch. 14; p. 146, 6–9 says: νοσήματα, ὁπόσα κατάρρους καὶ ὑδέρους καὶ φθόας ὀνομάξομεν καὶ ὁπόσαι ἱεραὶ νόσοι, ἰατροὶ μὲν παύουσιν ἐπαντλοῦντές τι ἢ ποτίζοντες ἢ ἐπιπλάττοντες, γυμναστικὴ δὲ τὰ τοιαῦτα διαίταις ἴσχει καὶ τρίψει. In this connection we may also think of the ignis sacer, etc. Cf. Sticker (960).

[100]Callimachus (195), Aitia, p. 206, 12–19.

[101]Cf. ibid., p. 2 and particularly Eitrem's (318), p. 87 arguments.

seems to have suffered attacks of the same disease, viz., quartan fever. This is corroborated by the remark of an ancient commentator suggesting that Callimachus objected to naming the pestilential disease (which fits quartan fever rather than epilepsy) as "sacred."[102] In this connection it should not be overlooked that fevers, as Aristophanes proves, were not exempted from demoniac personification.[103]

In the case of leprosy, which late authors, especially Greek Fathers of the Church, termed a "sacred disease,"[104] we can imagine particular reasons for the designation. Many of these Christian theologians, like Gregory Nazianzen and John Chrysostomus, lived in regions where leprosy was rife. Leprosy was identified with the biblical *Zara'ath*, whose diagnosis was the task of the priests[105] and which was often considered a punishment for sin. To the oriental peoples it may therefore have seemed a sacred disease, so that the appearance of this name in Byzantine writings reflected oriental rather than Greek usage. An alternate explanation suggests that leprosy received the name of sacred disease among the Byzantine Christians after epilepsy had lost it. To them, epilepsy was the work of a demon, and they even called it "demon,"[106] whereas leprosy was a trial imposed by God which made the sufferer from it an object of divine preference and of Christian love.[107] It seems not impossible that oriental tradition and Christian revaluation concurred; at least this would explain why in the Latin West leprosy did not become a sacred disease.

It is important to realize that various diseases were called "sacred disease" in Antiquity, because this fact affords us an insight into an undercurrent of popular ideas which came to the fore in later days. But it is of equal importance not to be confused by this evidence. The instances are but few where the term is applied to other diseases than epilepsy. In the great majority of cases "the sacred disease" meant epilepsy for physicians as well as laymen.

While the magical conception named epilepsy "the sacred disease," Greek mythology supplied it with an eponym. In one of the gynecological books of the Hippocratic collection, where displacement of the uterus is discussed, the author says: "When the uterus is near the liver and the hypochondrium and produces suffocation, the woman turns up

---

[102] Scholia to Apollonius Rhodius (898), A, 1019; pp. 89-90: κατ' εὐφημισμόν. τὰ γὰρ μεγάλα τῶν παθῶν εὐφήμως ἱερὰ καὶ καλά φαμεν, ὡς καὶ τὰς Ἐρωύας Εὐμενίδας καὶ τὴν λοιμικὴν νόσον ἱεράν, ὡς καὶ Καλλίμαχος "ψευδόμενοι δ' ἱερὴν φημίξομεν."

[103] Aristophanes (51), *Wasps*, 1038 f.; cf. Lanata (608), p. 71.

[104] The passages have been collected by Dölger (289), p. 166 ff.

[105] Dölger, *ibid.*, p. 168, footnote 4, draws attention to the point that the Syriac text of Zacharias Scholasticus designates leprosy as "sacerdotal disease."

[106] See below, III-1.

[107] This theory has been proposed by Philipsborn (791) after Kukules (quoted by Philipsborn, p. 224) and Keenan (576), p. 18, had made suggestions in the same direction.

the white of her eyes, becomes cold (some become even livid), gnashes her teeth, saliva flows into her mouth, and she resembles the persons seized by the Herculean disease."[108] This description does not necessarily point to epilepsy; there is no mention of convulsions, and flow of saliva was part of the ancient picture of maniac frenzy. Those interpreting the Herculean Disease as epilepsy had much difficulty in explaining this name.[109] Some thought that the great labors imposed upon Hercules had made him subject to epilepsy.[110] Others denied that Hercules had really suffered from epilepsy and believed that the name of the powerful hero was meant to indicate the greatness of the disease.[111] The legends of Hercules do not speak of him as epileptic; they have him suffer an attack of maniac fury during which he slew his wife and children. Thus, with reference to the above passage, one of the early commentators of the Hippocratic writings could suggest that mania was meant, "because the hero had suffered from this malady only."[112] Euripides in the *Madness of Hercules* has the attack brought on by Lyssa, the goddess of raging madness; he calls Hercules a maniac, never an epileptic or a victim of the sacred disease. Assertions to the contrary notwithstanding,[113] there is no reason to assume that Euripides, or Seneca after him, tried to depict an epileptic.[114]

---

[108] Hippocrates (491), *On Diseases of Women*, I, ch. 7; vol. 8, pp. 32–34.

[109] For collection of passages cf. Roscher (867), col. 458 f.

[110] Dikaearchus quoted by Zenobius (775), IV, 26; vol. 1, p. 91. Diogenianus (775), V, 8; vol. 1, p. 250. Macarius (775), IV, 56; vol. 2, p. 172; cf. also Pseudo-Plutarch (809), *Proverbia Alexandrinorum*, 36; p. 166, 38–40.

[111] Cf. Galen (394), *In Hippocr. epid. VI, comment.* VI, sec. 6, c. 7; vol. 17 B, p. 341, also the scholium in Oribasius (754), vol. 3, p. 683. Substantially this is also the opinion of von Wilamowitz-Moellendorff (1099), vol. 1, p. 92, ftn. 170, who believes that Herculean disease meant as much as the "monstrous" (*ungeheuerliche*) disease, just as the name "Herculean stone" for the loadstone meant the amazing stone.

[112] Erotianus (327), *Vocum Hippocraticarum conlectio*, p. 75, 12 ff. Certain incurable skin diseases like the "Herculean Psora" [cf. Zenobius (775), VI, 49; vol. 1, p. 174, and Diogenianus (775), V, 7; *ibid.*, p. 250] and the "elephant disease," i.e., leprosy [cf. Aretaeus (49), ed. Hude, IV, 13; p. 87, 15], were also called after him. This variety of diseases corresponds to the fact that the various myths about the hero's life tell of his being affected by different diseases. Just as these tales may have originated independently, so the various diseases may have been called after Hercules without any interconnection.

[113] For instance, Dieterich (277), pp. 53 and 403, and Blaiklock (118).

[114] In Euripides (334), *Madness of Hercules*, 923 ff.; vol. 3, p. 202 ff., and Seneca's (911), *Hercules furens*, 930 ff., the hero is confused and has illusions during which he kills his wife and children. Then he falls to the ground and sleeps; finally he awakes cured, but without memory of the whole episode. Modern psychiatric literature from the nineteenth century on relates similar actions of epileptics, cf. below, IX–1c. However, the question is not how *we* may diagnose these conditions, but how the ancients diagnosed them. Euripides' Hercules, 1004–6, is hit with a stone by Pallas Athene, which stops him from killing his father and sends him to sleep. The sleep, therefore, does not follow naturally as in an epileptic attack. In *Iphigenia in Taurica*, 281 ff., Euripides (334) depicts Orestes as having illusions which make him attack cattle with his sword; then he falls down, his beard dripping with foam. But here too, line 377, Euripides ascribes all this to mania. Killing of cattle or man performed under the influence of illusions is a dramatic device at least as old as Sophocles' *Ajax*. If Euripides consciously used epileptics as a model, it is not clear why he did not declare Hercules smitten with the sacred

The most important statement, after Hippocrates, explicitly connecting Hercules with the sacred disease belongs to a compiler of uncertain date whose *Problems* are ascribed to Aristotle. One of these "Problems"[115] states that Hercules had been of a melancholy temperament and that the black bile had caused his mental derangement.[116] The author does not say that Hercules himself had suffered from epilepsy, but he counts epilepsy among the diseases that black bile could engender, and he believes that "the ancients" had called the afflictions of epileptics a sacred disease after Hercules. All this proves little for the original meaning of the term "Herculean Disease." However, the author propounds the thesis that all outstanding men had been melancholic, and this thesis, in the Renaissance, gave classical authority to the idea that great men were particularly prone to epilepsy.

In later times, especially since the rise of Christianity, other names of rather vague character can be found.[117] They will be discussed in connection with the Middle Ages, when they acquire importance. Now, however, we have to turn from the magicians to the attitude of the physicians proper. This leads us to that name for the disease which in medical literature has survived through the ages: Epilepsy.

## 4. PHYSICIANS AND MAGIC

The words "epilepsy" and "epileptic" are of Greek origin and have the same root as the verb *epilambanein*, which means "to seize" or "to attack." "Epilepsy," therefore, means "seizure"; "epileptic," "seized." In Greek, just as in modern speech, one would say of any disease that it had "seized" a man, and this terminology perhaps goes back to a very old magic conception according to which all diseases were believed "attacks" and seizures by gods or demons, as documented in Babylonian medicine.[118] Since epilepsy was the demoniac disease par excellence, the term gradually acquired a more particular meaning and came to signify epileptic seizure.[119] If this explanation is true, the process

---

disease. The fact that the Greeks called epilepsy a sacred disease and the existence of a monograph on it in the Hippocratic collection seem to have exerted an undue fascination upon modern scholars.

[115] Aristotle (55), *Problems*, 30, 1; vol. 2, p. 154. According to von Wilamowitz-Moellendorff (1099), vol. 1, p. 92, ftn. 170, the content of this problem is genuinely Aristotelian.

[116] As well as skin ulcers before his death. Cf. Apollodorus (40), *The Library*, II, 7, 7; vol. 1, p. 268.

[117] It is sometimes stated that *morbus detestabilis* was also a name for epilepsy. Cf. Dölger (286), p. 131, who refers to Apuleius' *Metamorphoses*, 9, 39, where it is said: "iners asellus et nihilo minus <ferox> morboque detestabili caducus." Butler (44), p. 87, translates this passage (rightly, as I think): "That wretched ass, for all that he is a lazy brute, has got a nasty temper and, what is worse, suffers from a cursed complaint."

[118] Cf. Sudhoff (971), p. 368.

[119] The Latin term *morbus sonticus* also suggests the development from a general to a more restricted meaning. As Gellius (63), *Noctes Atticae*, 20, 1, 27; p. 416, proves, *morbus sonticus*

must have taken place in very ancient times. For already in the Hippocratic collection, "epilepsy" and "epileptic" are used in the more technical books and are nowhere interpreted in a magical sense.[120] On the contrary, the ancients in trying to explain the etymology of "epilepsy" offer quite rational explanations. Epilepsy, they say, has its name because it "attacks" both senses and mind,[121] or, according to another late authority, because it "seizes" the senses of the victim.[122]

But though "epilepsy" and "epileptic" were used in some Hippocratic books as designations of epileptic attacks and of epileptic persons, the term *epilēpsiē* did not yet mean the underlying disease.[123] When referring to the latter, the physicians had to speak of the sacred disease (or the somewhat doubtful "great disease").[124] It is possible that the magic concept, with its personification of disease, held the advantage over the rational and observational approach.[125]

Our statement that the ancient physicians opposed the magical interpretation of epilepsy needs further qualification. The books of physicians and scientists, at least from the fourth century B.C. on, are full of remedies for epilepsy and of advice as to treatment which we nowadays call superstitious. Diocles of Carystus and Praxagoras of Cos, the two outstanding physicians of the fourth century B.C., recommended among other things: lichen of horses or mules, genitals of seals, testicles of the hippopotamus, and the blood of the tortoise or of the flatfish.[126] The story of the lizard swallowing his discarded skin because it grudges mankind this remedy for epilepsy, and that of the seal vomiting the rennet useful for the same purpose, when it is about to be caught, are both credited to Aristotle and his greatest pupil, Theophrastus.[127] Serapion of Alexandria, living about 200 B.C. and the founder of the so-called empiric school, called the lichen of horses a specific against epilepsy. Besides camel's hair and the gall and rennet of the seal, he gave a medicament which was composed of the feces of the land crocodile, the

---

in the law of the twelve tables connoted any grave and debilitating disease, while Pliny (806), *Nat. hist.*, 36, 142; vol. 5, p. 131, obviously uses it for epilepsy.

[120] Cf. Temkin (999), p. 318; I have also given, on p. 315, a list of the passages in the Hippocratic collection.

[121] E.g., Caelius Aurelianus (192), *Morb. chron.*, I, 4, par. 60: "Epilepsia vocabulum sumpsit quod sensum atque mentem pariter apprehendat."

[122] Alexander of Tralles (21), I, 15; vol. 1, p. 535.

[123] Cf. Temkin (999), pp. 314–19.

[124] This has been rightly pointed out by Grensemann (429), p. 5, for the author of *On the Sacred Disease*. As far as I can see, it holds good for the entire Hippocratic collection, which does not yet go beyond τὰ ἐπιληπτικά; cf. Temkin (999), p. 315.

[125] Halliday (810), p. 280, has referred to Sophocles, *Philoctetes*, 757, 766, as an example of the coming and going of a disease.

[126] Cf. Caelius Aurelianus (192), *Morb. chron.*, I, 4, par. 133 f.

[127] Aristotle (52), *On Marvellous Things Heard*, 835 A and B; pp. 262 and 266. Theophrastus (1011), p. 835, and Pliny (806), *Nat. hist.*, 8, 111; vol. 2, p. 63.

heart and genitals of the hare, and the blood of the sea tortoise, or the testicles of a boar, ram, or poultry cock.[128]

These and similar remedies obtain abundantly in the medical literature of later times. From the first century A.D. on, the use of human blood and other human organs is also recorded in the medical literature preserved. Celsus says that some people have freed themselves of the disease by swallowing the blood of a stabbed gladiator.[129] His contemporary, Scribonius Largus, also reports various ways in which blood has been used against the disease and says that epileptics eat a piece from the liver of a gladiator, and this is given them nine times. But he adds: "This, and whatever is of the same kind, falls outside professional medicine—although it has apparently helped in some cases."[130] This sentence shows that Scribonius Largus—and the same is true of Celsus— admits the possibly salutary effects of such cannibalistic remedies but thinks that the professional physician is not allowed to use them. Pliny, whose books abound in the most superstitious advice, much of it gathered from Greek authorities, gives the name of a midwife who recommended rubbing the patient's feet with menstrual blood as an excellent method for arousing epileptics.[131] It can by no means be objected that these practices were believed in only by superstitious Romans or midwives. Even Galen admits that human bones may have a curative effect. "I know," he says, "that some of our people have cured epilepsy and arthritis in many cases by prescribing a drink of burned (human) bones, the patients not knowing what they drank lest they should be nauseated."[132] Some physicians, at least, did not confine themselves to the reporting of such material, and the very extreme was reached by those who approved of calling in magicians with their incantations![133]

All this goes to show that the attitude of the ancient physicians toward magic treatment of epilepsy was not uniform. In the time of the Hippocratics, magic was attacked vigorously. But from the fourth century B.C. on a change took place. Only in the works of Soranus, the

---

[128] Cf. Deichgräber (259), p. 166. Muth (726), p. 142 f., thinks that feces were prescribed by the ancient physicians in their eagerness to find remedies against the disease whose natural character had just been revealed to them. I find this hard to believe.

[129] Celsus (212), *De medicina*, III, 23, 7; vol. 1, p. 338. Cf. Dölger (288), p. 204 ff.

[130] Scribonius Largus (907), *Conpositiones*, 17; p. 11, 19–22: "Item ex iecinore gladiatoris iugulati particulam aliquam novies datam consumant. <Hoc> quaeque eiusdem generis sunt, extra medicinae professionem cadunt, quamvis profuisse quibusdam visa sint."

[131] Pliny (806), *Nat. hist.*, 28, 83; vol. 4, p. 171. *Ibid.*, 28, 7, Pliny tells of one Artemon who prescribed water drawn at night and drunk from the skull of a murdered and unburned man. I do not know whether this Artemon was a physician or a magician.

[132] Galen (394), *De simplicium medicamentorum temperamentis ac facultatibus*, XI, 18; vol. 12, p. 342.

[133] Caelius Aurelianus (192), *Morb. chron.*, I, 4; p. 315: "Alii vero etiam ligamenta probaverunt, et magos adhibendos, atque eorum incantationes" etc.

greatest representative of the methodist school, do we find an outright refutation of such remedies as have been related. The other extreme, that of physicians recognizing magicians and incantations, was probably rare too—at least among scientific physicians. For as far as the latters' works are preserved, incantations do not appear. The majority of the physicians accepted various remedies from popular or magicians' practices. In doing so they probably were not always conscious of the magical background but justified their procedure by apparent experience and rational explanations.

As the lack of such prescriptions in the Hippocratic collection shows, they must have originated outside scientific medicine. In many of them the magical motive can scarcely be doubted. But once in use, they were recommended as having helped in many cases, and this claim to successful experience was more difficult to refute than magical theories proper. Even the author of the book *On the Sacred Disease* did not entirely deny that the magicians' proscription of the various dishes might be effective. All he did was to impute to the magicians that, in order to avoid responsibility, they had banned such dishes as might be harmful to sick persons.[134] Soranus, too, whom we mentioned as the most radical opponent of superstition among the later physicians, did not altogether deny the effect of blood upon epilepsy. He argued that its use rested on bad observation, in that blood was not beneficial but, on the contrary, utterly dangerous.[135]

For the understanding of the therapy of epilepsy down to modern times, it is of the greatest importance to realize how difficult it is to judge a remedy solely on the basis of experience. Even nowadays it often takes years to prove or disprove the effectiveness of a drug. A vast number of observations made under rigid control by many independent observers are an indispensable condition for the establishment of therapeutic facts. But as long as critical statistics did not—and could not— exist, the limited experience of the individual physician was the highest criterion, yet one which by necessity must lead to doubtful results. Small wonder, then, that the sect of the empiricists, the very physicians who based medicine on experience alone, was among the chief victims of credulity.[136] The empiricists rejected scientific speculation "because nature is incomprehensible,"[137] and once the incomprehensibility of nature's actions was accepted, it was easy to admit that she might possess occult powers which, acting through certain drugs and amulets, could bring about the most miraculous cures. The same idea was also

---

[134] Hippocrates (489), ed. Jones, vol. 2, pp. 141–43.

[135] Caelius Aurelianus (192), *Morb. chron.*, I, 4, par. 128 ff.

[136] Cf. Neuburger (730), vol. 2, p. 17; Baumann (88), p. 30.

[137] Celsus (212), *De medicina*, Prooem. 27; vol. 1, pp. 14–16.

acceptable to scientists who believed that the things of nature might exert "sympathetic" or "antipathetic" influences upon each other. Thus, it happened that these remedies were called "sympathetic," "natural," or "empirical." Their use formed a special branch of medical assistance. Late in the sixth century A.D., Alexander of Tralles said: "The skilful [physician] must help in every way, employing natural [remedies], scientific reasoning, and technical method; and he must, so to speak, set everything in motion that is apt quickly to free the patient from a long disease and misery."[138]

Even physicians who believed in a natural causal explanation of the phenomena of nature could not resist the claims of alleged experience. But if they employed the same remedies and amulets, they tried at least to find a scientific explanation. An illustrative example of the inadequate attempt at critical observation and subsequent explanation is found in the writings of Galen. Talking about the root of the peony, he says: "On the whole its effect is very drying, so that I do not entirely relinquish the hope that it may have been reasonable to rely on it to cure epilepsy in children, even if used as an amulet. And I know a child that had not been attacked at all for eight months since wearing the root. When, however, somehow the amulet slid off, he was immediately seized. And when another one had been hung around his neck, he again felt perfectly well. But for experiment's sake it seemed better to me to take it off again; and when I had done so, and he was seized by convulsions again, I hung a big, fresh part of the root around his neck. And from that time on the boy was absolutely healthy and was no longer seized by convulsions. It was now logical [to assume] either that certain particles of the root fell out, were sucked in by inspiration, and did thus heat the affected part—or that the air itself was tempered and changed by the root."[139]

The connection of magic practices, rational explanation, and empiricism makes it very hard, or even impossible in many cases, to find out what had first led to the use of a drug. The peony, for instance, which for many centuries was one of the principal drugs used against epilepsy, had both an empirical and magic connotation. The Hippocratics had used it in the treatment of fever[140] and various gynecological complaints,[141] but on the other hand, it was also surrounded by a magic lore.[142]

---

[138] Alexander of Tralles (21), I, 15; vol. 1, pp. 571-73.

[139] Galen (394), *De simpl. med. temp. ac facult.*, VI, c. 3; vol. 11, p. 859 f.

[140] Cf. Hippocrates (491), ed. Littré, vol. 7, p. 266.

[141] Cf. *ibid.*, vol. 7, pp. 314, 320, 350, 352, 358, 426; vol. 8, pp. 82, 118, 130, 308, 382 (hysterical suffocation!), 448, 458, 502.

[142] Cf. Aelianus (10), *De nat. anim.*, 14, 27, where it is said to cure the disease which is caused by the moon. Cf. also Delatte (263), p. 3 ff., and Marzell (673), col. 1698 f.

Besides the materia medica proper, the substances which were believed to provoke an attack in epileptics, and thus to establish the
diagnosis of the disease, were of an equally equivocal character. Alexander of Tralles mentions them, together with the practice of putting the
patient into a goat's skin, plunging him into the sea, and observing
whether he sank or not; if the former, the diagnosis was positive.[143]
Plutarch related that the Spartan women, in order to find out whether
an infant was worth rearing, washed it all over with undiluted wine,
which would make epileptic and sickly ones fall into convulsions but
strengthen the healthy ones.[144] These diagnostic substances were
chiefly such things as jet, asphalt, horn, lamp wick, goat's liver, which
were burned before the patient. Most of them, as has been shown in the
case of jet, had a definite magical character. But some scientists attributed their effect to the bad odor, fatal for epileptics, and the late
Aristotelian philosopher, Alexander of Aphrodisias, added a strictly
physical explanation: "For the thickness of the particles of the odors,"
he writes, "carried up through the nose, thickens and condenses the
psychic pneuma, which is already thick and cold, and renders the
psychic pneuma unfit for functions of the soul. Now the body, if not
supported by the soul, is overcome by its own weight and falls
down."[145]

Even the influence of the moon itself was admitted and explained
physically by philosophers and physicians. Galen believed that its effect
on the periodicity of epileptic attacks depended on "the greater or
smaller share it received from the sun"; its effects were weak at half
moon, but strong at full moon.[146] On the basis of similar principles
which can be traced back to earlier philosophers, Antyllus, an older
contemporary of Galen and one of the greatest surgeons of Antiquity,
wrote: ". . . the moon rather moistens [the bodies]. And for this reason
it makes the brain relatively liquid and the flesh putrid and renders the
bodies of people who live in a clear cold air moist and dull and, for the
same reason, stirs up heaviness in the head and epilepsies."[147]

If one tries to sum up the attitude of the Greek physicians toward
"superstitious" beliefs and practices concerning epilepsy, one comes to
the following conclusions: After definite opposition on the part of the

---

[143] Alexander of Tralles (21), I, 15; vol. 1, p. 559.

[144] Plutarch (812), *Lycurgus*, 49 E; vol. 1, p. 254.

[145] Alexander of Aphrodisias (530), *Problems*, II, 64; vol. 1, p. 73, 28–34: ἡ γὰρ
ἀναφερομένη διὰ τῶν ῥινῶν παχυμέρεια τῶν ἀτμῶν παχύνει καὶ πιλοῖ τὸ ψυχικὸν πνεῦμα ἤδη
πρόσληψιν ἔχον παχύτητος καὶ ψυχρότητος καὶ ἀνεπιτήδειον ποιεῖ τὸ ψυχικὸν πνεῦμα τῇ ψυχῇ
πρὸς ἐνέργειαν. μὴ ὀχούμενον οὖν ὑπὸ ψυχῆς τὸ σῶμα τῷ οἰκείῳ βάρει ἐλεγχόμενον
καταπίπτει.

[146] Galen (394), *De diebus decretoriis*, III, 2; vol. 9, p. 903. Cf. also the scholium to Galen
(392), *In Hippocr. progn.*, p. 206, apparatus.

[147] Oribasius (753), *Collect. med.*, IX, 3; vol. 2, p. 7, 12–16. Cf. also Stahl (950), p. 257.

Hippocratics, the later physicians from the fourth century on became more and more inclined toward a practical compromise. In their majority they remained hostile to belief in a demoniac etiology, and they themselves did not use incantations. Yet with few exceptions they admitted the effectiveness of amulets and miraculous remedies as well as the influence of the moon. But it must be added that as far as can be judged from the fragmentary remains of their works, all these factors played only a subsidiary role and were separated from the rational explanation and treatment of the disease.[148]

---

[148] For this whole section cf. Edelstein (313), p. 205 ff., and below, II-3c.

# II
# Epilepsy in Ancient Medical Science

To trace the complete pathogenesis of a disease is one of the ideals of modern medical research. If successful, it states the etiology of the disease and explains its clinical picture on the basis of the underlying anatomical and physiological processes. In the case of epilepsy this ideal has not yet been reached, and it is doubtful whether it will be realized. For the existence of a "disease" epilepsy has become questionable, and many physicians are inclined to consider it a syndrome rather than an independent morbid entity.

This distinction between symptomatic epilepsy, i.e., a syndrome which might be associated with various diseases, and the possible existence of an "essential" or "genuine" *disease*, epilepsy, is, however, of relatively modern origin and was of little importance in Antiquity. The word "epilepsy" was used to connote both the disease and the single attack. From the times of Hippocrates on, physicians were well acquainted with the fact that the attacks had a tendency to repeat themselves, and epilepsy was therefore classified among the chronic diseases, while the individual attacks were considered paroxysms of the disease.[149] It was by the character of the attack that the disease was defined. "Epilepsy is a convulsion of the whole body together with an impairment of the leading functions,"[150] a definition found in several later authors,[151] obviously describes an attack, and whenever a

---

[149] Cf., e.g., Aretaeus (49), ed. Hude, III, 4; p. 38, 12–13.

[150] I.e., psychic functions.

[151] Cf. Fuchs (383), p. 598, footnote. Paulus of Aegina (778), ed. Heiberg, III, 13; vol. 1, p. 152, 18–19. Similarly Galen (394), *De symptomatum differentiis*, c. 3; vol. 7, p. 58 f., and *De locis affectis*, III, 9; vol. 8, p. 173.

fit corresponding to this or a similar description was observed, the patient was called an epileptic. This fact is of the utmost importance for the history of epilepsy, not in Antiquity only but in later periods as well. It makes it obvious that diseases such as eclampsia infantum, eclampsia gravidarum[152] were also called epilepsy. This in turn immediately explains why in Antiquity epilepsy in early childhood was considered such a frequent event as even to justify the synonym of "children's disease."[153]

Although at the present time there does not yet exist any general agreement about the pathology of epilepsy, all workers in the field are at least convinced that research has to proceed on scientific as well as clinical lines. But this was not the case in Antiquity, when scientific considerations were rejected by many physicians. The principles of medicine differed essentially according to the philosophy of the medical sect. In the time after Hippocrates, three main sects were formed, the dogmatic, empiric, and methodist. Of these, the dogmatists believed in the necessity of scientific research, for they thought systematic anatomical and physiological studies necessary in order to find the underlying or "hidden" causes of disease. The empiricists, on the other hand, whose sect was founded at the end of the third century B.C., doubted the possibility of ever finding these "hidden" causes and confined themselves to experience and the observation of such "evident causes" as heat, cold, hunger, satiety. The methodists, finally, the youngest of the three, were organized in the beginning of the first century A.D. The most radical adherents of this sect rejected causal thinking altogether and classified diseases according to some common features. Too much excretion proved a *status laxus*, too little a *status strictus*, and a mixture of both a *status mixtus*. Again, diseases might be acute or chronic and might pass through the stages of "increase," "constancy," or "diminuation." Later methodists, however, like Soranus, did not restrict themselves to such narrow principles but paid attention to causal factors too.[154]

These philosophical differences made the development of a pathology on generally accepted lines impossible in Antiquity. Only among the dogmatists can anatomical and physiological research into the nature of the disease be expected, and the dogmatists among themselves were divided into the followers of many competing systems. These theoretical differences were, of course, also reflected in the classification and treatment of epilepsy. Galen, for instance, distinguished three

---

[152] Cf. below, II-1a.

[153] Cf. below, II-1a.

[154] For characteristics of the three sects as well as for further more detailed literature on the subject cf. Edelstein (313).

types of the disease according to the different organs from which it
originated, and these types were to be diagnosed and treated accordingly. But for the methodists such an anatomical division was not binding and was replaced by considerations about the *status* which epilepsy
represented.

The pathology of epilepsy, then, and its rational therapy, have a
definite historical development, dependent on the traditions of sects
and the establishment of theories. To a certain extent this historical
development can still be traced, notwithstanding the fact that by far
the greater part of the ancient medical books has been lost.

This is not the case, however, concerning the observation of symptoms and the use of various therapeutic procedures. The medical literature of any period is an imperfect source for its actual clinical knowledge, and no textbook can record the multitude of varying signs which
are observed in practice. This is especially true where the bulk of the
literature is lost. It would be misleading to assume that observations
were first made at the time when they are first mentioned.[155] Description of a stage of tonic convulsion in the epileptic attack, for example,
is first found in a late writer of the Christian era; yet it must have been
known to earlier physicians. The same can be said of therapeutic procedures which have no obvious relation to a definite pathological
theory and are not recorded under an inventor's name. They may have
been used for hundreds of years before being mentioned in one of the
books that have come down to us.

It will consequently be advisable to study the medical literature of
the ancients from three points of view:

First: What they actually knew about epilepsy. Here it will be best
to record their clinical observations systematically according to the
arrangement followed in modern textbooks and without paying strict
attention to a chronological order.

Second: What they believed about the disease, that is, their pathological theories as far as they can be traced from the time of the
Hippocratics to the last of the ancient Greek writers.

Third: How the ancient physicians fought the disease.

To a certain extent, of course, the division of the first two parts is
artificial, for even observations are never quite free from tradition and
beliefs, as is especially true of etiological factors, even though their
discovery was deemed the result of experience. A certain synthesis of
these two parts will result from the third point of view, where it will be
possible to discuss how far the therapy was rational and how far it was
traditional and empiric.

---

[155] Cf. Baumann (88), p. 22.

## 1. THE CLINICAL PICTURE

### a. Etiology

Etiology, relating the *causes* of a disease, has by necessity a theoretical character. Usually there are many "causes" or "conditions" involved which all together form the complete "etiology," and these conditions may be more or less open to observation. The ancient distinction between "hidden" and "evident" causes reflects a difference which is especially important in a disease like epilepsy. The author of *On the Sacred Disease*, himself, discussed various factors which entered into a full explanation of the origin as well as the symptoms of epilepsy. He gave an account of the predisposition for the disease, of its anatomical basis, and finally of the causes provoking the single attacks. Theories about the "hidden" anatomical and physiological causes had necessarily a highly hypothetical character and will be discussed in the next chapter. Of the predisposing and provoking causes, on the other hand, such as heredity, constitution, age, sex, season, physical and mental strain, many could be observed directly, and as far as they were not bound to any specific theory they will be discussed here.

It was commonly recognized that epilepsy occurred most frequently in the early period of life,[156] especially at teething.[157] Its appearance for the first time after the age of twenty was deemed exceptional,[158] although some authors stated that it was characteristic of adolescence.[159] The possibility of its being congenital was also recognized[160] and the author of *On the Sacred Disease* even went as far as to maintain its hereditary character.[161] Curiously enough, his is the only statement of this kind to be found in the remains of ancient literature, and this seems no mere chance. For he maintained that *all* diseases were hereditary, that the sacred disease formed no exception, and that it was, therefore, just as capable of a natural explanation as were the others. His isolated statement, therefore, represents a dialectic argument against magic beliefs rather than the early recognition of the hereditary character of epilepsy.[162]

---

[156]Cf. Paulus of Aegina (778), ed. Heiberg, III, 13; vol. I, p. 152, 27 f. Caelius Aurelianus (192), *Morb. chron.*, I, 4, par. 60.

[157]Cf. Caelius Aurelianus, *ibid.*, par. 70.

[158]Cf. Hippocrates (491), *On the Sacred Disease*, ch. 10; vol. 6, p. 380, 15–16; Grensemann (429), p. 78, 10.

[159]Cf. Hippocrates (491), *Aphorisms*, III, 29; vol. 4, p. 500. Celsus (212), *De medicina*, II, I, 21; vol. 1, p. 94. Galen (394), vol. 17 B, p. 642, 16 ff., in his commentary on the Hippocratic aphorisms, criticized this statement.

[160]Cf. Hippocrates (491), *Prorrhetic*, II, 5; vol. 9, p. 20.

[161]Hippocrates (491), *On the Sacred Disease*, ch. 2; vol. 6, p. 364, 15; Grensemann (429), p. 68, 4.

[162]Cf. Temkin (999), p. 285 f.

The disease was thought to occur more often in men than in women,[163] and, besides the sexual distribution, sexual life in general was connected with it in many ways. The epileptic attack was compared to the sexual act, and both Hippocrates and Democritus were credited with the saying that "coitus is a slight epileptic attack."[164] Generally, the age of puberty was considered decisive in the course of epilepsy, since in many cases the epileptic attacks would stop at this period; otherwise, the disease would become incurable. Consequently, some physicians attributed the cause of a cure at this age to the first practice of intercourse and even did "violence to the nature of children by unseasonable coition"[165] in order to hasten this beneficial event. But most authorities rejected this idea, thought coitus harmful for epileptics, and advised abstinence from it, some even going as far as to recommend castration as a treatment.[166]

Conflicting as were the ideas about the influence of normal sexual life on epileptics, disturbances in this sphere were deemed an etiological factor. Galen counted untimely intercourse among the causes of epileptic seizures,[167] and the Hippocratic corpus included cessation of the menstrual flux.[168] Consequently, good menses were believed to prevent epilepsy in women.[169] Epileptiform seizures in pregnant women (eclampsia) were also observed and attributed to the uterus. "It has been seen in a pregnant woman that [epilepsy] arose from the uterus— but stopped after delivery."[170]

The climatic factor was carefully considered with respect to geographical position, seasons, wind, and rain. In cities, it is stated, which are exposed to cold winter winds but sheltered from southern and warm winds, cases of the so-called "sacred disease" would be rare but severe.[171] On the other hand, the children in such cities as stand under the influence of warm summer winds but are sheltered from the north winds would show attacks of "convulsions and difficult breathing which people believe . . . to be a sacred disease."[172] The dependence of

---

[163] Cf. Celsus (212), *De medicina*, III, 23; vol. 1, p. 334.

[164] Cf. Daremberg (754), vol. 1, p. 668.

[165] Aretaeus (50), ed. Adams, p. 473 (Adams' translation).

[166] All the references for this paragraph can be found in Daremberg (754), vol. 1, pp. 667-68.

[167] Galen (394), *De locis affectis*, V, 6; vol. 8, p. 341.

[168] Hippocrates (491), *Coan Prenotions*, 511; vol. 5, p. 702.

[169] Cf. Galen (394), *De venae sect. adv. Erasistr.*, c. 5; vol. 11, p. 165.

[170] Paulus of Aegina (778), ed. Heiberg, III, 13; vol. 1, p. 152, 25-27: ὤφθη δέ ποτε καὶ ἀπὸ τῆς ὑστέρας ἐπί τινος γυναικός, καθ' ὃν ἔγκυος ἐγένετο χρόνον, μετὰ δὲ τὴν ἀπότεξιν ἀπεπαύετο.

[171] Hippocrates (492), *Airs, Waters, Places*, ch. 4; p. 58, 25.

[172] *Ibid.*, ch. 3; p. 57, 25-27. For the reading of this and the above passage cf. Temkin (999), pp. 307-8.

the attacks on the character of the wind is also emphasized by the author of *On the Sacred Disease*, who, moreover, connects the various provoking causes, such as temperature, season, and wind, with the age of the patient. Sudden chilling after previous warming of the head and sudden change from south to north wind are bad for children, change of wind, especially one involving the south wind, for adults. To aged people spring and, above all, winter are most dangerous: spring, when the head has been exposed to the sun, winter, when they have warmed themselves at the fire and have then gone out into the cold or vice versa. Summer, on the other hand, since it lacks sudden changes, is comparatively safe for them.[173] Here, as everywhere in this book, however, the data are not stated as mere facts of observation but are made to conform with the author's theory of the dependence of epileptic attacks on the state of the brain. More generally, spring[174] and autumn[175] were held favorable to the occurrence of epileptic seizures, and the influence of the spring must have been generally accepted, since even a man like Soranus, who as a methodist did not pay too much attention to etiological factors, said that although attacks might occur at all times they were very frequent in spring.[176] In addition it was contended that epilepsy belonged to the diseases met during rainy periods.[177]

One of the characteristic features of ancient medicine is the emphasis placed on regimen as an etiological as well as a therapeutic factor, but it must be remembered that the ancient meaning of the word "regimen" was very broad and covered all the necessities of daily life, such as food and drink, sleep, and exercise, both physical and mental. Many internal diseases were attributed to mistakes committed in one or all of these spheres, and epilepsy was no exception. Galen stated that all cases of epilepsy which began at the time of adolescence were caused by dietetic errors.[178]

Regarding food, a great number of dishes were considered harmful, and their avoidance, as will be seen later, formed a chief part of the treatment of the disease. In general, all digestive trouble was believed to

---

[173]Hippocrates (491), *On the Sacred Disease*, chs. 10-11.

[174]Hippocrates (491), *Aphorisms*, III, 20; vol. 4, p. 494. Celsus (212), *De medicina*, II, I, 6; vol. 1, p. 88.

[175]Hippocrates, *l.c.*, III, 22; vol. 4, p. 496. Celsus, *l.c.*, II, I, 8; vol. 1, pp. 88-90. Galen (394), vol. 17 B, p. 624, in the commentary on this aphorism, attributes the cause to the daily changes of temperature during this season.

[176]Caelius Aurelianus (192), *Morb. chron.*, I, 4, par. 71.

[177]Hippocrates, *l.c.*, III, 16; vol. 4, p. 492. Celsus, *l.c.*, II, I, 12; vol. 1, pp. 90-92. Galen (394), vol. 17 B, p. 643, in his commentary, mentions exposure to sun and rain among the causes which might engender epilepsy in adolescents. Kobert (587), p. 20, interprets aphorisms III, 16 and 22, as referring to ergotism.

[178]Galen, *l.c.*

be one of the prime factors.[179] In the first place, this referred to actual difficulties in the digestion of food, but in certain cases, where the stomach was impaired, prolonged abstinence from food might also bring on attacks.[180]

Equal if not greater attention was paid to the consumption of wine. Great quantities of wine, far from heating the drinker, were thought to cause "cold" diseases.[181] Drunkenness, therefore, was one of the causes[182] of epilepsy, and this opinion was shared by physicians of quite different scientific views, e.g., Diocles of Carystus[183] and Soranus.[184] According to the latter, drunkenness in the wet nurse was likely to cause epileptic convulsions in the child.[185]

In certain people, exercise might engender epilepsy[186] and so might lack of exercise.[187] Hence, it will be found that among the therapeutic regulations the amount and method of exercise receive careful consideration.

To sleep on the earth might induce the disease in adolescents,[188] and to go to sleep on one's back might provoke attacks.[189] No less a scientist than Aristotle drew the general comparison that "sleep is similar to epilepsy and in some way, sleep is epilepsy."[190] Thus, the two physiological functions of sleep and sexual intercourse,[191] which both belong to the sphere of "regimen," were likened to the same disease, notwithstanding their different character.

Among the psychic causes, overwhelming fright[192] and anger[193] were recognized as factors in children; particularly, fright caused by something invisible or fear when someone shouted.[194] Under this category must also be mentioned various sensual impressions, for instance bad

---

[179] Cf. Galen (394), *De locis affectis*, V, 6; vol. 8, p. 341. Caelius Aurelianus, *l.c.*, par. 61.

[180] Cf. Galen (394), *De venae sect. adv. Erasistr.*, c. 9; vol. 11, pp. 241-42.

[181] Cf. Galen (394), *De temperamentis*, III, 2; vol. 1, p. 661.

[182] Cf. Galen (394), *De locis affectis*, V, 6; vol. 8, 341, and *De morb. caus.*, c. 8; vol. 7, pp. 13-14.

[183] Cf. Caelius Aurelianus, *l.c.*, par. 131.

[184] *Ibid.*, par. 61.

[185] Soranus (938), *Gynaeciorum*, II, 27; p. 74; translated in Soranus (937), p. 101. Generally speaking, epilepsy could be the consequence of spoiled milk, *ibid.*, II, 38; pp. 81 and 110 respectively.

[186] Cf. Galen (394), *Commentary on Hippocrates' Aphorisms*, III, 20; vol. 17 B, pp. 617-18.

[187] Cf. Galen (390), *De sanitate tuenda*, I, 8; p. 20, 1-11; for translation see Galen (396), p. 27. This passage is completely based on Galen's theory of innate heat and the humors; it is important because here Galen numbers epilepsy among the catarrhal and rheumatic diseases.

[188] Cf. Galen (394), *Commentary on Hippocrates' Aphorisms*, III, 29; vol. 17 B, p. 643.

[189] According to Diocles of Carystus; cf. Wellmann (1077), pp. 182-83.

[190] Aristotle (53), *On Sleep and Waking*, 457 A, 8-9.

[191] Cf. above.

[192] Caelius Aurelianus, *l.c.*, par. 61.

[193] Cf. below.

[194] Hippocrates (491), *On the Sacred Disease*, ch. 10.

smells[195] and the sight of whirling wheels.[196] Even philosophers like Plutarch knew of such provoking circumstances and compared the fatal influence of dizzy heights on epileptics to the moral maxim that evil would not be concealed by an elevated wordly position.[197]

All these and a few other "dietetic" factors in the broadest sense of the word were summarized by Galen when he said: "Sometimes, however, he [i.e., the epileptic] will necessarily encounter frost and violent heat, strong winds and strenuous baths, repulsive food and whirling wheels, lightning and thunder, sleeplessness and indigestion, distress and anger and weariness and similar things of which the chief characteristic is that they stir up and trouble the body violently, remind it of the disease, and produce a paroxysm."[198]

In marked contrast to the multitude of "dietetic" factors, other diseases were rarely considered the cause of epileptic fits. It was recognized that persistent attacks of vertigo might develop into epilepsy, and it was stated that melancholics were apt to become epileptic. Pathological conditions of the stomach, which were made responsible for certain forms of epileptic attacks, must be considered theoretical postulates, and the same is true of constitutional types as predisposing factors. Some of the dietetic irregularities, such as drinking, indigestion, irregularities of sexual life, might, of course, be mentioned again in this connection, especially the cessation of the menstrual flux. This latter finds its more general counterpart in the prognosis that when people who suffer from periodic hemorrhoidal bleedings become thirsty, and hemorrhage does not set in, they will die in an epileptic attack.[199] The fatal case of a two-months-old child, who suffered convulsions and epileptic seizures after skin eruptions and red swellings on various parts of the body had subsided,[200] is one of the few other instances of preceding illness.

This raises the question whether injuries to the skull had been observed as giving rise to subsequent epilepsy. The Hippocratic surgeons mention the occurrence of convulsions as a fatal sign of such injuries, and they assign them to the side opposite to that where the trauma or operation had taken place.[201] The fact that cramp had seized both hands of a man who had been hit by a stone on the bregma and who

---

[195] Cf. above, I–4.

[196] Apuleius (43), *Apologia*, 45.

[197] Plutarch (813), *To an Uneducated Ruler*, 782 E; vol. 10, p. 68.

[198] Galen (391), *Advice for an Epileptic Boy*, p. 181.

[199] Hippocrates (491), *Coan Prenotions*, 339; vol. 5, p. 656, and *Prorrhetic*, I, 131; vol. 5, p. 556. Cf. Temkin (999), p. 313 f.

[200] Hippocrates (491), *Epidemics*, VII, 106; vol. 5, p. 456.

[201] Hippocrates (491), *On Wounds in the Head*, chs. 13 and 19; vol. 3, pp. 234 and 254. *Coan Prenotions*, 184 and 488; vol. 5, pp. 624 and 696. *Prorrhetic*, I, 121; vol. 5, pp. 550–52. Case histories are given in *Epidemics*, V, 27, 28, and 50; vol. 5, pp. 226, 228, and 236, and *Epidemics*, VII, 35; vol. 5, pp. 402–4.

had died, in spite of belated trephining, was explained by the location of the injury in the middle of the head.[202] But in these instances the authors speak of "convulsions," not of epilepsy, and the convulsions occur a few days after the injury.[203]

### b. Definitions

"Epilepsy is an illness of various shapes and horrible," said Aretaeus,[204] thus summing up knowledge that had long found expression in the different descriptions and classifications of the symptoms. Even the shortest definitions of the disease, based only on the main features of the attack, show this variety. One of these definitions, viz., "epilepsy is a convulsion of the whole body together with an impairment of the leading functions," has been cited already. According to a statement whose authenticity is very suspect, it goes back to the Alexandrian physician Erasistratus[205] (third century B.C.), and in later times it acquired almost canonical value. Here epilepsy was among the convulsive disorders, and the important addition of "impairment of the leading functions" served to distinguish it from other convulsions. "Yet if there is not only convulsion of the whole body, but also interruption of the leading functions, then this is called 'epilepsy,'" said Galen.[206] To others, however, the convulsions seemed entirely accidental. "Epilepsy," wrote the author of the pseudo-Galenic *Medical Definitions*, "is a seizure of the mind and the senses together with a sudden fall, in some with convulsions, in others, however, without convulsion. Besides, in these patients froth flows through the mouth when the evil is abating and past its height."[207] Here the loss of consciousness and the sudden collapse stand in the foreground.

Accordingly, some physicians distinguished two different types of epilepsy: one in which the patient seemed to be overcome by a deep sleep—this type was likened to apoplexy,[208] and a second where he showed convulsions.[209] Others, however, combining the two added a third: the patient was first seized with convulsions and passed then into a deep sopor.[210]

---

[202] Hippocrates (491), *Epidemics*, V, 27; vol. 5, p. 226.

[203] Cf., however, the theories of Asclepiades and Soranus below, II–2b.

[204] Aretaeus (50), ed. Adams, p. 296 (Adams' translation).

[205] Cf. Fuchs (383), p. 598.

[206] Galen (394), *De symptom. differ.*, c. 3; vol. 7, pp. 58–59.

[207] Galen (394), *Definitiones medicae*, 240; vol. 19, p. 414. Celsus (212), *De medicina*, III, 23; vol. 1, pp. 332–34, has substantially the same definition.

[208] Caelius Aurelianus (192), *Morb. chron.*, I, 4, par. 61: "Quarum prima gravior iudicatur, siquidem est similis apoplexiae."

[209] Cf. Caelius Aurelianus, *ibid.*, and Anonymus Parisinus (1000), p. 140.

[210] Cf. Caelius Aurelianus, *ibid.*

These definitions, which were based on the clinical symptoms of the attack, were supplemented by an anatomical classification relative to the part primarily affected. According to Galen, the attack might originate from the brain directly, or the brain might be affected either by the stomach or by any other part of the body. The distinction of the three types chiefly rested on theoretical grounds, but partly it was also based on differences in the aura preceding the actual attack.

In accordance with these various definitions, the detailed descriptions of the epileptic attack as given by the authors vary greatly. Instead of discussing every description separately, it will be best to consider them as accounts of the various types of seizures which were observed and recorded by the ancients. We shall now summarize the observations concerning the epileptic attack and shall then discuss the course of the disease, its diagnosis, and prognosis.

### c. Aura

"Aura" nowadays means subjective symptoms at the onset of an attack. This word, taken from the Greek, originally meant a "breeze." It was introduced into medical terminology not by a physician but by a patient. When still a young man, Galen, together with other physicians, visited a thirteen-year-old boy. The patient told them that the condition originated in the lower leg, and that "from here it climbed upwards in a straight line through the thigh and further through the flank and side to the neck and as far as the head; but as soon as it had touched the latter he was no longer able to follow." When the physicians asked him what exactly rose up to the head, he could not tell. But another youth, who was a better observer, said "that it was like a cold breeze."[211]

Obviously, then, "aura" at first connoted one particular type of sensation with which the attack began, and the broadening of its meaning was the work of much later periods. Besides the "breeze," however, the ancients themselves knew many other premonitory signs, tactile, sensory, motor, and psychic. But they grouped them differently. One of the Hippocratic authors described patients who, while without fever, suffered from headache, noises, dizziness, slow speech, and stiffness of the hands. He expected them to be seized by an apoplectic or epileptic attack or to lose their memory.[212] Some centuries later Soranus (or rather his later Latin paraphraser, Caelius Aurelianus) gave the following list of symptoms which he thought characterized the onset of epilepsy as well as of any other disease originating in the meninges:

---

[211] Galen (394), *De locis affectis*, III, 11; vol. 8, p. 194: . . . οἶον αὔραν τινὰ ψυχρὰν ἔφασκεν εἶναι τὴν ἀνερχομένην.

[212] Hippocrates (491), *Coan Prenotions*, 157; vol. 5, p. 618.

"Heaviness and giddiness in the head, an inner noise, which is felt in the occiput too, tension in the eyes, ringing in the ears[213] or difficulty in hearing; and together with the vertigo, dimness of the eyesight or something hanging down before the eyes, as it were, either similar to the spots of marble which the Greeks call 'armarygmata' or 'marmarygas,' or similar to spider webs or to very thin clouds or to very small flying animals like gnats. The patients also perceive tiny sparks, so to speak, or fiery circles borne around before their eyes. The tongue is not flexible, and at the same time muscles twitch, and they have pains in the back between the shoulders. There also follow rigor of the throat and a concomitant precordial distention together with yawning, sneezing, flow of saliva, and aversion to food or immoderate appetite. Continuous sleeplessness or a very deep and unprofitable sleep, troubled dreams, and difficult digestion of food. Erection of the genital without evident reason and frequent delight in sexual intercourse. Sometimes also loss of semen during sleep, which the Greeks call 'onirogmon.' The mind is anxious and troubled, and they are readily roused to anger for no major reason. There is forgetfulness for what has been done shortly beforehand and a ready disposition for things causing gloom."[214]

All these signs, according to Soranus, might be observed at the very onset of the disease as well as before a recurring attack. Moreover, certain additional symptoms in epileptics announced the repetition of the seizure: "They are listless and go about their accustomed tasks with sluggish movements; they have a feeling of heaviness and are sleepy and depressed. Their complexion is unnatural, and the veins distended; their eyes have a sort of distortion, their gaze is lowered. In fact, it is difficult for the patient to raise his eyes, that is, to look upward; and if he tries to do so, he is soon discouraged and lowers the pupils of his eyes again.[215] And if they turn the head to the other side with a sudden movement, they experience giddiness, trembling, and torpor, together with contraction of, or pain in, the fingers, or heaviness of the thighs and the extremities of the hands and feet."[216]

It will be noticed that these lists of premonitory signs included some of longer duration as well as some which might immediately precede the seizure. Aretaeus tried to separate these two groups.[217] The former, he thought, included stupor, vertigo, tension of the members, fulness and swelling of the veins of the neck, aversion to food, much vomiting of phlegm, flatulence, high diaphragm. But "when the term of the attack

[213] For this symptom cf. also Celsus (212), *De medicina*, VI, 7, 8; vol. 2, p. 238.

[214] Caelius Aurelianus (192), *Morb. chron.*, I, 4, par. 62 f. with some adaptations from Drabkin's (192) translation.

[215] Drabkin's (192) translation (adapted).

[216] Caelius Aurelianus, *l.c.*, par. 69.

[217] Cf. Baumann (88), p. 19.

comes nearer, red or black lights or both together appear in arcs before the eyes, similar to the rainbow. The patients feel their ears ringing, they smell bad odors, are irritable, and become angry without reason."[218] The writers on physiognomy also had something to contribute, particularly concerning the eyes. Eyes deviating upward were one sign of "the so-called sacred disease." If, in addition, there was quivering (nystagmus?), an epileptic attack was imminent.[219]

Galen and his successors, however, stressed the classification of premonitory signs according to the supposed starting point of the seizure. Such signs as heaviness of the head, dizziness, weak sight, and dullness would indicate the brain as the primary seat of the disease.[220] Sensations in the region of the stomach would point to the latter organ as primarily affected.[221] But then the disease might also originate from any part of the body. It was in this case, according to Galen, that the "aura," i.e., the "breeze," would be felt ascending from that part to the head. Aretaeus, who recognized nerves distant from the head as a possible origin, gave a slightly different description: "Wherefore the great fingers of the hands, and the great toes of the feet are contracted; pain, torpor, and trembling succeed, and a rush of them to the head takes place. If the mischief spread until it reach the head, a crash takes place, in these cases, as if from the stroke of a piece of wood, or of stone; and, when they rise up, they tell how they have been maliciously struck by some person."[222]

Various motives made the ancients pay attention to the premonitory signs. Manipulations, such as ligatures, might postpone the attack which announced itself in a limb.[223] The place of origin, whether or not the seizure started from some distant part, was believed prognostically significant.[224] Besides, realization of the approaching attack might save the patient from danger, giving him time to choose a place where he could fall "securely and without disgrace."[225]

So well known, indeed, was the existence of premonitory signs and of the advantages accruing therefrom that Seneca could use this knowledge as a parable for moral reflections. "People," he wrote, "who are wont to be seized by epilepsy, know that the evil is approaching if the

---

[218] Aretaeus (49), ed. Hude, I, 5, p. 3, 9–12.

[219] Adamantius and similarly Pseudo-Polemon, Foerster (368), p. 315.

[220] Alexander of Tralles (21), I, 15; vol. 1, p. 537.

[221] Alexander of Tralles, *ibid.* Paulus of Aegina (778), ed. Heiberg, III, 13, 3; vol. 1, p. 155.

[222] Aretaeus (50), ed. Adams, p. 244 (Adams' translation).

[223] Aretaeus (49), ed. Hude, I, 5; p. 4, 2. The parallel with Jacksonian epilepsy is obvious; see below, p. 305.

[224] Cf. Hippocrates (491), *Prorrhetic,* II, 9; vol. 9, p. 28. Cf. also Temkin (999), p. 305. Celsus (212), *De medicina,* II, 8, 29; vol. 1, p. 146.

[225] Caelius Aurelianus, *l.c.,* par. 68.

warmth has left the extremities and an uncertain light and trembling of the sinews are present, if memory slips and the head whirls." He then described their attempts to avoid the oncoming attack and added: "It is useful to know one's disease and to suppress its powers, before they spread."[226]

### d. The Epileptic Attack

Whether forewarned or taken by surprise,[227] the patient falls to the ground, unconscious and not susceptible to pain. When he regains consciousness he does not remember what happened to him during the fit.

These are the features common to all forms of epileptic attacks, whereas all further symptoms depend on the type of fit. If no convulsions are present,[228] the patient lies pale and motionless in a deep sleep approaching a state of torpor, his mouth is open, he breathes slowly and noisily, and his pulse is big.[229]

Whereas the "apoplectic" type shows but a simple clinical picture, the "convulsive" type is described in much more detail. In the Hippocratic writings the descriptions are sketchy, emphasizing the main symptoms only. The patient is dumb and loses consciousness, being insensible to sound, sight, and pain. His body is drawn and twisted on all sides; in particular, his hands are cramped, his teeth clenched; he kicks with his legs and shows distortion of the eyes. Foam flows from his mouth, he suffocates and may pass excrements.[230] In addition, coldness of the legs and hands, possible lividity, turning upward of the white of the eyes, palpitation of the heart, and profuse sweating are among the symptoms, and these make an epileptic and a hysterical attack very similar.[231]

In later medical literature we find more comprehensive accounts of the epileptic paroxysm with a more detailed analysis of its course and its symptoms, some physicians even trying to separate the various stages of the seizure. After the fall to the ground, Aretaeus distinguishes three main periods: manifestation, abatement, cessation. The manifestation is characterized by insensibility and tonic and clonic convulsions. While it is on the increase, suffocation with its concomitant signs appears and, at the end, erection of the genital. During the abatement, the patients

---

[226] Seneca (910), *On Anger*, III, 10, 3-4; pp. 278-80.

[227] Caelius Aurelianus (192), *Morb. chron.*, I, 4, par. 67 f. Theodorus Priscianus (1006), *Logicus*, 15; p. 147, 15.

[228] The description of this type has been combined from the Anonymus Parisinus (1000), p. 140, and Caelius Aurelianus, *l.c.*, paragraphs 61 and 64.

[229] The characterizations of the pulse are not the same in the different authors. Caelius Aurelianus, *l.c.*, gives "big" as the only characteristic. The Anonymus Parisinus, *l.c.*, describes it as "big, retarding and lethargic." Pseudo-Rufus (879), *Synopsis of the Pulse*, ch. 6; pp. 227-28, calls it "big, empty, and usually constant and rapid."

[230] This description is combined from Hippocrates (491), *On the Sacred Disease*, ch. 7, and *On Breaths*, ch. 14.

[231] Hippocrates (491), *On Diseases of Women*, I, ch. 7 and II, ch. 151; vol. 8, pp. 32 and 326.

unconsciously discharge urine, excrements, and semen, and finally a flow of froth ends the suffocation. Then they arise, the evil having ended. But during the following cessation they still have various signs of physical and psychic discomfort.[232]

Curiously enough, it is a late Latin author, Theodorus Priscianus, whose chapter on epilepsy pictures the course of an attack in a way similar to the grand mal of the modern textbook. After various premonitory signs the patient falls down, stretched out or twisted, and in this condition he remains for some time. After these tonic convulsions he passes into the stage of clonic convulsions and a condition where he appears to be sleeping.[233] The attack is followed by complete amnesia.

Considering the great variety in the appearance of epileptic fits, it is no wonder that the accounts of the various physicians are not quite identical. But if all the symptoms they describe are put together, the sum total shows a thorough acquaintance not only with the main features as mentioned in the Hippocratic collection but with finer details as well.

Besides stridor, moaning, and the uttering of confused sounds,[234] the initial cry, too, was observed.[235] Regarding the behavior of the seized person, Aretaeus compared it to the sight of an ox whose throat had been cut: arms cramped, the head drawn forward, backward, or to the shoulders, and the legs kicking in all directions.[236] Special attention was paid to the convulsive movements in the region of the face: the cheeks tremble,[237] and the whole face is swollen,[238] red, and distorted,[239] the mouth is dry[240] with the tongue protruding,[241] and when the teeth are clenched the tongue is hurt[242] or a piece of it is even bitten off.[243] The lips are either pursed tightly or retracted as in a smile,[244] the eyebrows and the skin of the forehead stretched or contracted as in a frown,[245] the eyelids raised and quivering.[246] The eyes are either turned in-

---

[232] Aretaeus (49), ed. Hude, I, 5; pp. 4-5.

[233] Theodorus Priscianus, l.c., p. 148, 3-4: "et veluti dormientes cum sonitu pectoris gravius comprimuntur." Cf. Baumann (88), p. 25.

[234] Cf. preceding footnote and Caelius Aurelianus, l.c., par. 65.

[235] Paulus of Aegina (778), ed. Heiberg, III, 13; vol. 1, p. 153, 8-9. The cries of the patients discussed in ch. 1 of On the Sacred Disease can also be interpreted as initial cries.

[236] Aretaeus, l.c., p. 4, 7 ff.

[237] Aretaeus, ibid., p. 4, 21-22.

[238] Anonymus Parisinus (1000), p. 140.

[239] Caelius Aurelianus, l.c., par. 64 f.

[240] Aretaeus, l.c., p. 4, 14.

[241] Aretaeus, ibid. Caelius Aurelianus, l.c., par. 65. Anonymus Parisinus, l.c., p. 140.

[242] Ibid.

[243] Aretaeus, ibid. Anonymus Parisinus, ibid.

[244] Aretaeus, l.c., p. 4, 22-24.

[245] Ibid., p. 4. 18-21.

[246] Ibid., p. 4, 16.

ward,[247] or glassy and immobile first, then twisted and distorted.[248]
The veins of the head stand out[249] and, with the increasing attack, the
head takes on a livid discoloration and the blood vessels of the neck
become swollen too.[250]

An upward jump may sometimes be observed in the precordial
region,[251] while the abdomen is contracted.[252] Respiration stops and is
resumed at intervals.[253] The pulse, which may show a similar phenomenon,[254] is irregular during the whole course of the attack;[255] as to its
other qualities, it is "strong, and quick, and small in the beginning;—
great, slow, and feeble in the end."[256] But here agreement was not
reached. One anonymous writer believed a big and hollow pulse characteristic for a convulsive seizure,[257] whereas Galen differentiated according to the strength of the attack. If it is moderate, a certain tension of
the artery will be the only noticeable sign; if it is more violent, the
pulse appears uneven, tense, and relatively small, feeble, and thin. In a
vehement attack, finally, the pulse will be feeble, frequent, and
quick.[258]

In addition to the amnesia, the authors also record various other
symptoms which appear after the patients have roused themselves and
have regained consciousness. They are weak, pale, and languid, move
lazily, yawn, and the head feels heavy.[259] The distortion of the eyes
and protrusion of the veins on the forehead may still continue, and in
some cases there is mental aberration, and they do not recognize their
friends.[260] Apart from their physical discomfort, they are "spiritless,
and dejected, from the suffering and shame of the dreadful
malady."[261]

### e. The Course of the Disease

The isolated epileptic paroxysm is an acute affliction.[262] But more
often than not it will repeat itself, and the disease will take on a chronic

---

[247] *Ibid.*

[248] Anonymus Parisinus, *l.c.*

[249] *Ibid.* and Caelius Aurelianus, *l.c.*, par. 65.

[250] Aretaeus, *l.c.*, p. 4, 24-25.

[251] Caelius Aurelianus, *l.c.*, par. 65.

[252] Anonymus Parisinus, *l.c.*

[253] Caelius Aurelianus, *l.c.*, par. 65.

[254] *Ibid.*

[255] Anonymus Parisinus, *l.c.*; Aretaeus, *l.c.*, p. 4, 29.

[256] Aretaeus (50), ed. Adams, p. 245 (Adams' translation).

[257] Pseudo-Rufus (879), *Synopsis of the Pulse*, ch. 6; p. 228, 2-4.

[258] Galen (394), *De pulsibus ad tirones*, c. 12; vol. 8, pp. 487-88.

[259] Aretaeus (49), ed. Hude, I, 5; p. 5, 11-12. Caelius Aurelianus, *l.c.*, par. 66.

[260] Caelius Aurelianus, *ibid.*

[261] Aretaeus (50), ed. Adams, p. 246 (Adams' translation).

[262] Aretaeus discusses the epileptic attack among the acute diseases, but ranges epilepsy among the chronic diseases.

form; consequently, after the cessation of the first attack, the physician will still suspect its latent presence in the body.[263] The development of the disease may announce itself by the premonitory signs which mark the onset of a typical fit. In particular, two pathological conditions, nightmare and vertigo, were seen closely related to epilepsy. In the book *On the Sacred Disease*, nightly terrors have already been mentioned as a form of the disease attributed to Hekate and the Heroes.[264] And although a later author, Soranus, discusses nightmare in a separate chapter, he nevertheless calls it a forerunner of epilepsy.[265] If it is not cured but becomes worse, epilepsy will follow.[266] Posidonius, a physician of the fourth century A.D., also calls it a "threatening symptom and preface" of epilepsy or mania, or apoplexy and adds: "What epileptics suffer in their attacks when awake, sufferers from incubus undergo in their sleep."[267]

Vertigo, likewise, if incurable, may be the beginning of epilepsy,[268] and where the latter exists, it is present too.[269] Soranus mentions that sufferers from vertigo may also fall suddenly and get up very quickly. But he differentiates it from an epileptic attack, since it does not bereave the patient of his senses nor affect him with a convulsion.[270] According to Aretaeus, however, "ignorance of themselves and of those around" is among the characteristic features of the condition.[271] The Greeks themselves said that the "ancients" had called vertigo a "little epilepsy,"[272] which all goes to prove that minor attacks were known to them, although they were often confused with other forms of dizziness and nausea.[273]

A typical case of chronic epilepsy would begin in childhood and, provided it was not cured or did not disappear at the time of puberty, it would increase and become worse and worse.[274] The attacks would repeat themselves with or without any definite periodicity. The inter-

---

[263] Caelius Aurelianus (192), *Morb. chron.*, I, 4; par. 82.

[264] Cf. above, I-3.

[265] Caelius Aurelianus (192), *Morb. chron.*, I, 3, par. 55: "Est autem supradicta passio epilepsiae tentatio."

[266] *Ibid.*, par. 59.

[267] Aetius (11), *Libr. med.*, VI, c. 12; p. 152, 13-14: οὐκ ἔστιν ὁ καλούμενος ἐφιάλτης δαίμων, ἀλλὰ μελέτη καὶ προοίμια ἐπιληψίας ἢ μανίας ἢ ἀποπληξίας. *Ibid.*, lines 25-26: ὅσα γὰρ οἱ ἐπίληπτοι ἐπὶ τοῖς παροξυσμοῖς πάσχουσι, ταῦτα οἱ ἐφιαλτικοὶ καθεύδοντες. See below, footnote 276.

[268] Aretaeus (49), ed. Hude, III, 3; p. 38, 3-5.

[269] (Pseudo) Galen (394), *Introductio seu medicus*, c. 13; vol. 14, p. 740.

[270] Caelius Aurelianus (192), *Morb. chron.*, I, 2, par. 52.

[271] Aretaeus (50), ed. Adams, p. 296 (Adams' translation).

[272] Caelius Aurelianus, *l.c.*, par. 51: "Veteres denique parvam epilepsiam vocaverunt."

[273] Aretaeus, *l.c.*, p. 296, adds to his description of vertigo: ". . . and, if the disease go on increasing, the limbs sink below them, and they crawl on the ground; there is nausea and vomitings of phlegm, or of yellow or black bilious matter" (Adams' translation).

[274] Galen (394), *In Hippocr. epid. VI, comment.*, V, sect. 5, c. 26; vol. 17 B, p. 288 ff.

vals between the attacks might be very long, perhaps twelve months; or
shorter, so that the fits could recur in the same month or even in the
same day.[275] They might take place during sleep[276] and, according to
Aristotle, in many persons the disease originated in their sleep and did
not attack them while awake.[277]

The intervals themselves often were not free from disturbances,
especially dizziness and the various symptoms enumerated, together
with the premonitory signs.[278] And if the disease became chronic, the
whole personality of the patients would be affected. They became
"languid, spiritless, stupid, inhuman, unsociable, and not disposed to
hold intercourse, nor to be sociable, at any period of life; sleepless,
subject to many horrid dreams, without appetite, and with bad digestion; pale, of a leaden color; slow to learn, from torpidity of the understanding and of the senses; dull of hearing; have noises and ringing in
the head; utterance indistinct and bewildered, either from the nature of
the disease, or from the wounds during the attacks; the tongue is rolled
about in the mouth convulsively in various ways."[279] Finally, persons
who had been epileptic from youth would reach a mental state comparable to the stupor of extreme drunkenness.[280] The epileptic slave,
Thallus, is described as falling down three or four times a day with
limbs convulsed, his face is ulcerated, forehead and occiput bruised, his
eyes look dull, his nostrils are distended, his feet are weak, he cannot
stand long, for he reels, "tending to the disease as to sleep."[281]

### f. Prognosis and Complications

A severe epileptic fit may kill the patient immediately.[282] This is
especially the case when the disease is not yet chronic[283] or if the

---

[275]Caelius Aurelianus (192), *Morb. chron.*, I, 4, par. 67.

[276]Diocles of Carystus [Wellmann (1077), p. 182] warned that δύσπνοια ... καὶ πνιγμοὶ καὶ
ἐπιληπτικὰ καὶ ἐξονειριασμοί threatened those sleeping on their backs. According to Plato
(802), *Timaeus*, 85 B; p. 228, attacks during sleep were more easily stopped than those during
the waking state. Professor H. J. Drossaart Lulofs (personal communication) kindly drew my
attention to possible confusions between nocturnal epileptic attacks and nightmares and to
Galen's comment on the passage in the *Timaeus*. Galen (389), *Compendium Timaei Platonis*,
22; p. 30 (Arabic text) says: "And when the phlegm mingles with the black bile and is poured
out into the head, the disease which is called the divine (*al-'ilāhīyu*) arises therefrom. And [of]
the genus of this disease [also are] the manifestations occurring during sleep. Obviously he [i.e.,
Plato] means by 'the manifestations occurring during sleep' the disease which recent physicians
call 'incubus'" (see also Latin translation and comments on p. 90). Neither Galen nor "the
recent physicians," it seems, claimed identity of epilepsy and incubus. Cf. above, footnote 267.

[277]Aristotle (53), *On Sleep and Waking*, 3, 457 A, 9-11; p. 336.

[278]Caelius Aurelianus, *l.c.*, par. 66.

[279]Aretaeus, *l.c.*, p. 297 (Adams' translation).

[280]Aristotle (55), *Problems*, 30, 1; 953 B, p. 156.

[281]Apuleius (43), *Apologia*, 43, 30; cf. *ibid.*, 44.

[282]Hippocrates (491), *On the Sacred Disease*, ch. 7; vol. 6, p. 374, 13 ff.; Grensemann
(429), p. 75, 14.

[283]Celsus (212), *De medicina*, III, 23; vol. 1, p. 334.

attack extends into the second day.[284] Small children are in danger of
their lives when a severe attack overcomes them while the south wind is
blowing.[285] If the disease makes its first appearance in old age, it is
usually fatal,[286] above all if the attack occurs in winter.[287] It also
carries death when it appears in dropsical persons.[288]

On the whole, however, the life of the epileptic is little endangered
by the disease. Yet there are certain complications which can develop
after the fit, above all distortions and paresis of certain parts. During
the attack, especially if the evil had set in in an acute form, the eyes
would be distorted, and the epileptic might continue to squint afterwards.[289] The question which interested philosophers of the Aristotelian school, viz., why in man, of all animals, squinting occurred, was
answered tentatively by the statement that man alone suffered from
epilepsy.[290] Besides squinting, nystagmus of one or both eyes could
also have its cause in epilepsy,[291] and so might more serious eye
trouble,[292] even blindness.[293] Distortions too were apt to befall the
region of the face and neck[294] or the sides,[295] with consequent weakness of the part.[296] A hand could become paretic[297] or atrophied,[298] or
a foot or a whole leg paralyzed.[299]

Children were the preferred victims of such complications, and besides those mentioned they might also evince tumors below the neck, a
voice which sounded thin, a chronic dry cough, frequent stomach pain
without diarrhea, thick varicose veins in the region of the stomach, and

---

[284]Caelius Aurelianus (192), *Morb. chron.*, I, 4, par. 87. This may have referred to *status
epilepticus*.

[285]Hippocrates (491), *On the Sacred Disease*, ch. 8; vol. 6, p. 374, 21 ff.; Grensemann
(429), p. 75, 1.

[286]Hippocrates (491), *Prorrhetic*, II, 9; vol. 9, p. 28, 22 ff.

[287]Hippocrates (491), *On the Sacred Disease*, ch. 9; vol. 6, p. 378, 1-4; Grensemann (429),
p. 77, 4.

[288]Hippocrates (491), *Coan Prenotions*, 445; vol. 5, p. 684 (eclamptic form of uremia?).

[289]Caelius Aurelianus, *l.c.*, par. 64: ". . . vultus contortio vel oculorum sequetur, quae saepe
perseverans etiam post accessionem strabos fingit aegrotantes; atque contrario quibus tarda
fuerit correctio, naturalis visus simulant aequitatem." Cf. also Hippocrates (491), *Epidemics*, II,
5, 11; vol. 5, p. 130. *Prorrhetic*, II, 10; vol. 9, p. 28. Anonymus Parisinus (1000), p. 140.

[290]Aristotle (55), *Problems*, 31, 26 and 27, 960 A; vol. 2, p. 198.

[291]Celsus (212), *De medicina*, VI, 6, 36; vol. 2, 222.

[292]Hippocrates (491), *Prorrhetic*, II, 10; vol. 9, p. 28.

[293]Hippocrates (491), *Epidemics*, II, 5, 11; vol. 5, p. 130. Aretaeus (49), ed. Hude, III, 4; p.
38, 20-21, says quite generally that any sense might be disabled.

[294]Hippocrates (491), *On the Sacred Disease*, ch. 8; vol. 6, p. 376, 4; Grensemann (429), p.
75, 4.

[295]Hippocrates (491), *Prorrhetic*, II, 10; vol. 9, p. 30.

[296]Hippocrates (491), *On the Sacred Disease*, ch. 8; vol. 6, p. 376, 6-7; Grensemann (429),
p. 75, 4-5.

[297]Aretaeus (49), ed. Hude, III, 4; p. 38, 20.

[298]Hippocrates (491), *Prorrhetic*, II, 10; vol. 9, p. 30, 5.

[299]*Ibid.*

enlarged testicles.[300] Old people, on the other hand, if they survived the onset of epilepsy at all, according to the author of *On the Sacred Disease*, would become paralyzed on one side.[301]

Concerning the chances of recovery, it was of the utmost importance at what age the disease first put in an appearance. Epilepsy dating from birth is obstinate.[302] Yet, as a rule, it may cease if it appears before puberty,[303] and this latter period itself, as has been mentioned above, often brings relief from the disease.[304] Apart from this change of age, change of place and habit of life is also beneficial for juvenile epileptics.[305] Even epilepsy which started at adolescence need not persist, provided that the regimen is suitable.[306] But if it began before puberty and extended right through this period, then, indeed, it is bad in the extreme.[307] It is even worse than if it had started between twenty-five and forty-five years of age,[308] though as a general rule epilepsy originating after the age of twenty-five lasts until death.[309] In these chronic cases the attacks become more and more frequent but are easily overcome, and, although the disease is now incurable, the patient grows old together with it.[310] A third unfavorable possibility is presented where the attack has no localized onset. The hands and feet are the best points of departure, the sides relatively better than the head, which latter is the worst.[311]

On the whole, it can be said that the epileptic's chances of complete recovery were viewed with pessimism, especially when the disease had taken on a chronic form. What the chances of successful treatment were believed to be will be discussed later. But apart from artificial treatment, nature offered one powerful preventive of and remedy for the disease. "People who are seized by quartan fever are not seized by the

---

[300]Hippocrates, *ibid.*, where "dropping of the omentum" is also listed. Swelling of the testicles is also mentioned in *Epidemics*, II, 5, 11; vol. 5, p. 130, which adds pains in the loins and "raising of the breasts." This list is identical with that in *Crises*, 44; vol. 9, p. 290, which refers to "chronic" epilepsy.

[301]Hippocrates (491), *On the Sacred Disease*, ch. 9; vol. 6, p. 378, 2-6; Grensemann (429), p. 77, 3. This statement, however, is largely based on the author's pathological speculations.

[302]Hippocrates (491), *Prorrhetic*, II, 5; vol. 9, p. 20.

[303]Hippocrates (491), *Aphorisms*, V, 7; vol. 4, p. 534. Celsus (212), *De medicina*, II, 8, 11; vol. 1, p. 136.

[304]Cf. above, II-1e.

[305]Hippocrates (491), *Aphorisms*, II, 45; vol. 4, p. 482.

[306]Cf. Galen's (394) commentary on Hippocrates' aphorism V, 7; vol. 17 B, p. 792.

[307]Hippocrates (491), *Prorrhetic*, II, 9; vol. 9, p. 28.

[308]*Ibid.*

[309]Hippocrates (491), *Aphorisms*, V, 7; vol. 4, p. 534. Celsus (212), *l.c.*, II, 8, 29; vol. 1, p. 146. Anonymus Parisinus (1000), p. 140.

[310]Hippocrates (491), *On the Sacred Disease*, ch. 11; vol. 6, p. 382; Grensemann (429), p. 79, 1 and 6. Celsus, *l.c.*, III, 23, 1; vol. 1, p. 334.

[311]Hippocrates (491), *Prorrhetic*, II, 9; vol. 9, p. 28. Celsus, *l.c.*, II, 8, 29 and II, 8, 11; vol. 1, pp. 146 and 136.

great disease. If, however, they are seized [i.e., by epilepsy] first, and quartan fever supervenes, they are released [i.e., from epilepsy]."[312] This Hippocratic dictum, which was also referred to spasms in general,[313] was taken up by later physicians as well,[314] and Rufus of Ephesus gave it an almost religious turn. A physician able to cure by wilfully provoking fever ought, indeed, to be considered a god! But, alas, humans did not possess such power, which was reserved to gods alone. Then he related the story of Teucer, the Cyzican, whom the god Asclepius asked whether he was willing to be cured from his epilepsy by exchanging it for another smaller evil. Upon Teucer's consent the god gave him quartan fever, and the epilepsy stopped.[315]

### g. Diagnosis

If the physician witnesses an epileptic attack, recognition of the disease is comparatively easy.[316] During the intervals a diagnosis is much more difficult. Then the physician might try to question the patient about any of the signs preceding attacks or occurring during the intervals.[317] Apart from this anamnestic method, which to a certain extent depended on the cooperation of the patient, possible residues of former attacks, such as squinting, atrophy, or paresis of extremities, might point to the disease.[318] But sometimes it was imperative to reach a diagnosis, even if the patient did not offer any objective signs and did not cooperate. This was especially the case when the question concerned a slave offered for sale.

The ancient Babylonian law of Hamurabbi contained a paragraph in which it was said that a slave could be returned and the money given back if *bennu* appeared within the month after the purchase.[319] The word *bennu* has been interpreted as meaning epilepsy,[320] though unfortunately the translation is not beyond doubt.[321] At any rate, in the

---

[312]Hippocrates (491), *Epidemics*, VI, 6, 5; vol. 5, p. 324.

[313]Hippocrates (491), *Aphorisms*, V, 70; vol. 4, p. 562.

[314]Galen (394), *In Hippocr. epid. VI, comment.* VI, sect. 6, c. 7; vol. 17 B, p. 341 ff.

[315]Oribasius (753), *Collect. med.*, 45, 30; vol. 3, p. 192, 3 ff. According to von Wilamowitz-Moellendorff (1102), p. 122, footnote, Teucer was a Greek historian and contemporary of Rufus.

[316]Caelius Aurelianus (192), *Morb. chron.*, I, 4, par. 70.

[317]*Ibid.*

[318]Hippocrates (491), *Prorrhetic*, II, 10; vol. 9, pp. 28–30.

[319]Cf. Edwards (316), p. 45.

[320]Sudhoff (971), p. 360.

[321]From the use of *bennu* in other texts it is not quite possible to get a clear picture of the disease; cf. Thompson (1017), p. 816 and (1016), p. 147. If it is really identical with the disease šu Dingir. Ra, then its symptoms would be: "he blasphemes the gods, speaks wantonly, strikes everything he sees" [Thompson (1018), p. 452, and (1016), p. 147, footnote]. But this description suggests mania rather than epilepsy. Kinnier Wilson (582), p. 202, thinks of a heart condition. On the other hand, the identification of Sumerian *antašubbû* (see above footnote 2)

fourth century B.C. a law existed in Athens providing that "when a party sells a slave, he shall declare beforehand if he has any blemish; if he omit to do so, he shall be compelled to make restitution."[322] The example given of such a "blemish" is epilepsy,[323] and Greek business documents from Egypt prove the commercial importance of this point by the clause that the validity of the sale of the slave can be questioned if he proves a sufferer from the "sacred disease."[324] In one document from 359 A.D. the period of probation is stipulated as six months following the purchase.[325]

In his *Laws* Plato proposed detailed provisions for the process of restitution in such cases. "If a man sell a slave who is suffering from phthisis or stone or strangury or the 'sacred disease' (as it is called), or from any other complaint, mental or physical, which most men would fail to notice, although it be prolonged and hard to cure,—in case the purchaser be a doctor or a trainer, it shall not be possible for him to gain restitution for such a case, nor yet if the seller warned the purchaser of the facts. But if any professional person sell any such slave to a lay person, the buyer shall claim restitution within six months, saving only in the case of epilepsy,[326] for which disease he shall be permitted to claim within twelve months. The action shall be tried before a bench of doctors nominated and chosen by both the parties; and the party that loses his case shall pay double the selling price of the slave. If a lay person sells to a lay person, there shall be the same right of restitution and trial as in the cases just mentioned; but the losing party shall pay the selling price only."[327]

This passage gives a good summary of some general opinions concerning epilepsy. Like several other diseases, it is chronic and hard to cure. It may not reveal itself for a whole year and would easily be hidden to the layman.[328] But not so to the physician. He cannot even claim restitu-

---

with *miqtu* (from Accadian *mqt*, "to fall") and with *bennu* supports the interpretation of the latter as epilepsy.

[322] Hyperides (522), *Against Athenogenes*, p. 19 (Kenyon's translation).

[323] This is implied by the passage: "Moreover, an epileptic slave does not involve in ruin all the rest of his owner's property" etc. (*ibid.*, Kenyon's translation). Cf. Westermann (1088), col. 911.

[324] Cf. Sudhoff (971), pp. 363–65 and Sudhoff (967), pp. 142–49. In view of the additional evidence given by the passages in Hyperides, Plato, and Apuleius (cf. below), the interpretation of "sacred disease" as epilepsy can scarcely be doubted.

[325] Cf. Sudhoff, *l.c.*, pp. 365 and 145. For similar Assyrian and Babylonian documents cf. *ibid.* (971), p. 357 ff.

[326] Plato (803), *Laws*, XI, 916 B; vol. 10, p. 398: πλὴν τῆς ἱερᾶς.

[327] Plato (803), *Laws*, XI, 916 A – C; vol. 10, p. 399 (Bury's translation).

[328] The *Corpus iuris civilis* (240), *Digesta*, XXI, 1, 53; p. 277 says: "Qui (i.e., slaves) Tertiana aut quartana febri aut podagra vexarentur quive comitialem morbum haberent, ne quidem his diebus, quibus morbus vacaret, recte sani dicentur." Cf. Abt (2), p. 186, who quotes some more passages referring to epilepsy.

tion, and disputed cases come up to him for decision, for he is believed capable of recognizing the disease in any stage.

This motive explains the existence of more drastic methods of "testing" epilepsy[329] by provoking an attack artificially. The rotation of a potter's wheel before his eyes would make the epileptic feel giddy and might be the cause of a seizure.[330] Fumigation with kindled jet was one of the recorded experiments by which the physicians tested the health of "slaves exposed for sale."[331] This latter practice definitely connects such procedures with the economic motive, and it was probably for the same reason that other ill-smelling substances, as well as various "sympathetic" or "natural" diagnostic agents, were employed by the physicians.[332]

### h. Differential Diagnosis

It has been pointed out that any epileptiform seizure could be diagnosed as epilepsy, and that consequently many diseases which nowadays are differentiated from it were not so distinguished in Antiquity. Some of the supposed complications of epileptic fits suggest a different origin, especially the occurrence of distortions or paresis of certain parts. When it is said, for instance, that in children a subsequent crookedness of the mouth, of an eye, the neck, or a hand, may have a beneficial effect, since it spares them further attacks,[333] cases of infantile hemiplegia, infantile paralysis, etc., could be involved. Among the hemiplegias described as following epileptic attacks in old people, cerebral hemorrhages or emboli probably numbered among the actual causes, though Galen emphasized that epileptic attacks in contrast to apoplexy were *not* followed by paresis.[334]

In theory at least, epileptic attacks were clearly distinguished from local and general convulsions. According to Galen, participation of the whole body and loss of consciousness marked the epileptic fit, and the intermittent form of the attacks was contrasted with the continuous form of tetanus.[335] In accordance with a strict use of terminology, patients sometimes were described as seized by "epileptic convulsions,"[336] and a remedy was designated "for epileptics and those who

---

[329]Galen (394), *De simpl. med. temp. ac facult.*, XI, c. 1, 11; vol. 12, p. 336: ἐλέγχειν τε τοὺς ἐπιλήπτους. Cf. also above, I-2.

[330]Apuleius (43), *Apologia*, 45.

[331]*Ibid.* (Butler and Owen's translation, p. 106).

[332]Cf. above, I-4.

[333]Hippocrates (491) *On the Sacred Disease*, ch. 8; vol. 6, p. 376; Grensemann (429), p. 75, 4.

[334]Galen (394), *De locis affectis*, IV, 3; vol. 8, p. 231 f.

[335]Galen, *ibid.*, III, 9; p. 173.

[336]Hippocrates (491), *Epidemics*, VII, 46; vol. 5, p. 414: ἐπιληπτικοῖς σπασμοῖς; cf. Temkin (999), pp. 318-19.

are convulsed periodically."[337] The latter example is worth remembering, since it shows that even periodic convulsions were not necessarily identified with epilepsy. But not always was attention paid to clear distinctions. The Hippocratic statement about the beneficial effect of quartan fevers in one passage refers to epilepsy and in another one to convulsions, both passages being otherwise identical.[338] Or, again, the Hippocratic collection mentions various symptoms, optic disturbances and loss of consciousness among them, as indicating the approach of *convulsions.*[339] Early physicians, such as the Hippocratic authors, are likely to have used the words epilepsy and convulsions more interchangeably than later authors, especially Galen, who favored terminological clarity.

Above all others, diseases arising from the uterus seemed to the ancients to be worth comparing with epilepsy. The Hippocratic Corpus had drawn parallels between the closely similar features of epileptic and "hysterical" attacks, and most of the later physicians followed suit. It was necessary to note the differences too. Celsus went very far in this respect. He said that a disease originating from the uterus sometimes made women so weak that it prostrated them as in epilepsy. "Yet," he added, "this case is different in that the eyes are not distorted, nor does saliva flow forth, nor are the nerves convulsed: it is but a deep sleep. And in some women this returns often and for life."[340] This statement is interesting because what actually remains is not more than the description of a fainting fit, and the comparison with epilepsy obviously alludes to the "apoplectic" rather than the "convulsive" type. The lack of convulsions in "hysterical suffocation" is also noted as a distinguishing feature by Aretaeus,[341] while Soranus emphasizes the absence of a flow of saliva and of a big pulse.[342] But Celsus' statement is also important as a further example that the ancients not only avoided identifying all types of recurrent falling fits with epilepsy, but even tried to define the characteristic differences.

Although it was recognized that epilepsy tended to impair the mind, signs and symptoms differentiating epilepsy from mental diseases were

---

[337]Oribasius (753), *Eclogae medicament.*, 2; vol. 4, p. 186, 27-28: Ἄλλο ἐπιληπτικοῖς καὶ τοῖς περιοδικῶς σπωμένοις etc.

[338]Cf. above, II-1f.

[339]Hippocrates (491), *Prorrhetic*, I, 112 and 113; vol. 5, p. 546. *Coan Prenotions*, 82, 222, 252, and 258; *ibid.*, pp. 600-2, 632, 638, and 640.

[340]Celsus (212), *De medicina*, IV, 27; vol. 1, p. 446: "Interdum etiam sic exanimat, ut tamquam comitiali morbo prosternat. Distat tamen hic casus eo, quod neque oculi vertuntur nec spumae profluunt nec nervi distenduntur: sopor tantum est. Idque quibusdam feminis crebro revertens perpetuum est."

[341]Aretaeus (49), ed. Hude, II, 11, p. 33, 2-3.

[342]Soranus (938), *Gynaeciorum*, III, 27; p. 110, 9-10. Cf. also Caelius Aurelianus (192), *Morb. chron.*, I, 4, par. 12. In this connection attention has to be drawn to Hippocrates (491), *On Regimen in Acute Diseases*, append. 35; vol. 2, p. 522, which seems to be another example of the synonymous use of "convulsive" and "epileptic"; cf. Diepgen (272), p. 234.

not detailed. In ancient medical literature epilepsy and mental diseases, such as melancholy and mania, were clearly separated in the descriptions of their clinical symptoms. Uncertainty involved those premonitory signs which epilepsy shared with mania and other diseases, which, according to Soranus, originated from the meninges. Some physicians thought they noticed differences in sleep and pulse, observations the validity of which was denied by Soranus himself.[343]

## 2. THEORIES

The history of ancient theories about epilepsy is easily divided into three periods: the Hippocratic period, the time of the medical sects, and the period dominated by Galen and his followers. The physicians and philosophers of the fifth and fourth centuries B.C. gave many different explanations of the disease; by contrast little is known about the development during the following four centuries. Shortly before Galen a certain stabilization seems to have been reached, owing to the eclectic tendencies of the time. Methodists like Soranus inclined toward a solidary pathology, yet their interest in scientific speculation was but slight and, therefore, of little consequence. The scientists among the physicians belonged to the dogmatic school, and with minor variations they accepted a humoral theory which they traced back to Plato and the name of Hippocrates. This theory was systematized by Galen in the late second century, and his followers, the Greek physicians of the third to the seventh centuries, further simplified it and brought it into a rigid form. We shall, therefore, first discuss the speculations of the fifth and fourth centuries, then give a brief outline of the development down to the second century A.D. Then we shall attempt a description of the Galenic theory and its interpretation by the later physicians.

### a. The Fifth and Fourth Centuries

One of the most astonishing features of ancient medical speculation is the attitude of the Greek philosophers and physicians toward diseases involving consciousness and the mind. The resistance of these early thinkers to magic beliefs is nowadays praised as one of their greatest achievements. Whereas it is relatively easy to understand that purely somatic illnesses were explained as consequences of purely somatic processes, it remains a cause for wonder that they attempted a theory of psychic afflictions which was not only rational and natural but was mainly based on somatic factors. This materialistic bias laid the foundation for a medical tradition interpreting all diseases as disturbances of the body. In the case of epilepsy, this attitude found expression in the fact that the disease was numbered among the afflictions of the body and that both its somatic and psychic manifestations were traced back

---

[343]Caelius Aurelianus (192), *Morb. chron.*, I, 5, par. 148 f.

to the same underlying causes. The Hippocratic authors as well as Plato and Aristotle all shared this belief, though their explanations varied widely in the details. Three books of the Hippocratic collection present theoretical arguments, and each differs from the other two. The book *On the Sacred Disease* ranks first, both as to thoroughness and future significance. Its goal and general character have already been outlined, and it has been stated that the author sought to convince his lay audience that epilepsy was a natural disease, curable by natural means if treatment was begun early. This motive directed his arguments and compelled him to leave no feature of the disease unexplained.[344]

Like all other diseases epilepsy too, according to this author, arises through heredity, since in the production of semen diseased parts of the parental body send off diseased seed. Moreover, epilepsy befalls phlegmatics only, never cholerics.[345] This humoral principle, together with the statement that the causes of epilepsy as well as of the other "greatest" diseases are to be found in the brain, forms the cornerstone of the theory.

In order to make the pathogenesis of the disease understandable, the author gives a brief sketch of his anatomical and physiological concepts. The human brain is double, a delicate membrane dividing it in the middle. From the entire body many fine veins run to the brain, which is, moreover, connected with two thick vessels from the liver and the spleen. The liver vein has two parts. One is called "hollow vein" and extends to the foot, whereas the other penetrates the diaphragm and lung, sending branches to the heart and the right arm. In its further upward course it divides at the ear, the chief part going to the brain, but the ear, eye, and nose receive branches too. Apart from the fact that the vein from the spleen is thinner, its course on the left side corresponds to that from the liver on the right.[346] These vessels are the breathing organs of the body. They draw the air into themselves, spread it via the small vessels over the whole organism, cooling the organism, and then let the breath out again. The breath is thus continually moving up and down; if in some part of the body it is segregated from the rest and forced to stand still, that part becomes powerless.[347]

After these necessary explanations, the author now returns to the pathology of epilepsy, tracing the germ of the disease back to the fetus. In this stage of its development all parts of the body undergo a process

---

[344]Cf. Temkin (999). In the following outline of Hippocratic theories I shall largely confine myself to references to chapters, since I have dealt with questions of detail in the above-mentioned article and in the preceding pages.

[345]Hippocrates (491), *On the Sacred Disease*, ch. 2. For the theory of heredity contained here cf. Lesky (635), p. 109 ff.

[346]*Ibid.*, ch. 3.

[347]*Ibid.*, ch. 4.

of purification. If such purification is entirely absent in the brain the person will be a phlegmatic, and if he does not catch up in early childhood by the formation of ulcers and slimy discharges, then, indeed, he is in danger of becoming an epileptic.[348]

There is still the possibility that the excess phlegm from the brain may turn to the lung and heart or to the abdomen, causing palpitation, asthma, etc., or diarrhea.[349] But if these roads are blocked, the cold phlegm rushes into the vessels and causes the symptoms of the epileptic attack by obstructing the vessels, cooling the blood and making it stand still, and by interfering with the movements of the breath. Ordinarily, the air is taken to the brain first and to the members afterwards, supplying them with intelligence and movement.[350] For the brain, as the author makes clear in subsequent chapters, is the central organ for all psychic phenomena. When the air, in the respiratory process, reaches the brain, it deposits here its intelligence content and then goes on to the other parts. Therefore the brain serves as the rational interpreter and messenger as long as it partakes of the breath.[351] But if the air is cut off from the brain and the vessels, the person becomes dumb and unconscious; suffocation arises, which by its violence makes the excrements pass. The lung, being cut off from the breath, foams and effervesces and causes frothing at the mouth. The small vessels of the eye beat vehemently, and so the eyes become distorted; in the legs the incarcerated breath causes cramp and pain and makes the patient kick. In the hands, however, the blood stands still, and they become powerless and cramped. In case the flux is violent, the cold phlegm will congeal the blood, and the patient will die. Otherwise, it will be dispersed into the vessels and mixed with the blood, air will be taken in again, and the attack end.[352]

The volume of the vessels changes with the age, and so does the quality of the blood; the flux may be of variant strength and may affect one side only, and the wind will blow from different directions. All these factors, as the author shows at length, decide the outcome of the attack and account for possible ensuing complications.

Change of winds and of temperature and, in children, fright and fear are the chief provoking causes of the attacks. The mechanism involved is one of change in the consistency of the brain and of the phlegm. If in children, for example, the head is warmed, the phlegm melts, and if then the brain is suddenly cooled, the phlegm is separated and flows

---

[348]*Ibid.*, ch. 5.
[349]*Ibid.*, ch. 6.
[350]*Ibid.*, ch. 7.
[351]*Ibid.*, chs. 14-17.
[352]*Ibid.*, ch. 7.

downwards. In chronic adult epileptics, where the wind is the main provoking factor, the brain is so moist that the phlegm cannot be segregated, and it remains moist in spite of the increasing frequency of the attacks. The skulls of epileptic goats give immediate proof of this contention. If they are split open, the brain appears moist, hydropic, and of evil smell. Finally, the phlegm causes parts of the brain to melt, turn into water, and wash around the rest of the brain. When this stage is reached, the disease becomes incurable.[353]

Disregarding such details as seem strange to the modern reader, one will have to admit that this first monograph on epilepsy comprises all points essential for a complete pathology. The morbid anatomy and physiology of the disease, together with its predisposing causes, are considered as carefully as the causes provoking the single attacks and the mechanism of their action. In his hypothesis that the air carries intelligence to the brain, which acts as the interpreter, the author was probably dependent on the philosopher, Diogenes of Apollonia.[354] However this may be, in ascribing a central role to the brain the author met with the theory of the disease as presented by Plato. According to Plato, the most divine part of man's soul revolved in the head, and when "white" phlegm mingled with black bile disturbed its circulation, the "sacred disease" resulted.[355] Although the book *On the Sacred Disease* expressly excluded cholerics from epilepsy, Plato's view of black bile as a causal factor was partly corroborated by another Hippocratic writing.[356] When the breath is shut off in the vessels and black bile and pungent fluxes flow forth, cramp will appear if the flux has reached the heart, liver, or vein. And in case the surrounding parts are attacked by the flux and the latter dried up by the stagnating breath, epilepsy will follow.[357]

To the modern reader Plato's short note may seem negligible, but not so to men like Galen who considered him as great an authority for philosophy as he thought Hippocrates for medicine. Thus, it can be understood that a late Greek text said: "The cause of the affliction [i.e., epilepsy] is, as Plato and Hippocrates say, phlegm and black bile."[358]

The theories described are not the only ones of their period to come down to us. In the book *On the Sacred Disease* it is the phlegm which

---

[353]*Ibid.*, chs. 8-13.

[354]Cf. Taylor (995), p. 604. Wellmann (1080) considered Alcmaeon as the main source, a theory which is rejected by Pohlenz (816), p. 93. The relationship to Diogenes of Apollonia is stressed by Miller (701). Michler (697) sees influences of Diogenes and of Alcmaeon as does Grensemann (429), pp. 27-30.

[355]Plato (802), *Timaeus*, 85 A-B; pp. 228-30.

[356]*On Regimen in Acute Diseases* (Appendix). Cf. Taylor (995), p. 604.

[357]Hippocrates (491), *On Regimen in Acute Diseases*, Append., ch. 5; vol. 2, pp. 404-6.

[358]Galen (394), *Introductio seu medicus*, c. 13; vol. 14, p. 739.

causes the disease by interfering with the breath. In the Hippocratic work *On Breaths* the breath is the morbid agent. The condition of the mind depends on the condition of the blood; if this is agitated the mind is deranged. Now in epilepsy much air is mixed with the blood and obstructions in the vessels arise. Consequently, the passage of the blood is impeded and becomes irregular. These irregularities account for the convulsions and distortions of the body as well as for the loss of consciousness. The air rises to the mouth, carrying along the finest part of the blood, and so the foam is produced. But the attack provides for its own abatement. Warmed by the exertions of the body, the blood in its turn warms the air, which is dispersed, and with its departure from the body the attack ends.[359]

The book *On the Sacred Disease* is the only one to explain the disease as well as the single attacks of epilepsy. All the other explanations refer to the attack only. This is also true of the theory held by Plato's greatest pupil, Aristotle, who believed that food produces an evaporation into the veins which rises upward, turns, and descends again. This process underlies the phenomena of sleep,[360] and it also explains certain diseases, epilepsy among them. In a certain way, sleep is an epileptic seizure, and for this reason the disease as well as the attacks often originate during sleep. If much vapor[361] is carried upward, it makes the veins swell on its descent and thus compresses the respiratory duct.[362]

Aristotle's influence upon the development of ancient and medieval biology can scarcely be overrated. The above vapor theory of epilepsy will be found in Galen and elsewhere. However, it contrasts with the idea expressed in the pseudo-Aristotelian *Problemata*, where epilepsy is characterized as a melancholic disease, i.e., engendered by black bile.[363] The latter statement not only agreed with the *Timaeus* but also with the Hippocratic saying that "Most melancholics usually also become epileptics, and epileptics melancholics. One or the other [condition] prevails according to where the disease leans: if towards the body, they become epileptics, if towards reason, melancholics."[364] Moreover, the physicians Diocles and Praxagoras, who are said to have been influenced by the philosopher and who at least shared his view of the heart as a psychic organ, propounded a different theory: "Praxag-

---

[359]Hippocrates (491), *On Breaths*, ch. 14; vol. 6, p. 110 ff. On other editions of the text and detailed interpretation cf. Temkin (999), pp. 302-5.

[360]Aristotle (53), *On Sleep and Waking*, 456 B; pp. 334-36.

[361]*Ibid.*, 457 A 12; p. 338: πνεῦμα, i.e., literally "breath." But according to the context the vapor must be meant.

[362]*Ibid.*, pp. 336-38. From the text it remains doubtful whether this explanation of epilepsy refers to children only or to epileptics in general.

[363]Aristotle (55), *Problems*, 30, 1, 954 B; vol. 2, p. 164.

[364]Hippocrates (491), *Epidemics*, VI, 8, 31; vol. 5, pp. 354-56.

oras says that epilepsy is engendered in the region of the aorta by the aggregation of phlegmatic humors in it. These, formed into bubbles, block the passage of the psychic pneuma from the heart, and thus the pneuma makes the body shake and convulse. And when the bubbles have disappeared, the attack is over."[365] These are not Praxagoras' own words, but the report of a later anonymous writer who used the terminology of his own time.[366] Perhaps Praxagoras did not use the expression "psychic pneuma," which in the following centuries meant an air-like substance serving as the material substratum for the mental functions. At any rate, so much seems certain, that for Praxagoras the phlegm was the humoral agent which caused the initial disturbance. The same is true for Diocles, for the anonymous source continues: "Diocles also believes in an obstruction in the same place, and, as regards the remainder of the process too, he is of the same opinion as Praxagoras. It is true he omitted the specific cause, but, in his account of the disease, he says that it must be referred to obstacles to the pneuma which were difficult to overcome."[367] It is also related that where the disease was due to the constitution of the body, Diocles advised purging of the thick humor which he called "phlegm."[368]

The period of approximately 100 years from the time of the Hippocratic authors to the end of the fourth century shows a confusing multitude of different and even conflicting theories. It is scarcely possible to see any straight development. At best it can be said that phlegm as an etiological factor was recognized by a relative majority. But as to the seat of the disease, nothing had been decided.

### b. Third Century B.C.—Second Century A.D.

In the beginning of the third century B.C. Alexandria became the center of research for Greek medicine, retaining this status until the seventh century A.D. It was here that Herophilus and Erasistratus, the heads of the dogmatic school, performed human dissections. Both these men were greatly interested in the anatomy of the nervous system, and to them is owed what has been called "the discovery of the nerves."[369] It means the detachment of the functions of sensing and moving from nutrition and from the blood and blood vessels and their assignment to a special anatomical system connected with the brain. Herophilus gave an account of the brain which, in its chief points, must have been identical with Galen's later description. *Calamus scriptorius* and *tor-*

---

[365]Temkin (1000), p. 139 and Steckerl (952), p. 80.

[366]Cf. Temkin, *ibid.*, p. 143.

[367]*Ibid.*, p. 139, and Steckerl (952), p. 80.

[368]Cf. Caelius Aurelianus (192), *Morb. chron.*, I, 4, par. 131. Cf. also Wellmann (1077), pp. 29 and 140.

[369]Solmsen (935).

*cular (Herophili)* are terms coined by him and indicative of his neurological researches. Erasistratus is credited with the distinction between motor and sensory nerves. At first he believed that the nerves originated from the meninges of the brain, but in later times he corrected this error. He described the ventricles of the brain and thought them full of psychic pneuma.[370] The works of Herophilus and Erasistratus have been lost, and the fragmentary remarks contained in the writings of later authors give but scanty data. It is not known whether Herophilus ever expounded any theories on epilepsy at all, and the short passage from Erasistratus dealing with the subject and quoted by Galen shows no connection with his investigations into the nervous system. Erasistratus believed that in normal life the veins contained blood only, the arteries being filled with "pneuma." When pathological conditions prevailed, the amount of blood in the veins might increase and a "plethora" result. This plethora in its turn would cause various diseases, according to its anatomical localization. "In some cases it tends toward the liver; in some, however, toward the bowel; in others to epileptic afflictions; in still others to the joints."[371] Everybody should, therefore, take adequate precautions against the form of disease from which he usually suffered. "For he who is subject to epileptic attacks should not take the same precautions as one inclined to blood-spitting; rather should the former exert himself unsparingly . . . Likewise, one inclining to epilepsy should be made to fast without mercy and be put on short rations, but should beware of too much bathing and things causing a powerful change."[372] Although the passage emphasizes the dependence of every form of plethora on the organ affected, this organ is not mentioned in the case of epilepsy.

In some respects, Erasistratus' principles were shared by Asclepiades (c. 100 B.C.), the chief forerunner of the methodist school. At least, both Erasistratus and Asclepiades tended to a mechanical conception of biological processes which the latter, influenced by Epicurean philosophy, developed into an atomistic system of solidary pathology. Of Asclepiades it is said that he explained epilepsy as the result of a blow and of the rending of the membrane covering the brain or as the result of great fear. This view was reported and accepted by Soranus, who numbered epilepsy among the diseases arising from the meninges, and who added "contusion" as a further mechanical cause.[373] But to him,

---

[370]Cf. Wellmann (1076), col. 343.

[371]Galen (394), *De venae sect. adv. Erasistrateos Romae degentes*, c. 8; vol. 11, p. 239.

[372]*Ibid.*, pp. 239–40.

[373]Caelius Aurelianus (192), *Morb. chron.*, I, 4, par. 61: "Fit plerumque vel nascitur ex vinolentia aut indigestione aut contusione vel, ut Asclepiades, percussu atque divisura membranorum quae cerebrum tegunt, aut nimio timore." *Ibid.*, par. 62: ". . . etiam ceterarum passionum quae ex membrana cerebri oriuntur . . ."

as a methodist, a detailed anatomical explanation was of relatively little interest. For therapeutic purposes he thought it more important to know that epilepsy represented a state of stricture, that it affected the whole nervous system, especially the head, and to realize its chronic character and the rhythm of its paroxysms and remissions.[374] To the modern pathologist who sets such high store by mechanical explanations, it would certainly be interesting to know more about the views of the ancient mechanists who centered around the philosophy of Democritus and Epicurus. Unfortunately, nothing more definite is known. Even Lucretius, the most famous interpreter of Epicurean philosophy, remains vague in this respect. Without calling the disease by name, he gives a detailed description of its attack, but his chief aim is the demonstration of the vulnerability and mortality of the soul:

> And, moreover,
> Often will some one in a sudden fit,
> As if by stroke of lightning, tumble down
> Before our eyes, and sputter foam, and grunt,
> Blither, and twist about with sinews taut,
> Gasp up in starts, and weary out his limbs
> With tossing round. No marvel, since distract
> Through frame by violence of disease . . .
>
>     *     *     *     *     *
>
> Confounds, he foams, as if to vomit soul,
> As on the salt sea boil the billows round
> Under the master might of winds. And now
> A groan's forced out, because his limbs are griped,
> But, in the main, because the seeds of voice
> Are driven forth and carried in a mass
> Outwards by mouth, where they are wont to go,
> And have a builded highway. He becomes
> Mere fool, since energy of mind and soul
> Confounded is, and, as I've shown, to-riven,
> Asunder thrown, and torn to pieces all
> By that same venom. But, again, where cause
> Of that disease has faced about, and back
> Retreats sharp poison of corrupted frame
> Into its shadowy lairs, the man at first
> Arises reeling, and gradually comes back
> To all his senses and recovers soul.[375]

Soranus, living at the beginning of the second century A.D., is the last physician of any originality to lean toward a solidary pathology of epilepsy. The other theories of this century are all of a humoral character and Galen's is by far the most important among them. But before

---

[374] *Ibid.*, paragraphs 72–73.
[375] Lucretius (653), *Of the Nature of Things*, III, 487–509; p. 110 (Leonard's translation).

entering upon a detailed discussion of his views it will be advisable to mention those of Aretaeus and Apuleius. Aretaeus may have lived before Galen;[376] Apuleius was his contemporary. The theories of all three of them have certain points in common and show the growing consolidation in the scientific thinking of the ancients.

The remarks of Aretaeus are few, emphasizing the main points only. Epilepsy takes its origin from the head, either directly or by stimulation of peripheral nerves which have a sympathetic relation to the head.[377] This latter is the case when the attack is preceded by sensations and contractions in the extremities.[378] Besides, in some rare cases the abdomen is a possible starting point.[379] Now, according to the humoral system, "cold and moist" are the qualities of phlegm. Aretaeus does not expressly cite phlegm as the responsible humor, but from various remarks it can be inferred that he attributed significance to it. Some of his therapeutic efforts are directed toward the evacuation of phlegm, especially from the head,[380] and it is "thick and cold phlegm" which at the end of the attack can be drawn forth from the mouth.[381]

Apuleius, on the other hand, speaks as a philosopher rather than as a physician. Accused of having practised magic on a slave and on a woman, he defends himself with the contention that they were brought to him by a physician who wished to have his opinion.[382] In the attempt to prove the purely scientific interest of his examination, he launches upon an explanation of the disease based upon the authority of other philosophers—mainly Plato and Aristotle. Plato, he says, had taught that if a whitish and humid moisture flowed forth upon the outside of the body it would produce cutaneous eruptions upon the chest.[383] This would save the patient from epilepsy, which, however, resulted if this humor turned inside and were mixed with black bile. Then it would pervade all veins, would spread over the brain, and debilitate the "regal" part of the soul; for it would "cover and disturb its divine ways and wise passages." If this occurred during sleep the harm would be comparatively small, "since it troubles the sated moderately with a premonitory strangulation of epilepsy. But if it has increased to such an extent as to fill the head of people awake, they become insensible with a sudden clouding of the mind and fall down,

---

[376]The dating of Aretaeus is uncertain. Kudlien (600) has tried to put him into the first century.

[377]Aretaeus (49), ed. Hude, I, 5; p. 3, 15–18.

[378]Ibid., p. 3, 18 ff.

[379]Ibid., VII, 4; p. 153, 13 ff.

[380]Ibid., p. 152, 30.

[381]Ibid., I, 5; p. 5, 3.

[382]Apuleius (43), Apologia, 48, 1 ff.

[383]Ibid., 50, 1–10.

the body ready to die and the soul standing idly by."[384] Now he, Apuleius, had asked the woman whether her head felt heavy, the neck numb, whether her temples were pulsating and the ears ringing, in order to find out whether the disease had penetrated the head. The right side of the body being the stronger, her admission that the noise was louder in the right ear was a sign that the disease had penetrated the body through and through, and that the hope for recovery was but small. For Aristotle had written in his *Problems* that "in those epileptics in whom the disease starts from the right side, the cure is more difficult."[385]

The latter statement is not to be found in the pseudo-Aristotelian *Problems* which have come down to us. And the original statement in Plato's *Timaeus* has been elaborated by Apuleius into a much more detailed account. The theories of both Aretaeus and Apuleius are of a fragmentary character inasmuch as they do not explain all phenomena of the disease. But they contain elements of the comprehensive theory of epilepsy which was presented by Galen.

### c. Galen

For the understanding of Galen's teachings on epilepsy certain essential aspects of his whole work have to be considered.[386] Galen firmly believes that the ideal physician has to be a philosopher, and he sees himself as a true pupil of both Hippocrates and Plato. He writes commentaries on Plato's *Timaeus* and on many Hippocratic books. To him, Hippocrates is the founder of the theory of the four qualities and the four humors. Consequently, he explains disease in terms of the four humors: Blood, Phlegm, Black and Yellow Bile, and of the qualities: cold, warm, moist, and dry. But he is also an heir of the great scientific tradition of Aristotle and the Alexandrian physicians, whose findings he studies, criticizes, and advances by dissections and experiments of his own. Integrating these trends, he arrives at a theory of nervous disorders which is based at once on anatomical knowledge and traditional speculation.

An agnostic in those metaphysical questions which he believes of no consequence to scientific problems, Galen confesses ignorance about such questions as the immortality of the soul.[387] On the other hand, he is convinced that "the soul itself has its domicile in the substance of the brain, where reasoning originates and the memory of sensual perceptions is stored."[388] Now sensibility and voluntary mobility of the body are functions of this rational soul, and to fulfil these functions the soul

---

[384]*Ibid.*, 50, 10–21.

[385]*Ibid.*, 51, 2–12.

[386]For Galen's "System" as a whole cf. Siegel (924), particularly pp. 308–15, which deal with epilepsy.

[387]Galen (395), *Quod animi facultates corporis temperamenta sequantur*, c. 3; p. 36, 12–16.

[388]Galen (394), *De locis affectis*, III, 9; vol. 8, pp. 174–75.

needs instruments. The first instrument is the psychic pneuma in the ventricles of the brain—especially the third and fourth ventricles—and this psychic pneuma, through the spinal cord and the nerves, accepts sensations and carries the soul's commands to the voluntary muscles.

These principles suffice for the understanding of Galen's theory of epilepsy. He emphatically asserted that all epileptic attacks were due to affections of the brain.[389] However, the brain could be affected primarily and directly, or indirectly from another part of the organism. In the first case, epilepsy was the outcome of an "idiopathic" or "pro-topathic" disease of the brain.[390] In the second case, the involvement of the brain was "sympathetic." As used by Galen, the term "sympathetic" did not imply anything mysterious. It meant that the brain, though healthy in itself, had become involved in a disease process which started outside it.

In its systematized form, Galen's explanation of epilepsy as an idiopathic or protopathic disease of the brain presented itself as follows.

When convulsions occurred in an isolated part of the body, the cause must lie in an injury of the corresponding nerve. When the whole body was convulsed with the exception of the facial muscles, "the common principle of all the nerves below the face is affected." Presumably, this meant the cervical part of the spinal cord.[391] Where the face also was involved, the brain itself must be affected, since anatomy taught that the muscles moving the eyes, the skin of the forehead, the cheeks, and the root of the tongue derived their nerves from the brain.[392]

Starting from a Hippocratic aphorism that convulsions arose from repletion or from depletion,[393] Galen offered a mechanical explanation of convulsions. Muscles contracted by being drawn toward their origins. This movement was initiated by the nerves, and here Galen apparently had in mind an actual pulling motion on the part of the motor nerves that communicated itself to the muscles. Under normal conditions, our will, "posted at the beginning of the nerves in the brain," imparted motion to the primary nerves.[394] But convulsions took place involuntarily, and Galen arrived at the cause which replaced the will as the originator of motor action by comparing the nerves with the chords of a lyre. These chords, he maintained, were stretched when the surround-

---

[389]*De locis affectis*, III, 11; vol. 8, p. 193. For the following cf. also Brock's (163) translation from this chapter.

[390]On this terminology cf. *De locis affectis*, I, 3; vol. 8, p. 30 f.

[391]Galen (394), *De locis affectis*, III, 8; vol. 8, p. 169. *De symptomatum causis*, I, 8; vol. 7, p. 145: "In convulsions of the whole body, without derangement [of the mind] or torpor, the disease is of the cervical cord, just as the damage is of a nerve moving the part whenever a hand or leg or one muscle is forcibly stretched out or convulsed."

[392]Galen (394), *De locis affectis*, III, 8; vol. 8, p. 170.

[393]Hippocrates (489), *Aphorisms*, VI, 39; vol. 4, p. 189: "Convulsions occur either from repletion or from depletion. So too with hiccough" (Jones' translation).

[394]Galen (394), *De locis affectis*, III, 8; vol. 8, p. 171.

ing air was dry or wet. Extreme humidity made them swell into a sodden abnormal mass. Dryness, on the other hand, made the chords contract (Galen here used the added example of skins dried in the sun or leather thongs dried by a fire). In either case, the chords were now subject to tension or, as Galen said, they were "stretched." In the lyre this could even lead to the breaking of the chords. Transferred to the nerves, humidity caused their repletion, whereas dryness brought about their depletion. Toil, sleeplessness, want, anxieties, a "dry and burning fever," all suggested dryness and depletion. Repletion suggested itself in persons given to drink, heavy eating, and idleness.[395]

The explanation offered so far covered localized or generalized convulsions, such as took place in tetanus. It was not sufficient for epilepsy, though epilepsy too was a convulsion of all parts of the body. But epileptic convulsions appeared at intervals, and the mind and the senses also suffered. Consequently, epilepsy must have its origin higher up, in the brain itself.[396] Mental diseases, such as senile dementia[397] and melancholy, which were also located in the brain, arose when the substance itself of the brain was deteriorated by a humor.[398] In epilepsy, however, another explanation must be sought, for since the attack lasted but a short while, it could not result from an alteration of the cerebral substance.[399] Moreover, the seizure passed quickly. Galen thought it probable that in epilepsy a thick humor, gathering in the cerebral ventricles, blocked the passage of psychic pneuma. Thereupon "the beginning of the nerves shakes itself to push away what distresses it."[400]

In Galen's theory, the production of the thick humor accumulating in the cerebral ventricles and obstructing the psychic pneuma constituted the "idiopathic" basis of this form of epilepsy. It also explained the psychic symptoms. The generalized convulsions were then produced by the shaking of the origin of the nerves. This shaking was a biological reaction to the impediment in the brain, a response to a molestation, patterned after the human desire to rid itself of any irritation.[401] Both elements of this theory, the primary disease of the brain, and the ensuing convulsions, were elaborated further.

Galen was not satisfied with the simple statement that the obstruction in the cerebral ventricles was formed by a thick humor. The humor

---

[395]*Ibid.*, pp. 171–73.

[396]*Ibid.*, III, 9; p. 173.

[397]*De symptomatum causis*, II, 7; vol. 7, p. 201.

[398]*De locis affectis*, III, 9; vol. 8, pp. 177–78.

[399]*De symptomatum causis*, II, 7; vol. 7, p. 201.

[400]*De locis affectis*, III, 9; p. 173; also *In Hippocr. de humoribus comment.* 1, 1; vol. 16, p. 52.

[401]On Galen's theory of irritation cf. Temkin (998), pp. 306–18.

might consist of phlegm or of black bile. All phlegmatic humors were characterized by a preponderance of "cold and moist," whereas the melancholic humors were characterized by "cold and dry."[402] Epilepsy might be caused by the thick variety of either one of them, and since they had the quality of "cold" in common, epilepsy, in any case, was a "cold" disease.[403]

Galen's teleological explanation of the epileptic convulsions as a purposeful shaking of the beginning of the nerves was supplemented by his mechanistic theory of convulsion: the origin of every nerve was soaked, and the result was similar to what happened in convulsions from the spinal cord. Dryness and depletion, on the other hand, were ruled out as etiological factors in epilepsy. The quick onset of the attack argued against them; moreover, they would leave unexplained the concomitant loss of sensation and the impairment of reason and memory.[404]

This theory then was to account for epilepsy as an idiopathic disease of the brain. The affliction began in early childhood, and most epileptics belonged to this group.[405] But in a limited number of cases the original lesion was located somewhere else, and the epileptic attacks were the result of a "sympathetic" affliction of the brain. Galen tried to explain such sympathetic involvement, of which he distinguished two possibilities, on quite natural grounds. The first possibility, which he studied in the case of the grammarian, Diodorus,[406] consisted of a primary impairment of the cardia.[407] In persons with an abundance of bile and weakness of the stomach, ichors might accumulate and give rise to exhalations which affected the brain and might cause epilepsy.[408] Or epilepsy (and a number of other disorders) was brought on by atony of the cardia. The latter was extremely sensitive because of its abundant supply of nerves. Through its association with nerves and thus with the brain, a weak cardia, in persons with weak nerves and a weak brain, led to epilepsy, or torpor, coma, catalepsy, derangement, and melancholy.[409]

According to the second possibility the primary lesion lay in the extremities or any part of the body. These were the cases where the patients noticed the upward movement of the "aura," i.e., the breeze.

---

[402]*De locis affectis*, III, 9; vol. 8, p. 175.

[403]*De tremore, palpitatione, convulsione et rigore*, c. 6; vol. 7, pp. 608 and 618.

[404]*De locis affectis*, III, 9; pp. 173-74.

[405]*Ibid.*, III, 11; vol. 8, p. 193. *In Hippocr. epid. VI, comment.* I, 5; vol. 17 A, p. 825.

[406]*De venae sect. adv. Erasistrateos Romae degentes*, c. 9; vol. 11, p. 242.

[407]*De locis affectis*, V, 6; vol. 8, pp. 338 and 340 f. Galen (390), *De sanitate tuenda*, VI, 14; p. 196 f.

[408]Galen (390), *De sanitate tuenda*, VI, 10; pp. 186, 32-187, 4.

[409]Galen (394), *De symptomatum causis*, 1, 7; vol. 7, pp. 127-37.

Here again Galen thought that some qualitative change or a "pneumatic substance" spread over the body till it finally reached the brain, just as the poison from the bite of a scorpion or spider affected the whole organism.[410] Galen's explanation of epileptic attacks which were brought on by sympathetic involvement of the brain seemed to be supported by his observations. He noticed that in these cases the convulsions were comparatively weak and in their rhythm resembled a hiccup. A hiccup he thought to be caused by the action of "biting" substances upon the cardia. Here again the epileptic convulsions were an attempt on the part of the roots of the nerves to remove what had been inflicted upon them.[411]

Altogether, then, Galen distinguished three forms of epilepsy:

1. Epilepsy due to an idiopathic disease of the brain.
2. Epilepsy due to sympathic involvement of the brain originating from the cardia.
3. Epilepsy due to a sympathetic involvement of the brain originating from any other part of the body.

This is a general outline of Galen's ideas as they present themselves in the many scattered passages where he deals with epilepsy. The same ideas are expressed by the Greek Galenists of the following centuries. Aetius of Amida, Alexander of Tralles, and Paulus of Aegina, the leading physicians of the sixth and seventh centuries A.D., acknowledge the distinction of the three types of epilepsy. And the Iatrosophists of this period, the teachers of medical theory who interpreted Hippocrates and Galen to the students, are likewise dependent on Galenic principles. They scarcely propound any views which cannot be found in the Galenic writings. One of their more original contributions is Theophilus' explanation of the Hippocratic statement that epilepsy is numbered among the diseases of spring. Some people, he thinks, eat bad food during autumn and winter, thus engendering bad humors. During winter the cold keeps these humors deep in the body. But then comes spring, which causes the accumulated humors to flow forth. They are passed on to the head in the form of vapors, and if they happen to be phlegmatic in nature, the result is epilepsy.[412] Yet even this example shows nothing but an elaboration of the principles which Galen had used in explaining epilepsy due to sympathetic involvement of the brain.

---

[410]*De locis affectis*, III, 11; vol. 8, pp. 194-95. Cf. Brock's (163) translation, p. 222.

[411]*De locis affectis*, III, 11; vol. 8, pp. 198-200.

[412]Dietz (278), vol. 2, p. 369. Similarly Theophilus (1009), *De corporis humani fabrica*, IV, 4; p. 132 f., where he discusses the four kinds of *pneumata* arising from the four humors.

## 3. TREATMENT

### a. Indications and Aim of Treatment

The Greek physicians approached the treatment of epilepsy without undue illusions. Even the most optimistic among them, like the author of *On the Sacred Disease*, acknowledged inveterate cases as incurable.[413] Aretaeus gave expression to a prevailing opinion when he said: "But if the mischief lurk there until it strike root, it will not yield either to the physician or the changes of age, so as to take its departure, but lives with the patient until death."[414]

It was, therefore, of great importance to treat the patient before the disease had become chronic. The best chances of treatment were offered when the attacks started from the hands and feet and the patients were young and fond of work, not mentally impaired nor sufferers from apoplexy.[415] If epilepsy appeared in old people, they were helped best if left alone; in these cases the physician's assistance was of little avail.[416] These Hippocratic principles were repeated by Celsus 400 years later.[417] Others supplemented them by experimental tests: e.g., it was believed that an epileptic who vomited a drink of acacia was incurable.[418]

Prevention, of course, is the first treatment, and the most promising at that. "For it is easier," said Soranus, "to prevent what is threatening than to expel what is present."[419] With this general maxim he justified his advice concerning such people as seemed to be inclined toward epilepsy without manifesting the disease. Epileptics themselves also tried to prevent the development of the attack when they felt its onset. They would use some customary remedy, remove anything of offensive smell or taste, and apply fomentations to combat the feeling of cold and stiffness.[420] In those cases, however, where the attack began in a definite part of the body, they would pull at this part and have it bound and stretched with the result, as Aretaeus states, of chasing the attack away for one day.[421] But physicians too, besides applying drugs, would bind the extremity if it was the starting point for the "aura."

---

[413]Hippocrates (491), *On the Sacred Disease*, chs. 2 and 11; vol. 6, pp. 364 and 382; Grensemann (429), pp. 67, 3 and 79, 6.

[414]Aretaeus (50), ed. Adams, pp. 296–97 (Adams' translation).

[415]Hippocrates (491), *Prorrhetic*, II, ch. 9; vol. 9, p. 28.

[416]*Ibid.*

[417]Celsus (212), *De medicina*, II, 8, 29; vol. 1, p. 146.

[418]Cf. Galen (394), *De remediis parabilibus*, II, c. 2, 8; vol. 14, p. 402.

[419]Caelius Aurelianus (192), *Morb. chron.*, I, 4, par. 95.

[420]Seneca (910), *On Anger*, III, c. 10, 3; p. 280.

[421]Aretaeus (49), ed. Hude, I, 5; pp. 3, 23–4, 5.

This procedure, said by Galen to have been successful, recommended itself in analogy to the treatment of a poisonous bite and on the supposition of an ascending pneumatic substance.[422]

If the ancient physician did not undertake the treatment of epilepsy light-heartedly, neither did he easily trust the result of his endeavors. There were, of course, differences in outlook, dependent on the personality of the physician. Galen, for instance, often boasts of successful cures of epilepsy,[423] whereas Soranus warns against believing in the effectiveness of treatment, unless the patient meets the following conditions: he must pass the usual times of attack without any inconvenience, his sleep must be undisturbed, he must enjoy perfect health as to the functions of body and mind, showing good appetite, digestion, and color. Even then he will have to avoid any of the possible provoking causes, for "on a slight impulse the body repeats what it just seemed to have abandoned."[424] But though the patient may not have got rid of his epilepsy, the physician ought, nevertheless, to continue treatment. He will at least provide partial relief, preventing frequent attacks of long duration or in public places and distress of mind following the attacks.[425]

Realization that the ancient physicians were well aware of their limitations helps us to understand why many of them had recourse to "sympathetic" remedies, some even allowing the intervention of magicians. It throws light on the courage of a man like Soranus, who, in spite of his therapeutic pessimism, rejected anything irrational or superstitious.

### b. Methods and Theory of Treatment

The author of the book *On the Sacred Disease* advised the use of drastic measures against epilepsy,[426] including drugs[427] and dietetic prescriptions.[428] But, as the ancients already noticed with disapproval,[429] he does not give any details concerning his method. The only

---

[422]Galen (394), *De locis affectis*, III, 11; vol. 8, pp. 197–98. The need for preventing the development of epilepsy or of the epileptic attack was so generally recognized that it could serve as a simile for one of Plutarch's theological reflections. God, he thought, often punished evil-doers for therapeutic reasons "just as in epilepsy, removing the evil before it has taken possession." [Plutarch (813), *On the Delays of the Divine Vengeance*, 20, 562 D; vol. 7, p. 264.] Cf. Rabbow (834), p. 69.

[423]E.g., Galen (394), *De locis affectis*, V, 6; vol. 8, pp. 340–41. Cf. also his *Advice for an Epileptic Boy*, Galen (391), p. 188.

[424]Caelius Aurelianus, *l.c.*, par. 114.

[425]*Ibid.*, par. 115.

[426]Hippocrates (491), *On the Sacred Disease*, ch. 18; vol. 6, pp. 394–96; Grensemann (429), p. 88, 5.

[427]*Ibid.*, ch. 2; p. 364; Grensemann, p. 66, 3.

[428]*Ibid.*, ch. 18; p. 396; Grensemann, pp. 88–90.

[429]Caelius Aurelianus (192), *Morb. chron.*, I, 4, par. 131.

therapeutic measure against epilepsy recorded in the Hippocratic collection refers to the case of a man who had been seized by epileptic convulsions after having anointed himself in winter before the fire in a bath. Complete abstinence from food and drink was prescribed, and a cure was effected.[430]

In the fourth century, Diocles treated epileptic patients according to the underlying cause. If this was to be found in the physical constitution, he advised purging of phlegm and, in addition, diuretic remedies, walking, and exercise. If, however, the disease had been brought about by drunkenness or eating meat, he recommended phlebotomy. Together with bloodletting, he used some kind of pills which, according to Soranus, upset the stomach and caused vomiting after meals. Other prescriptions were: the drinking of vinegar, provocation of sneezing before going to bed, wormwood, centauria, and the lichen of horses or mules.[431]

Praxagoras of Cos advised a treatment similar to that of his approximate contemporary, Diocles. Among other things, he prescribed shaving of the head, rubbing, and the application of a vinegar poultice. He made his patients eat the meat of lamb, young he-goats, pigs, and young dogs, and recommended holding the breath. At the beginning of an attack the parts involved were compressed and rubbed with various substances, such as the genitals of the seal; the parts were also cauterized and incised.[432]

By the end of the fourth century B.C. then, the methods used for the treatment of epilepsy were dietetic, surgical, and pharmacological. Very little is known, however, about therapeutic efforts during the following pre-Christian centuries. The scanty references to Erasistratus[433] and Asclepiades[434] are not very suggestive; by far the most interesting account refers to one of the founders of the empirical school, Serapion. It differs from the other accounts mentioned in that it does not constitute a mere list of dietetic prescriptions and other remedies, but takes the form of a definite regimen. Serapion anoints the neck of the patient with vinegar and rose oil and the rest of the body with olive oil. Then the patient takes his exercise, drinks vinegar-honey, and rests. Toward evening he takes a walk, rests, walks, takes a bath, and, while

---

[430]Hippocrates (491), *Epidemics*, VII, 46; vol. 5, p. 414.

[431]Caelius Aurelianus, *l.c.*, paragraphs 131-33. Cf. Wellmann (1077), pp. 140 and 152.

[432]Caelius Aurelianus, *l.c.*, par. 133 f.

[433]Cf. Galen (394), *De venae sect. adv. Erasistrateos Romae degentes*, c. 8 and 9; vol. 11, pp. 239-45. Erasistratus exposed people inclined to epileptic seizures to strenuous exercise, hunger, and scanty food, but warned of frequent baths.

[434]Cf. Caelius Aurelianus, *l.c.*, par. 136. Asclepiades confined bleeding to cases with convulsions; in addition he prescribed enemas or suppositories, fumigations, injections of vinegar into the nose, and made the patients roll around on muslin. He forbade meat and wine but encouraged coitus.

resting again, drinks of a decoction of hyssop containing vinegar and honey and partakes of food. So much for the daily regimen. One or two days preceding the attack (provided that the attacks follow a definite rhythm), the patient is either bled or purged with medicaments: sometimes with emetics (e.g., white hellebore), sometimes with cathartics (e.g., with scammony or black hellebore). In addition, Serapion prescribes superstitious remedies which he believes to be specifics[435] and uses odoriferous substances and enemas.[436]

This treatment seems to have been very popular. A whole group of physicians between 300 B.C. and 100 A.D. used it with more or less important modifications, and this group included the names of both dogmatists and empiricists.[437]

In the writings of the later ancient physicians the treatment of epilepsy by a dietetic regimen, including the regulation of exercise, sleep, evacuations, always plays an important role. There exist countless differences between the various regimens, differences in detail which seemed of utmost importance to the ancients. Whether or not the patient ought to be bled and at what time, when food should be given to him after the attack, whether he should hold his breath at times or not—all these questions and many others of the same kind aroused controversy, not only between the various schools but even between members of the same sect. Modern medicine is not "dietetic" in the sense of the ancients, and we have little practical knowledge of the therapeutic value of the minutiae of their cures. To us they often seem irrelevant and indeed appear to confuse the lines of historical development. Nevertheless, such lines exist, in theory at least, and are noticeable in the differences between the dogmatist and methodist principles of treatment. The dogmatic treatment was supposedly based on the pathology of the disease, and since the latter was mostly a humoral one, the therapy aimed at dispelling the noxious humor and preventing its accumulation. Often the therapeutic data are so scanty that the connection between pathology and therapy is not very clear,[438] but with Aretaeus and Galen a coordination between theory and regimen becomes more obvious.

In his description of the symptoms and causes of epilepsy Aretaeus distinguished between the acute epileptic paroxysm and the chronic

[435]Cf. above, p. 22.

[436]Cf. Caelius Aurelianus, l.c., paragraphs 137–39. Cf. Deichgräber (259), p. 165 f.

[437]Cf. Caelius Aurelianus, l.c., par. 139 ff.

[438]With the exception of Diocles, whose use of phlegmagogues and diuretics corresponds to his assumption of phlegm as the cause of epilepsy. Of Rufus of Ephesus, the most important dogmatic physician at the end of the first century A.D., a few fragments report that he prescribed food which was apt to make the body dry and evacuate the stomach. He praised an ointment of ground and pulverized peony mixed with rose oil for an epileptic child. Tepid water to drink instead of wine, and lukewarm baths were also good for epilepsy and the same he said of bear's gall. Cf. Rufus of Ephesus (879), pp. 460 and 461.

disease. In his therapy he follows the same division. For the paroxysm he applies venesection, clysters, ointments, cupping, in order to rouse the patient. Besides, he provokes vomiting: in small children by mechanical means, in older ones by emetic draughts of varying strength.[439] In his cure of the chronic form he distinguishes between cases where the head is the primary seat and those where the middle parts of the body (intestinal tract) bring on the disease. Consequently, in the first category, procedures such as bleeding at the elbow and forehead, cupping, cutting of arteries before and behind the ears, trephining and cauterization of the skull, application of rubefacients to the head, and purging with strong phlegmagogues prevail. In the second group, on the other hand, besides bleeding and cupping, emphasis is laid upon the use of remedies which help digestion and have a heating, drying, and diuretic effect, above all castoreum and theriacs.[440]

Beyond these remedies, Aretaeus prescribes a definite regimen for epileptics, guided by the maxim that nothing must be left to chance, and everything promising the slightest benefit must be done. In particular, the patient must avoid sensations that may provoke an attack. His sleep ought to be of moderate length. Afterward the bowels should be moved and winds and phlegm evacuated. He should take long walks, keeping to a straight route where the air is fragrant. Gestation[441] is also advised and is followed by a quiet walk and rest. Then the patient should perform exercises with his arms, neck, and shoulders, and his hands and head should be rubbed—all this being calculated to attenuate his physique.[442]

The food and beverage which the patient is to be allowed for his meal are also selected according to similar principles. Thus, the bread ought to be relatively dry; of herbs, those which are acrid, attenuating, and diuretic are preferred; much cucumber and melon is forbidden since they are "cold and moist." During the active treatment, at least, the patient ought to abstain from all meat; only when his strength is regained should he partake of light and digestible meats, e.g., fowl or hare. The meal is followed by walks and harmless entertainment. Wrath and sexual intercourse are bad, and "since the disease is cold and moist,"[443] the patient ought to live in a warm and dry country.[444]

The dietetic treatment of epilepsy as based on pathological considerations finds its fullest development in the writings of Galen. The kind of remedies to be used follows from the nature of the disease, and

---

[439]For a more detailed account cf. Adams' translation of Aretaeus (50), pp. 399–400.

[440]Cf. *ibid.*, pp. 469–71. On theriacs and epilepsy cf. Watson (1066), pp. 22, 46, and 52.

[441]I.e., being carried in a litter or carriage.

[442]Cf. *ibid.*, pp. 471 f.

[443]Aretaeus (49), ed. Hude, VII, 4; p. 155, 30.

[444]Cf. Aretaeus (50), ed. Adams, pp. 472–73. Aretaeus' medicinal therapy in connection with his theories has been discussed by Stannard (951), who mentions epilepsy on p. 47.

the right place of their application is determined by the physician's knowledge of the actions and the use of the bodily parts.[445]

Galen, as has been seen, distinguished three types of epilepsy.[446] But in his therapeutic considerations, the two kinds of sympathetic epilepsy play but a small role since he considers them rare occurrences.[447] For that type which arises from some part of the body accompanied by the ascending "aura," he refers to the practices of other physicians who purged the patient, bound the limb, and applied a medicament of thapsia or mustard to it.[448] In a case of sympathetic epilepsy originating from the cardia and caused by bile, he prescribed the following treatment: The patient ought to keep his digestion in good order. Every day at around nine or ten o'clock in the morning he ought to eat some carefully prepared wheat bread in order to prevent an attack due to an empty stomach. If necessary, he should drink diluted and slightly astringent white wine, which would strengthen the stomach without burdening his head. Twice or three times a year he should be purged with bitter aloes, which relieves the stomach of excess material, while at the same time strengthening the other functions.[449]

Galen's chief attention was directed to the first type, that of "idiopathic" epilepsy, the pathology of which he had described in such detail.[450] To this type he referred when speaking of epilepsy in general. But on his own admission the pathological details were not important for the direction of the treatment. Here it sufficed to know that the brain was the affected place, a viscous and thick humor being collected in the ventricles, and to recognize the nature of this humor.[451] This latter point was simplified further. To all practical purposes he assumed that idiopathic epilepsy was the result of a cold and moist dyscrasia of the brain[452] leading to the collection of a thick phlegm in its ventricles, and that consequently it was a phlegmatic disease[453] and of a cold and moist nature.

This theory of the nature and seat of epilepsy not only motivates many of Galen's therapeutical prescriptions but also helps him to explain its spontaneous cure in puberty and by quartan fever. At the time of puberty the body acquires a drier and warmer temperature than it

[445]Galen (394), *Methodus medendi*, XIII, 21; vol. 10, p. 932.

[446]Cf. above, II-2c.

[447]Galen (394), *In Hippocr. epid. VI, comment.*, I, 5; vol. 17 A, p. 825.

[448]*De locis affectis*, III, 11; vol. 8, p. 198.

[449]*Ibid.*, V, 6; p. 340.

[450]Cf. above, II-2c.

[451]*De locis affectis*, III, 9; vol. 8, p. 175.

[452]*In Hippocr. epid. VI, comment.*, I, 5; vol. 17 A, p. 825.

[453]*In Hippocr. epid. VI, comment.*, V, sect. 5, c. 26; vol. 17 B, p. 289: ... τὴν ἐπιληψίαν καὶ τὰ ἄλλα ὅσα φλεγματικὰ νοσήματα ...

had before,[454] which will obviously counteract the character of the disease. Quartan fever, on the other hand, especially if chronic and accompanied by shivering, will, by its heat, render the thick humor thin and may even evacuate it. The shivers, moreover, will change the moist and cold temperament into a warmer one and expel the phlegm by the resultant sweating, vomiting, or movement of the bowels.[455] Galen even believes epileptic convulsions to have a possibly salutary effect, since they will shake and warm the body and thus partly expel the noxious material, partly drive it into another and less important part of the organism.[456]

It is not known whether Galen advised special treatment for the epileptic attack, but he was well aware of the difference between slight and incipient cases on the one hand and chronic cases on the other. For example, he stated that the "attenuating diet" alone would cure mild and incipient epilepsy completely, yet would also prove helpful in chronic cases.[457]

In the treatment of chronic epileptics the evacuation of the phlegmatic humor was one of his chief aims.[458] This evacuation was performed either by the use of purgative medicaments[459] or by bleeding from the lower arm[460] or the thigh.[461] Galen was very confident of the effectiveness of this treatment, maintaining that he had cured epilepsy by this method and had hereby incurred the hatred of his colleagues.[462] The proper time for the purgation he considered to be the beginning of spring,[463] and people inclined to epileptic attacks should also be bled at this time.[464] But the bleeding would prove successful only if the patient were willing to lead a temperate life afterward. Excesses in eating and drinking would quickly make undigested humors accumulate and thus spoil the effect of the evacuation. Therefore, the physician ought to accept only such patients as would promise obedience to his dietetic regulations, and having bled them in the beginning of spring, he should

---

[454]*In Hippocr. aphor. comment.*; vol. 17 B, p. 791. *In Hippocr. epid. VI, comment.*, I, 5; vol. 17 A, p. 825.

[455]*In Hippocr. epid. VI, comment.*, VI, sect. 6, c. 7; vol. 17 B, p. 342. The text of this passage is corrupt; cf. Wenkebach (1083), p. 35.

[456]Galen (392), *In Hippocr. de victu acut. comment.*, IV, 27; p. 296, 21-27.

[457]Galen (390), *De victu attenuante*, c. 1; p. 433, 13-16.

[458]Galen (394), *In Hippocr. aphor. comment.*, vol. 18 A, pp. 79 and 80-81. *Quos, quibus catharticis medicamentis et quando purgare oporteat*, c. 1; vol. 11, p. 345.

[459]*Quos, quibus* etc., *ibid.*, p. 349. *In Hippocr. de humoribus comment.*, I, 12; vol. 16, p. 125.

[460]*In Hippocr. de humoribus comment.*, *ibid.*, p. 136.

[461]*De curandi ratione per venae sectionem*, c. 19; vol. 11, p. 307.

[462]*De purgantium medicamentorum facultate*, c. 5; vol. 11, p. 341.

[463]*Quos, quibus* etc., c. 1; vol. 11, p. 345.

[464]*In Hippocr. de humoribus comment.*, III, 33; vol. 16, p. 483.

prescribe exercises and a wholesome diet.[465] Evacuation by phlegmagogues and bleeding were furthermore helped by rubbing, which
according to Galen had the same, though a milder, effect.[466] Apart
from such active measures, chief emphasis was laid upon a proper
regimen, including exercises and assisted by various drugs.

Preserved among Galen's writings is a letter written to the father of
an epileptic boy in which Galen gives a detailed schedule of treatment.[467] Although Galen had never seen the boy, he had discussed the
case with the attending physician, and upon the father's insistence he
laid down the following rules of conduct: First, he emphasized the
necessity of avoiding everything which might possibly provoke an attack. If, nevertheless, a paroxysm occurred, the boy had to stay at
home on a very light diet. At the beginning of spring the boy ought to
be purged and his life ordered as follows: He should rise early, take a
moderate walk, and apply himself to his usual studies. Then he should
walk to the gymnasium where he would meet his master of exercises,
who would be charged with the details, but as a general principle the
exercises would be calculated to warm up the body in order to expel
excess material and should aim at strengthening the head and the
cardia.[468] Galen considered rubbing of equal benefit. First the boy
ought to be rubbed with muslin from the arms down to the legs. This,
he thought, would divert the noxious material. Care should be taken in
rubbing the head, lest it lead to an accumulation of humors. It should,
however, be rubbed energetically and the hair combed after the boy
had calmed down from the exercises, but the usual bath should be
omitted.

Lunch followed next, preceded by an aperitif and consisting of bread
together with vegetables and the like. For drink he might take vinegar
in which honey had been diluted. Galen considered this drink almost a
remedy for epilepsy, especially if the juice of squills had been added to
it. The heavier dishes were left for dinner. He went through many kinds
of vegetables and foods, discussing their merits and possible disad-
vantages in great detail. "Speaking generally," he said, "I recommend
abstinence from daily or immoderate use of such food as engenders
unhealthy humors, or as causes constipation or flatulence, and is hard
to digest. Such food, if taken constantly or more than is advisable at a
time, usually causes harm, not in this disease only, but in all other
diseases too."[469] In particular, he warns of food which might engender

[465]*De curandi ratione per venae sectionem*, c. 7; vol. 11, pp. 271-73.

[466]*De venae sect. adv. Erasistrateos Romae degentes*, c. 9; vol. 11, p. 241.

[467]*Advice for an Epileptic Boy*. For the following cf. my translation of this little treatise, Galen (391).

[468]In *De sanitate tuenda*, V, 10, Galen (390), p. 156, 7-11 specified that bowing, bending, and rolling around on the ground should be avoided, whereas walking, moderate running, and hanging from a bar ought to be encouraged.

[469]Galen (391), *Advice for an Epileptic Boy*, p. 185.

phlegmatic humors, of which category he thinks mushrooms to be the worst. On the other hand, he believed that the boy "may have plenty of such food as contains something sharp and pungent, and which does not obviously engender bad humors nor has a smell which might affect the head."[470] For the latter reason he excluded wine, mustard, etc. Although Galen did not view favorably foods such as apples and pears, he nevertheless allowed their occasional consumption, for he said: "I prefer to concede to children many such foods as, although not beneficial, do not do much harm if eaten openly and at the right time and with the necessary moderation, lest at the wrong time they might be compelled by vehement desire to eat more and greedily."[471]

After lunch the boy takes a short rest, then a leisurely walk and resumes his studies. Having finished them, he walks again and takes his dinner, consisting of bread and other foods, including meat, fish, and pulse. Again, all kinds of meat and fish are reviewed carefully. The principles of their selection are the same as those mentioned above. Birds, except waterfowl, are freely admitted, whereas the more fleshy parts of quadrupeds are excluded. Fish living near rocks are the best; oysters, snails, cheese, and the like belong to the same objectionable category as mushrooms.

Galen ends his letter with detailed instructions for the use and preparation of his "squill remedy." It should be taken after the purgation which has to take place in early spring, and every day before the boy leaves for the gymnasium. "And," he adds, "if the disease is not very severe and hardened, it may be hoped that it will cede completely in forty days through this drug; indeed, I have cured innumerable children in this way without having to use hellebore. But it is necessary to drink wormwood once or twice after the purgation and before using the drug."[472] Then follow careful instructions for the preparation of the "vinegar-honey" and for the extraction of the juice of the squills. As the last quotation shows, Galen set no little trust in the efficacy of this remedy. Yet he emphasizes that it is not the drug itself which ensures success, but its appropriate use by the well-trained physician in the right quantity and at the right time. This remark shows that for the Greek physicians who cured by diet, drugs were considered important in the framework of a rational treatment but not as independent remedies.

With Galen the treatment of epilepsy according to dogmatic principles reached its highest development. It found its counterpart in the therapy of Galen's older contemporary, Soranus, the great representative of the methodist school. This school, in contrast to the dogmatists,

---

[470]*Ibid.*

[471]*Ibid.*, pp. 186–87.

[472]*Ibid.*, p. 188.

based its therapeutic activities not so much on pathological theories as on a carefully planned and methodical treatment, arranged as far as possible according to intervals of three days and extending over a definite period. The cure should take the "status" of the disease into consideration, which in the case of epilepsy was the *status strictus*,[473] and would therefore chiefly rely on relaxing measures. Furthermore, in chronic epilepsy as in chronic diseases in general it would try to retune the body by treatment consisting of two cycles. During the "recuperative" cycle the strength of the patient would be built up, while during the "recorporative" cycle the physician would try to change his whole physique by a very active medication.

Some of these principles can already be recognized in a group of authors who were more or less closely connected with the methodists: Themison, their main forerunner, Celsus[474] the Roman encyclopedist, and the so-called "Anonymus Parisinus." Among them it is Celsus who, by reason of the authoritative role he played during the Renaissance, deserves some attention. His treatment provided for the acute attack, the chronic, and the hopeless form. Since the epileptic will regain consciousness spontaneously, he thinks it unnecessary to arouse him artificially.[475] Phlebotomy is requisite in those attacks only which are not accompanied by convulsions. All patients, however, should be purged by enemas or black hellebore. Next, their heads ought to be shaved and anointed with oil and vinegar and, three days after the attack, food of medium quality should be given. All provoking factors like heat, cold, and drunkenness must be avoided and food be given every second day, till a fortnight has passed since the attack. At this time the disease is no longer acute, and if it continues it has to be treated as chronic. Now the patient has to be evacuated three or four times with white hellebore. During the intervals he follows a daily regimen including rubbing and walking. If he has not yet been restored, his head will be shaved again and anointed, he will take a shower of salt water, and will drink castoreum in water on an empty stomach. This is also the time for more heroic procedures: the patient ought to be bled at the ankles, incisions should be made at the occiput and cupping instruments applied, and the patient should even be cauterized at the occiput and topmost vertebra, so that from these two points "the pernicious humor may evacuate."[476] If all this has been of no avail the case is hopeless, and exercise, rubbing, and a careful diet are all the physician can do to alleviate the disease.[477]

---

[473]Cf. above, p. 58.

[474]For Celsus' relation to the methodist school cf. Temkin (997).

[475]The "Anonymus Parisinus," on the other hand, uses various remedies such as skin irritants and sternutatives to rouse the epileptic; cf. Temkin (1000) pp. 141–42.

[476]Celsus (212), *De medicina*, III, 23, 7; vol. 1, p. 338.

[477]*Ibid.*, c. 23; vol. 1, pp. 332–38.

In its general outline the therapeutic method of Soranus shows definite similarity to Celsus' plan, although it is much more detailed. Even the treatment of the acute attack is divided into several stages: the beginning of the attack,[478] the status,[479] and the after-treatment.[480] A special paragraph is devoted to the care of babies. They ought not to be cupped, but kept warm, and following the paroxysm they should receive goats' milk, considered especially nourishing. The wet nurse too must keep to a strict regimen and if sick she should be dismissed, particularly if she is epileptic herself or suffering from cachexia.[481]

The treatment of chronic epilepsy is regulated according to the paroxysms and the latent periods of the disease.[482] The former require the same kind of attention as the acute attack but are followed, during the quiet interval, by a "cyclic" therapy.[483] The first recuperative cycle is intended to rebuild the patient's strength by dietetic measures. It is followed by the recorporative cycle, which is either "partial" or "complete."[484] The partial recorporative cycle provides for eating of sharp things, local manipulations at the head, like combing of the hair, shaving of the head, and cupping, chewing of pepper, sneezing with hellebore, the application of rubefacients, and prescriptions of phlegmagogues![485] The total recorporative cycle consists above all in the proper administration of hellebore,[486] which might be repeated two or three times.[487] Besides, the patient will take hyssopus, origanum, and thyme, drugs which in Soranus' opinion make body and humors thin. He will also travel and perform more strenuous work and exercises.[488]

A comparison of the treatment of epilepsy as practiced by the three medical sects down to the second century A.D. raises the question of the real influence of pathological theory on therapeutic activities. It will be realized that between dogmatists and empiricists a divergency of therapeutic procedure scarcely existed, since physicians of both schools used the regimen introduced by Serapion.[489] The differences appear greatest if the procedures of these two schools are contrasted with those of a

---

[478]Caelius Aurelianus (192), *Morb. chron.*, I, 4, par. 73 ff.

[479]*Ibid.*, par. 76: "Cum statum sumpserit accessio . . .," i.e., when the attack has reached its height, at which it may stay for some time. The "status" as used here is not identical with the modern concept of *status epilepticus*, though the latter term may go back to the old term. Cf. below, IX-1a.

[480]*Ibid.*, par. 80.

[481]*Ibid.*, paragraphs 77-80.

[482]*Ibid.*, par. 96.

[483]*Ibid.*

[484]*Ibid.*, par. 97.

[485]*Ibid.*, par 98; "apophlegmatismum adicientes."

[486]*Ibid.*, par. 99 ff.

[487]*Ibid.*, par. 111.

[488]*Ibid.*, par. 112.

[489]Cf. above, p. 67 f.

methodist like Soranus. But even here the practical differences were slighter than the fundamental discrepancies in the theory would have led one to expect. For even Soranus used the therapeutic measures which were advised by representatives of the other schools: rubbing with oil, exercise, light food, phlebotomy, and purging with hellebore.

In some instances the differences seem to be individual rather than factional. This is especially true of one of the most interesting surgical operations, that of trephining. Themison, the chief forerunner of the methodists, advised (a) incisions in the occiput in the form of the Greek letter "X"; (b) circumscript cauterization of the head leading to desquamation of the bone; and (c) perforation of the skull at the bregma.[490] The two latter operations were apparently combined by the dogmatist, Aretaeus, who said:

"It is also necessary to apply burning heat to the head, for it is effective. But first one should perforate the bone as far as the diploe—afterward one should use wax salves and plasters, until the meninx separates from the bones. With the trephine one must cut the bare [bones] all around (even if they show a slight resistance before they separate spontaneously) until, at last, one comes upon the black and thick meninx of these [patients]. And when, under the courageous treatment of the physician, the wound has suppurated—or cleaned itself—and turned into a scar, the patient has escaped from the disease."[491]

If this translation is correct[492] (unfortunately, the difficult wording of the text does not put it beyond doubt), the procedure was as follows: The substantia compacta of the parietal bone was perforated and a cautery applied to the diploe and tabula interna. Then cooling ointments were used till the scorched bones began to separate from the dura mater. These bones were removed by the trephine, whereupon the dura mater, thickened and blackened as a result of the cauterization, lay bare. Finally, the wound was healed either by first or second intention.

---

[490]Caelius Aurelianus, l.c., par. 143: "... utitur etiam [i.e., Themison] localibus adiutoriis, et quidem multis pro differentia, et quibusdam falsissimis, ut est sub occipitio accurata divisura, quam chiasmum vocari diximus, et ferro circumscripta in capite cutis ustura qua testa squamulis despumatur, item medium testae, quod Graeci bregma appellant, terebri perforatione ..."

[491]Aretaeus (49), ed. Hude, VII, 4; p. 153, 2-9: χρεὼν καὶ πῦρ φέρειν ἐς τὴν κεφαλήν · ἀνύει γάρ. τετρῆναι δὲ χρὴ πρῶτα τὸ ὀστέον μέχρι διπλόης, ἔπειτα κηρωτῆσι καὶ ἐπιπλάσμασι χρέεσθαι, ἔστ᾽ ἂν ἡ μῆνιγξ τῶν ὀστέων ἀποστῇ · τερέτρῳ χρὴ περικόπτειν τὰ γυμνά, κἢν ἐπὶ σμικρὸν ἀντέχῃ μέχρι αὐτομάτου ἀποσπάσιος, ἕως ὅτε μέλαινά κοτε τουτέων καὶ παχείη εὑρεθῇ ἡ μῆνιγξ. καὶ ἐπὴν ἐς μύδησιν ἢ καὶ κάθαρσιν τοῦ ἰητροῦ εὐτόλμως ἀκεομένου ἐς ὠτειλὴν ξυμβῇ τὸ τρῶμα, ὥνθρωπος ἐξῆλθε τῆς νούσου.

[492]Adams' (50), p. 469, translation is slightly different from mine; his interpretation of the passage seems, however, to be the same. For in his commentary on Paulus of Aegina (779), vol. 2, p. 249, he writes: "Aretaeus directs us, in cases of cephalaea and epilepsy, to perforate the bone as far as the diploe, and afterwards to burn it until the dura mater is separated from the bone."

The performance of arteriotomy was likewise recommended by both the late methodist, Theodorus Priscianus,[493] and the dogmatist, Aretaeus. According to the latter, all the arteries before as well as behind the ears ought to be cut.[494] Soranus, distrustful of such drastic procedures, rejected arteriotomy, cauterization, and perforation of the skull,[495] and confined himself to the milder operations of scarification and cupping. But the Galenist, Alexander of Tralles, also tried to avoid arteriotomy, trephining, cauterization of the skull, and other remedies "which to many become a punishment rather than a cure."[496]

All this leads to the conclusion that even conflicting theories did not quite prevent similar therapeutic measures. What seemed to be good was accepted, even if differently accounted for.

From the third century A.D. on, the therapy of epilepsy is no longer guided by any new theories. The great compilers of this time accept the Galenic theory of epilepsy and much of his therapeutics as well. This, however, does not prevent them from including cures which seem to hail from methodist sources. There is little originality in their therapy—except, perhaps, some new prescriptions—and to a great extent they copy older sources, sometimes almost verbally. This latter point is best illustrated by Aetius of Amida. He first gives a short outline of the Galenic pathological views.[497] This is followed by a lengthy passage which contains a few further pathological remarks, the statement that the regularity or irregularity of the attacks depends on the character of the diet, and the therapy, first of the acute attack, then of the chronic disease.[498] Posidonius, who lived at the end of the fourth century A.D., is given as the source for the whole passage,[499] and it is of course possible that his works, which are now lost, contained the two therapeutic parts as well. But he was not their original author. Oribasius, his approximate contemporary, also gives the therapeutic paragraphs,[500] and the old Latin translation of Oribasius' *Synopsis* ascribes them to Philumenos,[501] a physician of the early third century A.D. There are indications that they are still older. The first paragraph, dealing with the treatment of the acute case, shows a definite similarity

---

[493]Theodorus Priscianus (1006), *Logicus*, 15; p. 149, 11-12.

[494]Aretaeus (49), ed. Hude, *l.c.*, p. 152, 27-28.

[495]Cf. above, footnote 490.

[496]Alexander of Tralles (21), I, 15; vol. 1, p. 575.

[497]Aetius (11), Sermo sextus, c. 13; p. 153.

[498]*Ibid.*, pp. 153, 19–155, 2.

[499]*Ibid.*, p. 153, 18, Kudlien (599), pp. 422-24 has tried to identify this Posidonius with the Stoic philosopher of the first century B.C.; Flashar (363), p. 121 f., has offered strong reasons against such an identification.

[500]Oribasius (753), *Ecl. med.*, 37; vol. 4, p. 199 f. and *Synopsis* (755), VIII, 3; p. 245 ff. Cf. also Paulus of Aegina (778), ed. Heiberg, III, c. 13, 2; vol. 1, p. 153 ff.

[501]Oribasius (754), vol. 6, p. 206.

with the corresponding passages in Aretaeus, and even the latter's originality has been questioned![502] The paragraph about the cure of chronic epilepsy, on the other hand, in one manuscript is ascribed to Rufus of Ephesus.[503] If this latter ascription were correct it would be remarkable enough. For this treatment represents a regular cure extending over many days and is strongly reminiscent of the methodist procedure.

Lacking in originality as these late writers were, they achieved a certain uniformity in therapeutic procedures. Thus, they became important and authoritative for later times, even down to the eighteenth century.

### c. The Problem of Pharmacology

The treatment of diseases by diet was the most rational part of ancient therapeutics. It tried to strike at the root of the disease, not only at its symptoms, and it showed the closest connection with scientific pathology. In regulating food, drink, sleep, and exercise the physician was dealing with facts of everyday life. The dietician could feel himself master of his art: he effected cures without the invocation of supernatural powers or reliance on occult properties. This makes it understandable why the author of the book *On the Sacred Disease*, who opened his treatise with an attack upon magic, in the final chapter stressed the superiority of dietetic treatment.

The Greek physicians also tried to establish a scientific pharmacology and to explain the actions of the various drugs by their "qualities." Galen, above all others, laid down rules how these qualities could be recognized. Once the quality of a disease was known, it would be treated with drugs of the opposite qualities. Epilepsy, being "cold and moist," would need heating and drying substances, and since it was caused by a thick phlegm, the physician would prescribe phlegmagogues and "sharp" drugs able to "cut" the viscous humor. In this way, as has been shown in the preceding paragraphs, a coordination of dietetic and pharmacological treatment was effected, and the efficacy of the regimen was enhanced by a rational use of drugs.

Yet a discrepancy between dietetic and pharmacological therapy remained, for in their materia medica very few of the ancients freed themselves from superstition. This fact, the reasons for which have been stated above,[504] finds an illustration in the *Materia medica* of Dioscurides, the most famous of the ancient pharmacological writers.

---

[502]Cf. Wellmann (1079), p. 54 ff.

[503]Rufus (879), p. 360.

[504]Cf. above, I–4.

Altogether, forty-five substances are mentioned for epilepsy.[505] Eighteen of these show no immediate connection with magic, and their supposed pharmacological action corresponds to the current pathology of the disease: cardamum (heating),[506] the fruit of the balsam tree (heating),[507] dried figs (heating),[508] whey (mildly evacuating),[509] gum ammoniacum (heating, etc.),[510] black hellebore (cathartic, removes phlegm and bile),[511] hippophaiston (used to remove water and phlegm),[512] black bryony (diuretic),[513] plantain (styptic, drying),[514] mustard (heating, etc.),[515] tree fungi (styptic, heating),[516] hartwort (heating),[517] fruit of cow parsnip (evacuates phlegm from abdomen),[518] laserwort (removes flatulence and is sharp),[519] sagapenum (sharp),[520] galbanum (heating, etc.),[521] oxymel (dispels thickness),[522] cassidony wine (dispels thickness and flatulence).[523] At least thirteen substances whose effects Dioscurides often cites with the qualification "said to" are definitely superstitious: hare's rennet,[524] stomach and blood of the weasel,[525] ass's liver,[526] ass's hoof,[527] lichen of horses,[528] liver of the he-goat,[529] amulet of stones found in the stomach of swallows at the waxing moon,[530] seal's rennet,[531] blood of the land turtle,[532] stork's

---

[505]To which have to be added asphalt, onyx, and lignite whose fumes serve to "diagnose" epilepsy, and human milk which is considered unsuitable for epileptics.

[506]Cf. Dioscurides (282), ed. Wellmann, vol. I, p. 10, 19.

[507]*Ibid.*, p. 25, 17—26, 3.

[508]*Ibid.*, p. 117, 14.

[509]*Ibid.*, p. 144, 12.

[510]*Ibid.*, vol. 2, p. 101, 7.

[511]*Ibid.*, p. 308, 1.

[512]*Ibid.*, p. 305, 7.

[513]*Ibid.*, p. 332, 6.

[514]*Ibid.*, vol. 1, p. 199, 5.

[515]*Ibid.*, p. 220, 7.

[516]*Ibid.*, vol. 2, p. 2, 8.

[517]*Ibid.*, p. 67, 5.

[518]*Ibid.*, p. 89, 1.

[519]*Ibid.*, p. 95, 10.

[520]*Ibid.*, p. 97, 10.

[521]*Ibid.*, p. 99, 14.

[522]*Ibid.*, vol. 3, p. 16, 3.

[523]*Ibid.*, p. 29, 7.

[524]*Ibid.*, vol. 1, p. 128, 1.

[525]*Ibid.*, pp. 130, 11 and 130, 14.

[526]*Ibid.*, p. 134, 3.

[527]*Ibid.*, p. 134, 8.

[528]*Ibid.*, p. 134, 13.

[529]*Ibid.*, p. 135, 2.

[530]*Ibid.*, p. 138, 9. Such stones are recommended for lunatics and epileptics in the epitome of the Orphic lapidary, ed. Mély (681), p. 169, 12.

[531]*Ibid.*, p. 150, 22.

[532]*Ibid.*, p. 161, 8.

dung,[533] scrapings from the selenite stone found by night at the waxing
moon,[534] and filings of iron sharpened on whetstone from Naxus.[535]

Of the remaining fourteen substances, ten are without any definite
magic connotation, although the manner of their action is not explained. They are: cancamon,[536] triphyllon,[537] fleabane,[538] cressa
cretica,[539] cestron,[540] violet,[541] white bryony,[542] frankincense,[543]
sulphurwort,[544] and squill vinegar.[545] In four, however, a superstitious
motive suggests itself: of cinquefoil[546] Dioscurides mentions that it is
also cut for expiation, religious service, and purification.[547] Frothy
poppy[548] acts as a "specific" emetic for epilepsy;[549] the "frothy" structure of the plant could have served as a signature, associating it with the
well-known frothing of the epileptic, and its other name of "heracleia"
connects it with the disease of Heracles. Bear's bile[550] and turtle's
bile[551] belong to the same category as do the other organic remedies,
although Dioscurides explains that all bile is pungent and heating.[552]
This is another example of a rationalization which tends to obscure the
original motives behind the use of drugs.

In sum, of the forty-five remedies for epilepsy mentioned by
Dioscurides, at least seventeen, i.e., over one-third, have a superstitious
connotation—certainly an impressive figure, and one which cannot be
explained by a personal inclination toward superstition. Galen documents clearly that it is the pharmacological rather than the dietetic side
of ancient medicine which tends toward magic beliefs. A perusal of the

---

[533]*Ibid.*, p. 163, 11.

[534]*Ibid.*, vol. 3, p. 100, 5-8. The "eagle's stone" (ἀετίτης πίθος), which was also credited
with antiepileptic properties, was not included originally in Dioscurides' work but was inter-
polated later from Aetius. Cf. *ibid.*, vol. 3, p. 100 f., footnotes.

[535]*Ibid.*, p. 102, 13-16.

[536]*Ibid.*, vol. I, p. 28, 13. Κάγκαμον is some kind of an Arabian gum; cf. Liddell and Scott
(640) *s.v.*

[537]*Ibid.*, vol. 1, p. 120, 9.

[538]*Ibid.*, p. 132, 9.

[539]*Ibid.*, p. 145, 10.

[540]*Ibid.*, p. 168, 16.

[541]*Ibid.*, p. 270, 11.

[542]*Ibid.*, p. 330, 18.

[543]*Ibid.*, p. 87, 4.

[544]*Ibid.*, p. 91, 11.

[545]*Ibid.*, vol. 3, p. 17, 17.

[546]*Ibid.*, vol. 2, p. 201, 14.

[547]*Ibid.*, p. 202, 1-2.

[548]*Ibid.*, p. 223, 12.

[549]*Ibid.*, p. 223, 11-13: καθαίρει δὲ δι' ἐμέτων ὀξυβάφου πλῆθος σὺν μελικράτῳ
λαμβανόμενος · ἰδίως δὲ ἡ τοιαύτη κάθαρσις ἐπιληπτικοῖς ἁρμόξει.

[550]*Ibid.*, vol. 1, p. 160, 12.

[551]*Ibid.*, p. 160, 14.

[552]*Ibid.*, p. 159, 15.

passages concerning epilepsy in his physiological, pathological, and dietetic works shows him a rational scientist and physician. It is mainly in the pharmacological books that one meets with such superstitious remedies as in Dioscurides.

Historically, pharmacological treatment probably preceded the dietetic, which developed during the fifth century B.C., the time of the Greek enlightenment. Drugs were more closely bound to tradition than was diet. But the marked difference between the dietetic and pharmacological treatment of epilepsy also suggests differences in the social standards of patients and physicians. It adds another facet to what was previously said about the relationship of ancient physicians to magic and superstitious practices.[553] The physicians whose therapeutic methods we have studied in the preceding paragraphs were philosophically and scientifically trained and stood at the top of their profession. Most of the patients whom they treated by diet belonged to the upper strata of ancient society. Only men free from the necessity of earning their daily bread and rich enough to choose their food, drink, and exercise could afford the luxury of a strict regimen. Poor people had to be treated differently.[554] They had to stake their hope on a drug that promised a quick cure or on some remedy—perhaps even an incantation—recommended to them by a friend or a quack.

It would certainly be a mistake to exaggerate this distinction between the dietetic and pharmacological treatment. There existed many educated people who put their trust in mysterious drugs. On the other hand, the pharmacologists often tried to rationalize the action of remedies of doubtful origin. Yet it is important to realize that a social factor was also involved in the views and therapy of epilepsy. This realization will prepare us for a changing attitude noticeable toward the end of Antiquity, when a new order of things began to emerge.

---

[553]See above I–4.

[554]Cf. Edelstein (314), p. 256 ff. and (313), p. 303 ff.

# PART TWO

# THE MIDDLE AGES

# Epilepsy: The Falling Sickness

## 1. NAMES AND NOTIONS

Among the many names which were applied to epilepsy, one at least was taken from the most noticeable symptom, that of the fall of the patient. Apuleius used *caducus* as a synonym for epileptic,[1] and St. Augustine informs us about the "*caducarii*, by which name," he says, "it is common among us to call those whom epilepsy has smitten."[2] The disease itself is designated as *passio caduca*[3] and analogous names appear in the medieval literature of many European nations: "falling evil" or "falling sickness" in English, *fallendes Siechtum*,[4] *Fallsucht, falligs Wai*[5] in German, *Padavica* among the southern Slavs.[6] Even the late Hebrew term for epilepsy, *choli nophel*,[7] has the same connotation. All these names have the stamp of popular origin, for they appear relatively late in written documents and then from the pens of authors who use colloquial rather than learned expressions. In all probability, the older names, "sacred disease," "epilepsy," and *morbus comitialis*, were of popular origin too. But whereas the last two, as has been shown, became recognized medical terms, this was not the case with the "falling evil." Not that this designation was

---

[1] Apuleius (43), *Apologia*, 45, 20 and 51, 11.

[2] "Augustinus, De beata vita (ad med.): Isti homines, caducarii sunt, quo nomine vulgo apud nos vocantur quos comitialis morbus subvertit." Quoted from Dölger (287), p. 108, footnote 49.

[3] Isidorus (536), *Etymol.*, IV, 7, 5: "Haec passio et caduca vocatur, eo quod cadens aeger spasmos patiatur." Cf. *ibid.*, X, 61.

[4] Cf. Höfler (498), p. 648.

[5] Cf. Hovorka-Kronfeld (516), vol. 2, p. 213.

[6] *Ibid.*, p. 224.

[7] Cf. Preuss (822), p. 345.

strictly excluded from medical books. Early medieval as well as later works often refer to it and prescribe *ad accidiva, ad cadivos,* etc.[8] Even nowadays, *morbus caducus* is one of the synonyms for epilepsy. The chief difference lies rather in the fact that whereas "epilepsy" and the other classical names connoted more or less the same pathological state when they first appeared in literature as they do today, "the falling evil" referred to all kinds of morbid conditions characterized by a sudden fall of the victim.

Perusal of the literature of late Antiquity and the early Middle Ages shows, however, that "falling evil" was not the only term of a broad and badly defined nature applied to epilepsy. Byzantine medical books said that the people called this disease "demon" and "lunacy."[9] Latin texts of the seventh and perhaps even earlier centuries identified *caducus* with *demoniacus*[10] and prescribed a remedy "for epileptics, i.e., demoniacs and those suffering convulsion."[11] The epileptic was also popularly called *lunaticus,* as stated by Isidorus, the Bishop of Seville, who lived in the seventh century A.D.[12]

The names, *caducus, demoniacus,* and *lunaticus,* had several points in common. They began to play a role in late Antiquity. They were not coined by the physicians and for a long time not used by them, and they were not restricted to those conditions which the ancient physicians called epilepsy. These facts are suggestive of a change in the conception of epilepsy.

### a. Possession

The morbid conditions with which epilepsy in the Western world becomes increasingly associated from about the beginning of the Christian era are periodic ecstasies, raptures, and prophetic trances comprehended vaguely under the name of possession.[13] The victim is within the power of a supernatural being whose will he must obey. In a more limited sense, possession is ascribed to the intrusion of a god, demon, or ghost into the body of a hitherto normal individual who now behaves like a willing or reluctant instrument of the intruder. The forms

---

[8]Cf. Jörimann (565), pp. 22 and 42.

[9]Leo Philosophus (326), *Conspectus medicinae,* p. 115: Ἐπιληψία ἐστὶν, ὡς εἴρηται ἐν τῷ τρίτῳ τῆς διαγνωστικῆς, ὅταν πεσών τις ἐξαίφνης σπᾶται καὶ ἀφρίξῃ ὅπερ λέγουσιν οἱ ἰδιῶται δαίμονα καὶ σεληνιασμόν. Similarly Theophanes Nonnus (1008), *Epitome,* ch. 36; vol. 1, p. 144 f. Gregorius Nyssenus (426), *De beatitudinibus,* oratio VII; 1284 D, seems to use δαίμων almost synonymously with possession.

[10]*Corpus Glossariorum Latinorum* (238), vol. 4, p. 27, 29: "Caducus demoniacus"; cf. *ibid.,* pp. 215, 12; 492, 16; and vol. 5, p. 355, 43.

[11]Pseudo-Apuleius (39), *Herbarius,* 131, 4; p. 224: "Ad epilempticos, hoc est daemoniosos et qui spasmum patiuntur. . . ."

[12]Isidorus (536), *Etymol.,* IV, 7, 6: "Hos etiam vulgus lunaticos vocant, quod per lunae cursum comitetur eos insidia daemonum." One glossary of the ninth century (238), vol. 4, p. 315, 23, gives the following definition: "Caducus uecors daemoniacus lunaticus."

[13]Cf. Oesterreich (749), and Rosen (872), *passim* and especially pp. 42-62.

in which possession expresses itself vary from crude convulsions by which an evil spirit seems to torment its victim (see Fig. 1) to the exalted state of inspiration when a deity reveals past and future through the mouth of the prophet.

Since possession is connected with definite assumptions regarding the activities of supernatural powers, its manifestations change with the opinions of the times; it has a history of its own. A mere belief in the existence of gods, demons, and ghosts does not suffice to create the behavior of possession. Though *On the Sacred Disease* speaks of attacks by such powers, it does not state that they had entered the bodies of the victims, and it does not refer to exorcisms. Widespread belief in intrusive possession in ancient and classical Greece is altogether problematic.[14] On the other hand, where such a belief is strong, a neurotic person will easily behave "like one possessed," as did Charcot's hysterical patients who came from the less enlightened strata of French society.

With the extension of oriental religions and demonologies, the occurrence of intrusive possession became increasingly accepted in the West, and during the Middle Ages and Renaissance it was rarely doubted. This posed the question whether a person afflicted with the falling evil was possessed or was suffering from epilepsy as a natural disease. The question was difficult to decide, for in either condition the sufferer was attacked at intervals, while in between he might appear normal, and the attacks could look very much alike. He fell to the ground, distorted his limbs in convulsions, foamed at the mouth, ground his teeth, and finally fell into a coma-like sleep. Epileptics, moreover, could have dreamy, visionary states preceding, following, or replacing the convulsive attack and possibly associated with powerful excitement.[15]

There are no clear traces of confusion of epilepsy and possession in classical Antiquity, possession playing a minor role in philosophical thought. When physicians did discuss it, they did so under a heading different from epilepsy. Praxagoras of Cos, the contemporary of Aristotle, is said to have been alone among the ancients to mention divine possession. In accordance with the rational medical attitude, he gave it a physiological explanation and placed its seat in the region of the heart and of the aorta.[16] So strong was this ancient rational tradition that even later medical texts through the early Middle Ages down

---

[14] See Smith (932), who, in my opinion, has succeeded in casting doubt upon a pervasive belief in intrusive possession in ancient Greece. Whether the belief was absent altogether, I am unable to decide.

[15] Cf. below the pertinent chapters in the sections on the Renaissance and the late nineteenth century.

[16] Steckerl (952), p. 81, fragm. 71: Πραξαγόρας τοῦ ἐνθεαστικοῦ πάθους μόνος τῶν ἀρχαίων ἐμνήσθη φάσκων περὶ τὴν καρδίαν αὐτὴν εἶναι καὶ τὴν παχεῖαν ἀρτηρίαν.

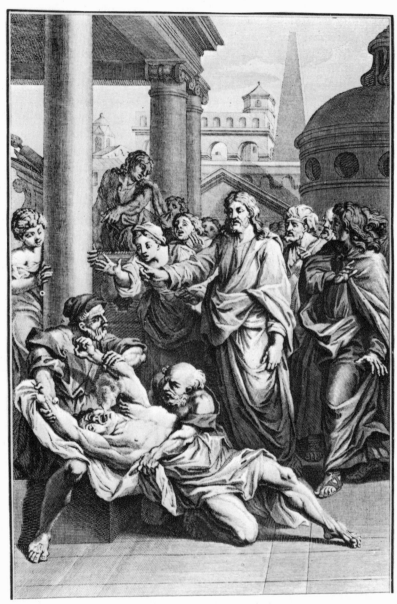

Fig. 1

Possession.  Bible of 1720, Jesus driving out an
unclean spirit. (O. Rosenthal, *Wunderheilungen
und ärztliche Schutzpatrone in der bildenden Kunst*,
Leipzig, F. C. W. Vogel, 1925, table 21.)

to the eleventh century treated it in a detached naturalistic way. Theodorus Priscianus (fourth century A.D.) thought that the same cure as he prescribed for madness and epilepsy should also be applied to those suffering from divine possession.[17] Paulus of Aegina (seventh century A.D.) dealt with it in his chapter on madness.[18] Most interesting in this connection is the group of closely related early medieval books which have come down under the titles of *Passionarius Galeni*, and *Esculapius*, and parts of which are also contained in a collection of medical glosses. Expounding on *Enteasmos*, the glosses define it as a dangerous form of madness, the sufferers from which hear music, dance, and wound themselves or others with the sword.[19] These descriptions refer to the bacchantic orgies of old and to certain practices of raving heathen priests, such as the worshippers of Cybele, of whom Aretaeus said that they "cut their limbs in holy phantasy, as if thereby propitiating peculiar divinities. . . . This madness is of divine origin[20] . . . . " They foreshadow the tarantism and dancing mania of the later Middle Ages.

But side by side with the ancient tradition the conception broadens. Thus, for example, the same medical glosses distinguish between two kinds of epilepsy. Those afflicted with the first kind fall down suddenly, are unconscious, and suffer from convulsions or tremor of hands, feet, and neck. Those afflicted with the second kind, whom the crowd calls "demoniacs," froth and tremble, but their limbs are not convulsed. The latter, moreover, are partly conscious, whereas the former are completely senseless.[21] Such statements belong to the time when the vague name of "falling evil" competed with the older and better defined terms for epilepsy.

The older texts, it is true, tell us about magic and popular beliefs according to which epilepsy is caused by the gods and ghosts, especially by the goddess of the moon, but their medical and philosophical authors are far from identifying themselves with these beliefs. And since it is mainly through the medium of well-educated writers that we

---

[17]Theodorus Priscianus (1006), *Logicus*, c. 17; p. 152, 6: "hanc curam etiam entheasticis adhibere debebimus."

[18]Paulus of Aegina (778), ed. Heiberg, III, 14; vol. 1, p. 156, 20–22.

[19]*Glossae medicinales* (416), pp. 29–30: "Enteasmos: species est maniae periculosa."

[20]Aretaeus (50), p. 304, (Adams' translation). The behavior of the prophets of Baal, who "cried aloud, and cut themselves after their manner with knives and lancets, till the blood gushed out upon them" (1 Kings 18:28), also fits into this picture. Cf. Rosen (872), p. 51.

[21]*Glossae medicinales* (416), p. 33: "Epylemsiae genera sunt duo. una est talis, in qua cadunt subito nescientes et contractionem manuum pedumque et cervicis vel tremorem patiuntur, alia vero est, in qua spumant et tremunt et non contrahunt membra, cum ceciderint, quos vulgus demoniacos dicit; et hii quidem ex parte sentiunt, illi vero omnino sine sensu sunt." A preceding version (*ibid.*, p. 32) distinguishes between those with tremor and sleep and others without tremor and sleep. The former, who are said to be seized by a demon, are incurable, while the latter can be cured.

obtain information about the popular opinions, the latter are obscured to our view. For the educated class of pagan society, imbued with the teaching of the philosophers, looked with disdain upon the display of violent emotions, including those of religious life. To the philosopher, excesses seemed of the nature of disease, and Aristotle had already compared incontinence to epilepsy.[22] Among the Stoics anger and its evil consequences were a favorite topic for moral reflection.[23] The trembling, moving, and yet paralyzed limbs of an angry man reminded Philodemus (first century B.C.) of the same symptoms in epileptics.[24] Plutarch thought it best to remain calm or if angered to flee, hide oneself, and regain one's composure, just as if one felt the approach of an epileptic attack.[25]

Such people, if confronted with a case of possession and its pretended cure by exorcism, would not so easily be impressed as to confound it with a natural disease like epilepsy. The more credulous among them would admit that "there are more things in heaven and earth . . . than are dreamt of in our philosophy," while the more sceptical would laugh off the whole tale. An example is presented by one of Lucian's (second century A.D.) dialogues, where the superstitious Platonist, Ion, and his sarcastic opponent meet: " 'You act ridiculously,' said Ion, 'to doubt everything. For my part, I should like to ask you what you say to those who free possessed men from their terrors by exorcising the spirits so manifestly. I need not discuss this: everyone knows about the Syrian from Palestine, the adept in it, how many he takes in hand who fall down in the light of the moon and roll their eyes and fill their mouths with foam; nevertheless, he restores them to health and sends them away normal in mind, delivering them from their straits for a large fee. When he stands beside them as they lie there and asks: "Whence came you into his body?" the patient himself is silent, but the spirit answers in Greek or in the language of whatever foreign country he comes from, telling how and whence he entered into the man; whereupon, by adjuring the spirit and, if he does not obey, threatening him, he drives him out. Indeed, I actually saw one coming out, black and smoky in colour.' 'It is nothing much,' I remarked, 'for you, Ion, to seek that kind of sight, when even the "forms" that the father of your school, Plato, points out are plain to you, a hazy object of vision to the rest of us, whose eyes are weak.' "[26] This case, where the pretended

---

[22] Aristotle (56), *Ethica Nicomachea*, VII, 8; 1150 B, 32-35: "for wickedness is like a disease such as dropsy or consumption, while incontinence is like epilepsy; the former is a permanent, the latter an intermittent badness." (Ross' translation)

[23] Cf. Rabbow (834).

[24] Philodemus (792), *De ira*, col. IX, 1-4.

[25] Plutarch (813), *On the Control of Anger*, ch. 5, 455 C; vol. 6, p. 106. Cf. also Seneca, above, II-1c, and Rabbow (834), p. 69.

[26] Lucian (652), *The Lover of Lies*, 15-16; vol. 3, p. 345 (Harmon's translation).

demon speaks in Greek or a foreign language while the patient lies on the ground, is typical of "possession." The epileptic, during the attack, would not speak, a fact already established in the Hippocratic book *On the Sacred Disease* and presumably known to the educated of the time.

"The Syrian from Palestine" probably did not refer to Jesus. Yet Lucian's story illustrates the manner in which an enlightened pagan might have reacted to the account which the Gospel gives of Jesus' treatment of the lunatic. This account reveals the attitude which was spreading in the West together with the new religion, which was a movement of the common people. St. Mark, ix, 14–29 (with the parallel versions of St. Matthew, xvii, 14–20 and St. Luke, ix, 37–43) tells the story of a man who appeals to Jesus with the words: "Master, I have brought unto thee my son, which hath a dumb spirit; And wheresoever he taketh him, he teareth him: and he foameth, and gnasheth with his teeth, and pineth away . . . ." Jesus demands that the boy be brought before him, "and when he saw him, straightway the spirit tare him; and he fell on the ground, and wallowed foaming. And he asked the father, How long is it ago since this came unto him? And he said, Of a child. And ofttimes it hath cast him into the fire, and into the waters, to destroy him . . . ." Upon the father's assertion that he believed, Jesus "rebuked the foul spirit, saying unto him, Thou dumb and deaf spirit, I charge thee, come out of him, and enter no more into him. And the spirit cried, and rent him sore, and came out of him: and he was as one dead . . . . But Jesus took him by the hand, and lifted him up; and he arose."

This biblical story became of the greatest importance for many centuries to come. Neither Jesus nor the father of the boy calls him an epileptic. In the parallel report of St. Matthew the father describes the son as "lunatic," but both he and Jesus agree that the child is possessed by an unclean spirit, which in the end is actually driven out. The child shows all the main symptoms of epilepsy recognized by the ancient physicians.[27] The "spirit" *cries* (epileptic cry) but is otherwise *dumb and deaf*. During the attack the boy foams, grinds his teeth, is convulsed; the attacks have dated from childhood, and the boy may fall into fire or water, thus endangering his very life. After the attack he falls into a state of coma.

The diagnosis of this kind of "lunacy" as epilepsy suggests itself so readily[28] that it was made by no less a theological authority than

---

[27]Cf. Hobart (496), pp. 17–20.

[28]For recent literature and interpretations of this case cf. Van der Loos (1045), p. 397 ff.; Lennox (632), vol. I, chose Rafael's presentation of the boy in the *Transfiguration* as a frontispiece, and Gowers, according to Critchley (246), p. 34, as well as Vogel (1051a), p. 441, also diagnosed epilepsy. Long ago Charles Bell (96), p. 160 f., had pointed out that this picture did not agree well with "real" convulsions. "In the same painter's great picture of the Transfiguration, in the Vatican," Bell wrote, "there is a lad possessed, and in convulsions. I hope I am not

Origen († 254 A.D.).[29] But Origen was not interested in the medical interpretation of the biblical account. He followed the word of the Gospel and claimed a demoniac origin of lunacy in opposition to the naturalistic explanations of the physicians. "Physicians," he wrote, "may offer natural theories since according to their view it is not an unclean spirit but a bodily affection which presents itself." To this he opposed his own view uncompromisingly: "We, however, also believe the Gospel in the point that this disease [i.e., lunacy], in those affected with it, is obviously brought about by an unclean dumb and deaf spirit."[30] Origen's explanation was followed by many Greek as well as Latin Fathers of the Church.[31] This was a decisive break with pagan Antiquity. Now the popular belief, which in epileptics, just as in the possessed, saw nothing but demoniacs, had formed itself into a body of opinion.[32]

### b. Lunacy

The association of epilepsy with the moon was so widespread that sometimes an epileptic was defined as one seized by "the disease of the moon."[33] But the same popular opinion as attributed epilepsy to the

---

insensible to the beauties of that picture, nor presumptuous in saying that the figure is not natural. A physician would conclude that this youth was feigning. He is, I presume, convulsed; he is stiffened with contractions, and his eyes turned in their sockets. But no child was ever so affected. In real convulsions, the extensor muscles yield to the more powerful contractions of the flexor muscles; whereas, in the picture, the lad extends his arms; and the fingers of the left hand are stretched unnaturally backwards. Nor do the lower extremities correspond with truth; he stands firm; the eyes are not natural; they should have been turned more inwards, as looking into the head, and partially buried under the forehead. The mouth, too, is open, which is quite at variance with the general condition, and without the apology which Domenichino had. The muscles of the arms are exaggerated to a degree which Michael Angelo never attempted; and still it is the extensors and supinators, and not the flexors, which are thus prominent." Doose (292), p. 191, thinks that the boy's attitude makes him appear insane or hysterical rather than epileptic.

[29] Origenes (756), *Comment. in Matth.*, t. 13, 4; col. 1104: Εἰ δὲ οἱ πρῶτοι θέμενοι τὰ ὀνόματα τοῖς πράγμασι διὰ τοιοῦτόν τι ὠνόμασαν τὸ τῆς ἐπιληψίας πάθος σεληνιασμὸν, ἢ μὴ, καὶ αὐτὸς ἐπιστήσεις. Cf. Dölger (287), p. 96.

[30] *Ibid.*, 13, 6; col. 1105 f.: Ἰατροὶ μὲν οὖν φυσιολογείτωσαν, ἅτε μηδὲ ἀκάθαρτον πνεῦμα εἶναι νομίζοντες κατὰ τὸν τόπον, ἀλλὰ σωματικὸν σύμπτωμα, καὶ φυσιολογοῦντες τὰ ὑγρὰ λεγέτωσαν κινεῖσθαι τὰ ἐν τῇ κεφαλῇ, κατά τινα συμπάθειαν τὴν πρὸς τὸ σεληνιακὸν φῶς, ὑγρὰν ἔχον φύσιν · ἡμεῖς δὲ οἱ καὶ τῷ Εὐαγγελίῳ πιστεύοντες, ὅτι τὸ νόσημα τοῦτο ἀπὸ πνεύματος ἀκαθάρτου, ἀλάλου, καὶ κωφοῦ ἐν τοῖς πάσχουσιν αὐτὸ θεωρεῖται ἐνεργούμενον, etc. Cf. Dölger (287), p. 96.

[31] Cf. Dölger, *l.c.*

[32] Dölger, *l.c.*, p. 98, rightly says: "Die Erklärung des Origenes setzt voraus, dass er überhaupt keine Mondsucht im natürlichen Sinne annimmt, was bei Ärzten und beim Volke als solche bezeichnet wird, ist ihm in Wirklichkeit dämonische Besessenheit." It must, however, be emphasized that Origen was primarily interested in the interpretation of lunacy. It is, therefore, not impossible that he recognized other forms of epilepsy for which a natural explanation was acceptable. Even the physiological explanation of lunacy itself did not disappear from theological literature as can be seen from Euthymius Zigabenus (337), who in col. 188 conforms with the current medical views and in col. 488 follows Origen.

[33] Bekker (95), vol. 1, p. 255: Ἐπίληπτον: τὸν ἐπιλήψιμον τῷ τῆς σελήνης πάθει. Cf. Dölger, *l.c.*, p. 95.

moon also blamed it for other periodical disorders, especially those affecting the mind.[34] The early medieval glosses which, as has been mentioned, devoted a paragraph to certain pathological forms of divine possession said that some people called its victims "lunatics."[35] The term "lunatic" was, therefore, no mere synonym for "epileptic," but comprised all such abnormal states as manifested themselves in more or less regular periodical attacks.[36] The very comprehensiveness of the term explains its different meanings in various languages. In English it signified the sufferer from fits of insanity and later on an insane person in general.[37] In German, on the other hand, the terms *Mondsucht* and *mondsüchtig* remained rather vague but would now chiefly be understood as referring to lunambulism, that is, sleepwalking under the influence of the moon.

The various ideas which connected epilepsy, madness, possession, and similar states with the moon and other stars can be glimpsed in the astrological literature of the day, which goes back to the later centuries of pagan Antiquity. This material, however, must not be expected to yield clear medical information; it rather proves the complexity of the subject.

The astrological work of the Greek poet who wrote under the name of Manetho gives a good example of two different types of presumed lunar influence. He first describes people born under the conjunction of the moon with the sun in the western sign. They will be faint, subject to raging madness, poisoned, sick of soul, always near death.[38] Next he refers to the fate of those born under the conjunction of the full moon with the planet Saturn. They are completely *lunatic*,[39] seized by a god, and full of prophecies. A similar fate awaits persons born under the combined influence of the moon and Mars, or of Venus and Saturn;[40] they too become "lunatic in their minds,"[41] although in the latter case the moon does not exert its influence at all. As this instance shows, the

---

[34] Origenes, *l.c.*, col. 1108 f.: Ἔστι γοῦν ἀκοῦσαι τῶν γενεθλιαλόγων, τὴν αἰτίαν πάσης μανίας, καὶ παντὸς δαιμονιασμοῦ ἀναφερόντων ἐπὶ τοὺς τῆς σελήνης σχηματισμούς.

[35] *Glossae medicinales* (416), p. 30: "isti sunt, quos lunaticos alii vocant, inmissione vel iracundia deorum est," etc.

[36] Cf. Stahl (950), p. 256 ff.

[37] Cf. Oxford Dictionary (723), vol. 6, 1, *s.v.* "lunacy" and "lunatic."

[38] Manetho (663), *Apotelesmatica*, IV, 537–40; p. 84:
Μήνης δ' Ἡελίῳ σύνοδον κατὰ κόσμον ἐχούσης
ζωιδίῳ δύνοντι, βροτῶν γένος ἔσσετ' ἀμυδρόν,
ἢ καὶ λυσσαλέῃ μανίῃ δεδαμασμένον αἰεί,
φαρμακτόν, νοσόθυμον, ἀεὶ θανάτοιο πάρεδρον:

[39] *Ibid.*, 545 ff.; p. 84:
ἢν δὲ Σεληναίη κατέχῃ πάμμηνα κέλευθα
συνδέσμου Κρονικοῖο, σεληνιόωντα φανείη
φῦλα βροτῶν etc.

[40] *Ibid.*, 77–83 and 214–17; pp. 75 and 78.

[41] *Ibid.*, 81; p. 75: ... σεληνάξων τε νόοιο; *ibid.*, 217; p. 78: νοῦν τε σεληνάξοντα.

moon is by no means the only heavenly body to cause the falling evil and kindred conditions. Paulus of Alexandria ascribes to Mars the power of afflicting people with "falling fits."[42] Some Greek astrological authors use this term in a sense which may imply epilepsy. For example, Vettius Valens, a contemporary of Galen, says that Saturn and Mars in lower culmination make people weak-sighted or liable to falling fits, or make them conjurors of God or of the dead and adepts of hidden secrets. When these planets exert their influence upon the moon they create maniacs, ecstatics, persons liable to fall, and prophets.[43] However, "falling fits" are not necessarily identical with epilepsy; they can form some unclear morbid entity of their own. Thus, it is said of Mercury that he makes the following diseases: mania, ecstasy, melancholy, epilepsy, "falling fits," etc.[44] What exactly these "falling fits" mean is not clear, and a story told by Lucian may illustrate how vaguely such words were used: A man had a daughter who was not only hideous but, in addition, the right side of her body was parched and the eye lost; she was a squinting and unapproachable monstrosity. This man lost his fortune, but what worried him most was how to get his daughter married. Even when he had been rich nobody would take one who looked so wretched, "and who was even said to fall down at the waxing moon."[45]

There is no essential difference between Greek astrological literature and its Latin counterpart. Under certain conditions "and when the moon has an evil position," says Julius Firmicius Maternus, the Latin author of the most comprehensive astrological work composed in the fourth century A.D., "it makes people convulsed or lunatic or liable to falling fits."[46] In other passages he talks about lunatics and epileptics[47] and mentions "sacred diseases,"[48] without defining the latter. Such "sacred diseases" are also mentioned in a Latin astrological text of uncertain, though probably early, date. Here it seems that they were not thought identical with epilepsy. For the unknown author writes that in

---

[42]Paulus Alexandrinus (780), *Eisagoge*; fol. L 4 verso: ὁ δὲ οὗτος ὁ ἀστὴρ ἡμέρας μὲν ἐπὶ τοῦ τόπου τυγχάνων, ἐπινόσους καὶ πτωματιζομένους ἀποτελεῖ.

[43]Vettius Valens (1047), *Anthol.*, II, 36; pp. 112, 33–113, 2.

[44]*Catalogus cod. astrologorum* (209), vol. 2, p. 179: πάθη δὲ ποιεῖ μανίας, ἐκστάσεις, μελαγχολίας, ἐπιληψίας, πτωματισμοὺς etc. *Ibid.*, vol. 8, 4, p. 192, has the heading: "On maniacs and epileptics." Yet where epilepsy is actually mentioned in this chapter (p. 193), it appears coupled to possession, rather than insanity.

[45]Lucian (652), *Toxaris, or Friendship*, 24; vol. 5, p. 144: ἐλέγετο δὲ καὶ καταπίπτειν πρὸς τὴν σελήνην αὐξανομένην. For "falling fits" in older sources, cf. above, I-1 and I-3.

[46]Julius Firmicius Maternus (360), *Math.*, IV, 19, 30; vol. 1, p. 253, 25–26: "et si Luna male fuerit collocata, aut spasticos aut lunaticos aut caducos facit," etc.

[47]E.g., VI, 29, 16; vol. 2, p. 137, 7 f.: "... facient lunaticos epilempticos, et quorum mentem iratum vel malignum numen semper exagitet."

[48]IV, 14, 3; vol. 1, p. 225, 6–8: "Facit plerumque lunaticos aut sacrarum valitudinum vitia decernit, facit caducos et misera commotione dementes." Cf. also VI, 31, 63; vol. 2, p. 166, 6.

a certain constellation of the moon some people have "epilepsies or sacred diseases or suffer from stupefaction or ecstasy or are troubled by prophecies."[49]

Astrological ideas could be motivated in various ways, and for epilepsy at least three explanations can be found in ancient literature. There was first the pagan belief according to which epilepsy was a vengeance of the goddess of the moon. Next came the theory of the physicians who thought that the waxing moon heated the atmosphere surrounding the earth and consequently melted the brain, thus provoking an attack.[50] This was an astro-physical rather than astrological theory, and not dependent on magic or theological assumptions. The two views were linked by a third philosophical theory based upon the sympathetic relation between macrocosm and microcosm. Such an explanation was proffered by the anonymous Christian author[51] of a dialogue on astrology, called *Hermippus*. The moon, it was said, had the same cold temperament as the brain and was therefore able to inflict headache and epilepsy.[52] This happened when its moisture increased and a corresponding change took place in the brain. Since, however, in some people the cavities of the brain were not fitted for and sympathetic to this change, these afflictions were not brought upon all, nor were all patients attacked at the same time.[53] The Bishop Synesius (c. 400 A.D.) seemed to allude to similar ideas when in a chance remark he said that epileptics alone noticed the cooling effect of the moon.[54]

---

[49]Gundel (445), p. 82, 7-9: "Luna separata a Mercurio et Saturno coniunctionem faciens minima in diurna nativitate egenos centiculosos vel in sacris locis detentos facit. Quidam vero epilepsias vel sacras aegritudines vel per stupefactionem vel extasin passiones habent vel auguriis annexantur." Gundel, p. 354, connects this passage with the *Katochoi* and writes: "Damit ist das Problem der Katochoi dahin geklärt, dass es sich um Epileptiker handelt, die in den Tempel eingeschlossen werden und in ihren Zuckungen zu prophetischen Zwecken verwendet werden." I think that interpretation of the text does not bear out such a general conclusion. As in other astrological texts, the relation of epilepsy to other abnormal states remains rather unclear. Particularly, it is difficult to decide whether epilepsy in general or certain forms only were connected with prophetic trances; cf. below, V-2. A similar difficulty exists with regard to *epileptici* and *stellatici*. The passage on p. 78, 18-20: " . . . et nati laeduntur circa visum vel faciem vel stomatici fiunt vel in toto laesi vel partem aliquam corporis laeduntur vel divini fiunt vel epileptici, qui vocantur stellatici" sounds as if *stellatici* were synonymous with *epileptici*. In other places these two words seem to relate to different conditions. Thus p. 76, 12-13, reads: "Aliquando vero et a matre orphanitatem inducit et natos epilepticos divinos vel eos qui vocantur stellatici . . . " and p. 74, 16-17: "Sole et Venere in ascendente et Saturno in occidente vel in angulo terrae divinos facit et epilepticos vel eos, qui vocantur stellatici." For *Katochos* cf. Ganschinietz (397), whose contention, *ibid.*, col. 2530, that there existed a synonym δελφικὸν πάθος for epilepsy is, however, open to doubt. It is based on a Byzantine formula (1037) whose editor corrected τοῦ ἀδελφικοῦ (p. 374, 1) into τοῦ δελφικοῦ [πάθους] (p. 383).

[50]Cf. above, I-4.

[51]Possibly Joannes Katrarios of the early fourteenth century; cf. Kroll (596), col. 854.

[52]Anonymus Christianus (36), *Hermippus*, p. 19, 28-20, 1.

[53]*Ibid.*, p. 47, 16 ff.

[54]Synesius (322), *epist.* 154; p. 736-37: τῶν μὲν γὰρ ἐκ τῆς σεληνιακῆς αἰτίας ἀποψύξεων οἱ νοσοῦντες ἐπιληψίαν αἰσθάνονται μόνοι . . . .

There existed, however, a powerful Christian opposition to any of the just-mentioned astrological explanations of lunacy in general and epilepsy in particular. Obviously, Christians could not accept the existence of a heathen deity like the goddess of the moon. To them all pagan gods were demons, servants of Satan who tried to confuse the minds of men and to divert them from the true faith. On the other hand, the Gospel itself, where Jesus was reported to have driven out the demon from the epileptic boy, made the acceptance of a purely physical theory impossible. And yet there must be a connection with the moon; why else was the epileptic boy called a "lunatic"? To this question Origen gave an answer which became authoritative for many churchmen. He rejected the natural explanation of the physicians that the moisture in the head moved according to a certain sympathy with the light of the moon, which itself was of a moist nature.[55] No, as the Gospel said, the disease was caused by an unclean deaf and dumb spirit. But, he maintained, this spirit observed changes of the moon and acted accordingly, so that man might not put the blame upon the demon but upon the moon, which was God's creation and had no power over this disease.[56]

How powerful an influence this new theory exerted can be seen, not only from the names of the theologians who accepted it,[57] but also from the caution with which physicians had now to proceed. Illustrative in this respect is a remark regarding the lunar influence made by an Alexandrian medical commentator of about 600 A.D. "Neither has the affliction of epileptics divine wrath for the cause of its origin. Rather, epilepsy originates according to a certain lunar period— although I do not say that the wrath of God sends the disease to men through the motion of the heavenly bodies."[58]

### c. The Falling Evil

The confusion of epilepsy with mental disorders became marked during the long transition from Antiquity to the Middle Ages. We shall see later that an opposite trend tending to separate "natural" epilepsy from "possession" also came into existence at a rather early date. But on the whole the confusion prevailed, not only during the early part of the Middle Ages but during its later centuries as well.

---

[55] Cf. above, footnote 30.

[56] Cf. Dölger (287), pp. 96-97.

[57] Cf. ibid., p. 97 ff. As a brief statement of this belief we may quote Isidorus of Seville (536), Etymol., IV, 7, 6: "Hos etiam vulgus lunaticos vocant, quod per lunae cursum comitetur eos insidia daemonum."

[58] Stephanus (278), Scholia in Hippocr. prognosticon, vol. 1, p. 73: Καὶ τὸ τῶν ἐπιλήπτων δὲ πάθος οὐκ ἔχει θείαν ὀργὴν αἰτίαν τῆς γενέσεως, ἀλλὰ γίνεται ἡ ἐπιληψία κατά τινα σεληνιακὴν περίοδον, οὐ τοῦτο λέγοντός μου, ὅτι ἡ τοῦ θεοῦ ὀργὴ διὰ τῆς τῶν οὐρανίων κινήσεως ἐπιπέμπει τοῖς ἀνθρώποις τὸ πάθος.

This state of affairs revealed itself in various ways. Even in the more educated authors there are descriptions and explanations of certain conditions which it is hard to classify. This is the more remarkable since it involves writers who were acquainted with the medical literature of the time. St. Hildegard of Bingen (1098-1179), for instance, distinguishes two kinds of epilepsy. The first is associated with wrath, which sets the blood in motion, thus causing an ascent of smoke and humors which touch the brain and cause madness. When individuals of such a disposition are induced to anger aggravated by some worldly troubles, the devil will notice it and frighten them by his suggestions, whence their soul becomes tired, succumbs, and withdraws itself. As a result the body falls down and remains thus till the soul has regained its strength. People of this kind, according to St. Hildegard, have an angry look and wrathful movements. "And when they fall to the ground, they sometimes let forth a sound different from the natural voice. This aforementioned disease shows itself comparatively rarely and is difficult to check."[59] The other kind of epilepsy concerns people of unstable and easy morals. This again tires the soul and causes the body to fall down. But such persons have an attractive look and gentle gestures, and while they too may emit a sound when falling down, it is sad and natural; they expel much froth from their mouths, yet can easily be cured.[60]

St. Hildegard's two kinds may have been modeled after the two kinds described by Caelius Aurelianus and in the early medieval medical glosses.[61] But from her description it is scarcely possible to recognize any clinical entities. Rather, she sketches two imaginary types of "falling sickness" dependent on the moral character of the sufferers: the demoniacal agitation of the irascible and the more pitiful helplessness of the moral weakling.

The role played by the devil in the wrathful type of epilepsy deserves some attention. Here St. Hildegard expresses a view, fundamental for the medieval conception of demoniac influence upon men, which survived far down into modern times. The devil does not cause the epileptic attack by his own power. He exerts his influence when the body is off balance, the humors being stirred up and the brain affected. When his victim is thus disposed, he can act upon the soul "by the breath of his suggestion."[62] For the devil is essentially a spiritual being. His time

---

[59]St. Hildegard (883), *Causae et curae*, p. 156, 13-16: "Et cum in terram cadunt, aliquando vocem extra naturalem vocem emittunt. Et iste praefatus morbus rarius ostenditur et difficile compesci potest."

[60]*Ibid.*, p. 156.

[61]Cf. above, footnote 21.

[62]*Ibid.*, p. 156, 6-8: "Et cum isti aliquando in iram moventur et quibusdam saecularibus angustiis aggravantur, hoc diabolus videns etiam flatu suggestionis suae eos terret;" etc.

of action arrives when the psychic organs are in a pathological state. This was one of the prevalent theological explanations of the interplay between physical disease and demoniac power.

Dante, about 200 years after St. Hildegard, has given a short but impressive picture of what we had best call "the falling evil." The passage occurs in the *Inferno*,[63] where it is used as a comparison, and in Longfellow's translation it reads:

> And as he is who falls, and knows not how,
> By force of demons who to earth down drag him,
> Or other oppilation that binds man,
> When he arises and around him looks,
> Wholly bewildered by the mighty anguish
> Which he has suffered, and in looking sighs.[64]

The term "oppilation" (*oppilazion*) probably refers to the Latin *oppilatio*, commonly used by medieval physicians to designate the blocking up of the ventricles of the brain in epilepsy.[65] The relation to epilepsy was already noticed by Benvenutus de Rambaldis de Imola,[66] but as a whole the picture might refer to all kinds of epileptiform attacks.[67]

If such was the attitude among the educated, it is no wonder that the more popular medieval testimonies are even more ambiguous. Again, the names which were given to the disease serve as a good indication of the breadth of the underlying conceptions. It would be a tiresome task to list all of the popular medieval names, many of which still form part of the vocabulary of folk medicine.[68] It is, moreover, not always possible to tell with certainty how these names originated. Such designations as *schweres Gebrechen*,[69] *schwere Not*,[70] in German, or the corresponding *nuzda* (distress) among the Ruthenians[71] were probably taken from the severe character of the disease. The expression, *la male passion*, which occurs in the old French *Roman de Renart*,[72] can perhaps be explained on similar grounds. The superstitious fear of calling

---

[63] Dante (253), *Inferno*, 24, 112–17; p. 224:
> E qual è quel che cade, e non sa como,
> per forza di demon ch' a terra il tira,
> o d'altra oppilazion che lega l'omo,
>
> quando si leva, che 'ntorno si mira
> tutto smarrito de la grande angoscia
> ch' elli ha sofferta, e guardando sospira.

[64] Dante (254), p. 78.

[65] Cf. Casini's commentary to Dante (253), p. 224, footnote 114.

[66] Cf. Longfellow's notes (254), p. 172.

[67] Casini's commentary to the passage (253), p. 224, footnotes, rightly refers to possession as well as epilepsy.

[68] For more complete lists cf. Höfler (498), Hovorka-Kronfeld (516), and Kanner (573).

[69] Cf. Wittich (1109), *Libellus*, fol. 19$^V$.

[70] *Ibid.*, fol. 23 r.

[71] Cf. Hovorka-Kronfeld (516), vol. 2, p. 223.

[72] Cf. Auerbach (62), p. 220.

an evil by its right name may account for the French designation *le beau mal*, which appears in a document of the year 1404.[73] But the majority of these names can be arranged according to three categories: those which developed from classical tradition, those which had their origin in the heathen past of the people now converted to Christianity, and finally those which were connected with Christian ideas.

We have already met with various instances of the first group. Two more examples may be added as illustrations of the present argument. It will be remembered that the ancient physicians had noted vertigo as a symptom related to epilepsy. Now from the Latin *vertigo* (or rather its accusative form, *vertiginem*) the form *Avertin* and its parallel, *Esvertin*, were derived in old French and were introduced into the pathological vocabulary.[74] The old novel *Aucassin et Nicolette* says the following of a pilgrim:

> L'aute jour vis un pelerin
> Natif de Limousin,
> Couché dedans son lit
> Du mal de l'Esvertin.[75]

Whether this really alludes to epilepsy would be difficult to say. In a French document of 1382 the term appears together with other characteristics of the "falling evil," where a person is described as ". . . besgue, fol, lunatique, malade, et cheant souvent du mal d'Avertin."[76] In a document of the fifteenth century, however, the conception is more concrete. Here a child is mentioned which was "entachié d'une maladie d'Avertin de teste, nomée goute, dont il cheoit voulentiers par intervalles."[77]

In this latter example *goute* is given as a synonym, and the development by which "gout" came to comprise the meaning of epilepsy is interesting to follow. *Gutta*, in Latin, originally meant a drop. Then, in the early Middle Ages its meaning was extended to that of a little river, and as a medical term it designated a flux or catarrh.[78] Now it was used as a designation for all kinds of diseases, including gout in the modern sense.[79] In order to distinguish between these various diseases, qualifying adjectives were sometimes added, and one of these forms was *gutta*

---

[73] Du Cange (301), vol. 5, p. 518: "André Guibretea qui paravant pou de temps avoit esté détenu et cheu du mal caduc, appellé vulgairement le Beau mal." The Greeks had the same euphemistic designation for the disease (cf. above, Part One, footnote 102), but there is hardly any direct connection between the two.

[74] Cf. Tobler-Lommatzsch (1025), col. 730. Du Cange (301), vol. 1, pp. 98–99, however, explains it as "Morbus qui a sensu avertit."

[75] Du Cange, *l.c.*, p. 99.

[76] Du Cange, *l.c.*, and Tobler-Lommatzsch, *l.c.*

[77] Du Cange, *l.c.*

[78] Cf. Du Cange (301), *s.v. Gutta*, and D'Arnis (59), col. 1092.

[79] Cf. Lessiak (637), p. 113.

*cadiva* or *gutta caduca*, which meant epilepsy. As an author of the
eleventh century said, it was so called "because it causes falling."[80] The
same expression was introduced into the English vernacular where it
appeared as *falling gout*.[81] The Latin form too was used in popular
medical texts but degenerated into the scarcely recognizable *Gout
cayve*.[82]

The German equivalent for gout, *Gicht* or *Vergicht*, similarly connoted a host of various diseases, including epilepsy and all kinds of
convulsions. But this word was of Germanic derivation and originally
connoted trembling and palsy.[83] It, therefore, belongs to the second
group of names which were rooted in the pagan past of the European
nations. It goes together with another German expression, found under
various forms as *Frais*, *Fraisch*, etc., and which included epileptic fits in
children as well as whooping cough and skin diseases![84] The ancient
Germans believed that an evil nocturnal demon caused fright (*Eiss*) in
children and that the epileptiform attack was a consequence of this
fright (*Vereissen* = *Fraisen*).[85] Some evil spirit or black demon must
also have been blamed by the Ruthenians when they called epilepsy the
black disease (*cornaja boljiżn* or *čornaja slabost*).[86]

The popular desire to connect epilepsy with supernatural powers
found its Christian counterpart in the association with certain saints. In
some cases a saint was even directly or indirectly believed the cause of
the disease. *The Book of the Saints of the Ethiopian Church* relates
how St. Thomas was slain and buried, the king's son being a witness to
the execution. Suddenly, a devil seized the king's son, who fell down in
an "epileptic fit" and was only cured after his servants, strong in faith,
had put dust from the saint's grave over him.[87] Again, of St. Lupus it
was told that an envious bishop gave expression to his thoughts at St.
Lupus' grave. As a punishment he became epileptic but recovered after
having repented.[88] Either on account of this legend or for some other
reason the *Morbus St. Lupi* was used as a synonym for the falling
evil.[89]

[80]Robertus de Tumbalenia, quoted by Du Cange (301), vol. 4, p. 142: "... illa molestia
arripitur, quam Medici Epilepsiam ... dicunt, vel Sacrum morbum ...; nos vero vulgariter
Guttam Caducam, ex eo quod cadere faciat, vocamus."

[81]Cf. Oxford Dictionary (723), vol. 4, 2, p. 316.

[82]This is the plausible explanation as given by Schöffler (896), p. 53. Prescriptions for the
*gowt cayne* and *gowte gayue* are published by Müller (718), pp. 106-7, and Dawson (257), p.
135.

[83]Cf. Höfler (498), p. 189 f.

[84]*Ibid.*, p. 165; Lessiak (637), p. 136.

[85]Höfler (497), p. 476 f.

[86]Cf. Hovorka-Kronfeld (516), vol. 2, p. 222.

[87]Budge (183), *The Book of the Saints of the Ethiopian Church*, vol. 3, p. 935.

[88]Cf. Kerler (578), p. 84 f.

[89]Du Cange (301), vol. 5, p. 517: "... Morbum beati Lupi, seu aliter caducum, sustinere
saepius dicebatur." A Dutch priest of c. 1500 mentions the "penitence of St. Cornelius,"

The two saints whose names became most popular as designations for the disease were St. John and St. Valentine. Especially in France *le mal Saint-Jean* was a common expression. Why, exactly, St. John was brought into this connection is as little known as whether the name related to St. John the Baptist or St. John the Evangelist.[90] One theory finds an explanation in the story that the head of St. John the Baptist fell to the ground when he was decapitated.[91] According to another suggestion, St. John originally was the patron saint of the dancing mania, that curious psychic epidemic which gripped thousands of men and women and made them dance till they fell down in exhaustion. Later on St. Vitus became the specific saint of this neurosis, whereas St. John was relegated to epilepsy. Even if this theory cannot be proved, it points to an important circumstance. Victims of St. Vitus' dance showed certain similarities to epileptics when their limbs jerked and when they collapsed snorting, unconscious, and frothing.[92] It is probable, therefore, that *le mal St. Jean*, apart from epileptics, included sufferers from the dancing mania and perhaps from chorea too. This would find further confirmation in the fact that St. Willibrord is also numbered among the patron saints of epilepsy. He was the founder of the monastery of Echternach, the famous goal of the dancing procession first held in the thirteenth century to celebrate the deliverance of the district from an outbreak of St. Vitus' dance.[93]

The name of *St. Valentins* (or *St. Veltins*)-*Sucht*, on the other hand, seems to have originated in Germany. Apparently, it was due merely to a phonetic analogy. This at least is quoted as Luther's contention, who said that the legend of the saint contained no reference to the disease. Therefore, he would lay a bet that St. Valentin acquired this honor simply because his name and the German word *fallen* sounded identical.[94] And since again the falling down was the leading symptom, the name extended to apoplexy too, a condition not clearly distinguished from epilepsy. Even physicians did not always consider them two different pathological entities and sometimes called epilepsy a minor apoplexy.[95] A more popular writer, Konrad von Megenberg († 1374),

---

probably as a synonym for epilepsy and kindred convulsive diseases. Here the name refers to the power of the saint to inflict and cure the disease. Cf. Diepgen (273), p. 104, footnote 3.

[90]Cf. Bloch (122), p. 164, footnote.

[91]Cf. Littré (641), vol. 3, p. 178.

[92]Cf. Hecker (469), p. 144.

[93]Cf. Bargheer (79), col. 1173, and Kerler (578), pp. 85–86.

[94]Höfler (498), p. 764: "1516, Luther, 10 Geb.–Pred. VII, 75: zum dritten haben sie St. Valentin der 'fallenden' Sucht zum Patron gesetzt; nun liest man ja Nichts in seiner Legende, dass er mit dieser Krankheit zu thun gehabt; drum wollte ich schier wetten, St. Valentin komme zu der Ehre bloss des Namens halben, dass sein Name und das deutsche Wort 'fallen' gleich lauten." Cf. also *ibid.*, p. 717. I have not been able to trace this reference in Luther's works. If, however, this explanation is correct, then the Ruthenian designation of epilepsy as *slabistj swjentego Walentego*, cf. Hovorka-Kronfeld (516), vol. 2, p. 223, must be due to German influence.

stated quite plainly that there were "two falling evils of which one is called apoplexy, the other epilepsy."[96] Thus in the mind of the medieval laity the "falling evil" embraced a wide range of different diseases from the apoplectic stroke to the somatic manifestations of neuroses and psychoses. At the same time it was suspected to be the work of demons or devils or, in rare cases, of divine wrath. This conception of epilepsy must be remembered when considering the more practical attitude toward the disease.

## 2. CURE AND PREVENTION

### a. Magic and Superstition

The means which medieval man used in fighting epilepsy were rational and superstitious on the one hand, magic and religious on the other. The rational cure made use of diet and drugs, following the tradition of ancient rational treatment. Other remedies and procedures, such as observation of the phases of the moon, the use of human blood and bones, of amulets, of plants and precious stones, are superstitious from our point of view. But many of the medieval writers explained their effect on a rational basis. Here again they followed the ancient theory of astral influence and of the efficacy of empiric remedies which acted through their substance or through natural, though hidden, forces. In this latter sense Gilbertus Anglicus (thirteenth century) said of epilepsy: "Mark you, empiric [remedies] are very helpful in this disease."[97]

Laymen and physicians alike advised the use of superstitious remedies, and the leading Arabic medical textbooks were no exception. Amulets of peony[98] and of stones[99] were recommended by them, just as they had been recommended by classical as well as early medieval authors. Among the Salernitans, Platearius (twelfth century), for example, tells of an "experiment" by his father who prescribed a drink of blood, extracted by scarification, together with a raven's egg.[100] Some of the scholastic physicians abound in this kind of superstition

---

[95] Cf. below, footnote 221.

[96] Konrad von Megenberg (591), *D. Buch der Natur*, V. 52; p. 409, 30-33: "daz selb öl oder diu salb ist guot für daz paralis und für diu zwai vallenden lait, der ainz apoplexia haizt und daz ander epilencia," etc. Soranus' distinction of the apoplectiform and convulsive forms of epilepsy [cf. Caelius Aurelianus (192), *Morb. chron.*, I, 4, par. 61] is the forerunner.

[97] Gilbertus Anglicus (412), *Compendium medicinae*, fol. 111[r]: "Nota empirica in hac egritudine multum iuvare."

[98] Cf., e.g., Alí Ibn Abbās (22), *Practica*, V, 21; fol. 215[V]ff. Avicenna (71), *Canon*, lib. III, fen 1, tract, 5, c. 11; p. 492.

[99] Rhazes (843), *Continens*, fol. 13 verso: "Alchindus dixit quod lapis alcalcal suspensus ad collum curat epilepsiam." Cf. also Abulqasim's remark as quoted below, footnote 122.

[100] Platearius (915), *Practica brevis*, fol. 172[V]: "Experimentum patris mei circa epilepsiam. iii Ɜ sanguinis a spatulis extracti per scarificationem cum ovo corvi dentur in fine accessionis egro adhuc stupido," etc.

and scarcely any of them is free of it. And yet, how careful one must be in the interpretation of their actual beliefs is demonstrated by a passage from Antonius Guainerius (early fifteenth century).[101] He furnishes examples of "sacred medicine,"[102] as he calls such superstitious prescriptions: to give a frog's liver, to smear the patient's mouth with blood, to kill a dog and let the patient have its bile, and to let the person who first saw him fall urinate into his own shoe(?), stir the urine, and give it as a drink to the patient. Certain people, the author says, who believe themselves philosophers, wonder that this disease should require such prescriptions. The reason is that all diseases which are caused by some poisonous agent require "some occult quality" which is contrary to them. This being the case in epilepsy, remedies must be offered which contain such an "occult quality" as may be found in frog's liver, dog's blood, or human urine. "For how many properties are contained in things which as yet are unknown to us!" So far, there is nothing remarkable in this statement. But he also foresees the question why it should be necessary to put the urine into a shoe, and why this act should be performed by the person who first saw the patient fall. The answer is that this increases the belief in the medicament and consequently its effectiveness. "And thus it comes that we perform so many ceremonies in medicine." If then it were to be said that he wrote in the manner of old wives, and if it looked to the reader like witchcraft, nevertheless, nothing, he contended, was stated without reason based on natural principles.[103]

In theory, at least, there was a distinction between superstitions, supernatural magic, and religious acts. Remedies, however superstitious

---

[101] On him cf. Thorndike (1021), vol. 4, pp. 215 ff., and Lennox (627).

[102] This expression finds an analogue in Theodorus Priscianus (1006), *Logicus*, c. 15; p. 149, 15–18: "nam quam plurimi sapientiores etiam fysicorum adiutoria providerunt, in quibus, ut etiam nos in nostro libello fysicorum comprehendimus, magna et veluti religiosa remedia procurarunt."

[103] Antonius Guainerius (438), *Tractatus de egritudinibus capitis*, VII, fol. 12[r-v]: "Sed ad sacram medicinam veniendo dicunt quidem quod si a vena auris sanguis extrahatur: et ex eo os patientis illiniatur: mox a paroxismo surgit.... Item cum epilepticus ceciderit: canem unum statim interfice: et fel patienti quoquo modo poteris tribue. Item si is qui primo casum viderit in proprio sotulari minxerit: et postea agitaverit: ac si eum levare vellet: deinde urinam illam cum sotulari illo potui dederit liberabitur ex toto.... Mirantur quidam dico putantes se philosophos quod illa passio per descripta debeat amoveri: pro quo scito quod nulla venenositas a calido frigido succo vel humido solum pellitur: sed est necesse ut aliqua qualitas occulta huic venenositati contraria in re pellente reperiatur. Cum ergo epilepsia ratione venenositatis producatur: necesse est pellentem eam oppositam illi qualitatem occultam aliquam habere: que in iecore rane: sanguine canis vel in urina hominis seu in aliquo alio inesse potest. Quot enim proprietates rebus insunt que adhuc nobis existunt incognite. Sed dices cur primum ergo urinam ponis sotulari: cur istas ceremonias adiungis. videlicet qui primo casum viderit sic faciat: cur non omnes alii hec faciant. Et tu debes respondere quod hoc fit ut illi medicine quecunquam illa fuerit: maior fides attribuatur. Quanto enim infirmus maiori cum affectione medicamina sumit: tanto avidius natura illa recipit et multo meliorem ceteris paribus operationem efficit: quam si cum illa affectione reciperet. Et hinc est quod tot cerimonias in medicina facimus.... Si quedam (?) ergo in hoc meo opusculo deinceps ad modum vetularum descripsero: pensa non ab re me hic illa descripsisse. nam etsi tibi forsan praecantationes ap-

they may appear to us, were not yet considered supernatural if attributed to natural, though hidden, properties of things. They belonged to
the realm of "natural magic" as distinguished from supernatural
magic.[104] Religious help, on the other hand, consisted above all in
prayer to God and in fasting. Jesus himself, when expelling the demon
from the epileptic boy, had said to the disciples: "This kind can come
forth by nothing but by prayer and fasting."[105] To this were added
such religious ceremonies as were recognized by the church and performed under its supervision. Everything, however, that depended on
the interference of *supernatural* powers without keeping in the framework of the theological system was considered illicit magic.

Arnald of Villanova († 1311), a physician deeply interested in
theology,[106] can be cited as a witness for the above-mentioned
opinions. A believer in astrology and alchemy, in his book on epilepsy[107] he emphasizes the dependence of the disease on the constellation of the stars and especially the moon.[108] Likewise, he recommends
the use of all kinds of queer substances, including animal organs and
precious stones, and he attributes the effect of these things to various
natural causes. They may, therefore, be applied as long as no magic
characters or even divine symbols and prayers are involved.[109] Arnald
of Villanova is vehement in his denunciation of conjurors and augurs;
together with Origen, he thinks it better to be ignorant than to learn
from demons.[110]

His view that even divine words, if carried on the body, would represent magic amulets agreed with the opinion of more rigorous church-

---

pareant: nihil tamen est sine ratione positum quam tibi ubi opus esset ex principiis naturalibus
assignarem. Sed cum hoc sit philosophi declarare huic meo opusculo esset impertinens."

[104] In order to evade a confusion of terms, I use "magic" in the latter sense only.

[105] St. Mark, 9: 29 and St. Matthew 17: 21.

[106] Cf. Diepgen (276).

[107] This treatise appears in Arnald of Villanova's work under the title *Arnaldi De Villa Nova
De Epilepsia*. It shows some differences of view with the chapter on epilepsy contained in
Arnald's *Breviarium*, and may not be genuine. I am, however, not able to decide this question,
and the discrepancies are not great enough to exclude authorship by the same man. An English
translation of the chapter in the *Breviarium* has been published by Von Storch (1054).

[108] Arnald of Villanova (58), *De Epilepsia*, c. 1; col. 1603: "Ex quibus omnibus liquide
patet acute videntibus, quod hic languor caducus iure hoc lunaticus sortiatur a Luna." Pagel
(762), p. 255, mentions the lunar influence on epilepsy in the framework of Arnald's astrological theories.

[109] *Op. cit.*, c. 25; col. 1629: "Haec autem sunt de genere animalium terrae nascentium,
mineralium, et lapidum duntaxat absque omni caractere, et superstitionibus applicentur, ut
nullum eorum colligatur cum Symbolo divino, vel oratione Dominica, et similibus. Nec tamen
his et similibus tangantur, et suspendantur ad collum, vel ad aliud membrum patientis, vel
quocunque alio modo portentur. Res enim convenientes curationi de generibus his sunt materia
calidarum, vel causarum salubrium corporis humani operantium in his, in idipsum a sua substantia materiali, et a sua quantitate, et a sua specie tota."

[110] *L.c.*: "Repellantur igitur ignominiosi incantatores, coniuratores, spirituum invocatores,
divinatores, et augures in ministerio medicinali humani corporis domestici, et ministri iam facti
diaboli, de Deo diffidentes, et summum Medicum Iesum Christum, regnantem in coelis, occi-

men like St. Eligius, who thought them "fraught, not with the remedy of Christ, but with the poison of the Devil."[111] Similar sentiments were voiced in the sixteenth century by physicians like Johann Weyer, under the influence of the Reformation and Counter Reformation.

But the impression prevails that on the whole these theoretical distinctions did not carry much weight in the practical attitude of the period toward epilepsy. The broad mass of the people, as can be seen from popular prescriptions, put their trust in superstitious remedies to which were added magic signs and rituals or, quite as often, Christian symbols and rites. The priests, on the other hand, very often helped in such performances and adapted themselves to the popular demand.[112] Even the physicians, though to a minor extent, indulged in similar practices.

The medical literature on epilepsy of the early Middle Ages, though full of superstitions, is yet comparatively free from downright magic and religious influence. This is particularly true of the early period of Salernitan writings, where a sound ancient tradition prevailed and dietetic and pharmacological measures stood in the foreground. A change can be noticed from the time of Constantinus of Africa on († 1087). This author advises the parents of an epileptic to take the patient to church during the second week following Whitsuntide and let him hear Mass on Friday and Saturday.[113] On Sunday the priest or a religious-minded man should write down the part of the Gospel "where it is said: 'this kind of demon is not cast out but by prayer and fasting.' And whether he be an epileptic or lunatic or demoniac, he will be freed."[114] The substance of this passage was repeated by later physicians,[115] and Bernard of Gordon (1303 A.D.) made the priest not only recite the biblical passage but also write it down to be carried by the patient as an amulet.[116] A Salernitan doctor, Petroncellus, whose dates

---

dentes: nempe, secundum Originem, melius est ignorare, quam a daemonibus discere, et melius est a physicis discere, quam a divino quaerere divinationem, quod per homines daemonibus reverentia fiat, sed gentilium ritus divinum credit esse per qualemcunque spiritum profertur."

[111] Quoted from Payne (781), p. 112.

[112] Cf. Franz (376), vol. 2, p. 498 ff.

[113] For interpretation of these dates, cf. Diepgen in his edition of Gualterius Agilon (12), p. 109, footnotes.

[114] Constantinus Africanus (235), *Pantegni*, lib. V practicae, c. 17; fol. 99$^r$: "Si patrem habet aut matrem ducat eum ad ecclesiam in die quattuor temporum: et audiat missam in sexta feria similiter in die sabbati faciat: die dominico veniente sacerdos vel vir religiosus scribat evangelium ubi dicitur: Hoc genus non eijicitur nisi in oratione et ieiunio: sive sit epilepticus sive lunaticus vel demoniacus curabitur absque dubio. Et notandum quod ex incestuosis coniugationibus natis non valet."

[115] Cf. Gualterius Agilon (12), *Summa medicinalis*, p. 109 and Bernard of Gordon (106), *Lilium medicinae*, fol. 119$^{r-v}$.

[116] Bernard of Gordon, *l.c.*: "Et postea quod ille sacerdos postquam devote et per intentionem legerit supra caput evangelium, scribat, et quod portetur ad collum, curat perfecte proculdubio."

are not certain,[117] thought antimony helpful, either alone or taken with holy water and with the Lord's Prayer repeated three times.[118]

These few examples may suffice to show that medieval physicians conformed to the practices of the time and that they were much more susceptible to magic and religious practices than their great classical forerunners had been. To this must be added Arabic influences, exemplified in the relation between Abulqasim (c. 1000 A.D.) and Matthaeus Ferrarius (fifteenth century). Abulqasim numbers five "efficient causes" of epilepsy. Four of these are the usual humors and vapors; but the fifth eventuality is that epilepsy "is caused by some outside agent whose mode [of action] is not known, and it is said that it is caused by demons."[119] More instructive, however, than this reference to demons is Abulqasim's account of how he himself came to believe in a demoniac form of epilepsy. He had long been doubtful of symptoms which pointed to such a cause, till the matter had recently been demonstrated to him. Among the many forms of the disease he had seen was that of people who fell down, whose appearance changed, who talked in a tongue formerly unknown to them and read books, wrote, and talked about scientific matters of which they had hitherto been ignorant. Finally, they recovered, although the reason for this remained obscure. The cause of the phenomenon had escaped him until in some books, which Hunain ibn Ishaq had translated under the name of Galen, he had come across the statement that diseases befell men in the following ways: either through some dietetic mistake, or through their sins and crimes, or through "the accursed demons who are called 'allahin ablis.' "[120] If in such cases medical treatment failed, the patients had better be left to the mercy of their Creator.[121] In conformity with

[117]According to Bloedner (123), he lived in the twelfth century.

[118]De Renzi (840), vol. 4, p. 293: "Solum antimonium sumtum curat, et si cum aqua benedicta, quam greci in Epifania benedicunt, sumatur cum dominica oratione cantata tribus vicibus in nomine patientis arrepta; vel succus vel herba peonie data potenter valet."

[119]Abulqasim (4), Liber theoricae nec non practicae, fol. 34r: "... aut causatur ex re extranea cuius modus ignoratur et dicitur quod est a causa demonum."

[120]Cf. below, footnote 121, where Abulqasim mentions four possibilities. I can, however, distinguish three only, and so, apparently, did Matthaeus Ferrarius (352), who, in quoting Abulqasim, says, Practica, fol. 45r: "et hoc est bene notandum quod egritudines tribus modis invadunt homines ex aliqua causarum: ut ex malitia regiminis cibi et potus et ex peccatis et praevaricationibus: et ultima causa ex maledictis demonibus qui dicuntur alabin etc."

[121]Abulqasim (4) l.c., fol. 34v: "Signa ex causa demonum inquit auctor semper dubitans eram super hoc donec nuper mihi demonostrative patuit. Vidi enim hanc aegritudinem multis modis. Quod est quia sunt aliqui invite corruentes et quorum forma transmutatur et locuntur aliena lingua quam prius ignorabant loqui et legunt alaūa (!) et alios libros quos minime sciebant et scribunt et locuntur multa de tractatibus scientiarum quarum nihil viderant nec intellexerant, et ultimo sanantur, nec cum hoc praecesserit eos aliquid propter quod debet eis huiusmodi advenire nec permutata fuit ipsorum naturalis complexio nec ipsorum cognitio et intellectus. Causam ignoravi huius accidentis donec studens in quibusdam libris quos interpretatus est hanen filius ysaac nomine G[aleni] inveni enim in ipsis quod dicitur, quod aegritudines invadunt homines quatuor modis, id est ex aliqua causarum ex malicia regiminis cibi et potus ex

these views, Abulqasim mentions an amulet that would protect people from the attacks of demons.[122]

Matthaeus Ferrarius quotes this story from Abulqasim, mentioning his name[123] and having little of his own to add to it.[124] The type of demoniac disease which Abulqasim here describes has all the classical signs of "possession." It is remarkable that Abulqasim not only became converted to the prevalent belief in "possession," but that he ranged it among the signs and causes of epilepsy. Thus, Abulqasim and those following him came very near the popular concept of the "falling evil." However, this attitude was an exception rather than the rule.

Constantinus of Africa, for example, noticed the similarity between epilepsy, lunacy, and demoniac possession and proposed the following test to decide the nature of the evil: A formula commanding the demon to recede would be spoken into the ear of the patient. If he were lunatic or demoniac, he would be in a deathlike state for an hour. Afterward he would be able to tell anything he might be asked. If, however, he did not fall down, this would prove him an epileptic.[125] This passage shows the belief in the demoniac nature of some cases of the falling evil, but at the same time it suggests that epilepsy was not necessarily attributed to such influence. In another work Constantinus

---

peccatis et praevaricationibus et ex maledictis demonibus qui dicuntur allahin ablis. In quarum curatione si nostra ingeniatio defecerit et ipsarum causae a nobis decisae sint relinquite opus creatori eorum, non est operum miserator magis quam ipsorum creator, et quia occulta est medicis causa huius aegritudinis et eorum cognitio circa eam deficit recusarunt eius curationem tractare, sed non est dubium penes me quod hoc est de antiquis scientiis quae hodie occultatae sunt hominibus."

[122] *Ibid.*, fol. 35[r]: "et dixit alcabri quod in ventre galli reperitur lapis albus qui portatus suspensus omnes malignos spiritus et demones ab eo fugat et confert pueris qui timent in somno."

[123] Cf. particularly Matthaeus Ferrarius (352), *Practica*, fol. 45[r] and 48[r].

[124] It is, however, interesting that in his reference to demoniac epilepsy he refers to the recognized practices of the Church; fol. 48[r]: "tunc curandus est ut reconcilietur cum deo et practicetur in hoc illa scientia canonica extra de penitentiis. cum infirmitas non nunquam ex peccato contingat etc."

[125] Constantinus Africanus (234), *Pantegni*, lib. V practicae, c. 17; fol. 99[r]: "Est et aliud experimentum et est probatum: dic hoc nomen in aure suspecti patientis. Recede demon: quia dee fanoleri precipiunt. Si lunaticus vel demoniacus: ibi statim efficitur velut mortuus fere per unam horam: eo surgente interroga eum de quacunque re volueris: et dicet tibi: et si vero ceciderit scias audito hoc nomine esse epilepticum." The latter part of this passage is not quite clear and I have preferred the version of Gualterius Agilon (12), *Summa medicinalis*, p. 108: "Et notandum, quod epilenticus et lunaticus et demoniacus quodammodo sunt similes, ut ait Constantinus in practica sua capitulo de epilentia, et ad probandum, utrum cadens in terram sit lunaticus sive demoniacus sive epilenticus, fiat tale experimentum: Dic hoc nomen in aure suspecti: 'Recede demon! quod essimoloy precipiunt!' Si lunaticus sive demoniacus sit, efficiatur quasi mortuus fere per unam horam; eo surgente interroga eum, de quacumque re volueris, et dicet tibi, et, si non ceciderit audito hoc nomine, scias illum esse epilenticum." Whatever the original version may have been, the essential point is that the possessed and the epileptic react differently and that the former only has prophetic (?) gifts. John of Gaddesden (535), *Rosa anglica*, p. 45, was also acquainted with this passage: "Et nota quod Epilepticus, Lunaticus, Daemoniacus quodammodo sunt similes, ut testatur Constantinus 9. Practicae suae cap. 5. de Epilepsia."

Africanus made a statement which would tend to show that physicians, in opposition to the popular demonistic beliefs, were inclined to consider possession to be either epilepsy or madness. "The crowd," he says, "calls [epilepsy] 'divination' because it is an obscure disease, and they say that the sufferers from this disease are demoniacs. But of the physicians, some say that it is epilepsy, others mania."[126] This passage, together with the word "divination," was perhaps a translation from the Arabic.[127] However this may be, the fact remains that the leading medieval textbooks contain relatively few allusions to the supernatural character of epilepsy. Furthermore, in their discussions of nightmare, a condition related by them to epilepsy, they sometimes put their own natural explanation into clear contrast to the supernatural explanations of theologians and of the mass of the people.[128]

If, therefore, both laity and physicians indulged in the same doubtful practices, the reasons cannot always have been the same. Credulity, the unclear conception of the "falling evil," and the predominant belief in devils and demons account for the attitude of the people and the lower clergy. The same reasons also influenced some physicians. Others, perhaps the majority, may not have paid much attention to the nice distinction between "hidden causes of nature" and a hidden power of magic words and actions, and made use of both. But there was also a third

---

[126]Constantinus Africanus (235), *De melancholia*, lib. I; vol. 1, pp. 289-90: "Epilepsia est ergo humiditas carens, et ventriculos cerebri implens, non ex toto tamen prohibens animam actionem monstrare suam, quoadusque natura oppilantem materiam digerat. Unde antiqui hanc passionem apoplexiam vocaverunt minorem. . . . A vulgo divinatio appellatur, quia morbus est absconsus, dicentes demoniacos esse hunc morbum patientes. Sed medicorum alii dicunt esse maniam."

[127]The dependence of *De melancholia* of Constantine of Africa on the *Maqālat fī l-mālikhō-liyā* by Ishāq ibn 'Amrān is discussed by Flashar (363), pp. 88-91, who cites additional literature on the subject. The term *divinatio* also appears in the Latin translation of the *Practica* of Serapion (915), fol. 8$^V$: "Haec autem egritudo multis nominatur nominibus ex quibus est fedemin: quoniam accidit plus pueris: et epilepsia. quoniam facit spasmum et constringit motus: et sensus: et divinatio. Unde putant quod ipse sit ex parte demonum. unde nocet membris principalibus. Et herculea ex nomine Herculis superbi quasi sit propter magnitudinem eius." The translations prove no more than the connection of epilepsy with divination in the West. The original meaning behind the term *divinatio* could be ascertained only on the basis of the Arabic and, possibly, Syriac texts. The whole complex of epileptic prophecy is discussed below in the section on the Renaissance. The name *fedemin* is a corruption of the Greek *paidion*, cf. below, footnote 168.

[128]In a paper on "Demonology and Medical Tradition in the Middle Ages" read before the Eleventh International Congress of the History of Medicine at Zagreb, 1938, I discussed this subject in more detail. I add a quotation from Geraldus de Solo (407), *Expositio*, fol. 34$^r$, which emphasizes the different theories of *incubus* held by theologians and physicians: "una theologorum qui dicunt quod causa huius passionis sunt demones qui sunt existentes in aere supra corpus humanum principaliter respiciunt cor. et quia cor non potest sustinere aspectum illius mali spiritus et ideo non potest moveri. et quia fumi vadunt ad caput ideo non possunt loqui nec sentire. alii dicunt quod est vetula vel merula quae vadit vel scandit ad aliud seculum et illa ponit se supra hominem et calcat et comprimit et illud nihil est. Alia est causa medicorum ponentium quod causae incubi sunt tres . . . " and then follows a discussion of the natural causes. The reserved attitude of medieval physicians toward the supernatural origin of disease was pointed out by Diepgen (271) in 1921. On the subject of impotence caused by sorcery cf. Hoffmann (504).

group, who merely prescribed what the faithful expected them to prescribe.[129] The result, in any case, was the same. The medical texts of
the later Middle Ages, i.e., from the eleventh century on, contain ample
instances of magic and religious therapy. They, therefore, constitute
one of the main sources of our knowledge of the various forms of
supernatural cures current during the Middle Ages and preserved in the
folk medicine of later centuries.

### b. Saints and Relics

With the spread of Christianity people began to expect help from
saints and relics. Early ecclesiastic writers report miraculous cures of
epilepsy wrought by holy men themselves or at their shrines. Because of
the broad interpretation of the falling evil, it is not always clear
whether the complaint was epilepsy in the medical sense or some other
disorder. This has led to the belief that such treatments owed their
reputation to cases where the patient suffered from a neurosis, easily
influenced by the suggestive power of saints, relics, and talismans.[130]
Plausible as this explanation is, it must not be unduly generalized, for
sometimes a chance remark by the writer gives a diagnostic hint in a
different direction. Among the many miracles reported by Gregory of
Tours (sixth century) is the story of a boy who suffered from an
epileptic disease, "so that usually in falling down and frothing, *he cut
his tongue with his own teeth.*" Treated by the physicians, the boy had
a free interval of a few months but subsequently suffered a relapse
which left him worse than ever. He was sent to the grave of St. Nicetius
and returned healthy, nor was he attacked by the disease again, "for it
was the seventh [year] since the restoration of the boy when the
bishop presented him to us."[131]
Laying aside the question of the actual effectiveness of this kind of
treatment, there can be no doubt about its popularity. The fact that

---

[129]The apocryphal *Letter to his Son on Incantations and Invocations*, which is to be found
among the alleged works of Constantinus Africanus (235), vol. 1, p. 317, shows that healing
through faith was explained on natural principles: "Cui inquam mens humana rem aliquam,
licet naturaliter non iuvantem, si prodesse certificat, ex sola mentis intentione corpus res illa
iuvat. Verbi gratia: Si quis incantationem sibi prodesse confidat, qualiscunque sit, eum tamen
adiuvat: Si enim, ut diximus, complexio corporis virtutem sequatur animae, necesse est taliter
rem se habere."

[130]Cf., e.g., Bloch (122), p. 418.

[131]Gregory of Tours (428), *Liber vitae patrum*, VIII, 8; p. 699, 1-9: "Phronimi igitur
Agatensis episcopi famulus epilentici morbi accentu fatigabatur, ita ut plerumque cadens ac
spumans, linguam suam propriis dentibus laceraret; et cum ei a medicis plurima fierent, acci-
debat, ut paucis mensibus interpositis, non tangeretur a morbo; sed iterum in redivivo cruciatu
ruens, peius quam prius egerat perferebat. Dominus vero eius cum vidisset tantas virtutes ad
sepulchrum beati Niceti fieri, dixit ad eum: 'Vade et prosternere coram sepulchro sancti, orans,
ut te adiuvare dignetur.' Qui cum iussa explesset, sanus regressus est, nec ultra eum hic adtigit
morbus. Septimus enim erat [annus] ab incolomitate pueri, quando eum nobis episcopus
praesentavit." Biting of the tongue usually is absent in purely functional epileptiform fits.
Gregory (427), *Hist. Francorum*, IV, 12; p. 148, 13-16, tells another interesting story of a

some saints lent their names to the disease and became its patrons is proof in itself. Pilgrimages were undertaken to the Priory of St. Valentine at Rufach in Alsace, where, at the end of the fifteenth century, a hospital for epileptics was built.[132] Contemporary woodcuts represent the pilgrims approaching the saint, a man and woman lying on the ground, and a swine, the symbol of the devil, standing at his right (cf. Fig. 2). St. Bibiana also was a patron of epilepsy, and the monastery dedicated to her in Rome formed another center of healing, famous for its herb, hulwort. The patients had to go through an elaborate cere-

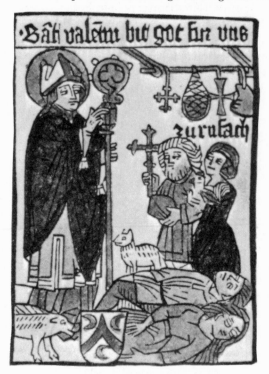

Fig. 2

St. Valentine, Patron of Epileptics.
Woodcut, c. 1480. (Sudhoff,
*Archiv für Gesch. d. Medizin, 6,*
1913, p. 452.)

---

bishop who became epileptic as a result of heavy drinking: "Denique Cautinus, adsumpto episcopatu, talem se reddidit, ut ab omnibus execraretur, vino ultra modum deditus. Nam plerumque in tantum infundebatur potu, ut de convivio vix a quattuor portaretur. Unde factum est, ut epylenticus fieret in sequenti. Quod saepius populis manifestatum est."

[132] Cf. Sudhoff (972), p. 450 ff.

mony in which the celebration of three Masses played an important part. Powdered hulwort was given them in the name of the Father, the Son, and the Holy Spirit at the end of each Mass. A visit to the grave of the saint finished the whole procedure. It was, however, not necessary to go to Rome, since the powder was exported and could be swallowed anywhere, accompanied by the same rites.[133]

Apart from those mentioned, there are many other saints who appear as patrons of epilepsy,[134] most of them of merely local fame. Among those who acquired a widespread reputation were the three wise men. St. Matthew tells how they followed the star to Bethlehem. "And when they were come into the house, they saw the young child with Mary his mother, *and fell down*, and worshipped him: and when they had opened their treasures, they presented unto him gifts; gold, and frankincense, and myrrh."[135] Probably due to their falling down before Jesus,[136] and perhaps as magicians credited with an insight into mysterious things,[137] the three wise men were connected with epilepsy. Certainly from the twelfth century on, perhaps even a little earlier,[138] their names were pronounced into the ear of the patient to arouse him from his paroxysm, or they were written on a piece of paper, on a ring, etc., and carried as amulets and talismans. Bernard of Gordon was the first physician to mention the custom, and he used a formula which became typical for centuries:

> Gaspar fert mirrham, thus Melchior: Balthasar aurum:
> Haec tria qui secum portabit nomina regum,
> Solvitur a morbo Christi pietate caduco.

Correctly spoken into the ear, the words, he did not doubt, would have an immediate effect.[139] There existed, of course, many variants of the procedure.[140] John of Arderne, for instance, gave the following advice: "Against Epilepsy write these three names with blood taken from the auricular [i.e., little] finger of the patient.—Jasper—Melchoir—Balthazar

---

[133] Cf. Franz (376), vol. 2, p. 500.

[134] Cf. the list given by Kerler (578), pp. 82–86.

[135] St. Matthew, 2: 11.

[136] Cf. Sudhoff (975), p. 384; Franz (376), vol. 2, pp. 505–6; Bargheer (79), cols. 1172–73; and Ohrt (751), col. 1180.

[137] Cf. Kehrer (577), vol. 1, p. 76.

[138] Cf. Kehrer, *ibid.*

[139] Bernard of Gordon (106), *Lilium medicinae*, fol. 119[r]: "Cum aliquis est in paroxismo, si aliquis ponat os supra aurem patientis, et dicat ter istos 3 versus, proculdubio statim surgit [follows the above formula]. Quod autem his dictis recte in foramine auris verum est, probatum est frequenter quod statim surgit. Et dicitur etiam si scribantur, et portentur ad collum quod perfecte curantur." Geraldus de Solo (407), *Expositio*, alludes to these verses as commonly known when he says, fol. 32[v]: "... ille versus Gaspar fert myrram thus melchior baltazar aurum," and again on fol. 33[v]: "... et portatio versuum communium ut: Gaspar fert etc."

[140] Cf., e.g., Sudhoff (975), p. 383 f., and Hovorka-Kronfeld (516), vol. 2, p. 214.

and put gold, frankincense and myrrh into a box. Let the patient say three paternosters and III Ave marias daily for the souls of the fathers and mothers of these three kings for a month and let the patient drink for a month of the juice of peony with beer or wine and if he be a child write with blood as before . . . on a murrha [i.e., a piece of porcelain or fine china] and let it be put in the beer and without doubt this remedy never fails."[141]

Draughts of peony juice, combined with the invocation of the three wise men, and the dispensing of hulwort at the monastery of St. Bibiana are instances of old magic plants accepted in a Christian age. The magic character of peony has already been mentioned.[142] As to hulwort, some anonymous Greek had advised the wearing of a cluster on the body "against the solitary sleep sent from heaven which some call a grave, sacred disease . . . others an evil lunar enchantment of the body."[143] Now such plants were connected with Christian symbols. Bartholomaeus, a Salernitan physician of the early twelfth century, tells how to proceed in gathering hulwort to be used as an ointment and amulet for epileptics and lunatics.[144] It must be done with great reverence; first the Gospel of St. John the Baptist, three paternosters, and three Ave Marias must be recited, gold and silver must be strewn around, one must pray to God that the patient may never have a relapse—then the plants may be gathered.[145]

Mistletoe also acquired a Christian lore.[146] It was said that David, while guarding his father's cattle, saw a woman collapse, suffering from the falling evil. Thereupon he prayed God to reveal a remedy to him. An angel appeared and told him that mistletoe worn on the right hand would prevent further attacks.[147]

---

[141]Quoted from Sir D'Arcy Power's translation of Arderne's (48), *De arte phisicali et de cirurgia*, p. 6.

[142]Cf. above, p. 13.

[143]*Anonymi carmen de herbis* (35), p. 177:

Δεῖ δέ σε καὶ περὶ σῶμα φορεῖν πολίοιο κόρυμβον
πρὸς τὸν ἀπαυλισμὸν τὸν ἀπ' αἰθέρος ὃν καλέουσιν
ἄνθρωποι χαλεπὴν ἱερὴν νόσον ἀμπλακιῶτιν,
οἱ δὲ σεληνιακὴν ἐπὶ σῶμα κακὴν ἐπιπομπήν.

[144]Bartholomaeus (840), *Practica*, vol. 4, p. 356: "Item polium herba teratur et sucus misceatur cum aceto syllitico et totus ante accessionem ungatur, et de hac ipsa herba in collo ligetur; valde iuvat eos, et si lunaticus erit, verum nunquam ei revertetur." I am not certain whether Bartholomaeus distinguishes between epileptics and lunatics and whether the ceremony applies to both or only to the latter.

[145]*Ibid.*: "Sed istud sic dictum fieri: Iste herbe debent colligi cum magna reverentia, et Evangelium Sancti Johannis Baptiste superius, et pater noster iij, et iij ave marie, et circundare eos auro et argento, rogando deum qui eas creavit, et invocando ut hanc virtutem tibi ostendat, et quicumque super se portaverit, nunquam ei revertetur, et postea colligantur."

[146]On the history of mistletoe cf. Kanner (572).

[147]Schönbach (897), p. 147 f., quotes the story from a German manuscript of the fifteenth century. Cf. also Ohrt (751), col. 1179, where the biblical story of the woman of Tekoah (II Samuel, 14: 4) who fell down before David and asked for his help is suggested as a possible source.

The name and memory of Christ were connected with cures of this kind. Gilbertus Anglicus gives a long prescription for the preparation of an ointment, reminiscent of the doings of Greek magicians as reported by the book *On the Sacred Disease*. Finally, before applying the ointment, he advises saying into the right ear of the patient: "Christ has conquered"; into the left: "Christ governs"; and into his face: "Christ commands."[148]

Even outspoken incantations against the falling evil made use of prayers and referred to Christ and the names of saints. On the other hand, the symbolism is often scarcely understandable and represents a variety of elements, some of them going back to much older times. A formula may here be mentioned which has aroused more than passing interest. It is a German *Fallsuchtsegen* which goes back at least to the eleventh century and which is so poorly preserved and so obscure in its meaning that many contradicting explanations have been offered.[149] Its Latin introduction and end, however, afford an insight into its ritual. It is entitled "Contra caducum morbum" and prescribes the following procedure: "Approach the patient who lies on the ground. And stepping from the left side to the right and thus standing over him say three times . . . ,"[150] whereupon there follows the German text which alludes to a bridge and a fight in which Adam's son slays the Devil's son.[151] Finally, in a mixture of Latin and German, it says: "And touch the earth with each hand and say a pater noster. Then spring over to the right, touch his right side with the right foot and say: 'Get up . . . God has so commanded you.' Do this three times, and you will presently see the patient rise healthy."[152] One passage of the formula mentions the unclean spirit whom the incantation probably intended to drive out.

As an example of the use of church lights—a very popular ingredient of antiepileptic ceremonies[153]—the following medieval English prescription may be named: Seven wax candles are made, and on each a day of the week is inscribed. Then they are lighted and Mass is sung. When Mass is finished the epileptic takes one of the candles and will from now on fast on the day indicated.[154] Finally, confession, church lights,

---

[148]Gilbertus Anglicus (412), *Compendium medicinae*, fol. 111^V: et dic sibi in aure dextra. Cristus vicit. in sinistra. Cristus regnat. in fronte. Cristus imperat. amen. postea inungantur ei predicta."

[149]The text is preserved in two manuscripts (*P* and *M*) of the twelfth and eleventh centuries. My translation follows *P* as given in Steinmeyer's (954) edition, p. 380 f. For interpretation cf. Steinmeyer, *l.c.*, and Ohrt (751), col. 1179 f.

[150]Steinmeyer (954), p. 380.

[151]For a restitution of the German text on the basis of *M*, cf. Krogmann (595).

[152]Steinmeyer, *l.c.*, p. 381: "et tange terram utraque manu. et dic pater noster. Post haec transilias ad dextram et dextro pede dextrum latus eius tange et dic. stant uf waz was dir. got der gebot dir ez. hoc ter fac. et mox uidebis infirmum surgere sanum."

[153]Cf., e.g., Hovorka-Kronfeld (516), vol. 2, p. 213.

[154]Cf. Müller (718), p. 107. A somewhat similar formula is cited by Cholmeley (220), p. 51 f.

reading of the Gospel, recitation of prayers could be combined in a very elaborate Mass for the epileptic, without superseding various kinds of remedies and charms.[155] The juxtaposition of religion, magic, superstition, and drug-lore in the treatment of epilepsy gives a more realistic impression of the reaction of medieval man to this disease than does the analysis of isolated tendencies.

In medieval England amulets against epilepsy acquired political significance in the form of so-called cramp-rings.[156] Apparently, it was a widespread custom to have rings against epilepsy made from gold or silver coins which had repeatedly been sacrificed to the Church and then redeemed.[157] It seems that Edward II had such rings made to enhance royal prestige. On Good Friday the king, advancing to the cross on his knees, placed a certain number of gold and silver pieces on the altar. Then these pieces were replaced by ordinary money and were used for making rings. Originally the significance of the rite consisted in the donation of the metal to the cross. But under Edward's successors it became a miracle in which the sacred majesty of the king and the royal touch played the decisive role. Even the ceremony itself changed; around 1500 the rings were fabricated in advance and then consecrated by the king. Legend tried to give the custom a venerable origin. Edward the Confessor had given his ring to St. John, who had approached him as a beggar. Under miraculous circumstances the ring had found its way back to the king, was kept at Westminster Abbey, and had the power of curing epilepsy.[158] Thus, legend tried to motivate the custom which ended rather abruptly with the death of Queen Mary.[159] The rings were believed to bestow immunity, not against epilepsy only but also against "all plots of Satan," and to give relief in every kind of disease.[160]

### c. Infection

The popular view of epilepsy as "contagious" goes back, as will be remembered, to Antiquity, when people used to spit before an epileptic and refused to eat and drink from the same dishes with him. The

---

[155] See Ogden (750), pp. 39–42 and 99.

[156] For the following I am accepting the interpretation given by Bloch (122), p. 159 ff.

[157] For St. Gall in Switzerland cf. Franz (376), vol. 2, p. 502.

[158] Cf. Crawfurd (243), pp. 166, 171, 179, and 182. But rings obtained in other ways, without royal consecration, were also believed to help against epilepsy, especially if inscribed with the names of the three wise men. Cf. Crawfurd, *ibid.*, p. 173, and Antonius Guainerius (438), *Tract. de egritud. cap.*, VII, 8; fol. 14$^r$, who gives the following instructions: "Fiunt item anuli quidam accipe de umbilico puelli noviter nati: et in anulo auri eum include: smeraldum vero desuper. Vel facias sic. accipe de pilis canis albi cum modico peonie radicis: ac radicis piretri: et illa anulo aureo includantur: smeraldus vero desuper. Vel facias sic. . . . Et si super hos anulos infrascriptum feceris. Gaspar fert myrrham thus etc. Fertur enim quod praescriptus versus super se portatus epilepticum cadere non sinit. Hi anuli in digito vel ad collum portati valent."

[159] Cf. Crawfurd, *ibid.*, p. 179.

[160] Crawfurd, *ibid.*, p. 183.

demon driven out of the epileptic boy by Jesus was also called an "unclean spirit" in the Gospel. "Unclean" in the meaning of the cult usually indicated an object whose presence or touch might prove disastrous. When early Christianity adopted the idea of demoniac possession, it often tended to include epileptics in this category. And when, furthermore, early churchmen and synods segregated the possessed from the faithful[161] and refused them oblation and the Eucharist,[162] the reasons were similar to those motivating the behavior toward epileptics in Antiquity: the possessed would desecrate the holy objects[163] and would infect the common plate and cup.[164]

All these restrictions show the conscious or unconscious dread of the sinister power lurking behind the possessed and epileptic. This fear, indeed, often was of a rather vague character. People were afraid of some evil which the *contagium* might bring upon them, but which need not necessarily be the same disease. The belief in the specifically infectious nature of epilepsy was, however, clearly voiced during the later part of the Middle Ages.

Berthold of Regensburg, a German preacher of the thirteenth century, attributed the infection of the falling evil to the contagious character of the patient's evil breath. He said that there were two diseases, leprosy and the falling evil, which even the greatest masters of medicine, Hippocrates, Galen, Constantinus of Africa, Avicenna, Macer, and Bartholomaeus could not cure.[165] Whoever had suffered from the falling evil for more than twenty-four years was without hope. "And when he falls down, lies on the ground, and froths—beware of him if you value your life! Let nobody go near him, for such a terrible breath comes forth from his mouth that the person into whose mouth this breath enters may acquire the same disease. Beware then lest you approach him when he is seized by the disease!"[166] Epilepsy was included among the infectious diseases enumerated in the verse of the so-called *Schola Salernitana*, where it was named *pedicon*.[167] This term

---

[161] Cf. Dölger (285), pp. 119 and 125 ff.

[162] Cf. *ibid.*, p. 125.

[163] Cf. *ibid.*, p. 113.

[164] Cf. Dölger (286), p. 135. Dölger emphasizes the survival of the ancient fear of epileptics in the attitude toward the possessed.

[165] Cf. Martin (671), p. 106.

[166] Martin, *ibid.*: "Swer die vallende suht hât über vier unde zweinzic jâr, dâ gên alle die zuo die dâ hiute leben, die künden den siechtum niemer gebüezen. Unde swenne er alsô hin vellet unde lît unde schûmet, sô hüetet iuch vor im als liep iu lîp si, daz sich ieman nâhen zuo im habe, wan im gêt ein sô griulich âtem ûz dem munde, daz er vil lîhte den selben siechtuom gewünne, swem der âtem in den munt kaeme. Unde dâ von sô hüetet iuch daz ir im iht nâhen komet innen des, daz in der siechtuom an gêt." In the eighteenth century, Tissot (1024), *Traitê de l'épilepsie*, pp. 5-6 mentioned "the unbearable cadaverous smell" of the froth of some epileptics.

[167] De Renzi (840), vol. 5, p. 71:
Febris acuta, phthisis, scabies, pedicon, sacer ignis,

is nothing but a variant of the Greek *paidion*, given as a synonym for epilepsy by Galen and other ancient writers and meaning "children's disease."[168] But many medieval authors, not knowing Greek and misled by a consonance, referred it to the Latin *pes*, i.e., foot, whence arose all kinds of etymological speculations. Some connected it with the epileptic's kicking of the legs;[169] others with an alleged evil smell of his feet.[170]

Layman and physician alike believed in the infectious nature of the breath. "Therefore, neither talk nor bathe with them, since by their mere breath they infect people," wrote a professor of the fifteenth century.[171] A combination of factors accounts for this strange view. At the bottom of it were the old superstitious fears of the epileptic and the association of demons with wind and breath. A current medical theory attributing the cause of the epileptic attack to the ascent of poisonous, horrid, and fetid vapors to the brain,[172] gave it a scientific justification.

The fear of catching the disease expressed itself in various ways. In Basel at the end of the fourteenth century the city council either ordered, or at least suggested, that epileptics as well as sufferers from other infectious diseases should not be allowed to sell food and drink and should be expelled from the city.[173] When, in 1510, stipulations

---

Anthrax, lippa, lepra, frenesis contagia praestant:
Iungitur ophtalmus, congelans lippus et arba.
Sudhoff (969), p. 224, thinks that the original form of these verses was:
Febris acuta, ptisis, pedicon, scabies, sacer ignis,
Antrax, lippa, lepra nobis contagia praestant.
Sudhoff, *ibid.*, p. 226 f., gives a short history of the diseases considered as contagious by the Arabs and then by medieval authors. He notes that Rhazes counts four such diseases. However, the early Arabic *Book of the Dakhíra* (933), 18, p. 7 already mentions seven contagious and seven hereditary diseases. In the translation of Meyerhof (693), p. 61, this passage reads: "What they (the Ancients) recommended is abstinence from intercourse with people who are suffering from contagious diseases which are in general seven: leprosy, scabies, small-pox ..., measles, ozaena ..., ophthalmia and the pestilential diseases. Moreover to beware of diseases which are hereditary from the parents, and which are also in general seven: leprosy, vitiligo, consumption ..., phthisis, melancholy, gout and epilepsy."

[168] On the doubtful Hippocratic origin of the term cf. Temkin (999), p. 308, footnote 105. The correct derivation of *pedicon* is already mentioned by Antonius Guainerius (438), *Tract. de egritud. cap.*, VII, 1; fol. 11ʳ: "Et quia passio hec pueros quammaxime deprehendit pedicon a quibusdam dicta est a pede grece quod est latine puer." I think that the Arabic synonym for epilepsy *'ummu s-sibyáni*, "mother of the boy," stands for *paidion*.

[169] Antonius Guainerius, *l.c.*, continues: "Vel ut aliis placet ab inordinata pedum motione: que in huius passionis paroxismo communiter fit." Geraldus de Solo (407), *Expositio*, fol. 29ᵛ: "Secundo vocatur peditio ab immoderato motu pedis in paroxismo."

[170] Cf. Martin (671), p. 105. According to Tissot (1024), *Traité de l'épilepsie*, p. 9, De Haen commented upon the bad smell of the epileptics' sweat. Mechler (679), p. 536, mentions a form *peditio* sometimes used in the seventeenth and eighteenth centuries.

[171] Siegmund Albich, whom I quote from Sudhoff (972), p. 454: "Igitur non loguimini cum eis nec balneamini, quia solo anhelitu inficiunt hominem." This does not refer to epileptics alone, but to all diseases which were believed infectious, including epilepsy. According to Aristotle (55), *Problems*, VII, 8, 887 A; vol. 1, p. 176, the breath of consumptives is infectious.

[172] Cf. the following chapter.

[173] Cf. Sudhoff (969), p. 220.

were made for the *Zwölfbrüderhaus* at Nürnberg, it was specified that a brother suffering from leprosy, epilepsy, or syphilis should be expelled.[174] Indeed, contact with epileptics was feared in the Middle Ages, as was contact with syphilitics in later centuries. This is documented by a lawsuit against one Jehan Jehannin in Dijon, in 1463, who was accused of having abducted a girl by the name of Jacote. In his testimony the accused stated that after the girl had told him that she had *le gros mal*[175] he let her alone, "being dismayed and having a horror of the disease."[176] The *gros mal* was the *morbus grossus*, the *grand mal*, i.e., epilepsy, believed to be of a contagious nature[177] and therefore to be avoided.

At the beginning of the sixteenth century, when contagious diseases were more accurately studied, the belief in the infectious nature of epilepsy was discarded by medical men. Fernelius, the most influential pathologist of the time, stated the new view in unmistakable terms: "A person who has taken poison or suffers from epilepsy cannot contaminate others, either by his breath or by his contact. For this reason these diseases are different from epidemic and contagious diseases."[178] But the belief was to reappear later on, although not in its original form. The infectiousness of epilepsy was again discussed in the eighteenth century, when it was observed that the mere sight of epileptics was sufficient to provoke seizures in the onlookers. But then, of course, another explanation was given—not the breath of the patient but the imagination of the spectator might engender the disease.

---

[174] Cf. *ibid.*, p. 222.

[175] Cf. Haustein (464), pp. 376 and 377.

[176] Haustein, *ibid.*, p. 377: "ladite fille luy deist qu'elle avoit le gros mal, parquoy luy tout espardu et ayant horreur du mal se ne monta et ne se travailla plus avant de la cognoistre charnelment."

[177] Du Cange (301), vol. 5, p. 517, quotes from a French document of 1415: "Dès le temps de sa nascion le suppliant a esté entachié d'une maladie contagieuse, que l'en appelle le grant Mal ou le mal S. Jehan." Cf. Haustein, *l.c.*, p. 381 ff., who has proved conclusively that the case of Dijon was epilepsy and not syphilis, as had been believed by previous historians.

[178] Fernelius (351), *De abditis rerum causis*, II, 11; p. 74: "Qui venenum hausit, aut comitiali morbo laborat, neque halitu neque contactu alios inquinare potest, qua ratione hi ab epidemiis et a contagiosis distant."

# IV
# Medieval Medical Theories

## 1. EARLY MIDDLE AGES

If one takes a broad view of the medical theories of epilepsy during the Middle Ages, they appear as mere variants of ancient theories, especially those of Galen. They are devoid of the provoking originality of the theological speculations of the time, and they are more often dimmed by confusion than guided by experience. Not that they lack differences of opinion and subtleties of conception, but these differences, based on the traditional system of the humors and the ancient neurology of the animal spirit, seem mere quibbling to the modern reader. It is for this reason that we shall neglect many of the finer arguments and emphasize the more obvious characteristics which mark the history of epilepsy during this epoch.

In the west of the Roman world the Middle Ages began much earlier than in its eastern part. Certain Latin pharmacological texts, like the so-called *Medicina Plinii* and the work of Gargilius Martialis, though still belonging to the third to fourth centuries, are already medieval in character. Nearly all the prescriptions for epilepsy in the former work are of a superstitious nature,[179] and the same is true of Quintus Serenus' medical poem. Yet the theories and descriptions of epilepsy recorded in this period of transition are still comparatively free from misunderstandings and corruptions. Such authors as Theodorus Priscianus and Caelius Aurelianus are valuable sources for ancient thought on epilepsy. Fragments preserved under the

---

[179] Cf. Pliny (pseudo) (808), *De medicina*, III, 21; p. 93 f.

names of Soranus and Caelius Aurelianus give short but clear and concise descriptions of the disease.[180] Even Cassius Felix, who wrote as late as 447 A.D., offers nothing but a recapitulation of ancient views. In summarizing his predecessors, he distinguishes two varieties of epilepsy: one accompanied by convulsions, the other marked by sleep.[181] At the same time he differentiates three pathological forms of the disease according to its point of origin: the brain, where the whole nervous system suffers from a melancholy humor and cold phlegm,[182] the stomach,[183] and any lower part.[184]

We may use this summary by Cassius Felix as a starting point from which to discuss the changes, both conceptual and terminological, effected soon afterward. The two varieties of the disease (convulsions or sleep) were given a new interpretation. The influence of the demoniac beliefs prevailing among the people and voiced by theological writers made one form of the disease represent natural epilepsy, while the other form constituted what was called demoniac possession,[185] although the texts are not very clear about the distinctive features of these two varieties.[186] The medical writers of the period took into account the demonistic concept of epilepsy, but they were careful to emphasize its popular character and not to identify themselves with it.[187] Their attitude was somewhat similar to that of the Hippocratics, who had talked about the "so-called sacred disease."

---

[180] Cf. Rose (870), p. 268, No. 207 and p. 231, No. 54.

[181] Cassius Felix (207), De medicina, c. 71; p. 168, 17-19: "et sunt distantiae passionis duae. aliquando enim sub diverso raptu membrorum efficitur, aliquando cum somno."

[182] Cassius Felix, l.c., p. 169, 1-3: "in his cerebrum patitur et omnis nervositas a cerebro descendens sub melancholico humore et frigido flegmate." Marcellus (666), De medicamentis, I, 6; p. 27, 2 ff., alludes to a similar concept when he advises evacuating the humor from the head through nose or mouth.

[183] L.c., p. 169, 3-4: "aliquando a stomacho patiuntur."

[184] Ibid., p. 169, 8-10: "etiam et vapor quidam in eis ab inferiore ventris parte super fertur, quo vapore mininga pulsata concutitur, et cadunt." It is interesting that Cassius Felix believes the vapor to affect the meninges. He seems to be combining Galenic and methodist views.

[185] Cf. above, p. 89.

[186] Esculapius (328), p. v: "Epilepticorum genera sunt duo. Unum genus cum tremore et somno: vel stertunt. Aliud genus sine tremore, et sine somno. Qui cum spasmo sunt, hoc est, tremore, non curantur: qui sine tremore sunt, curantur . . . qui cum tremore totius corporis, daemonem dicuntur (sic!) apprehendere." Gariopontus (399), Passionarius Galeni, fol. 3^v, on the other hand, describes the second variety as follows: "Aliud in quo spumant et stertunt: nec contrahunt membra cum ceciderunt: quos vulgus (sic!) demoniacos dicit." Cf. also Glossae medicinales (416), pp. 32-33.

[187] Cf. preceding footnote. Cf. also the Reichenauer Antidotarium published by Sigerist (927), p. 46, where the following effect is ascribed to the Antidotum gera: "Non facit augustiam neque festinationes aliquas et sanum reddit corpus et ad claritatem perducit, epilemticis et ad cadentes subito et ad contractionem patientes et linguam suam masticantes et salibam mittentes et de aliquo modo tenentes, hos uulgus demoniacos uocant." And Petrocellus (840), vol. 4, p. 288, writes: "Ad epilempsiam quae sic grece dicitur, Latini autem vulgo demoniacos vocant."

Another terminological change concerned the three pathological forms distinguished by Galen and his successors, which were now given separate names. Epilepsy as a general term connoted the disease as such, and in a restricted sense it also signified the idiopathic form located in the head. The form originating in the stomach was distinguished as "analepsy." The form arising from any other member of the body was now called "catalepsy." The new terminology is of Greek provenience, though apparently of Latin usage. St. Luke 9:51 speaks of Jesus' ascension, *analēpsis*, and the Greek term (not necessarily taken from the Gospel) now alludes to the vapors ascending from the stomach to the brain.[188] "Catalepsy," on the other hand, in ancient writings represented either the clinical picture which still carries this name or, more often, a disease with fever and pronounced mental disturbances.[189] In a medical catechism by Caelius Aurelianus the differences between catalepsy and epilepsy were clearly stated. Fever, it was said, is characteristic of catalepsy but absent in epilepsy, whereas the latter shows frothing from mouth and nose, a sign not to be found in catalepsy.[190] Even when catalepsy became a subdivision of epilepsy this difference was still retained for some time.[191] But in the later part of the Middle Ages it was forgotten. By then the Galenic theory had acquired fundamental importance and a terminological distinction of the three types must have been very convenient. Only at the time of the Renaissance when, under the influence of humanistic learning, medical terminology was purged, did these names disappear from the literature.

The inclusion of catalepsy among the types of epilepsy is one instance of nosological confusion. Another example is given by the fact that epilepsy and frenzy were thrown together. In the *Practica Petrocelli*, a pre-Salternitan medieval work of uncertain date, fever appears as

---

[188]Contemporary interpretations differed. Esculapius (328), p. 4, explained: "Analepsia dicta est, eo quod scissa, una parte capitis sensum praebet." A similar explanation was given in the *Glossae medicinales* (416), p. 7, 9-10, where, according to Heiberg's emendation, the passage reads: "analemsia autem dicta est eo, quod sanas partes capitis sensu privet." As a synonym for epilepsy, analempsia occurs in glossaries of the tenth and eleventh centuries; cf. *Corpus Gloss. Lat.* (238), vol. 3, pp. 510, 5 and 488, 76. Some early medieval texts give *anathemia* which, according to Heiberg (416), p. 7, footnote 6, is derived from ἀναθυμία, as a synonym for *analemsia*, and explain it by "ex anatemia stomaçi," i.e., "through an exhalation from the stomach"; cf. *ibid.*, p. 7, 6. I believe this to be the correct explanation.

[189]Cf. Baumann (90).

[190]Caelius Aurelianus, *De significatione diaeticarum passionum*, 57, in Rose (870), p. 231: "Quomodo discernis a catalepticis epilepticos? primo ex febre, quam necesse est esse in catalepticis. dehinc ex spumarum eruptione, quam necesse est esse in epilepticis per os atque nares, quod a catalepticis supra dicta vice alienum est ut ab epilepticis febris."

[191]Esculapius (328), p. 4: "Catalepsia passio est epilepticorum, cum uno signo epilepticorum, et febre. Quoniam epilepticis febris non est, sed spumas per os et per nares digerunt. Cataleptici vero non spumant, sed passio ipsorum a pedibus et tibiis inchoat," etc. It is, of course, quite possible that in making catalepsy a form of epilepsy, one of the original meanings of the word *catalepsis* (i.e., "grip") rather than the name of a disease has been used.

the only distinctive sign between epilepsy and phrenesis.[192] In the ancient texts this latter condition had never been put in the same category as epilepsy. Now the classification of the various nervous disturbances tended to become loose. This was the medical counterpart of the vague popular conception of the falling evil.

## 2. SCHOLASTICISM

A new period in the history of medieval medicine was initiated by two factors: the translation into Latin of many important classical and Arabic texts, and the organization of medical studies at medical schools and universities. Thus, from the end of the eleventh century on, the science of medicine entered upon a new phase, commonly called scholastic.

In the East, scholastic medicine had developed at a much earlier date. By about 500 A.D. medical studies were well organized at Alexandria. Hippocrates and Galen had become the leading authorities and had acquired the same importance in medicine as Plato and Aristotle in philosophy. The work of the Alexandrian teachers consisted above all in the interpretation of classical medical writings from the Galenic point of view, and it resulted in a firmly established system of Galenic medicine. The influence of Alexandria spread further east, and the Syrian and Arabic physicians acquired ancient medicine in its late, scholastic form. They cultivated this tradition, developed it considerably, and passed it on to the Western scholars. Until the end of the fifteenth century the Galenic doctrine was not seriously challenged, although modified in many details.

In our review of scholastic theories of epilepsy we shall not try to establish a chronological development. Limiting ourselves to those Arabic works which became known in the Occident through Latin translations, we shall not even separate the contribution of the Arabs from that of the Western doctors. By this procedure we shall avoid numerous repetitions and shall be able to present a somewhat clearer panorama of abstruse medical thought.

Partly from the older tradition, partly from observations of their own, the scholastic doctors were acquainted with the generalized convulsive epileptic attack as well as some of the other forms. Although not many observations of these other forms were recorded during the Middle Ages, they are not altogether missing. Bernard of Gordon, for

---

[192]De Renzi (840), vol. 4, p. 235: "Epilempticorum et alienatorum mentibus naribus iniecta anagalla que habet florem roseum, melle mixto, salutem restituit. Debes item noscere quia hec passio unam valitudinem habet, sed differt, quoniam epilempsia sine febre fit; alienatio, id est frenesis cum febre fit. Item hec passio cum frigdor contraxerit miringas, et pre habundantia humorum spiritus meatum facilem non habent, tunc demum mens errorem gignit."

instance, makes the following interesting statement: "And I have often seen that the attack was so short that the only thing necessary for the patient was to lean against a wall or something similar and to rub his face—and it ceased. Sometimes, however, he did not have to lean; he was seized by a confusion in the head and darkness in the eyes, and feeling it beforehand, he said an Ave Maria, and before he had finished the paroxysm had passed. He spat out once, and it was all over, but it came frequently during the day. There are some people who, after the paroxysm, have absolutely no memory of their falling down or of their affliction, while there are others who remember and feel ashamed."[193]

On the other hand, the scholastic physicians had taken over the Galenic distinction of the three types of epilepsy to which the early Middle Ages had applied such convenient terms: epilepsy, analepsy, catalepsy, according to the different anatomical origin of the attacks. But apart from this clearly recognized principle of localization,[194] the classification also involved two other aspects: viz., a consideration of the various forms of epileptic aura and a theory of the mechanism of epilepsy.

Galen had paid special attention to the gastric aura and to that particular form where a cold breeze seemed to ascend from an extremity to the head. The latter case had served him as an example for the origin of epilepsy from any part of the body. Paulus of Aegina, moreover, had mentioned epilepsy from the pregnant uterus, i.e., eclampsia,[195] and the authority of Paulus caused the Arabic, and then the Western, physicians to pay attention to this phenomenon.[196] It can be traced in all the leading textbooks of the period and was also carried over into modern medical literature.[197] The medieval physicians went further in this direction and discussed all possible organs of the body. But there was not always a "cold breeze" ascending from such organs.

---

[193] Bernard of Gordon (106), *Lilium medicinae*, fol. 117[V]: "Et vidi frequenter quod erat ita brevis, quod non oportebat, nisi quod appodiaret se ad parietem vel ad aliquod tale, et quod fricaret faciem et cessabat. Aliquando autem non indigebat appodiatione, sed veniebat sibi perturbatio in capite et caligo in oculis, et ipse praesentiens dicebat Ave maria, et antequam complevisset, transiverat paroxismus, et expuebat semel, et totum transibat, et veniebat frequenter in die. Et aliqui sunt, qui post paroxismum penitus non recordantur de casu, nec de afflictione, et aliqui sunt qui recordantur et verecundantur." Cf. Lennox (628), p. 381 f., who diagnoses this case as "a short psychic seizure."

[194] Antonius Guainerius (438), *Tract. de egritud. cap.*, fol. 11[V]: "Sed ratione loci triplicem denominationem recipit. Nam cum per causam propriam in cerebro existentem causatur: dicitur epilepsia: et si a stomacho analepsia: ab aliis vero membris catalepsia."

[195] Cf. above, p. 32.

[196] Serapion (915), *Practica*, fol. 8[r]: "Paulus vero degenti dixit se vidisse hanc aegritudinem accidisse ex matrice: et illud fuit in muliere pregnante: et postquam ipsa peperit quievit egritudo."

[197] Cf. Alĭ Ibn Abbās (22), *Theorica*, IX, 6; fol. 103[V]; Constantinus Africanus (235), *De communibus medico* etc., vol. 2, p. 248; Avicenna (71), *Canon*, lib. III, fen 1, tract. 5, c. 8; p. 486; Arnald of Villanova (58), *De epilepsia*, c. 18; col. 1622; Fernelius (351), *Pathologia*, VI, 16; p. 232.

Probably for this reason some writers reserved the term "catalepsy" for attacks originating in the more remote limbs,[198] whereas the majority included in this category attacks originating in all parts other than the stomach. More important, however, than proper classification was the question of how to diagnose the seat of the original lesion. Even physicians of the sixteenth century, famous for their keen observations, recorded symptoms indicating liver, spleen, kidneys, etc., as starting points of the disease. Petrus Forestus (1522-97) remarked that in epilepsy from the liver, pain in the right side would precede the attack, and signs of an affected liver would be present. If the affliction arose from the spleen, the patient would feel pain in the left side; if from the intestines, the pain would be located in that region, and the patient would pass more feces during the paroxysm; if from another part, e.g., fingers or toes, the patient would feel a vapor ascend.[199] This diagnosis, in as much as it was not purely imaginary, rested mainly on various premonitory signs. Accordingly, many authors claimed that premonition of the oncoming attack was restricted to those forms which affected the brain only indirectly.[200]

In setting down the three varieties of epilepsy, Galen had also distinguished between different mechanisms. Idiopathic epilepsy was caused by obstruction of the ventricles of the brain and of the roots of the nerves by cold and viscous humors. The roots of the nerves tried to shake off this obnoxious mass, which caused them to widen and shorten and thus to pull at the nerves. In contrast, epilepsy from a distal part was caused by the irritating effect of an ascending pneumatic substance or a qualitative change. Here, as the analogy with poisoning by a scorpion or a spider suggested, the noxious matter was negligibly small. In between there stood the sympathetic affection of the brain from the stomach.[201]

For the scholastic physician, there remained considerable room for speculation. Sometimes the problem was barely stated, the various classifications being placed side by side as had been usual in early medieval books. The Salernitan physician, Platearius, for instance, mentioned the three Galenic types as well as two clinical varieties, which he distinguished as "major" and "minor" epilepsy. The passage in

---

[198] Arnald of Villanova (58), *De epilepsia*, c. 1; col. 1602: "distinguitur etenim, cum arcem corporis id est caput vix noxiae materiae origo obsidet, epilepticam procreat valetudinem: cum vero viscera, intestina, generationis membra earumque delatoria pervaserit, ad analepticam vertitur aegritudinem: cumque illa membra morbida in artubus originatur remotis, catalepsia nuncupatur."

[199] Cf. Petrus Forestus (369), *Observationum* etc. lib. X, observ. 56; p. 385. Actually he but echoes what Bernard of Gordon had said long ago; see Lennox (632), p. 17 f.

[200] E.g., Geraldus de Solo (407), *Expositio*, fol. 29ᵛ-30ʳ: "... quando venit a cerebro non praesentitur paroxismus."

[201] Cf. above, II-2c.

which he described and explained this latter distinction is worth quoting, since it is reminiscent of the later distinction between "grand mal" and "petit mal," and because the explanation given is comparatively simple. "Major epilepsy," says Platearius, "is a complete obstruction of the principal ventricles of the brain. People suffering from it fall down quickly. The mouth and face are distorted, and there is also a trembling movement of the neck and of the whole body and clenching of the teeth. Sometimes they pass urine, feces, and seed involuntarily; they snore and froth and, when the froth has been wiped off, they froth again. Minor epilepsy is an incomplete obstruction of the ventricles of the brain. People suffering from it sometimes fall down; sometimes they do not fall down, but faint. The froth, once having been wiped off, does not reappear, and they are quickly relieved."[202]

These two species of "major" and "minor" epilepsy, satisfactory from a clinical point of view, were accepted by various physicians, though they were not always so clearly defined as by Platearius. But the pathological explanation did not fit well into the Galenic scheme. Another division, into "true" and "spurious" epilepsy, was more adequate in this respect. "True" epilepsy was usually identified with the "idiopathic" epilepsy of the Galenic nomenclature, i.e., with "epilepsy" in the restricted sense of the medieval doctors, whereas "spurious" epilepsy was believed to originate from any of the other parts of the body.[203] Apart from this anatomical difference, one also looked for different humors. Arnald of Villanova said that true epilepsy was engendered by phlegm, spurious epilepsy by black bile mixed with phlegm.[204] Gilbertus Anglicus believed true epilepsy to arise from phlegm, spurious epilepsy from the other humors.[205] Or it was possible to differentiate between material obstruction and the irritating effect of a "quality." According to this view, true epilepsy was caused by the amount of the material congesting the ventricles, while in spurious epilepsy the amount of humor might be negligible and a "quality" be

---

[202] Platearius (915), *Practica brevis*, fol. 172$^r$: "Maior epilepsia est oppilatio principalium ventriculorum cerebri ex toto: hac laborantes cito cadunt: os obtorquitur et facies: cum tremore cervicis et totius corporis: et dentium constrictione: quandoque urinam egestionem sperma involuntarie emittunt: stertunt et spumant: spuma abstersa iterum spumant. Minor epilepsia est oppilatio ventriculorum cerebri: sed non ex toto. hac laborantes quandoque cadunt: quandoque non cadunt: sed scotomiam patiuntur. Spuma semel abstersa non iterum subvenit: et isti cito relevantur." Cf. also De Renzi (840), vol. 2, p. 111.

[203] Cf. below, footnote 205.

[204] Arnald of Villanova (58), *Breviarium*, I, 22, col. 1071: "Epilepsia alia vera, quae fit ex phlegmate: non vera fit ex melancholia mista cum phlegmate."

[205] Gilbertus Anglicus (412), *Compendium medicinae*, fol. 109$^r$: "Distinguitur autem epilempsia. quia alia vera alia non vera. vera fit ex flegmate. notha fit ex melancolia vel sanguine. rarissime ex colera naturali. aliquando ex his mixtis." *Ibid.*, fol. 109$^v$: "si igitur fit ex flegmate et vicio ipsius cerebri dicitur epilempsia vera. si vero fiat ex aliis humoribus vel vicio inferiorum partium dicitur notha."

the chief agent, e.g., if the surrounding air or the humor were cold.[206] Along a similar line of reasoning, Avicenna assumed that an epileptic attack would occur without perceptible convulsion if some fine substance abounded in the nervous system and acted without much badness of quality.[207]

But all this was not enough. John of Gaddesden established three forms: minor, medium, and major epilepsy, to which he assigned the paradoxical synonyms: true, truer, and truest. According to this terminology, minor epilepsy occurred through an obstruction of the arteries (i.e., when the passages from the heart to the brain were blocked), medium epilepsy through obstruction of the nerves, and "major" or "truest" epilepsy because of an obstruction of the ventricles of the brain.[208] The reference to an obstruction of the nerves is understandable, since the Arabs had paid particular attention to it. They had sometimes differentiated between epilepsy caused by a spasm of the nerves and epilepsy from the brain, so that the former almost appeared as a separate species.[209] Following Galen, they had explained its mechanism on the basis of an influx of materia peccans into the origin of the nerves,[210] shortening their length but broadening their latitude and thus leading to convulsions.[211]

"Analepsy," the form that arose from the stomach, also needed more detailed explanation. Here Galen himself had been unclear. He had

<hr>

[206]Ioannes Anglicus (535), *Rosa anglica*, p. 40: "Dico Epilepsiam duplicem esse, veram, et non veram sicut et Apoplexiam. Vera Epilepsia est quae fit ex oppilatione non integra ventriculorum non principalium cerebri. Non vera est quae fit ex eorum constrictione vel retractione virtutis cerebri fugiendo quasi nocivum. Prima non fit sine materia oppilante; verum non a quacunque, sed cito veniente et cito recedente. Secunda potest fieri a sola frigiditate constringente, non ex frigiditate complexionali cerebri: quia tunc esset inseparabilis; aut difficulter separabilis. . . . Fit igitur a frigiditate exteriori ipsius aëris, vel a frigiditate humoris, qui humor plus laedit sua frigiditate, quam sua quantitàte. . . ."

[207]Avicenna (71), *Canon*, lib. III, fen 1, tract. 5, c. 8; p. 486: "Et multoties fit epilepsia sine spasmo sensato: et illud ideo, quoniam materia faciens ipsam, est subtilis, et operatur cum repletione, non cum malitia vehementi."

[208]Ioannes Anglicus, *l.c.*, p. 36: "Iuxta quod notandum, Epilepsiam triplicem esse: scilicet veram, veriorem, verissimam: vel minorem, mediam, maiorem. Prima fit propter oppilationem arteriarum, et est minor. Secunda propter oppilationem nervorum, et est media: tertia propter oppilationem ventriculorum cerebri non principalium, et est maior." Cf. also the English translation published by Lennox (629).

[209]Abī Ibn Abbās (22), *Theorica*, IX, 6; fol. 103ᵛ: "Et epilepsia alia ex cerebro fit: alia ex nervorum spasmo." Cf. also Constantinus Africanus (235), *De communibus medico* etc., IX, 7; vol. 2, p. 247 f.

[210]Since according to Constantinus of Africa, *l.c.*, p. 248, the nerves receive the materia peccans from the brain, the pathological basis of the differentiation between epilepsy from the brain and epilepsy from the nerves remains obscure.

[211]Avicenna, *l.c.*, p. 485: ". . . et eorum [i.e., of the nerves] repletio ex humore expulso ad ipsos in principio ipsorum facit, ut augmentetur eorum latitudo, et abbrevietur eorum longitudo." Bernard of Gordon (106), *Lilium medicinae*, fol. 117: "tunc illa materia profundatur in nervo et nervus distenditur secundum latum et curtatur secundum longum. . . . Curtantur enim nervi et contrahuntur versus originem ut melius possint expellere nociva secundum quod dicit Avicenna."

mentioned exhalations from ichors filling the stomachs of persons who suffered from an abundance of yellow bile. But he had qualified neither the nature of these ichors nor the action of the exhalations. Again, he had suggested that weakness of the cardia through its close association with the nervous system could lead to epilepsy, apparently without the ascent of vapors.[212] Late Greek commentators had tried to establish a more definite theory. "For epilepsy," said one of them, "also arises from yellow bile . . . when the stomach is stung and the nerves and their origin agitated."[213] But there existed no unity among medieval authors. Some attributed the disease to phlegm in the cardia.[214] Others, while not specific about the humor, emphasized that the materia peccans was not located in the cavity of the stomach but in its veins, arteries, and nerves and that through them a bubbling substance was carried to the brain.[215] In the sixteenth century such a view was opposed by Cardanus.[216] He said that neither a vapor nor any material ascended from the stomach. Rather, he thought that the same nerve as conveyed the feeling of hunger and thirst contracted and by contamination caused the brain to contract too.[217]

All this shows that there existed considerable divergence of opinion concerning the kind of humors involved in the various forms of epilepsy, as well as their mode of action and their relation to the vapors. Most medieval physicians agreed, however, that in one way or another any one of the humors might be a cause of epileptic attacks. Moreover, it was believed possible to ascertain the humor involved. The diagnosis was based on rather imaginary signs. If, for example, the patient had much viscous and frothy saliva, this would point to phlegm. If his whole behavior were that of a madman (melancholic in the terms of ancient psychiatry), a melancholic humor would lie at the root of the evil.[218] Or the inspection of the urine on the day which preceded or followed the attack might give the answer.[219]

---

[212] See above, p. 63.

[213] Theophilus (278), *In Hippocratis aphor. comment.*, vol. 2, p. 380: γίνεται γὰρ καὶ ἀπὸ ξανθῆς χολῆς ἐπιληψία, καθὼς καὶ ἐν τῇ διαγνωστικῇ εἴρηται, δακνομένου τοῦ στομάχου καὶ κραδαινομένων τῶν νεύρων καὶ τῆς ἀρχῆς αὐτῶν.

[214] Constantinus Africanus (235), *De communibus* etc., VI, 19; vol. 2, p. 160: "Epilepsia quoque ex humoribus nascitur phlegmaticis quae in ore sunt stomachi."

[215] De Renzi (840), vol. 2, p. 111: "Analempsia fit ex materia existente in stomacho non in concavitate ut quidam dicunt sed in venis, arteriis et nervis ipsius stomachi, per quorum medietatem materia ebulliens rapitur ad cerebrum."

[216] His authorship is, however, questionable; cf. below, V-1c, footnote 35.

[217] Cardanus (201), *De epilepsia*, lect. 9; vol. 10, p. 400: "Et cadit homo in morbum comitialem, non quod ab ore ventriculi elevetur vapor, aut materia aliqua, minime (ut ego existimo), sed quoniam nervus ille contrahitur; contracto nervo per coinquinationem, contrahitur etiam cerebrum: et sic morbus comitialis evenit."

[218] Cf. Avicenna, *l.c.*, cap. 9; p. 489.

[219] Gilbertus Anglicus (412), *Compendium medicinae*, fol. 110ᵛ: "Si urina erit grossa erit de flegmate. si citrina et parum livida: de colera rubra. si alba et tenuis vel nigra: de melancolia."

Opinions were divided over the question whether the humors acted directly or indirectly. This question arose on account of certain difficulties in explaining the differences between epilepsy and apoplexy and over the conflicting views of Galen and Aristotle.

Most medieval authors agreed that epilepsy and apoplexy were closely related, apoplexy being the more powerful affliction of the two.[220] Hence, some of them either called epilepsy a "little apoplexy"[221] or, vice versa, apoplexy a "powerful epilepsy,"[222] and a German writer, Konrad von Megenberg, conforming to the popular view, went so far as to establish two kinds of the falling evil, "of which one is called apoplexy, the other epilepsy."[223] The main difference was seen in the fact that in apoplexy the patient neither felt nor moved, whereas during the epileptic attack he at least moved.[224] To explain the differences, many physicians assumed that in apoplexy all ventricles of the brain were obstructed; in epilepsy the principal ventricles only[225] or, at any rate, but a few.[226] Which exactly these "principal" ventricles were was not always made clear. Galen had located epilepsy in the third and fourth ventricles, whereas Avicenna assigned the anterior ventricle to it, since the attack affected the sense of sight and hearing and the muscles of the face first.[227] The main question, however, was what caused this obstruction. According to Galen, the answer was: a thick

---

quae sequente die casus vel precedente poterunt experiri." Gualterius Agilon (12), *Summa medicinalis*, p. 108, formulated the following rule: "Regula: urina alba in colore, tenuis in substantia, cum circulo plumbei coloris sive lividi epilentiam de melancolia naturali significat."

[220]Constantinus Africanus (235), *Liber aureus*, c. 4; vol. 1, p. 170: "De epilepsia et apoplexia. Hae duae passiones non differunt, nisi quia apoplexia est fortior. Causa vero earum una et eadem est. . . ." According to Sudhoff (976), p. 177, the *Liber aureus* was edited by Johannes Afflacius.

[221]Gilbertus Anglicus (412), *Compendium medicinae*, fol. 109$^r$: "ideo a quibusdam apoplexia parva vocatur."

[222]Antonius Guainerius (438), *Tract. de egritud. cap.*, VII, 2; fol. 11$^V$: " . . . ideo nonnulli apoplexiam epilepsiam fortem vocant. Nam epilepticos quosdam mori vidi: quos ultimus paroxismus fuit apoplexie."

[223]Cf. above, p. 101 f.

[224]Gilbertus Anglicus, *l.c.*, fol. 109$^r$: "Differt autem [i.e., epilepsy] ab appoplexia: quia appoplexia omnes ventriculos replet et sensum et motum privat. Differt autem epilempsia ab epialte: quia epialtes quodam modo est ei contraria: in ea enim privatur motus et non sensus. Item differt a scothomia quia scothomia est diminutio spiritus visibilis. unde a quibusdam epilempsia momentanea vocatur." According to some medieval authorities, however, the epileptic not only moves but also feels. Cf. Alī Ibn Abbās (22), *Theorica*, IX, 6; fol. 103$^V$, and Constantinus Africanus (235), *De communibus medico* etc., IX, 7; vol. 2, p. 247: "Unde fit ut infirmus in epilepsia sentiat, et se moveat."

[225]De Renzi (840), vol. 2, p. 110: "Apoplexia est opilatio omnium ventriculorum cerebri cum privatione vel diminutione sensus et motus. Epilempsia est opilatio principalium ventriculorum cerebri cum diminutione sensus et motus. . . ."

[226]Alī Ibn Abbās, *l.c.*, fol. 103$^V$; Constantinus Africanus (235), *De communibus medico* etc., IX, 7; vol. 2, p. 247: "Causa enim quae epilepsiam facit, non est in omnibus cerebri ventriculis. Sed quidam oppilantur ventriculorum, et viae nervorum membra corporis moventium."

[227]Avicenna (71), *Canon*, lib. III, fen 1, tract. 5, c. 8; p. 486: "principium epilepsiae propinquum ex cerebro est; scilicet aut ex ventriculo eius anteriore, aut ex ventriculis aliis cum

and cold humor, i.e., phlegm or black bile. This opinion found
followers throughout the Middle Ages,[228] and it seemed indeed to be
supported by anatomical observations. The Arabs were acquainted with
the Hippocratic book, *On the Sacred Disease*, of which Rhazes had
given a résumé in the *Continens*. He had mentioned that, according to
Hippocrates, the brain of epileptic goats, sheep, and rams was full of
water having a fetid smell.[229] Avicenna had reported the same statement,[230] which had also found its way into the textbooks of Latin
writers.[231] The example proved stimulating. Valescus de Tharanta, a
surgeon of Montpellier (c. 1380), claimed to have dissected a sparrow
which had died of epilepsy and to have found moisture similar to what
Hippocrates had discovered in epileptic sheep.[232]

This view, supported by the authority of Hippocrates and Galen,
was, however, contradicted by the authority of Aristotle, who had
attributed epileptic seizures to evaporations from food.[233] Such a statement by the leading scientific authority was bound to carry considerable weight. The Galenic theory was contrasted with the Aristotelian
explanation,[234] which had, indeed, many points in its favor. Averroës
carried the vaporal explanation of epilepsy to its extreme. The chief
argument against the direct action of the humors was the failure to

---

eo: quoniam primum nocumentum quo impedit, contingit in sensu visus et auditus, et in
motibus lacertorum faciei, et palpebrarum: quamvis reliqui sensus, et membra mobilia in
nocumento communicent."

[228] E.g., Ibn Zuhr (529), *Theisir*, lib. I, tract. 9, c. 7; fol. 9ᵛ: "Epilepsia quidem tunc
efficitur quando humor grossus diffunditur et spargitur in cannalibus et meatibus cerebri, et
humor grossus esse non potest: nisi sit flegma aut melancolia. et quando praedictus humor
oppilat cannales seu meatus cerebri: tunc contrahitur cerebrum ut expellat a se nocumentum et
inde sequitur contractio totius corporis," etc.

[229] Rhazes (843), *Continens*, fol. 12ᵛ: "Et dixit Hypo[cras] in libro quem fecit de morbo
dei. quod hic morbus accidit ex humiditate malefaciente cerebrum: et manifestatur per
pecudes: quia cum accidit eis hic morbus si aperitur eorum cerebrum inveniretur plenum
humiditate." *Ibid.*: "Dixit Hypo[cras] in libro suo de epilepsia . . . Et dixit quod multotiens
accidit hic morbus capris: vel ovibus: et arietibus: et si videretur cerebrum eorum tempore
huius morbi: inveniretur plenum aqua fetidi odoris."

[230] Avicenna, *l.c.*, p. 485: "Et Hippoc. quidem dixit quod plurimae oves patiuntur epilepsiam: quumque in cerebris suis anatomizantur, invenitur in eis humiditas mala foetida."

[231] Gilbertus Anglicus (412), *Compendium medicinae*, fol. 109ᵛ: "unde ypo[cras] Oves
quae patiuntur epilepsiam cum a cerebris suis anathomizantur: invenitur in his humiditas mala
salsa fetida. et illa est ex mala digestione in cerebro."

[232] Valescus de Tharanta (1039), *Philonium*, I, 18; fol. 16ʳ: "Nam cum Hip. anathomizaret
oves epilepticas: inveniebat in cerebro earum humiditatem multam fetidam. Et ego
anathomizavi strutionem mortuum ex epilepsia: et inveni similem humidi." On the sparrow cf.
below, V-4b.

[233] Cf. above, II-2a.

[234] Serapion (915), *Practica*, fol. 8ʳ: "Generatur autem hec egritudo secundum intentionem
Galeni ex humore qui oppilat meatus ventriculorum cerebri. Humor vero iste grossus secundum
plurimum est viscosus flegmaticus: et fortasse est in modico declivis ad choleram nigram: et
secundum sententiam Aristotelis non generatur nisi ex ventositate grossa que oppilat meatus
ventriculorum cerebri: et prohibet ipsam subtilitatem penetrare et dare membris motum.
propter illud ergo epilepsia accidit subito et quiescit subito. Quod est: quia ventositas est velocis
motus."

explain the relatively quick ending of the attack. Viscous humors could not be dispelled suddenly; therefore, it was necessary to look for another agent. This other agent had been suggested by Galen himself in the case of epilepsy from the leg accompanied by a "cold fume" (as the Latin Averroës termed it). A fume might easily be dispersed, and therefore the assumption seemed justified that all forms of epilepsy were caused by fumes generated either in the brain itself or in some other organ.[235]

This theory made possible greater uniformity in the pathology of the various forms of epilepsy, an advantage which could be preserved even if one did not go quite as far as Averroës and abandoned the theory of an obstruction by humors altogether. The alleged anatomical observation of a fluid in the brain of epileptics could, for example, be explained in the following way: When the vapors reached the brain they were condensed and were subsequently precipitated, thus obstructing and hindering the passage of the animal spirits. The bad smell of this fluid was ascribed to the poisonous, horrible, and fetid character of the substance of which the vapors were constituted.[236]

Apart from a more uniform pathology and the possibility of understanding the quick end of the epileptic fit as contrasted with the paralysis remaining from the apoplectic stroke, the "vapor" theory had another advantage. Medieval physicians were aware of the equivocal use of the term "epilepsy," which sometimes connoted a symptom, sometimes a disease.[237] The theory of vapors helped to explain the relation of the chronic disease and its periodic attacks. Averroës had not excluded the humors entirely from the pathogenesis of epilepsy. Although they did not cause the attack directly, they were the material from which the vapors arose. Consequently, in the cure of the disease it was necessary to evacuate the noxious humors, which were either cold and

---

[235] Averroës (64), *Colliget*, III, c. 41; fol. 66[r]: "Et ob hoc dicendum est quod hec egritudo non fit nisi propter fumum qui generatur in ipsomet cerebro vel in alio membro: quod ipsum ei transmittit: sicut dicit Galenus de iuvene qui sentiebat quod quasi quidam fumus frigidus ascenderet ab uno membro ad cerebrum: et quando perveniebat illuc cadebat epilepticus."

[236] Bernard of Gordon (106), *Lilium medicinae*, fol. 122[v], says of the vapors: "possunt ascendere ad cerebrum, et potissime illi ex quibus fit epilepsia, cum sint venenosi, horribiles et foetidi, sicut patet in animalibus patientibus morbum caducum, cum anatomizantur, in quibus invenitur aquositas horribilis foetida, et quia talia petunt membra nobilia, ideo si iret ad cor causaret sincopim, et si ad cerebrum, epilepsiam, potissime quia evaporati in cerebro condensantur, et postea condensati, cadunt inferius et ita opilant, et impediunt transitum, spirituum," etc.

[237] E.g., Jacobus Foroliviensis (370), *Quaestionum*, particula II, qu. 59; fol. 158[r]: "Quarta difficultas. An epilepsia debeat dici accidens vel aegritudo et cetera. . . . Ad quartam potest dici, quod isto termino epilepsia auctores utuntur multum equivoce. Quandoque enim accipiunt pro illo contractivo motu, ita quod epilepsia supponat pro illo motu, et appellet impedimentum in sensu et motu voluntario, et sic est accidens virtutis motivae, ut patet. Quandoque sumitur pro illa privatione sensus et motus voluntarii vel impedimento, et connotat contractionem aliquam in aliquo tempore sui, et sic iterum est accidens. Quandoque autem sumitur pro illa contractione substantie cerebri, et ventriculorum eius ad expellendum et cetera. et sic est aegritudo

moist or cold and dry.[238] John of Gaddesden used this idea in the following way: The falling evil, he said, comprised the disease in itself and its manifestation, the paroxysm. The disease itself was due to a thick material; it was of long duration and represented a weakness, not a convulsion. But the paroxysm came on quickly and passed off quickly, since it was caused by vapors, which were thin compared with the material from which they arose. These vapors settled in the peripheral pores of the nerves and made them dilate. They did not occupy the central pores of the nerves and did not extend them; therefore, the paroxysm was not followed by paralysis.[239]

This does not exhaust the great variety of speculations about the relative significance of humors, vapors, and qualities. The individual authors were not even always consistent in their opinions, thus giving an opportunity for further argument and qualification. But in contrast to the confusing complexity of details, there also existed attempts at presenting a simple outline of the etiology of epilepsy. By distinguishing a few general causes, this goal could apparently be reached. As an example we choose Michele Savonarola (early fifteenth century), who in common with many scholastic physicians numbered three main causes: primitive, antecedent, and conjoint.

The primitive causes are identical with external causes, such as air, whereas the other two represent the internal causes.[240] Of these the antecedent causes precede the outbreak of the disease. Savonarola

---

saltem in receptaculo. potest etiam dici accidens, quia motus malus, et sic potissime describitur ab auctoribus." This scholastic discussion continued down into the Renaissance. Untzer (1038), *Hieronosologia*, pp. 12-13, for instance, wrote in 1616: "Controversia hic non levis exoritur, cui affectuum praeter naturam generi proprie Epilepsia sit accensenda. Sunt enim nonnulli, qui in Morborum classem, alii vero qui in symptomatum numerum illam collocandam censent." It was also realized in the Middle Ages that epilepsy might either appear alone or combined with other diseases. Matthaeus Ferrarius (352), *Practica*, fol. 44[r]: "Ultima distinctio: quedam talis complicatur cum aliis morbis vel totius: ut febribus: vel particularium membrorum: et quedam non: patet." It is, therefore, not surprising to find medieval authors describing two classes of epilepsy in children: one from bad diet, the other in acute fevers. Cornelis Roelans von Mechelen (859), *Liber de aegritudinibus infantium*, 10; fol. 100[r]: " . . . et est duplex una que provenit eis ex humiditatibus eorum malis maxime per indigestionem genitis aut quia malum sugunt lac et maxime si nutrix epilentica fuerit et evenit nulla presente febre. Alia est que accidit eis in febribus eorum acutis."

[238] Averroës (64), *Colliget*, III, 41; fol. 66[r]: "Et hoc accidens [i.e., quick end of attack] est sufficiens ad probandum quod causa huius egritudinis est ventositas fumosa sed ista ventositas necessario communicat humoribus frigidis et humidis: aut frigidis et siccis: et isti humores sunt isti vento ut materia. Et propterea curatur haec egritudo evacuando illos humores."

[239] Ioannes Anglicus (535), *Rosa anglica*, p. 37: "ideo dico, quod in morbo caduco duo sunt scilicet: morbus in se, et paroxysmus. Morbus in se est de materia crassa, et est longus, quia omnis morbus de materia frigida difficulter digeritur. . . . et ideo morbus in se materialis non est spasmus, sed mollicies . . . sed morbus formalis et paroxysmus eius cito venit, et cito recedit: et ideo est de ventositate, quae crassa est in se; subtilis tamen respectu materiae a qua elevatur; et est spasmus, quia ibi ventositas est in poris circumferentialibus non centralibus ipsius nervi, sicut est in paralysi; et ideo nervi extenduntur in latum et spasmus fit: et non extenduntur in longum: et ideo non fit paralysis ex paroxysmo."

[240] Cf. e.g., Quercetanus (833), *Tetras*, p. 18: "Causas tam gravis et horrendi affectus medici dividunt in externas seu primitivas: et internas, nempe antecedentes et conjunctas."

divides them into "complexional," where the whole body or the brain is morbidly cold and moist and gives rise to a thick vapor or bad humor, and "humoral," where some humor abounds in the stomach or elsewhere. The "conjoint" cause, such as the vapor, is connected with the manifestation of the disease.[241] This concept of different causes goes back to Antiquity, but as far as epilepsy is concerned it reached its highest development in the seventeenth century. We shall later have to come back to it.

Apart from humors and vapors, the medieval physicians recognized a third factor which might cause epilepsy. Alī Ibn Abbās stated that an obstruction in the brain could also be the result of a compression of the brain brought about by fracture of the skull and accompanied by severe pain.[242] Possibly this statement is nothing but a short résumé of the Hippocratic observation that convulsions may appear in fractures of the skull.[243] Taken over by Constantinus of Africa,[244] it had the great merit of associating epilepsy with fractures of the skull and compression of the brain, thereby directing the attention of later physicians to this important relationship.

Of equal importance was the realization that epilepsy might be inherited. This view was also taken over from ancient sources (probably the book *On the Sacred Disease*), but it was much more emphasized in the Middle Ages than it had been in the preserved writings of the ancients. Among the early Arabic authors epilepsy figured as one of the seven diseases "which are hereditary from the parents."[245] It was recognized as such by the Latin scholars too, but there was no clear distinction between its hereditary character and other causes which might lead to a congenital disposition. The main stress was laid upon the incurability of congenital epilepsy. "When a person is begotten during the time of menstruation[246] or from unclean seed, or if the

---

[241] Savonarola (891), *Practica maior*, tract. 6, c. 1, rubrica 20; fol. 71[V]: "Causae, Et in summa causae primitivae sunt illae quae dicentur statim in canone universalissimo. Antecedens vero complexionalis est mala complexio totius, aut cerebri frigida et humida, qua generatur ventositas grossa, vel malus humor. Humoralis est ipse humor sanguineus vel phlegmaticus, aut cholericus, aut melancholicus in stomacho vel alibi multiplicatus. Coniuncta est ipse vapor vel ventositas grossa, aut mala complexio simplex oppilans."

[242] Alī Ibn Abbās (22), *Theorica*, IX, 6; fol. 103[V]: "Haec autem opilatio aut ex flegmatico fit humore grosso et viscoso qui ad cerebri influit ventriculos accessionis eius hora aut humore colerico nigro et grosso: aut ex compressione quae cerebro ex ossis cranei fractura accidit: fitque cum eo dolor gravis."

[243] Cf. above, p. 35.

[244] Constantinus Africanus (235), *De communibus medico* etc., IX, 7; vol. 2, p. 247: "Hae oppilationes ex humoribus sunt phlegmaticis crassis et viscosis, in hora passionibus ad ventriculos descendentibus cerebri, aut ex crassis humoribus melancholicis, aut ex compressione cerebri cum franguntur ossa capitis."

[245] Cf. above, footnote 167.

[246] Cf. Wittich (1109), *Libellus*, fol. 20[r]; Albertus Magnus (19), *De animalibus*, XVIII, tract. 2, c. 9, 98; vol. 2, p. 1243, 34–38, mentions epilepsy among the diseases which may arise if the mother has much corrupt superfluous matter.

parents are epileptic, and if after his birth he falls into epilepsy, such a
person does not seem curable."[247] In the sixteenth century Fernelius
emphasized that the father, through his seed, would transfer to his
offspring any disease from which he was suffering at the time of pro-
creation, "so that the children follow their parents as heirs to their
diseases no less than to their estates."[248] Around that time, heredity as
a cause of epilepsy and as a hindrance to its cure could count on
popular understanding. The apothecary in John Haywood's *The Playe
Called the Foure PP* narrates:

> I dyd a cure no lenger a go
> But Anno domini millesimo
> On a woman yonge and so fayre
> That neuer haue I sene a gayre
> God saue all women from that lyknes
> This wanton had the fallen syknes
> Whiche by dissent cam lynyally
> For her mother had it naturally
> Wherefore this woman to recure
> It was more harde ye may be sure.[249]

A century later the remark was made: "And therefore it is a great
fortune to have had healthy parents and to be well born. Nay, the
human race would be very well served if healthy and sound people
alone would contract marriages, as Plutarch admonishes in his book on
the education of children."[250]

We may well ask ourselves whether these opinions found a counterpart in reality. If we can believe Hector Boece (d. 1536), it was customary among the ancient Scots to castrate men suffering from inheritable diseases, including epilepsy. "Heretofore in Scotland, saith
Hect. Boethius, if any were visited with the falling-sickness, madness,
gout, leprosie, or any such dangerous disease, which was likely to be

---

[247] Bernard of Gordon (106), *Lilium medicinae*, fol. 119$^r$: "Quando aliquis est generatus in
tempore menstruorum, aut ex immundis spermatibus, aut parentes sunt epileptici, deinde
genitus incurrat epilepsiam, talis non videtur curabilis," etc. Similarly Ioannes Anglicus (535),
*Rosa anglica*, p. 50.

[248] Fernelius (351), *Pathologia*, I, 11; p. 135: "Quocunque etiam morbo pater quum generat
tenetur, eum semine transfert in prolem: quandoquidem ex corpore universo (ut aliquando
demonstravimus) decisum semen, tum morbi tum causae eius vim in se continet. Sic senes et
valetudinarii, imbecilles: nephritici, arthritici, et epileptici filios vitiosa constitutione gignunt,
qua tandem in morbos similes, haereditarios id circo nuncupatos, incurrant, ut parentibus liberi
succedant, non minus morborum, quam possessionum haeredes."

[249] Quoted from Whiting (1096), p. 512.

[250] Beverovicius (108), *Schatz der Ungesundheit*, pp. 2-3: "Von den inwendigen seind uns
etliche durch den zeug, daraus wir gemacht seind, von unsern Eltern angebohren: daher die
Erbkrankheiten, als die Gicht, der Stein, die Schwindsucht, Fallende sucht und dergleichen,
entstehen. Und darüm ist es ein grosses glük; gesunde Eltern gehabt zu haben, und wohl
gebohren zu sein. Ja darüm würde dem Menschlichen geschlecht überaus wohl geholfen sein,
wan allein gesunde und wohlfahrende Leute, wie Plutarch, in seinem Buche von Erziehung der
Kinder, ermahnet, sich in den Ehstand begeben möchten."

propagated from the father to the son, he was instantly gelded; a woman kept from all company of men; and if by chance having some such disease, she were found to be with child, she with her brood were buried alive."[251]

Burton, who quoted this passage, also supplied it with an interesting commentary. He admitted that such a practice was against Christian principles, and yet he could not help complaining that abandoning it had resulted in the production of a degenerate race.[252] Leaving aside the question whether Boece's account contains any historical truth, we may infer that in the sixteenth and seventeenth centuries at least epileptics were not castrated to prevent diseased progeny. Whenever castration was practised, it was as a therapeutic measure, and as such it remained alive to the end of the nineteenth century. Another question concerns marriage and divorce laws for epileptics. Here the material is rather confusing.[253] Even in the late seventeenth century the theologians of Paris rejected a divorce plea by a woman against her epileptic husband, although the claimant had expressed her fear of bearing more children afflicted with the disease.[254] But in other cases it is not quite clear whether it was not the alleged infectious nature of epilepsy rather than its tendency to be inherited that was acknowledged as a reason for annulment or divorce.[255] In the early eighteenth century, the medical faculty of Leipzig still found it necessary to point out that epilepsy was not infectious, although it did not deny that marriage to an epileptic might prove injurious to the health of the partner.[256]

To sum up, it can be said that the Middle Ages added little to the physiological understanding of epilepsy. Yet at a time when the vague conception of the falling evil prevailed among the people and when even the educated were inclined to mistake a disease for demoniac possession, it was no small merit for the medieval physicians to have kept alive the tradition of epilepsy as a natural disease caused by natural factors.

---

[251] Burton (189), *The Anatomy of Melancholy*, Part 1, sec. 2, mem. 1, subs. 6; p. 39.

[252] *Ibid.*: "A severe doom you will say, and not to be used amongst Christians, yet more to be looked into than it is. For now by our too much facility in this kind, in giving way for all to marry that will, too much liberty and indulgence in tolerating all sorts, there is a vast confusion of hereditary diseases, no family secure, no man almost free from some grievous infirmity or other," etc.

[253] The historical material has been collected by Echeverria (310).

[254] Cf. Robinson (858), pp. 154–56.

[255] Cf. Echeverria, *l.c.*, pp. 348–52.

[256] Alberti (18), *Systema jurisprudentiae medicae*, tom. IV, p. 493: "Was die andere Frage betrifft: So ist zwar die Epilepsie nicht eben ein morbus contagiosus, und lehret die Erfahrung sattsam, dass mehrmalen eines von den Eheleuten mit der Epilepsie behaftet, obwohl der andere Ehegatte davon weder die Epilepsie bekommen, noch auch einigen Abbruch der Gesundheit dieserhalben verspühret;" etc. An English résumé is given by Echeverria, *l.c.*, p. 351.

# PART THREE

# THE RENAISSANCE

# V

# Theological, Philosophical, and Social Aspects

In retrospect, the medieval literature on epilepsy appears strangely complacent in its cultivation of contrasting views. On the one hand, there is the vague concept of the falling evil, strongly bound to demoniac beliefs and theological speculations. On the other hand, the physicians cling to the ancient idea of a definite natural disease. The sources that have been consulted reveal little effort to force an issue; the doctors rarely, if ever, discuss the theological aspects involved. They are even unwilling to rely solely on their own observations and consistent reasoning. Although clever in inventing new terms and auxiliary hypotheses, they cannot rid themselves of traditional definitions and explanations. Instead they often compromise by taking over as many of the older ideas as possible without attempting consistency.

Toward the end of the fifteenth century a change seems to take place. Physicians begin to discuss the possibilities of possession, magic, and witchcraft more freely. They are by no means uniform in their opinions, nor does scepticism prevail; some medical authors of the sixteenth and seventeenth centuries insist more strongly on the power of magic and witchcraft than had the average medieval doctor. But there is now a vigorous participation by medical men in debating these problems which arouse people in all Western countries.

A similar attitude prevails with regard to the purely medical aspect of epilepsy. During the sixteenth century some physicians break entirely with the traditional views. Others go back to Antiquity and to a Galenic pathology free from Arabic influences. In doing so, they are led back to the ancient ideal of observation, and a large body of new facts, both clinical and anatomical, is accumulated.

Nevertheless, much of what seems new during the two hundred years conveniently, rather than accurately, designated as the Renaissance is a new discussion of old problems rooted in the Middle Ages or in Antiquity. The various roots have to be traced in order to perceive the new developments.

## 1. THE THEOLOGICAL DEBATE

### a. The Debate on Possession

Few people in the time of the Renaissance doubted the existence of a personal power of evil. Catholics, Protestants, and Jews alike dreaded it and tried to evade and to combat it. Physicians and laymen recognized it as the opponent of God, yet deriving its power from God and exercising it by His permission to fulfil His ends. This power of darkness was Satan, the Devil, and usually he was believed to be helped in his sinister purpose by a whole host of devils or evil demons. Very conflicting views were held, however, regarding the sphere of influence granted to the devil, the ways in which he might attack mankind, and the means by which he could be defeated. Thus, a discussion arose whether devil and demons could really act as a physical force or whether their influence was restricted to the mind of man, whether they could act through the medium of sorcerers and witches, whether they were able to reveal the future, and whether they should be repelled by exorcisms and charms or by the strength of pure faith.

Such questions were of great concern to medicine, and in these controversies epilepsy often stood in the center of the debate because of its peculiar relation to the various forms of possession.

It will be remembered that already in the Middle Ages some physicians were inclined to consider possession as either epilepsy or madness, and scepticism toward the very existence of possession is sometimes evident in medical books of the sixteenth century. The elder Riolanus (1538–1606) speaks about the state of mind which the ancients called enthusiasm, i.e., divine possession. Quoting Aristotle, Riolanus explains this condition as a disturbance of phantasy by melancholic vapors. "Therefore," he says, "it is not necessary for us to have recourse to a demon as the last refuge of ignorance, since we have a natural cause."[1] He doubts that such people talk in foreign languages or prophesy; the harmony of their soul being disturbed, they say all kinds of things which make sense only in the phantasy of the listeners. Alsarius, whose book on the more common diseases of the head appeared in 1617,

---

[1] Riolanus (851), *Ad libros Fernelii de abditis rerum causis commentarius*, p. 134: "Itaque non est necesse, ut ad daemonem, tanquam ignorationis extremum perfugium, confugiamus, cum naturalem causam teneamus."

likewise takes a purely medical stand in favor of natural causes. There is no need to deny that sometimes God inflicts diseases for the punishment of human crimes, and perhaps an evil demon can affect man's complexion and dispose him to disease. But neither God nor demon operates without the intermediary of natural causes, with which alone the physician need be concerned.[2]

Nevertheless, physicians of the sixteenth as well as of the seventeenth century not only admitted the possibility of possession but considered it their task to distinguish it from epilepsy. In 1602 Jean Taxil, physician at Arles, maintained that it was scarcely possible to find any case in literature of a demoniac who was not epileptic.[3] By this statement Taxil, who sincerely believed in the Devil, did not mean to explain possession as a natural disease. He simply referred to the phenomenon "that in the fury of their affliction, they [i.e., the possessed] were seized by epileptic convulsions."[4] Taxil was not the only physician to point out the close relation between epilepsy and possession, and the Church too was well aware of it. The *Compendium maleficarum* related "the usual practice to determine whether the sick man[5] is possessed by a demon."[6] If the patients were possessed, one of the possible reactions would be that "they fall down as if dead, as though they were suffering from tertiary epilepsy, and a sort of vapour rushes up into their heads: but at the priest's bidding they arise, and the vapour returns whence it came."[7] To decide whether a person was possessed or suffering from a natural disease like epilepsy, physicians might be called in. One such case gave occasion to Andreas Caesalpinus (1516-1603) to write a whole treatise on the subject of demoniac power. Together with the theologians, philosophers, and physicians of the University of Pisa he had been summoned to be present while some nuns "who had been annoyed by demons" were exorcised by a priest. The experts were asked to indicate the signs by which it could be decided "whether the disease depended upon natural causes, such as vapors ascending from the uterus, by which many virgins are wont to be harassed, or black bile and other bad humors which sometimes harm the mind, sometimes the body, as it happens in epileptic convulsions and melancholic insanity,

---

[2] Alsarius (25), *De morbis capitis frequentioribus*, p. 270 f.

[3] Taxil (994), *Traicté de l'épilepsie*, c. 17: "Que les Daemoniaques sont Epileptiques;" p. 156 f.: "Que lon lise hardiment, à grande peine trouuera-on Daemoniaque qui ne soit Epileptique." On Taxil cf. also De Saussure (889).

[4] Taxil, *ibid.*, p. 155 f.: ". . . qu'à la fureur de leur mal, ils sont attaints des conuulsions Epileptiques."

[5] Not necessarily an epileptic.

[6] Guazzo (439), *Compendium maleficarum*, III, 2; p. 170 f. (Ashwin's translation).

[7] *Ibid.* (Ashwin's translation). "Tertiary epilepsy" refers to the form where the convulsions started from some part of the body accompanied by the feeling of a "breeze." Cf. below, footnote 13.

or whether another, supernatural cause were concealed which would by
no means obey the physician, nature's servant, but could be removed
by divine help only."[8]

How then did physicians proceed in the differential diagnosis between epilepsy and possession?[9] Constantinus of Africa, Gualterius
Agilon, and Joannes Anglicus had proposed a magic formula which
would distinguish between lunatics and demoniacs on the one hand,
epileptics on the other, and Abulqasim had pointed to some classical
features of "possession."[10] For the time of the Renaissance an illustrative answer to this question is given by a case described by Fernelius
(1485-1558).[11] This description was repeated by other physicians of
the period and may here be quoted from the English version of
Ambroise Paré's work, *Of Monsters and Prodigies*:

> Another young Noble man, some few years since, was troubled at
> set times with a shaking of the bodie, and as it were, a convulsion,
> wherewith one while hee would moov onely his left arm, another
> while the right arm, and also som times but one finger onely, som-
> whiles but one leg, somtimes the other, and at other times the whole
> trunk of his bodie, with such force and agilitie, that lying in his bed,
> hee could scarce bee held by four men; his head laie without anie
> shakeing, his tongue and speech was free, his understanding sound,
> and all his senses perfect even in the height of his fit. Hee was taken
> at the least ten times a daie, well in the spaces between, but wearied
> with labor: it might have been judged a true Epilepsie, if the under-
> standing and senses had failed.
>
> The most judicious Physitians who were called to him, judged it a
> convulsion, cosen-germane to the falling sickness, proceeding from a
> malign and venemous vapor impact in the spine of the back, whence
> a vapor disspersed it self over all the nervs, which pass from the spine
> every waie into the limbs, but not into the brain. To remoov this,
> which they judged the caus, frequent glysters are ordained, and
> strong purges of all sorts, cupping-glasses are applied to the be-
> ginnings of the nervs, fomentations, unctions, emplasters, first to
> discuss, then to strengthen and wear awaie the malign qualitie: These

---

[8]Caesalpinus (193), *Daemonum investigatio peripatetica*, c. 1; fol. 145 C: "Postquam
Reverendissime Antistes convocatis Pisanae Academiae Theologis, Philosophis, ac Medicis
curasti, ut religiosis quibusdam virginibus a Daemone vexatis, dum a Sacerdote adiurarentur,
interessent, quo signis optime notatis iudicarent, utrum morbus a causis naturalibus penderet,
ut sunt vapores ab utero ascendentes, quibus pleraeque virgines infestari solent, aut atra bilis,
caeterique pravi humores modo mentem modo corpus laedentes, ut in Epilepticis convulsionibus, et Melancholicis deliramentis contingit: an altera lateret causa supra naturam, quae
Medico naturae ministro nequaquam obediret, sed tantum divinis auxiliis tolleretur."

[9]Of course epilepsy was not the only disease to be distinguished from possession. Antonius
Benivenius (101), *De abditis nonnullis ac mirandis morborum et sanationum causis*, c. 8, for
instance, relates a case of a hysterical woman whose symptoms the physicians first explained by
an ascent of the uterus and of bad vapors affecting the heart and brain. When adequate
treatment did not bring relief and when she began vomiting nails, etc., they judged her possessed by an evil spirit.

[10]Cf. above, p. 106.

[11]Fernelius (351), *De abditis rerum causis*, II, 16; p. 89.

things doing little good, hee was sweated with bathes, stoves, and a decoction of *Guajacum*, which did no more good then the former, for that wee were all far from the knowledg of the true cause of his diseas: for in the third month, a certain devil was found to bee the autor of all this ill, bewraying himself by voice, and unaccustomed words and sentences, as well Latin as Greek (though the patient were ignorant of the Greek tongue): he laied open manie secrets of the by-standers, and chiefly of the Physicians, derideing them for that hee had abused them to the patients great harm, becaus they had brought his bodie so low by needless purgations.[12]

This account shows the following important features: The symptoms do not quite fit into the nosological scheme of the time. In particular, they do not agree with the definition of epilepsy, since the mind is not affected. Nevertheless, the physicians relate the case to epilepsy, give it a natural explanation, and treat it according to a rational plan. This is done for some length of time but without success. Then the devil shows himself by speaking a language which the patient himself does not know and by making astounding revelations to the bystanders.

Any aberration from the usual clinical picture was suspicious. Caesalpinus pointed in particular to the form of epilepsy which arose from an extremity accompanied by a "breeze."[13] Another symptom of malign influence was the futility of rational treatment. The matter was clear beyond doubt if the patient's behaviour could not be explained on a natural basis at all, especially if he began to speak or understand foreign languages or if he prophesied.

These were the rules commonly applied. A great deal depended, of course, on the individual physician. Anything unusual might immediately arouse the suspicions of the superstitious mind. Many epileptics must have been taken for demoniacs. Other physicians, like Johann Weyer, might investigate any possibility of fraud and simulation before they were ready to admit the presence of the devil. But the discussion was not restricted to these points. A heated argument arose over the question whether the actual *disease* epilepsy could be brought about by the powers of hell.

### b. The Debate on Witchcraft

Epilepsy in itself was such a strange phenomenon that some superhuman agency was frequently assumed. Even an outstanding surgeon, Fabricius Hildanus (1560–1634), in a letter to Dr. Wertenberg, ad-

---

[12] Paré (773), p. 668 (Johnson's translation).

[13] Caesalpinus (193), *Daemonum investig. peripat.*, c. 22; fol. 166 C-D: "Omnino videretur tertia illa species Epilepsiae, quam Medici tradunt a membris extremis excitari aura quadam ad caput repente, nisi aura remearet unde discessit, accersireturque imperio sacerdotis. Solent autem sacerdotes in pedem sinistrum relegare." Cf. above, footnote 7.

mitted: "I agree with you in declaring that something divine can be observed in epileptics, since experience has not seldom taught me this. For very often something lies hidden in the bodies of epileptics which is above our power of comprehension."[14] For many of the uneducated, epilepsy was still a sacred disease.

Some theologians and physicians also believed that epilepsy might sometimes be brought about by witchcraft. The *Malleus maleficarum*, the classical textbook of witch hunting published in the eighties of the fifteenth century, reports cases of epilepsy inflicted "by means of eggs which have been buried with dead bodies, especially the dead bodies of witches,"[15] and Caesalpinus repeats this story.[16] Since it was believed that every kind of disease could be caused by witches,[17] epilepsy was not necessarily excepted, and the fact that diseases had natural causes need not exclude demons from instigating them.[18] The physician Franciscus Valesius and others made the demon act as an external cause of disease, setting the inner, material causes in motion.[19] The presence of phlegm, black bile, and other pathogenetic humors therefore need not be denied. Even in the case of possession it could be admitted that a melancholy temperament might make the victims predisposed to it. On this basis Valesius said that the demon "brings epilepsy, paralysis and such maladies by a stoppage of the heavier physical fluids, obstructing and blocking the ventricle of the brain and the nerve-roots."[20]

The following case, which occurred in the practice of Martin Ruland (1532–1602), a physician close to the Paracelsian school, contains some instructive points. A man forty years old had suffered from attacks of "epilepsy and mania" for a period of six years. The attacks occurred twice yearly and the epileptic paroxysms were so strong "that the man lay prostrate upon the ground as though dead." Having regained his strength but not yet his reason, "he fled to forests, fields,

---

[14] Fabricius Hildanus (338), *Opera*, p. 352: "In epilepticis divini quippiam observari posse, tecum assero, cum idipsum non raro me edocuerit experientia. Saepissime enim nonnihil quod captum nostrum superat, in corporibus Epilepticorum delitescit."

[15] Institoris (532), *Malleus maleficarum*, Par. II, Quest. 1, c. 11; p. 137 (Summers' translation).

[16] Caesalpinus, *l.c.*, c. 10; fol. 155 A-B.

[17] Caesalpinus, *l.c.*, c. 22; fol. 166 A: "Omne igitur genus morbi ex maleficiis inferri posse superius ostensum est. . . ."

[18] Guazzo (439), *Compendium maleficarum*, II, 8; p. 105: "Avicenna and Galen and Hippocrates deny that it is possible for any diseases to be brought upon man by demons; and their view is followed by Pietro Pomponazzi and Levin Lemne, not because they did not believe that the demons, which they acknowledged to be evil, wished to cause disease, but because they held that every disease is due to natural causes. But that is no good argument: for is it not possible for sicknesses to spring from natural causes, and at the same time possible for demons to be the instigators of such sicknesses?" (Ashwin's translation).

[19] *Ibid.*, p. 106: ". . . Franciscus Valesius, who says that the demon is the external cause of sickness when he comes from without to inhabit a body and bring diseases to it; and if the sickness has some material source he sets in motion its inner causes." (Ashwin's translation).

[20] *Ibid.*

and other places in a state of madness, running this way and that, until his reason was restored and he returned home."[21] Ruland had no doubts about the etiology of the case. A witch who lived in the same place had been supplied by the devil with a poison by means of which she had caused the disease. Having been arrested and tortured, the woman confessed, and before her execution she was ordered by the magistrate to undo the evil she had caused. "But the devilish woman says that it was not in her power to effect a cure and that (whatever her power might be) it was not possible to do so because of the length of time, because the poison had already spread throughout the particles of the whole body and because the diseases[22] had already affected its roots."[23] Thereupon the man asked Ruland's help and he cured him by bloodletting, a special sternutatory, and a strong cathartic.

Yet even the *Malleus maleficarum* admitted that epilepsy, because of its deep roots in the physique of the patient, offered very considerable difficulties to an explanation by witchcraft. "For although greater difficulty may be felt in believing that witches are able to cause leprosy or epilepsy, since these diseases generally arise from some long-standing physical predisposition or defect, none the less it has sometimes been found that even these have been caused by witchcraft."[24] This statement, which insisted that epilepsy had *sometimes* been traced to witchcraft, implicitly admitted that usually this was not the case. Indeed, if one expects epilepsy to be frequently mentioned as a result of the machinations of witches, one is likely to be disappointed. Whatever the mass of the people may have thought, the learned supporters of the theory of witchcraft strengthened rather than weakened the belief that epilepsy, as long as it did not show any atypical features, was a natural disease. Just because "certain convulsive movements of an epileptic appearance"[25] were counted among the characteristic symptoms of sickness brought on by witchcraft, and just because possession resembled epilepsy, it was necessary to acknowledge the differences between the natural disease and supernatural afflictions. Otherwise, the

---

[21]Rulandus (880), *Curationum* etc. centuria sexta, curatio 100; pp. 132-33: "Tobias Vueidner pileo annos quadraginta natus, Epilepsia et mania per sexennium correptus singulis annis paroxysmo epileptico bis ita affligebatur, ut instar mortui humi prostratus iaceret. Viribus refocillatis, ac principibus facultatibus a causa morbifica aliquantulum levatis, ratione tamen adhuc intercepta in sylvas et loca campestria aliaque amens aufugit, ultro citroque discurrens, quoad ratione in integrum restituta domum se contulisset."

[22]Ruland obviously considered the epileptic paroxysm and the subsequent confused state to be two different diseases.

[23]*Ibid.*, pp. 135-36: "Verum diabolica mulier, penes se non esse mederi, nec (quamvis valeret) ob temporis longitudinem, veneno iam per totius corporis particulas diffuso, morbis etiam radices iam agentibus, illud praestare posse pronunciat."

[24]Institoris (532), *Malleus maleficarum*, Par. II. Quest. 1, c. 11; p. 136 (Summers' translation).

[25]Guazzo (439), *Compendium maleficarum*, III, 2; p. 170 (Ashwin's translation).

conflict between a theological and medical diagnosis would have become too great.

Even as it was, such a conflict existed. Backed by the authority of Hippocrates, a group of physicians stressed the natural character of epilepsy against all popular and theological assumptions. Foremost among them were Hieronymus Gabucinius (fl. 1550),[26] Johann Weyer (1515–88),[27] and Levinus Lemnius (1505–68), the last of whom advanced views which were later on adopted by the representatives of Enlightenment. Commenting upon his superstitious contemporaries, he wrote: "Since therefore the cause of the Falling-sicknesse is so Evident, I would perswade the ignorant people to think of no other cause of this disease, than the motion of the humours, that men may not fear so much, when they see their mouths draw awry, their cheeks swoln, and strutting forth with a frothy humour: and should not be dismaid to come near them, and lend them their help. For so are all those that stand by and are fearful, amazed, when they see them rending themselves, and beating their heads and bodies against posts, that they think there is no hopes of them, and so cause them to be buried before their Souls are departed from them. For I have found it in our own dayes, and in former Ages also, that some have broken the Coffin, and lived again. Wherefore it is fit a Law should be made, that those who are to take care of the dead bodies should not presently put them into their coffins, whom they think to be dead, especially those that are strangled by the Apoplex, Epilepsie, or rising of the Mother; for oft-times their soul lies within them, and they live again."[28]

The difficulty which epilepsy presented to the believers in witchcraft helped the defenders of witches. They could easily presume the natural character of the disease and could base their arguments upon it. Just as in Antiquity Apuleius had unmasked the pretended victim of his magic art as an epileptic, so now Johann Weyer could reveal alleged cases of possession as epilepsy and thus refute the accusation of witchcraft.[29]

### c. The Debate on Magic and Superstitious Treatment

The time from the end of the fifteenth to the latter half of the seventeenth century presents a rather confusing picture of the evaluation of magic and superstitious remedies for epilepsy. It is confusing because of the many contradictory attitudes and because of the appar-

---

[26]Hieronymus Gabucinius (388), *De comitiali morbo*, fol. 2$^v$: Sed quorsum haec tam multa? ut ostenderem nullum plane morbum sacrum esse; nullumque praecantationibus auferri posse," etc. For Gabucinius cf. also Streeter (964).

[27]Cf. Weyer (1094), *De praestigiis daemonum*, II, c. 19.

[28]Lemnius (625), *The Secret Miracles of Nature*, II, 3; p. 93 (anonymous translation). For the Enlightenment cf. Ackerknecht (5).

[29]Cf. above, I-1, and Weyer, *l.c.*, V, 28.

ent lack of a progressive development. Very broadly speaking, it can be said that during the first half of the sixteenth century belief and beginning scepticism were both represented, that strong doubts were expressed during the second half of the century, whereas a reaction set in during the seventeenth century. Paracelsus and the school of hermetic medicine, with their inclination toward a mystic concept of the disease, tended most toward a magic treatment. But it has to be added at the very outset that scarcely any physician down to the end of the seventeenth century rejected "natural" remedies altogether. Even Johann Weyer expressly remarked that he did not want to take away faith in "natural" ligatures and amulets,[30] and even at the beginning of the eighteenth century human blood and bones were still recommended by reputable physicians. Radical reforms in these matters were not effected before the time of enlightenment.

Comparatively early a certain scepticism toward too promiscuous a use of empiric remedies was expressed. Laurentius Phriesen, in the German *Spiegel der Artzney*, first follows the traditional pattern when he says: "Now I will indicate how you should treat these diseases. First by a methodical medical cure, then by many nice experiments of creditable teachers, some of which I have experienced myself."[31] But after giving some examples of such "nice" experiments he adds: "There are many more empiric artifices which some people describe but from which I refrain. If a thing has no credible cause I do not think much of it. Leave it to the herbalists and adventurers. My advice is that you should always employ reason and not believe in experiment."[32] Others felt that certain experiments were even harmful. Cardanus (?),[33] in his lectures on epilepsy, mentions various old tests by which epilepsy could presumably be diagnosed but adds the very sensible remark: "In my opinion it would be much safer to give up this trial lest the disease come on again and thus be spurred on."[34] The same author shows a lack of trust in many superstitious medicines which is very remarkable for his time.[35] Although he does not dismiss them entirely, he often

---

[30]Weyer, *l.c.*, V, 20; col. 578: "Nullam tamen hic fidem ligaturis, periaptis et amuletis physicis subtractam volo."

[31]Laurentius Phriesen (795), *Spiegel der Artzney*, fol. 80r: "Nun wil ich dir anzeigen wie du dise kranckheiten wenden sollest. Zum ersten durch ein ordenlichen process der artzney, darnach mit vil schönen experimenten von glaubhafftigen lerern, und auch zum teil von mir erfaren."

[32]*Ibid.*, fol. 80v: "Sunst seind noch vil empörischer künstlin, so etliche schreiben, die lass ich sein. Wann was nit glaubhafftige ursach hat, da halt ich nit von. Lass das selbig den wurtzelgrabern, und abenteürern. Ist mein rath, das du alweg mit sinnen wurbest, und nit glaubest dem experiment."

[33]Cf. footnote 35, below.

[34]Cardanus (201), *Tractatus de epilepsia*, lect. 8; vol. 10, p. 398: "Meo iudicio longe tutius esset dimittere hanc experientiam, ne morbus iteratum accederet, et hoc modo incitaretur."

[35]There is, therefore, doubt whether the *Tractatus de epilepsia* really hails from Cardanus, who, in his consilium *Pro epileptico*, vol. 9, p. 61 ff., is much less sceptical.

tries to substitute a rational explanation and, more important, refuses credence where he does not find sense.[36] This is best illustrated by his remarks on the alleged usefulness of human bones, especially those of the skull. He thinks that there is nothing occult in bones, merely the manifest qualities of drying, etc. "Therefore I cannot see why human bones should be of more help than other bones. . . . Besides, some modern physicians in addition refer particularly to the bones of the human skull.[37] For they believe that since this disease is in the head, therefore, by similitude, the bones of the head help more than other bones, because of their conformity. Thus they take them by preference; without, however, any reason, according to my opinion."[38]

How belief in supernatural agents could at the same time be combined with a sceptical attitude toward the cruder forms of occult therapeutics is illustrated by Fernelius. He does not doubt demoniac possession, the existence of divine and magic cures, or the efficacy of remedies which act "by their whole substance." But in between these two categories he finds many prescriptions of a vain and superstitious nature. "These are such as wee cannot truly say of them, wherefore and whence they have the faculties asscribed to them: for they neither arise from the temperament, neither from the other manifest qualities, neither from the whole substance, neither from a divine or magical power. . . . Such like old wive's medicines and superstitious remedies are written figures and characters, rings, where neither the assistance of God or Spirits is implored. Let me ask you, is it not a superstitious medicine to heal the falling sickness, to carrie in writing the names of the three Kings, Gaspar, Melchior, and Balthasar, who came to worship Christ?"[39]

Since Fernelius rejected the medieval charm to which the last lines allude,[40] it is little wonder that the men who led the fight against the persecution of witches, Johann Weyer in Germany and Reginald Scot (†1599) in England, referred to it with obvious scorn. Weyer thought this and similar charms the invention of evil men who thereby wanted

---

[36]Cf. especially lecture 9.

[37]This may refer to Paracelsus and his school; cf. below, footnote 189.

[38]*Ibid.*, lect. 10; vol. 10, p. 402: "Addunt quidam quod ossa humana maiorem adhuc habent virtutem: sed quoniam nos credimus in ossibus nullam esse qualitatem occultam, sed solum illas manifestas exsiccandi, subtiliandi, et calefaciendi. Ideo non possum videre, quare magis iuvent ossa humana quam alia ossa; praeterea Galenus hoc non dicit, et solum exhibet ossa suilla, ossa pedum suis. Addunt praeterea medici quidam moderni; et dicunt quod praecipue inter humana ossa cranei, existimantes quod quomodo iste morbus est in capite, ita etiam per similitudinem ossa capitis plus iuvent quam alia ossa, quoniam enim sunt conformia, ideo potius ea sumant, nulla tamen ratione meo iudicio."

[39]Quoted from Paré (773), *Of Monsters and Prodigies*; p. 669 (Johnson's translation). Here again Paré repeats Fernelius (351), *De abditis rerum causis*, II, 16; p. 90.

[40]Fernelius, *l.c.*, gives it in full. For the complete Latin form cf. above, III-2b. Abraham Fleming (d. 1607) translated it into English verse used by Scot (906), *The Discoverie of Witch-*

to insult God and to defile medicine.[41] Reginald Scot found even stronger words against such incantations, of which he gives many examples. "There be innumerable charmes of conjurers, bad physicians, lewd surgians, melancholike witches, and couseners, for all diseases and greefes; speciallie for such as bad physicians and surgions knowe not how to cure, and in truth are good stuffe to shadow their ignorance, whereof I will repeate some. *For the falling evill*. Take the sicke man by the hand, and whisper these wordes softlie in his eare, I conjure thee by the sunne and moone, and by the gospell of this daie delivered by God to *Hubert, Giles, Cornelius,* and *John,* that thou rise and fall no more,"[42] etc.

But as belief in magic did not exclude rejection of superstitious cures, so scepticism did not prevent keeping up the old customs. Riolanus, who called demons "the last refuge of ignorance,"[43] repeated the charm of the three wise men after Valescus, whom he esteemed as "an author not to be despised."[44] Augier Ferrier (1513-88)[45] frankly admitted that he did not ascribe any real significance to superstitious procedures. Yet he made use of them (like others before him) because the patients believed in them and because their belief would effect the cure. For him a Latin verse held true, which Scot cited in English translation:

> Not hellish furies dwell in us,
> Nor starres with influence heavenlie;
> The spirit that lives and rules in us,
> Doth every thing ingeniouslie.[46]

---

*craft,* XII, 9; p. 132:
> Gasper with his myrh beganne
> these presents to unfold,
> Then Melchior brought in frankincense,
> and Balthasar brought in gold.
> Now he that of these holie kings
> the names about shall beare,
> The falling yll by grace of Christ
> shall never need to feare.

[41] Weyer (1094), *De praestigiis daemonum,* V, 8; col. 530: "Huc pertinent superstitionum et verborum ignotorum, quibus utrum bene aut male preceris ignoras, monstra: haud dubie a malis inventa hominibus, et pro libidine excogitata, quae cum Dei contumelia in sacrosanctae nostrae medicinae conspurcationem calumniamque furtim irrepsere. cuiusmodi hi usurpantur rhythmi contra epilepsiam: Gaspar fert," etc.

[42] Scot, *l.c.,* XII, 14; p. 138. The latter incantation is also cited by Weyer, *l.c.*

[43] Cf. above, footnote 1.

[44] Riolanus (851), *Particularis methodi medendi liber,* I, sect. 1, tract. 1, c. 16; p. 431: "Valescus auctor non contemnendus affirmat se multoties expertum epilepticos mox resurgere, si ter in aurem haec insusurrentur. Gaspar fert mirrham," etc.

[45] Cf. Scot, *l.c.,* XII, 12; p. 136 f.

[46] *Ibid.,* p. 137. The translation is by Abraham Fleming. The Latin text runs:
> Nos habitat non tartara, sed nec sidera coeli
> Spiritus in nobis qui viget illa facit.

## 2. THE EPILEPTIC AS A PROPHET

Prophesying was the real touchstone between the natural disease, epilepsy, and the involvement of supernatural powers. In the present context, prophecy means the knowledge of past, present, or future events through means not accessible to normal beings, whereby normal includes not only mental and physical normality but also conformity with the laws of orthodox religion.[47] Was there a connection between epilepsy and prophecy? This question allows a relatively simple positive answer as long as it is limited to the belief in the existence of prophesying epileptics. The question becomes complicated as soon as it reaches the level of interpretation, for here the theological presumptions of the time were involved, as well as its philosophical ideas about the relationship of body and mind.

### a. Prophesying Epileptics

Meric Casaubon (1599–1671), a scholar and divine living in Puritan England, related the following event that took place in Germany in 1581. A baker had mercilessly beaten his apprentice without sparing the head, "so that the Boy fell sick upon it of an Epilepsie: whereof he had divers terrible fits, and was twelve dayes speechlesse." In the course of time, the fits disappeared, only to be replaced by "ecstasies"

> in which he would continue two, three, four hours, without either sense or motion. As soon as he was out of a fit, the first thing he would do, was to sing divers songs and hymns, (though it was not known that he had ever learned any,) very melodiously. From this singing he would now and then passe abruptly to some strange relations, but especially of such & such, lately dead, whom he had seen in Paradise; and then fall to singing again. But when he was perfectly come to himself, and had left singing, then would he sadly and with much confidence maintain, That he had been, not upon his bed, as they that were present would make him believe; but in heaven with his Heavenly Father, having been carried thither by Angels, and placed in a most pleasant green, where he had enjoyed excessive happinesse, and had seen things that he could not expresse; &c. The same Boy when he foresaw his fit coming upon him, he would say, that now the Angels were ready to carry him away.

A physician of the same town first gave it as his opinion that the ecstasies and visions were symptoms of a melancholic disease "occasioned by the Epilepsie," but that the concurrent operation of the Devil could not be excluded regarding the prophesies. Later the doctor appar-

---

[47]This definition is supposed to conform to the concept of prophecy of the time. It is similar to that given by Walzer (1065), p. 206, for Al-Fārābī.

ently changed his mind and attributed the prophesies to plain fraud on the part of the clever young rogue.[48]

Prophesying epileptics seem not to have been rare during the period.[49] Historical examples and explorers' tales added to the number known. Jean Taxil mentioned "the Sibyls who were convulsed, fell down, frothed and were tormented when possessed by the Devil"; he referred to Saul, who frothed, threw himself about, stormed, and finally fainted when seized by the evil spirit, and he listed heathen priests who prophesied because of devilish possession, while the accompanying symptoms proved them true epileptics.[50]

So far, Taxil said nothing remarkable. Plato had attributed the prophetic power of the Sibyl to divine inspiration,[51] and what was divine to the pagan was devilish to the Christian. Saul's condition while prophesying at Ramah was to be diagnosed as status epilepticus, even three hundred years after Taxil.[52] The reference to heathen priests fits a number of ancient examples, for instance the priests of Baal and the Corybantes, the priests of Cybele. Then, however, Taxil adds an interesting remark. The behaviour of the heathen priests could be observed in Taxil's own day among the priests of the Tupinambos and Margayats [?]. According to Leri,[53] they really were seized by epilepsy when the devil tormented them during their attempts to reveal the future.

Today, those priests would be included in the broad category of shamans. Shamans of arctic Europe had been described by Olaus Magnus (1490-1558), and citing him Daniel Sennert (1572-1637) left no

---

[48]Casaubon (205), *A Treatise Concerning Euthusiasme*, ch. 3; p. 93 f. On Casaubon see Hunter and Macalpine (521), who on p. 145 f. reprint this narrative.

[49]A story similar to that above is to be found in Grässe (422), vol. I, p. 95. It concerns a certain Hans Kurtzhalss who, in 1574, became ill of the "the falling evil" and was paralyzed in hands and feet. Finally, he began to shout "like one possessed," prophesied, talked the Bavarian dialect, called everybody—even strangers—by name, and denounced witches so that many of them were brought to punishment. He also preached the Lord's wrath, announced the day of judgment, and admonished people to do penance.

[50]Taxil (994), *Traicté de l'épilepsie*, c. 17; p. 155 f. "J'appelle doncques en tesmoing ce que i'ay dict cy deuant des Sibylles, comme elles conuulsoient, tomboient, escumoient, et se tourmentoient lors qu'elles estoient endiablées. Saül à l'escripture Saincte, quand par la permission diuine, il fust saisi de l'esprit maling, que faisoit-il? Il escumoit, il se demenoit, il tempestoit, et en fin pasmoit. Nul ne doubte que les Prestres des idolatres, parlants prophetiquement, ne fissent cela, par la force du Diable, qui les possedoit: mais alors de leurs propheties de quels accidens estoient-ils saisis? vrayement en tournant la bouche, escumant, tombant, et demenant leurs corps, ils monstroyent estre vrays Epileptiques. Encore void on cela de nostre temps aduenir en l'Amerique, parmy les Taupinambaux, et Margayats [?], car leurs Prestres, qu'ils appellent Garaybes [?], quand le Diable les tourmente, qui est lors qu'ils veulent à la Payenne, donner reuelation des choses futures, sont vrayement saisis d'Epilepsie: de L'Hery autheur de ceste histoire t'en asseurera."

[51]Plato (801), *Phaedrus*, 244 B; cf. Dodds (283), ch. 3, and on the Sibyls, Pollard (818), ch. 6.

[52]Preuss (822), pp. 356-58, to which cf. Rosen (872), p. 54.

[53]The explorer Leri (Taxil spells the name L'Heri) whose *Histoire d'un voyage fait en la terre de Bresil* had appeared in 1578. See above, footnote 50.

doubt that the Lapplanders who prophesied about things going on three hundred miles away did so by devilish power. Sennert classified them under "ecstatics," whom he defined as "persons who, for a long time, lie with their minds withdrawn from their bodies as it were and after awakening relate the marvellous things which they say they have seen and heard."[54]

Ecstasy, as such, was a condition different from epilepsy. The Aristotelian *Problems* had connected it with the melancholic type, and the divinatory ecstatic state played a great role in the history of melancholy, particularly in the Renaissance.[55] But the Hippocratics had already seen a relationship between melancholy and epilepsy, and, as Casaubon's narrative shows, divinatory ecstasy could be connected with epilepsy. Another link between epilepsy and prophecy was suggested by the synonym *divinatio* for the disease. Antonius Guainerius cited the case of a young epileptic given to prophesying. "I have seen a certain choleric young man who said that during his paroxysms he always saw wondrous things which he very much wished to set down in writing. For without doubt he expected them to come to pass. For this reason the ancients called this disease divination."[56] Guainerius' source for "divination" was the Syro-Arabic physician Serapion.[57]

The name of Serapion points to the East, and doctors of the Renaissance commonly believed that epileptic prophets were numerous among the Arabs. In all probability, this belief was supported by the legend that Mohammed himself, the founder of Islam, had been an epileptic. The preoccupation of the West with this legend has been so great and it is so illustrative of the complexity of the history of epilepsy that it needs more than passing consideration.

Among the Arabs of Mohammed's time, the *kāhin*, the diviner and soothsayer, was expected to be able to predict future events. Like the *shā'ir*, the poet of pre-Islamic times, he was believed to receive his inspiration from the *jinn*, the demons who could cause madness and

---

[54] Sennert (913), *Institut. medic.*, II, pars 3, sect. 2, c. 9; vol. 1, p. 401: ". . . Lappii, quos *lib.* 3 *de gent. Septentr.* Olaus Magnus, ceremoniis quibusdam adhibitis subito labi, et quasi exanimari scribit, ut anima quasi e corpore excessisse videatur, eosdemque postea horis 24. elapsis, ceu profundo somno expergisci, et quasi in vitam revocari, ad interrogata respondere, et quid de absentibus etiam per trecenta milliaria fiat, narrare, et indiciis additis fidem facere. Quae a Diabolica, et foedere cum Diabolo provenire planum est: ut et ea, quae Sibyllis plerisque, et oraculorum sacerdotibus contigerunt." *Ibid.* "Verum vulgo ἐκστατικοὶ dicuntur, qui quasi mente a corpore abstracti diu iacent, et postquam evigilant, mira, quae vidisse et audivisse se dicunt, narrant." Cf. Minder (702), p. 15.

[55] Cf. Aristotle (55), *Problems*, 30, 1 *passim*. The work by Klibansky et al. (585) offers a very thorough discussion on the connection of melancholy and prophetic states, and should be consulted for this and the following sections. For other examples of the connection of ecstasy and mental illness cf. below, footnote 84.

[56] Antonius Guainerius (438), *Tractatus de egritudinibus capitis*, VII, 1; fol. 11ʳ; see below, footnote 114. Cf. also Lennox (627), p. 484, and Lennox (632), p. 278 f.

[57] On Serapion as the source for the term *divinatio* see above, Part Two, footnote 127.

epilepsy.[58] Indeed one Arabic author, Alī b. Rabban aṭ-Ṭabarī (about 850) mentioned "the diviner's disease" as a popular synonym for epilepsy. His discussion of diseases of the brain began with the falling sickness (sar'un),[59] which he expressly identified with epilepsy. "And the people," he added, "call it the diviner's disease, because some of them prophesy and have visions of wondrous things."[60] The hallucinations of some epileptics (sufferers from temporal lobe epilepsy, as we would suspect) were thus compared to the visions of the kāhin. Here there is a possible link with divination as a synonym for epilepsy mentioned in Serapion. A person having visions could thus have been suspected of suffering from epilepsy, if other symptoms pointed to the disease. Was then Mohammed suspected of having been an epileptic?

The Koran makes it clear that Mohammed had a vision in which a trustworthy messenger appeared to him.[61] Then, in a series of inspirations, the archangel Gabriel,[62] as Mohammed believed, communicated to him words that were written down and that were later compiled as the Koran. Moreover, Sura 17,1 of the Koran glorified Allah, "Who carried His servant [i.e., Mohammed] by night from the Inviolable Place of Worship [Mecca] to the Far Distant Place of Worship [Jerusalem]."[63] Whether this flight from Mecca to Jerusalem was a dream, a hallucination, or a mystic experience is a moot question.

The biographical tradition, which began to be edited in the eighth century, tells of a remarkable occurrence in Mohammed's early youth, and it has been suggested that an epileptic fit was at the bottom of it.[64] While living under the care of his wet-nurse, Ḥalīma, Mohammed was approached by two men (angels) who split open his abdomen and re-

---

[58]Goldziher (417), p. 25. On the kāhin in general see Fischer (361). The Book of Al Dakhīra (933), 49; p. 22 compares "the hideous movements" of epileptics with those of persons seized by the jinn.

[59]Sar'un is usually translated with epilepsy. It is derived from ṣara'a, "to throw down," and is therefore in the semantic orbit of "the falling sickness." By using the latter translation I have allowed a greater margin for "the diviner's disease" than "epilepsy" would constitute. Sura II, 275 as well as Spitaler's (945), col. 535 (top) remarks seem to support my interpretation.

[60]Alī b. Rabban al-Ṭabari (23), Paradise of Wisdom, p. 138: "aṣ-ṣar'u wa-huwa 'afīlabsiyā, wa-sammāhu qaumun bi-l-maradi (text: wsm'h qaumun 'blmrḍ) l-kāhinīyi li'anna minhum man yatakahhanu wa-yaẓharu lahu l-ashyā'u l-'ajībatu." I cannot agree with Meyerhof (692), p. 22, that al-maraḍu l-kāhinīyu is a translation of ἱερὴ νοῦσος which Ibn Abī Uṣaibi'a (524), ed. Müller, p. 33,6, translates with al-maraḍu l-'ilāhīyu (cf. above Part One, footnote 9).

[61]Suras 53 and, particularly, 81, 20–25. I am here following Andrae (33), pp. 43–47 who considers Ibn Sa'd's account closer to the original events than Ibn Isḥāq's. For a different opinion cf. Nöldeke-Schwally (736), vol. 1, p. 78.

[62]Sura II, 197; Pickthall (796), p. 41: "Who is an enemy to Gabriel! For he it is who hath revealed (this Scripture) to thy [i.e., Mohammed's] heart by Allah's leave. . . ." Bell (99), p. 31 ff., stresses the difference between the initial visions and the later inspirations.

[63]Pickthall (796), p. 204.

[64]Muir (721), p. 6: "It was probably a fit of epilepsy; but Muslim legend has invested it with so many marvellous features as makes it difficult to discover the real facts." Whereas the clause is true, there is no evidence for the alleged probability of an epileptic fit.

moved a black clot of blood which they threw away (according to a parallel version, the blood was removed from the heart). Then they cleansed his abdomen with melted snow in a golden basin. They weighed him, and his weight surpassed that of a thousand of his people. When he was found, his color had changed, and Ḥalima's husband became frightened, thinking of some kind of demoniac affliction.[65] Whatever the real facts behind this legend may have been—if, indeed, there was a real event at all—they cannot be established now. To some extent this also holds true of Mohammed's inspirational states of which oral tradition tells. For instance, it was said that his face took on a dusky pale hue, that for an hour he resembled a drunken person, that sweat ran down from him like pearls. Sometimes Gabriel addressed him as man to man; sometimes the message came to him like the sound of a bell.[66] A vivid picture was drawn by his wife, 'Ā'isha, when she was suspected of infidelity and Mohammed awaited an inspiration from God about her guilt or innocence.

And, by God, the apostle had not moved from where he was sitting when there came over him from God what used to come over him and he was wrapped in his garment and a leather cushion was put under his head. . . . Then the apostle recovered and sat up and there fell from him as it were drops of water on a winter day,[67] and he began to wipe the sweat from his brow, saying, "Good news, 'Ā'isha! God has sent down (word) about your innocence." I said, "Praise be to God," and he went out to the men and addressed them and recited to them what God had sent down concerning that.[68]

In the Koran, Mohammed employed the *saj'*, the rhymed prose used by the *kāhin*,[69] and he thus gave good reason for being ranged within this class of persons, familiar in his milieu. His unbelieving compatriots considered him all kinds of things, a liar, a sorcerer, a *kāhin*, a *shā'ir*, or a man possessed.[70] Mohammed rejected these accusations as well as the imputation of receiving his message from a *jinn*.[71] Even one of his enemies is reported to have denied that Mohammed showed the signs of possession, viz., "choking, spasmodic movements and whispering."[72]

---

[65]Ibn Saad (528), *Biographie Mohammeds bis zur Flucht*, p. 70 (of the Arabic text); Ibn Isḥāq (525), *The Life of Muhammad*, pp. 71-72.

[66]Ibn Saad (528), *l.c.*, p. 131 f. (of the Arabic text).

[67]Mohammed sweated, although the day was cold.

[68]Ibn Isḥāq (525), *The Life of Muhammad*, (Guillaume's translation) p. 497. This was the origin of Sura 24, 11.

[69]Goldziher (417), pp. 68-71, and Archer (47), p. 21.

[70]Ibn Isḥāq (525), *l.c.*, p. 130.

[71]Ahrens (15), pp. 53 and 140, has collected pertinent passages. He believes that Mohammed, to some degree, actually conformed to the customs of ancient Arabic mantic art. Goldziher (417), p. 4 f., already had pointed out formal parallels of this kind. See also Buhl (184), p. 154 f.

[72]Ibn Isḥāq (525), *l.c.*, p. 121.

Whatever he was called in the early days of his mission, in the Islamic tradition he was apparently never called epileptic.[73]

The Islamic tradition makes it quite clear that during his inspirational states Mohammed was in an abnormal condition. But the deviations from everyday behavior were treated as signs of Mohammed's truly prophetic status. Ibn Khaldūn (1332–1406) incorporated them into his elaborate theory of prophecy built up from ancient and Islamic sources.[74] While the tradition lacks evidence of obvious suppression of symptoms, elaborations certainly took place to underline the unusual character of Mohammed's mission.[75] The material was presented as with the eyes of believers. We are not dealing with entries in a medical case history, and all sifting of "what really happened" from "what was believed" is tinged by the interpreter's bias.[76]

As is to be expected, the positive bias of Islam was countered by an opposite bias in the Christian world. As to the origin of the diagnosis "epilepsy," everything points to Christian Byzantium, an empire that was not only hostile to Islam but at frequent war with the Arabs. Less than 200 years after Mohammed's death, the Byzantine historian Theophanes (died about 817) told a story which was bound to make Mohammed appear a fraud and to discredit the belief in his divine mission. According to Theophanes, Mohammed

> had the disease of epilepsy. And when his wife noticed it, she was very much grieved that she, being of noble descent, was tied to such a man, who was not only poor but epileptic as well. Now he attempts to soothe her with the following words: "I see a vision of an angel called Gabriel and not being able to bear the sight of him, I become weak and fall down." But she had a certain monk for her friend who had been exiled because of his false faith and who was living there, so she reported everything to him, including the name of the angel. And this man, wanting to reassure her, said to her: "He has spoken true, for this angel is sent forth to all prophets." And she, having received the word of the pseudo-prophet, believed him and announced to the other women of her tribe that he was a prophet.[77]

This is the story which was accepted by Western historians, theologians, and physicians.[78] The story has all the earmarks of religious

---

[73] Cf. Archer (47), pp. 18–19.

[74] Ibn Khaldūn (527), *The Muqaddimah*, vol. 1, pp. 184–245; also Rahman (836), and Walzer (1065), p. 206 ff.

[75] For instance the story of what happened to Mohammed's camel when the Prophet became inspired; cf. Ibn Saad (528), *Biographie Mohammeds bis zur Flucht*, p. 131 (of the Arabic text).

[76] I think that most medical analyses of Mohammed's life, e.g., by Bey (109), are subject to this criticism.

[77] Theophanes (1007), *Chronographia*, vol. 1, p. 334.

[78] Nöldeke (736), 1, p. 24, n. 5, lists some names and works of those who propagated the story. Of physicians, Gabucinius (388), *De comitiali morbo*, fol. 6$^r$ f., gives Coelius Rhodiginus (not mentioned by Nöldeke) as his source.

and political propaganda. Hence it was repudiated by Gibbon as "an absurd calumny of the Greeks."[79]

Whether accepted as true or not, in the Middle Ages and the Renaissance it contributed to the belief in the existence of prophesying epileptics. But the mere assurance of their existence did not suffice. The conditions of the time demanded an answer to the general question whether faith and reliance could be placed in prophesies emanating from disease and particularly from epilepsy. The task of answering fell upon philosophers and theologians, who drew on theories which Antiquity had bequeathed to them.

### b. Epilepsy and Prophetic Trance

Following the example of anthropologists, it has become customary to distinguish between shamanistic and mediumistic prophecy.[80] The essence of the shamanistic theory was the soul's ability to prophesy when dissociated from the body, and such dissociation could take place in sleep or in ecstatic states. Pythagoras, Empedocles, and others have been credited with practices that allowed them at will to enter a state of dissociation.[81] A fragment from a writing of the young Aristotle tells of a king whose soul for days was suspended in an ecstasy between life and death. Afterward, the king related what he had seen and foreseen, and it all proved true.[82]

Through Cicero, the shamanistic theory received a formulation that deeply influenced Latin medieval thinkers. "When sleep has removed the soul from association and contact with the body, then the soul remembers things past, perceives the present, and foresees what is to come. For the body of the person asleep lies like that of one dead, yet the soul is strong and alive."[83] In these or similar words, the notion of the soul liberated in sleep or ecstasy became current among the Neo-Platonists as well.

There is reason to assume that some people credited disease with inducing dissociation. An allegedly old Pythagorean belief allowed the soul to develop mantic power "in the ecstatic states of disease."[84] This

---

[79] Gibbon (408), *Decline and Fall*, ch. 50; vol. 2, p. 690. Gibbon emphasized the silence of Islamic commentators and characterized his own authorities, Ockley and Gagnier, as having espoused "the charitable side."

[80] See Dodds (283), pp. 70, 71, and 88 n. 42.

[81] Cf. Detienne (266), pp. 79–82.

[82] Cf. Walzer (1065), pp. 38–47. In the *Ethica Eudemia* (56), VII, 14, 1248 A-B, which, according to Ross (874), p. 21, belongs to his early works, Aristotle mentions melancholics in connection with persons who are guided by divine inspiration rather than by reason and who have an immediate insight into the present and the future.

[83] Cicero (222), *De divinatione*, I, 30, 63; p. 294.

[84] Photius (794), *Bibliotheca* 439 A 14–19: εἰ γὰρ κατὰ ποσόν τι ἡ ψυχὴ τοῦ σώματος ἐν τῷ ζῆν τὸ ζῶον χωριζομένη βελτίων γίνεται ἑαυτῆς, ἔν τε τοῖς ὕπνοις κατὰ τοὺς ὀνείρους καὶ ἐν ταῖς ἐκστάσεσι τῶν νόσων μαντικὴ γίνεται, πολλῷ μᾶλλον βελτιοῦται, ὅταν τέλεον χωρισθῇ ἀπὸ τοῦ σώματος. The passage is from a biography of Pythagoras which Immisch has ascribed to

notion was reinforced by a passage from Plato's *Timaeus*, which asserted that prophecy was given to man as a divine gift. Yet true and divinely inspired prophecy was possible "only when the power of [man's] intelligence is fettered in sleep or when it is distraught by disease or by reason of some divine inspiration."[85] Reason came into its own when the person was in his right mind again and when he interpreted his visions or had them interpreted by others. This was mediumistic prophecy,[86] and the Sibyl, the Delphic Pythia, and other divinely inspired persons of ancient legend and institutional life fell into this category.[87]

Thus, the theoretical possibility of making disease a source of prophecy, shamanistic or mediumistic, existed. The pseudo-Aristotelian *Problems* declared Sibyls, soothsayers, and inspired persons possessed of a hot melancholic temperament,[88] and the Stoics allowed bodily changes to cause a withdrawal of the mantic element from present reality, inducing in turn a heightened susceptibility for things to come, Posidonius even admitting true visions to the frenzied and melancholic.[89] Aretaeus, possibly influenced by Posidonius, assigned a particular status to sufferers from heart disease, who were "more acute in their senses, so that they see and hear better than formerly; they are also in understanding more sound and in mind more pure, not only regarding present things, but also with regard to futurity they are true prophets."[90]

Yet there existed much reluctance to derive prophecy from somatic disease. "Divination belongs to a healthy soul and not to a sick body," said Cicero's Stoic spokesman.[91] Two hundred years later, Apuleius'

---

Agatharchides; cf. Detienne (266), p. 78. The connection of ἔκστασις with mental illness is found in Hippocrates (e.g., *Aphorisms*, VII, 5) and Aristotle (*Categories*, 8, 10 A 1: μανική ἔκστασις), where it need not mean a trance. Cf. Dodds (283a) pp. 70-72 and *passim*.

[85] Plato (802), *Timaeus*, 71 E; p. 187 (Bury's translation, italics mine). Here and for the following cf. Dodds (283), ch. 3, and Rosen (872), who adduces much modern literature on possession and on prophecy. I am indebted to Professor Harold Cherniss for having drawn my attention to the difficulty inherent in the interpretation of *Timaeus*, and I present the passage without any attempt at co-ordinating it within the context of Plato's own thought. There is some similarity between this passage and Aristotle (56), *Ethica Eudemia*, VII, 14; cf. above, footnote 82.

[86] *Timaeus*, 72 A-B; p. 186, where Plato calls these others "the tribe of prophets." Cf. Dodds (283), p. 70.

[87] Plato (801), *Phaedrus*, 244 A-B.

[88] Aristotle (55), *Problems*, 30, 1; 954 E 35 ff.

[89] Plutarch (813), *De defectu oraculorum*, 431 B; vol. 5, p. 468; and Cicero (222), *De divinatione*, I, 36, 79; p. 79, which, however, is partly contradicted, *ibid.*, I, 37, 81; p. 314. Cf. Dodds (283), ch. 3, and Rahman (836), p. 36 ff. and the corresponding notes. For Posidonius [according to Klibansky et al. (585), p. 44] cf. Sextus Empiricus (920), *Against the Logicians*, I, 247; vol. 2, p. 132: μυρίοι γὰρ φρενιτίζοντες καὶ μελαγχολῶντες ἀληθῆ μὲν ἕλκουσι φαντασίαν, οὐ καταληπτικὴν δέ . . . .

[90] Aretaeus (50), II, 3; p. 271 (Adams' translation). According to Kudlien (597), p. 7 f., these patients belong in the category of persons facing death.

[91] Cicero (222), *De divinatione*, I, 38, 81; p. 314.

defense of himself was similarly based.[92] Still later, the Neo-Platonist Iamblichus (about 300 A.D.) asked: "What resemblance is there between melancholy, or the other frenzies roused by the body, and divine possession? What prophecy ever originated from the diseases of the body."[93]

A certain hesitation to believe in the frequent occurrence of prophecy is discernible in the philosophy of the older Aristotle. He conceded its possibility, especially in "ecstatics," an expression which probably covered the abnormal states of the media of Greek oracles.[94] He based his opinion on the freedom from ordinary sense perceptions in sleep, when the soul's sensitivity to slight movements was heightened.[95] His treatment of the matter rested on a physiological and psychological analysis which offered scientific arguments for the admission or rejection of natural prophecy, arguments which the Western schoolmen were later free to use.

Aristotle taught that actual and imagined sense perceptions were attributable to the same faculty, viz., the sensitive faculty, which acted as the imaginative faculty when the real objects had gone yet had left their impressions behind.[96] In sleep, in emotional states, or in disease, when the mind was not in control, man might be guided by what he imagined.[97] In this sense, dreaming belonged to the imaginative faculty;[98] in a severe faint, imagination could still be active; even those who looked dead were known still to utter words.[99]

Avicenna was following Aristotle when he wrote that "diseases which weaken the body and alienate the soul from reason and from discernment"[100] were among the conditions that allowed the imaginative faculty to present its products as real. In particular, Avicenna mentioned "the insane person,"[101] but by chance, intent, or misunderstanding, his Latin translator rendered this by "the epileptic."[102] Since

---

[92] See above, p. 9.

[93] Iamblichus (523), *De mysteriis*, III, 25; p. 159 f., and III, 26 f.; cf. Lloyd (642), p. 296. According to Klibansky et al. (585), p. 44, it was the mystic in Iamblichus who raised these objections.

[94] See further below, also above, footnotes 55 and 82.

[95] Aristotle (53), *On Prophecy in Sleep*, 2, 464 A 12–17. By "movements" (κινήσεις) Aristotle meant any changes including such physiological processes as lead to sense perceptions.

[96] Aristotle (53), *On Dreams*, 1, 459 A 15 ff. and 24 ff.

[97] Aristotle (53), *On the Soul*, III, 3, 429 A 5 ff.

[98] Aristotle (53), *On Dreams*, 1, 459 A 21.

[99] Aristotle (53), *On Sleep and Waking*, 3, 456 B, 11–16.

[100] Avicenna (68), *De anima* 4, 2; p. 172: *kamā yakūnu 'inda l-'amrādi llatī taḍ'ufu l-badana wa-tashghalu n-nafsa 'ani l-'aqli wa-t-tamyīzi.*

[101] *Ibid.*, p. 173: *al-'insānu l-majnūnu.*

[102] Avicenna (70), *Liber de anima*, pars 4, c. 2; p. 18, 40: "et propter hoc videt epilepticus et perterritus et dissolutus et soporatus imaginationes existentes qualiter vere videt in tempore salutis et etiam audit sonos." Cf. *ibid.*, index s.v. *epilepticus.*

Aristotle himself had likened the epileptic seizure to sleep,[103] one of the conditions in which the mind failed to restrain the imaginative faculty, the Latin translation, consciously or not, remained within the sphere of Aristotelian thought. At any rate, epilepsy was acceptable as a disease that could lead to natural ecstasy marked by visions.

In his commentaries on the pertinent Aristotelian writings, Thomas Aquinas elaborated on Aristotle's explanation of epilepsy. Regarding Aristotle's reference to imagination in the quasi dead, St. Thomas added: "And the same reasoning holds good concerning those laboring under the falling sickness who are quasi dead, and concerning other affections of this kind which by some grave affliction cause a defect of sensation. For no such person is asleep."[104] If the latter statement implied a difficulty in the face of Aristotle's explicit characterization of "sleep being in a certain way an epileptic seizure," St. Thomas did not comment on it. He dealt with the physiology of the epileptic attack at some length, and he did so twice. At one point he wrote: ". . . a certain disease, called epilepsy, which is the falling sickness, originates because of the copious evaporations that ascend to the brain," etc.[105] The second passage referred to Aristotle's discussion of heat as a cause of sleep and of the latter as a cooling process.[106] Sleep, St. Thomas explained, originated because of the cooling of the food vapors carried to the head by the veins. Their heaviness caused them to flow down, thus obstructing the paths of the spirits and of the natural heat, which served sensation. Sleep was the inability to feel. "And thus the natural heat that was carried upwards from the heart is diminished and is driven away from the peripheral parts [of the body] by the descending coldness of the vapor, and the persons fall down. This can be understood of the falling of those overtaken by sleep as well as of epilepsy. And man is said to fall, because he alone is an animal of erect stature, and

---

[103] Aristotle (53), *On Sleep and Waking*, 3, 457 A 8; cf. above, p. 34.

[104] Thomas Aquinas (1012), On *De somno et vigilia*, lectio V, p. 225 (col. 1): "Eadem ratio est de laborantibus morbo caduco, qui sunt quasi mortui, et aliis hujusmodi passionibus defectum sensus facientibus aliqua passione gravi. Nullus enim talis dormit." My attention was drawn to this commentary by Dr. E. E. Krapf in his review of the first edition of *The Falling Sickness* (see *Revista de Psiquiatria y Criminologia*, March 30, 1947).—There existed an ancient tradition which ascribed prophetic gifts to a man facing death. Socrates, convicted to die, told his judges that he wished to prophesy to them, "for I am now at the point where men are most given to prophesy: when they are about to die." [Plato (801), *Apology*, 30, 39 C; p. 136]. This was believed true too in severe illness with a fatal outcome [Cicero (222), *De divinatione*, I, 30, 63; p. 294] ; cf. above, footnote 90.

[105] *Ibia.*, p. 225 (col. 2): "Et est, quod quidam morbus, qui vocatur epilepsia, qui est morbus caducus, fit propter multas evaporationes ascendentes ad cerebrum. Talis morbus est similis somno, et est quodammodo somnus: quia cum deberet somnus naturalis fieri propter superabundantiam vaporum densorum descendentium et obturantium venas, intantum tumefiunt venae quod arteria, per quam fit respiratio vitae, intantum constringitur, quod pene deficit spiramen vitae, et ita fit per somnum morbus. Unde et frequentius dormientibus accidit talis passio, et raro vigilantibus."

[106] Aristotle (53), *On Sleep and Waking*, 3, 457 B 6 ff.

therefore he alone can properly be said to fall. And when he falls, his intellectual power is the first to be changed, and his imagination next. And this is especially true of epilepsy."[107]

Though Aristotle had little faith in the prophetic nature of dreams, he admitted that some persons in a trance might see what is to come. In this condition, the familiar processes did not obtrude themselves but were eliminated, so that these persons were now very sensitive to what was foreign and strange.[108] St. Thomas re-stated Aristotle's opinion of the prophesying power of "ecstatics" in their sleep with little addition of his own.[109]

What the schoolmen had received from the ancients had now to be harmonized with Christian theology, which rested on the Bible and a trust in prophecy from God. But not all prophecy was divinely inspired. "Prophecy," said Thomas Aquinas, "properly and simply so called, arises from divine revelation alone. Yet when the revelation is made by demons it can be called prophecy in a relative sense. Hence those to whom something is revealed by demons, are not simply called prophets in the Scriptures, but with some addition, for instance, *false prophets*, or *prophets of the idols*."[110] Prophesying in an obvious state of upset was suspicious in itself. According to Jean Bodin, the first distinguishing mark between prophecy from God and the enchantments of Satan was increased fury and madness on the part of those inspired by demons, "whereas those who are inspired by God are at that time more sensible than ever."[111] But ancient philosophy had left open the possibility of prophecy in a natural state of ecstasy which had to be differentiated from both divine and satanic rapture. St. Thomas defined

---

[107]Thomas Aquinas (1012), On *De somno et vigilia*, lectio VI, p. 227 (col. 2): "Et sic minuitur calor naturalis, et fugatur a partibus exterioribus per vaporis frigiditatem descendentem, qui calor sursum ferebatur a corde, et cadunt homines. Et hoc potest intelligi de casu somni sive epilepsiae. Et dicuntur homines cadere, quia solus homo est animal rectae staturae. Et ideo de solis illis proprie dicitur cadere. Et cum cadit, primo habet virtutem intellectivam alteratam, et deinde phantasiam. Et illud proprie de epilepsia est verum."

[108]Aristotle (54), *On Prophecy in Sleep*, 2, 464 A 24: τοῦ δ'ἐνίους τῶν ἐκστατικῶν προορᾶν αἴτιον ὅτι αἱ οἰκεῖαι κινήσεις οὐκ ἐνοχλοῦσιν ἀλλ' ἀπορραπίζονται· τῶν ξενικῶν οὖν μάλιστα αἰσθάνονται.

[109]Thomas Aquinas (1012), On *De divinatione per somnum*, lectio II, p. 243 (col. 2): "Determinat de divinatione in somnis a parte somniantium; dicens, quod extatici bene praevident de somnis; et causa est, quia non sunt solliciti solum circa proprios motus sed circa alienos: et ideo maxime percipiunt per somnia quae fiunt circa aliquos."

[110]Thomas Aquinas (1014), *Summa theol.*, 2.2, quaest. 172, art. 5; vol. 3, col. 1212 f.: "Et ideo prophetia proprie et simpliciter dicta fit per solam divinam revelationem; sed ipsa revelatio facta per daemones potest secundum quid dici prophetia [text: prohetia]. Unde illi quibus aliquid per daemones revelatur, non dicuntur in scripturis prophetae simpliciter, sed cum aliqua additione *puta prophetae falsi*, vel *prophetae idolorum*. Unde augustinus 12, super Genes. ad litt. cap. 19 circ. fin.: *Cum malus spiritus arripit hominem in haec*, scilicet visa *aut daemoniacos facit, aut arreptitios, aut falsos prophetas*."

[111]Bodin (128), *De la démonomanie des sorciers*, 1, 4; fol. 24^V: "Mais il y a deux choses bien remarquables pour la difference de la Prophetie de Dieu, et des enchantemens de Satan. La premiere est que ceux, qui sont inspirez des Daemons, sont alors les plus furieux et insensez, et ceux qui sont inspirez de Dieu, sont alors plus sages que iamais."

rapture as a state in which the soul of man was abstracted from the perception of things discernible by the senses. Three different causes could bring about this "abstraction": a corporal cause, as in people whom disease had bereft of their reason; a demoniac power, as in persons possessed; and divine power.[112] From what was said before, epilepsy might well fit into the first category.

By its very definition, epilepsy was a disease in which the functions of the senses were impeded. Consequently, it was possible to make the term epilepsy so comprehensive as to include nearly all trance-like states. On the authority of Gentile da Foligno, Matthaeus Ferrarius argued that the term epilepsy could be used for any state where the external senses were distracted. In the Christian world, he wrote, people whose minds had "transcended to heaven" belonged in this category, while among the Saracens they were called prophets.[113]

Antonius Guainerius used such ideas to defend the epileptic prophet against the charge of demoniac possession. The ancients, he explained, had called epilepsy "divination" because in epilepsy "when the obstruction is strong, all the external senses are fettered so that all their operations are largely idle. Therefore, the rational soul, unhindered by things outside itself, remains within its plain being, so to speak, and sometimes happens to perceive what the future holds. Thus, when the paroxysm has passed, they very often predict many things to come. The crowd, ignorant of the cause, believes this to be effected by the power of the demons."[114]

---

[112]Thomas Aquinas (1014), *Summa theol.*, 2, 2, quaest. 175, art. 1; vol. 3, col. 1234 f.: "Et ideo quando abstrahitur [i.e., anima hominis] a sensibilium apprehensione, dicitur rapi, etiamsi elevetur ad ea ad quae naturaliter ordinatur, dum tamen hoc non fiat ex propria intentione; sicut accidit in somno, qui est secundum naturam, unde non potest proprie raptus dici. Hujusmodi autem abstractio, ad quaecumque fiat, potest ex triplici causa contingere: uno modo ex causa corporali, sicut accidit in his qui propter aliquam infirmitatem alienationem patiuntur; secundo modo ex virtute daemonum, sicut patet in arreptitiis; tertio modo ex virtute divina. . . ."

[113]Matthaeus Ferrarius (352), *Practica*, fol. 44^V: "De hac difficultate [i.e., epilepsy without material cause] Gentilis multa dicit: sed summarie ponitur duplex distinctio. Una est quod epilepsia dupliciter sumitur. Uno modo large secundum quid nominis termini: quoaniam ut dicit Açaravius in principio capituli de epilepsia: intentio nominis est apprehendens sensus: sumitur igitur large pro qualibet distractione ab operationibus sensuum exteriorum: et hec sola imaginatio et fortis attentio vel consideratio facit ad epilepsiam: quia ad occupationem sensuum exteriorum: et ita in lege nostra dicit Gentilis tales sunt ad celestia transcendentes: et secundum sarracenos: ut dicit ipse prophete appellantur: qui sunt maxime attenti circa spiritualia: ita quod aliquando non sentiant etiam occurrente causa extrinseca ledente: et de hac non est sermo." Cf. below, footnote 115.

[114]Antonius Guainerius (438), *Tractatus de egritudinibus capitis*, VII, 1; fol. 11^r: "Divinatio autem a quibusdam dicitur: ut ille bonus Serapio inquit: quia eam ex parte demonum provenire putabant: sed eius pace illa eorum non fuit intentio: sed eam appellabant divinationem: quia in epilepsia in qua fortis fit oppilatio sensus omnes exteriores ita ligantur: ut fere ab omnibus eorum operationibus vacent: propter quod anima rationalis aliunde non impedita in suo simplici esse quasi remanet: quo fit ut quandoque futura deprehendat. amoto itaque paroxismo plurima persepe futura praedicunt: unde vulgares causam ignorantes demonum virtute hoc fieri putant: et hanc ob causam divinatio nonnulli veteres hunc morbum appellant. Et ego quemdam iuvenem cholericum vidi qui se aiebat in paroxismis semper miranda videre: quae

This was a clear assertion that the epileptic really could predict the future. Antonius Guainerius stood in a line of Neo-Platonic philosophers which went back to Averroës (1126-98) and Witelo (thirteenth century) and extended into the Renaissance. To show the increased functioning of the inner powers when the external ones were at rest, Averroës cited the example of persons in deep thought and of those born blind and deaf. Prophecy then might occur in a state similar to epilepsy, for when the inner powers were in the grip of strong motions, the external powers could be reduced to the point of loss of consciousness (syncope).[115]

Epilepsy, syncope, and divine rapture were all brought together in the Neo-Platonic philosophy of Agrippa of Nettesheim (1486-1535). He defined rapture as "an abstraction, alienation, and illumination of the soul, originating from God, whereby God draws the soul, which has fallen from the upper regions to the lower, back from the lower regions to the upper." Its cause, within us, was "a continuous contemplation of sublime things." By this supreme effort of the mind the soul was connected with incorporeal wisdom, while at the same time it was being withdrawn from sensible things and from the body. "And (as Plato says) this may go so far that sometimes the soul escapes the body and may be as though let loose."[116]

The connection between true rapture and epilepsy was established by Agrippa in a chapter "On rapture, ecstasy, and divination in those who are seized by epilepsy and fainting, and in the dying."[117] "In some manner," he declared, "fainting and epilepsy imitate rapture, and very often prophecies issue forth in them just as in a rapture. We read of

---

summe cupiebat litteris demandari. ille enim indubio futura esse sperabat. hanc igitur ob causam veteres divinatio hunc morbum appellant." Cf. above, p. 150. On Antonius Guainerius as a forerunner of Marsilius Ficinus cf. Klibansky et al. (585), p. 95 ff.

[115] Averroes (65), *Compendium libri Aristotelis de sompno et vigilia*, p. 114 f. "Et signum eius, quod virtutes interiores sunt perfectioris actionis apud quietem virtutum exteriorum, est quod illi qui multum cogitant intrant sue virtutes sensibiles intra corpus, ita quod accidit eis sompnus magnus; et ipsi etiam sponte faciunt quiescere sensus extrinsecos, ut melius cogitent. Et propter hanc causam illi qui nati sunt sine visu et sine auditu sunt perfectiores secundum virtutes interiores. Ideo prophetia venit in dispositione simili epilepsie: iste enim virtutes interiores, quando movebuntur forti motu, contrahentur virtutes exteriores, adeo quod forte accidet ex hoc syncopis." Cf. Thorndike (1021), vol. 5, p. 87 and (1020), p. 135, for Henri Bate of Melines (1246 to about 1310) who also associated epilepsy with prophecy.

[116] Agrippa ab Nettesheim (14), *De occulta philosophia*, p. cccxvii: "Raptus est abstractio, et alienatio et illustratio animae a deo proveniens, per quem deus animam a superis delapsam ad infera, rursus ab inferis retrahit ad supera. Huius causa est in nobis continua contemplatio subliminorum, quae quatenus profundissima mentis intentione animum incorporeae sapientiae coniungit, eatenus vehementioribus suis agitationibus ipsum a sensibilibus corporeque sevocat, et (ut inquit Plato) taliter quandoque quod nonnunquam corpus ipsum vel effugiat et quasi dissolvi videatur, quemadmodum Aurelius Augustinus narrat de sacerdote Calamensi (cuius supra meminimus)." The latter reference is to book 3, ch. 47; p. cccxxii: "sic sacerdos Calamensis (teste Aurelio Augustino) solebat sese suo arbitratu querula quadam harmonica evocare a corpore in raptum et extasim." The priest was from a town in Numidia.

[117] *Ibid.*, p. cccxvi. "De raptu et extasi, et vaticiniis quae iis qui morbo comitiali et syncopi corripiuntur, et quae agonizantibus contingunt."

Hercules and of very many Arabs who excelled in this kind of proph-esying."[118] Agrippa did not identify divine rapture and epileptic states; obviously their causes were different. Syncope and epilepsy only imi-tated divine rapture; but the imitation was close enough to allow the epileptic to prophesy—whether truly or not Agrippa did not make clear.

The epileptic prophet had a place in Renaissance thought, though this place was an ambiguous one. All epileptic visions could be regarded with suspicion, they could be explained naturally, or they could be accepted as truly prophetic even with the help of God or of demons. The resulting differences of opinion were great, but the lack of a con-sensus is hardly surprising in a time in which orthodox theology, Eras-mian tolerance, religious rebellion, burning of witches, and the practice of magic and hermetic philosophies existed side by side.

## 3. SOME SOCIAL ASPECTS

### a. Great Epileptics

Among the ancient books preserved, the Aristotelian *Problems* were the first to connect epilepsy and genius,[119] and very likely it was this source which suggested to Marsilius Ficinus that Hercules was an epilep-tic prophet. In 1602 Taxil said that Aristotle made a whole catalogue of famous epileptics in which he named Hercules, Ajax, Bellerophon, Socrates, Plato, Empedocles, Maracus of Syracuse, and the Sybils.[120] As a matter of fact these persons were considered melancholics by the author of the *Problems*, and although he believed epilepsy a melan-cholic affliction, it was Hercules alone whom he brought into definite connection with the sacred disease. Taxil's statement, therefore, was not exact, and there is no reason to assume that Empedocles, Socrates,

---

[118] *Ibid.*, p. cccxvii. "Syncopis etiam morbique comitialis raptum quodammodo imitantur, atque in ipsis saepissime sicut in raptu vaticinia proveniunt, quo quidem vaticinandi genere legimus Herculem Arabesque quam plures excelluisse." Here Agrippa seems to borrow from Marsilius Ficinus (356), *De vita triplica*, XIII, c. 2; fol. 217$^V$: "Sequitur vacatio quae fit per syncopam id est, per casum corporis semivivi: quando cordis defectu spiritus ad membra non mittuntur: et qui in membris sunt. retrahuntur ad cordis debilitati praesidium: quo in statu perinde ut in somno provenit vaticinium. Quo excelluisse Hercules dicitur, Arabesque permulti, qui comitiali morbo corripiebantur." Marsilius Ficinus apparently thought that in syncope the spirits no longer maintained communication between the sense organ and the heart so that sense perception stopped and the soul, withdrawn within itself, became prophetic. Agrippa of Nettesheim and Marsilius Ficinus are discussed at length by Klibansky et al. (585), pp. 254, 278, and 351 ff. Much of that discussion has a bearing on epilepsy too, but it seems that the demonistic elements in Agrippa's theory which Klibansky notices were not essential for Agrippa's explanation of epileptic rapture.

[119] Aristotle (55), *Problems*, 30, 1; vol. 2, p. 154.

[120] Taxil (994), *Traicté de l'épilepsie*, p. 137 f. ". . . ce philosophe [i.e., Aristotle] en faict un catalogue, proposant un Hercule, un Aiax, Bellerophon, Socrates, Platon, Empedocles, Maracus Siracusain, et les Sibylles, ausquels nous pourrions adiouster Iule Caesar, et Caligula Empereurs, Liuius Drusus, premier tribun du peuple Romain, Petrarche; et encore que ce detestable Mahomet, . . . et de nostre temps, noz practiciens nomment entre les grands Epilep-tiques, encores un Charles Quint, Empereur et Roy des Espaignes. . . ."

and Plato suffered from epilepsy. But regarding the names of later personalities mentioned by Taxil[121] and other physicians of the time, historical evidence is sounder. Of Drusus, the tribune of the Roman people, Pliny reports that he was cured of epilepsy by undergoing a treatment with hellebore on the island of Anticyra.[122] For Julius Caesar there is the testimony of Plutarch,[123] Suetonius,[124] and Appian,[125] which firmly established him among "the great epileptics." Petrarch refers to him,[126] and so, of course, does Shakespeare.[127] While the attacks are well attested for Caesar's middle age, there is some doubt about their appearance in his youth, and the idiopathic nature of the disease is not altogether certain.[128] The epilepsy of the Emperor Caligula is attested by Suetonius.[129] Petrarch's attacks began in old age and were probably caused by arteriosclerosis or some other disease.[130] The number of "great epileptics" known in the Renaissance also includes the Emperor Charles V and the poet Torquato Tasso. Their names are mentioned by contemporary physicians. Rondelet (1507-66), who was only seven years younger than Charles, alludes to the latter's sickness,[131] and Ballonius (1538-1616) cites the case of Tasso as confirmation of the Hippocratic view concerning the relation

---

[121] Cf. preceding footnote.

[122] Pliny (806), *Nat. hist.*, 25, 52; vol. 4, p. 77.

[123] Plutarch (812), *Caesar*, c. 17; vol. 7, p. 482. *Ibid.*, c. 53, pp. 566-68.

[124] Suetonius (977), *Julius Caesar*, 45; vol. 1, p. 62; cf. below, footnote 128.

[125] Appian (42), *The Civil Wars*, II, c. 16; vol. 3, p. 428.

[126] Dr. Thomas C. Benedek kindly has supplied me with a passage from Twyne's English version of Petrarch's *De remediis utriusque fortunae*. (*Physicke against Fortune*, translated by Thomas Twyne [London: Richard Watkyns, 1579], p. 302). Here "Reason" says: "Thou canst not fall into that [i.e., a trance] twyce. For none dyeth more than once: and whiche shoulde be the best kynde of death, there was somtyme disputation among certayne learned and notable men, at whiche was Iulius Caesar in presence, for empire and learnyng a most excellent personage: who also in his latter tyme, as some wryte of hym, used many tymes to faynt suddeynly, which question he in this manner determined, concludyng, that a suddeine and unlookedfor death, was of al the most commodious." The scholar Petrarch did not overlook the allegedly late onset of the fainting spells in Caesar's life.

[127] Shakespeare, *Julius Caesar*, Act 1, scene 2.

[128] Cf. Kanngiesser (574). Donnadieu (291) maintains that Caesar's epilepsy was pretended in order to impress people by the supernatural disease, the *morbus regius*. While it is true that a late Latin commentator (465), p. 645, 22 ff., identifies the *morbus regius* with the *morbus comitialis*, and although this identification is repeated in a doctoral thesis of 1571 (81), fol. B[1] "Ἐπιληψία, morbus . . . Regius item aliquibus (quod alias Icteri est nomen) . . . nominatur," it still remains very doubtful whether this is more than a confusion with the name for icterus. Esser (330), pp. 24-29 takes idiopathic epilepsy for granted, but he also adduces the material that points to a relatively late beginning of the attacks, e.g., the rumor that they first appeared in Corduba, related by Plutarch (812), *Caesar*, c. 17; vol. 7, p. 482, and Suetonius (977), book 1, ch. 45; vol. 1, p. 62: ". . . nisi quod tempore extremo repente animo linqui atque etiam per somnum exterreri solebat. Comitiali quoque morbo bis inter res agendas correptus est." Regarding the beginning and frequency of convulsive attacks, to which *comitiali morbo* seems to refer, the statement is not altogether clear. Dragotti (298) takes a somewhat skeptical view, also criticizing the diagnosis of Menière's disease which has been offered as an alternative.

[129] Suetonius (977), *Caligula*, 50; vol. 1, p. 480.

[130] For Petrarch cf. Dorez (788).

[131] Rondeletius (866), *Methodus curandi morbos*, I, 36; p. 172: "Haec annotavi, ut intelligerent studiosi epilepsiam fieri et a pituita tenui, et a spumosa, vel a bile flava, vel attenuata

of epilepsy and melancholy. Having been treated in vain for severe epileptic attacks by the physicians, Tasso was cured by nature herself. For he became mad, and when his madness disappeared, his epilepsy disappeared likewise.[132]

The knowledge that even great men might suffer from epilepsy culminated paradoxically in the belief that most epileptics were men of great intelligence.[133] This was an extension of the [Pseudo]-Aristotelian thesis that melancholy and genius went together. Rondelet said that epilepsy was more frequent in Florence than in other regions of Italy, chiefly because of the thin and very sensitive substance of the brains of the citizens, an assumption which he thought proved by their sharp-sighted cleverness and acute power of judgment."[134] The idea was stressed to an extreme in Campanella's *City of the Sun*. The inhabitants of this utopia were described as employing various remedies against "the sacred disease, from which they often suffer." And it was added: "This is a sign of great talent, wherefore Hercules, Socrates, Mohammed, Scotus, and Callimachus suffered from it."[135]

The lists of "great" epileptics compiled during the Renaissance contained names famous in the history of the West. So strong was the tradition that even in the nineteenth century, when new names were added, they were rarely chosen from among epileptics in other parts of the world. For instance, the epileptic emperors of Byzantium, Zenon (474-491), Michael IV (1034-41), and possibly others,[136] usually did

---

atra, aut eius ichoribus, vel a vaporibus acribus, vel ab odoratu, propter cerebri exactiorem sensum. Hinc efficitur, ut qui ingenii acumine pollent, huic morbo frequenter obnoxii sint, ut de Caesare, Mahumete, Carolo quinto Imperatore scriptum legimus."

[132] Ballonius (77), *Consil. medic.*, I, cons. 33; p. 124 f.: "Quod ne cui mirum videatur, huc celebris historia Equitis Torquati pertinebit. Hic cum crudelissimis Epilepsiae insultibus saepe decuteretur, suppetias nulla ex parte nactus est. At quod sua prudentia et consilio ars medica non consequitur, id instinctu solo bruto natura aptissime contigit. Nam eum furibundum reddidit, furendi tandem et brevi tempore finis fuit. Ab eo tempore epilepsiae molestias non sensit. Et illud est quod scriptis celebravit Hippocrates, *Epileptici fiunt melancholici, et contra.*"

[133] Taxil (994), *Traicté de l'épilepsie* (ch. 15), p. 137: "Que la plus part des Epileptiques sont hommes de grand entendement, et que là ou il y a beaucoup d'Epileptiques, là aussi y a beaucoup d'hommes de grand entendement."

[134] Rondeletius, *l.c.*, p. 173: "Frequentius in aliquibus regionibus morbus hic, quam in aliis grassatur, ut Florentiae magis est familiaris, quam in alia Italiae parte. Quod tribus de caussis accidere puto. Prima et potissima, est substantia cerebri tenuis et valde sensilis, ob quem sensum facilem hunc morbum incurrunt, ut melancholici dicuntur natura ingeniosi. Quod autem substantiam habeant subtilem, ostendit eorum civium perspicax ingenium et iudicium acre. Altera caussa esse potest victus ratio vaporosa et flatulenta. Tertiam esse puto, quod hic morbus sit hereditarius. Cum enim multi olim hunc morbum passi sunt, plures liberos ad eum suscipiendum idoneos procreant." Petrus Forestus (369), *Observationum* X, observ. 57, scholia; p. 386, quotes this passage from Rondelet and adds "ut Petrarchae contigit" (after "natura ingeniosi").

[135] Campanella (198), *La città del sole*, pp. 31-32: "[*Genovese*] ... Usano li bagni et olij all' usanza antica, e ci trovano molti più secreti per star netti, sani, gagliardi, si sforzano con questi et altri modi aiutarsi contro il morbo sacro, che ne patono spesso. *Hospitalario.*—Segno d' ingegno grande, onde Ercole, Socrate, Macometto, Scoto et Callimaco ne patirono."

[136] Jeanselme (562) mentions six epileptics on the throne of Byzantium. Apart from Zenon and Michael IV, they are: Michael V (1041-42), Isaac Comnenus (1057-59), John Vatatzes (1222-54), and Theodore II Lascaris (1254-58).

not appear on the lists of the nineteenth century. Historians, of course, knew about their diseases. Gibbon, in speaking of Zoe, the treacherous wife of Romanus III, who after her husband's death married Michael, wrote that her hopes were disappointed. "Instead of a vigorous and grateful lover, she had placed in her bed a miserable wretch, whose health and reason were impaired by epileptic fits."[137] But Michael IV, though a ruler, was little known in the West and not a great man, not even a paragon of evil. His exclusion, and that of others like him, suggests that interest centered on the diseases of the famous rather than on an objective psychological study of epileptics outstanding in political and cultural life.

### b. Beggars and Cheats

That epileptics were sometimes considered prophets or men of genius ought not to obscure the fact that during the Middle Ages and Renaissance, as well as in later centuries, epilepsy was looked upon as a heinous disease. "A plague upon your epileptic visage!" says Kent to the despised Oswald in King Lear.[138] Apart from the horror of the symptoms, the conviction that epilepsy was incurable must have contributed to its fearful reputation. That such a conviction existed among the laity is demonstrated by Berthold of Regensburg, who said that even the greatest physicians, including Hippocrates, could not cure the disease if it had lasted for more than twenty-four years. As for the physicians themselves, their views were not much different, in spite of the various kinds of treatment which they prescribed. They pretended to have tests by means of which they could ascertain whether a patient really had been cured. These tests were often identical with those used by the ancients to diagnose epilepsy, and indeed the same tests were still recommended for diagnostic purposes as well.[139] It has been pointed out that in Antiquity such procedures were motivated by the necessity of discovering diseases in slaves for sale; but with the practical disappearance of slavery in western Europe the need for such a quick diagnosis had also gone. Now goat's horn was burned to decide whether the patient had been completely cured.[140] This and other tests could

---

[137]Gibbon (408), Decline and Fall, ch. 48; vol. 2, p. 556. Michael IV's attacks are described in detail by Psellus (829), Chronographia, book 3, 22, p. 51, and book 4, where Psellus shows him as torn by regrets for his shameful actions.

[138]Shakespeare, King Lear, Act III, scene 2, 86. For a different interpretation cf. Friedlander (380), p. 116.

[139]Cf., e.g., Konrad of Megenberg (591), Das Buch der Natur, III, 12; p. 128, 16-18. Agricola (13), De natura eorum quae effluunt ex terra, II, p. 545.

[140]Arnald of Villanova (58), Breviarium, I, c. 13; col. 1075: "Item si vis scire an curatus sit epilepticus, an non, accipe cornu caprinum, vel lapidem achate, et pulverisa alterum eorum, et pulverem huius super carbones ardentes pone, et patiens fumum recipiat per os ex eis, et si non est perfecte curatus, statim cadit . . . si vero perfecte curatus est, non cadit." Cf. also Antonius Guainerius (438), Tractatus de egritundinibus capitis, VII, 3; fol. 12$^r$.

also be applied to find out whether an epileptic was curable at all. Laurentius Phriesen, for instance, advised the introduction of a needle into the ear. If the patient felt the prick, the case was hopeful, otherwise not.[141]

The desire to find out whether an epileptic was definitely cured was natural enough. However, during the Middle Ages the need of proof was sometimes accentuated by a more definite problem. The Church numbered epilepsy among the irregularities, i.e., the reasons which might prevent a person from taking orders as a priest.[142] It was important to know when an epileptic might be considered definitely cured and could consequently be ordained. The question was discussed at length among the canonists, and here again application of the various traditional tests was proposed.[143]

But the medieval physicians knew that in spite of everything chronic cases offered little hope. Bernard of Gordon described various signs and tests which were meant to decide the curability of the case, but he ended these descriptions with the following frank statement: "Nevertheless, I tell you, concerning epilepsy, that I have had in my treatment many people, young and old, rich and poor, men and women, suffering from almost every kind of epilepsy.—Yet I have not seen any one cured either by me or by another, except perhaps a child or when the disease had originated from a bad regimen and was not of long standing—yet I have been very careful in everything and the patients obedient. I am ignorant, but God has knowledge. And I say this for the following reason: When patients come to you, do not dishonor yourselves with empty and false promises in the treatment of epilepsy, since almost all epilepsy is eradicated with great difficulty—if indeed it can be eradicated."[144]

The epileptic was therefore considered a poor wretch, deserving pity, compassion, and special consideration. This being the case, certain people found it profitable to simulate epilepsy. One of the oldest cases of simulated epilepsy is described in an ancient Greek novel. A young girl, Antheia, is forced into prostitution; in order to evade such a fate

---

[141] Laurentius Phriesen (795), *Spiegel der artzney*, fol. 80ᵛ. Similarly, Arnald of Villanova, *l.c.*, col. 1076, where the nose is named instead of the ear.

[142] Cf. *Corpus iuris canonici* (239), vol. 1, col. 123. Similarly, among the Jews an epileptic was *ipso facto* excluded from the priesthood; cf. Preuss (822), p. 344.

[143] Cf. Zacchias (1115), *Quaest. medico-legal.*, p. 629 ff.

[144] Bernard of Gordon (106), *Lilium medicinae*, fol. 119ʳ: "Tamen dico vobis de epilepsia, quod ego habui in cura multos iuvenes, senes, pauperes, divites, viros, et mulieres, et fere de omni specie epilepsiae, et tamen nec per me, nec per alium vidi aliquem curatum, nisi esset puer, aut quod provenisset ex malo regimine, et quod non multum durasset, tamen fui diligentissimus in omnibus, et patientes obedientes, ego nescio, tamen deus scit. Et hic dico propter hoc, quod cum patientes venerint ad vos, nolite dehonestare vosipsos cum vanis et falsis promissionibus in curatione epilepsiae, quia fere omnis epilepsia cum magna difficultate eradicatur, dato quod eradicari possit."

she feigns an epileptic attack and invents the following tale: One night when she passed a new grave, the ghost of the buried man appeared and struck her on the chest. This blow, she claims, caused her malady.[145] In this case it would have been the awe and disgust inspired by epilepsy on which the girl counted when simulating the disease in self-defense. In the Middle Ages and the following centuries, the motive for simulating was mainly the desire to exploit the compassion felt by friendly people. How beggars used to imitate epileptic attacks has been described by Ambroise Paré, who speaks of "Such as falling down counterfeit the falling sickness, binde straitly both their wrests with plates of iron, tumble and rowl themselvs in the mire, sprinkle and defile their heads and faces with beasts bloud, and shake their limbs and whole bodie. Lastly, by putting sope into their mouths, they foam at the mouth like those that have the falling sickness."[146]

These beggars developed a jargon of their own and in sixteenth century England referred to epilepsy as the "Cranke." The story of such a "Counterfet Cranke" comes from Thomas Harman, who met the man in question in 1566. The pretended epileptic, whose picture Harman included (cf. Fig. 3), was clad in rags, his face was smeared with blood, and he gave the following fraudulent account of himself: " 'Syr,' saythe he, 'I was borne at Leycestar, my name is Nycholas Genings, and I haue had this falling sycknes viii. yeares, and I can get no remedy for the same; for I haue it by kinde, my father had it and my friendes before me; and I haue byne these two yeares here about London, and a yeare and a halfe in bethelem.' 'Why, wast thou out of thy wyttes?' quoth I. 'Ye, syr, that I was.' "[147] Harman exposed the impostor, who, of course, had never been in the hospital of St. Mary of Bethlehem. Yet the question whether he had been insane seems to prove that mere convulsions without impairment of mind would not have secured admission to the madhouse.

Beggars of this type were not confined to England and France. In Germany at the beginning of the sixteenth century, they were known as *Grantners*,[148] and a hundred years later we find them in Italy as *Accadenti*, one out of thirty-four classes of vagabonds.[149] Sometimes they cooperated with other criminals by simulating an attack in some public place; while the crowd gathered around, the companion would pick the pockets of the bystanders.[150]

---

[145]Cf. Rohde (861), pp. 414–15.

[146]Paré (773), *Of Monsters and Prodigies*, p. 672 (Johnson's translation).

[147]Cf. Harman (455), *A Caueat*, pp. 51 and 52.

[148]Cf. Ribton-Turner (845), p. 545.

[149]Cf. *ibid.*, p. 557 f.

[150]The case of such a "dummy chucker" who operated in London, as well as in this country, was published by MacDonald in 1880. The pretender used to cut his tongue with a

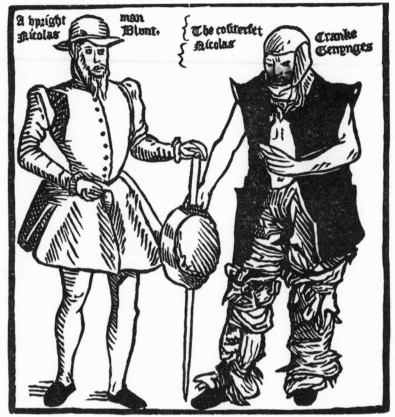

These two pyctures, lyuely set out,
One bodye and soule, god send him more grace.
This mounstrous desembelar, a Cranke all about.
Vncomly couetinge, of eche to imbrace,
Money or wares, as he made his race.
And sometyme a marynar, and a saruinge man,
Or els an artificer, as he would fayne than.
Such shyftes he vsed, beinge well tryed,
A bandoninge labour, tyll he was espyed.
Conding punishment, for his dissimulation,
He sewerly receaued with much declination [2]

Fig. 3

Beggar simulating epileptic. (Thomas Harman,
*A Caueat or Warening for Commen Cursetors
vulgarely called Vagabones*, ed. E. Viles and
F. J. Furnivall, Early English Text Society,
1869, p. 50.)

Begging and stealing were, of course, not the only motives for simulating epilepsy. The evasion of punishment and of torture also came into consideration. As late as the eighteenth century, Alberti reported a case which had been referred to the medical faculty of Halle for decision. While in jail and threatened with torture a woman had exhibited attacks and had claimed to suffer from epilepsy. After a thorough discussion of all the details, the faculty decided that epilepsy was out of the question, that the symptoms were feigned, and that therefore the torture would not endanger the woman's life.[151] Later, when universal military conscription was introduced in many European countries, the desire to evade service acted as one of the most powerful stimulants.[152]

The task of detecting feigned epilepsy was not an easy one. When the great French psychiatrist, Esquirol, once claimed that it was possible to discover any simulated case of epilepsy, his pupil, Calmeil, suddenly fell down with all the symptoms of a typical epileptic attack. Esquirol expressed his concern about the unfortunate young man, but the latter arose and proved to his master that he had let himself be deceived.[153] The methods used for the unmasking of feigned epilepsy were manifold and changed with the times. The simulant might not be thoroughly acquainted with the symptoms of the disease and might, for example, give himself away by closing his hands again after they had once been opened. He would, moreover, be eager to talk about his illness and to make it known to everybody, while the real epileptic would rather try to hide the fact. All such indications, however, were not reliable, since

---

knife and even risked serious falls in order to evade detection. He really succeeded in deceiving a great number of medical experts. Cf. MacDonald (655).

[151] Alberti (18), *Systema jurisprudentiae medicae*, tom. I, appendix pp. 104–7. On p. 209 of this volume Alberti cites literature on simulated epilepsy.

[152] Cf. Esquirol (329), *Des maladies mentales*, vol. 1, p. 315, and Bresler (150), p. 9. The unusual motive of feigning epileptic attacks in order to break a betrothal is the theme of Rudyard Kipling's (583a), *The Post that Fitted*. It tells the story of a subaltern, Sleary, who is in love with a girl called Carrie, yet too poor to marry her. Having been sent to the East, Sleary becomes engaged to Minnie Boffkin whose father obtains for him a remunerative political job: "Just the thing for me and Carrie." To induce Minnie to break the engagement, he imitates epileptic attacks, for which "Pears's shaving stick" provides the froth. The young lady returns the ring and

> Sleary bore the information with a chastened holy joy,—
> Epileptic fits don't matter in Political employ,—
> Wired three short words to Carrie—took his ticket, packed his
>       kit—
> Bade farewell to Minnie Boffkin in one last, long, lingering fit.
>
> Four weeks later, Carrie Sleary read—and laughed until she wept . . .
> Mrs. Boffkin's warning letter on the "wretched epilept." . . .
> Year by year, in pious patience, vengeful Mrs. Boffkin sits
> Waiting for the Sleary babies to develop Sleary's fits.

Critchley (246), p. 56, footnote, thinks that Kipling may have consulted Gowers on the poem, though it contains nothing unknown to the imposters of old.

[153] Cf. Trousseau (1032), *Clinique médicale*, p. 90.

the simulant might be sufficiently informed to avoid these and similar mistakes. More objective tests were needed, and for many centuries the physicians put their main trust in actual infliction of pain or at least in threats of painful operations. Thus, while the patient was supposedly unconscious the physician explained that castration or cauterization would have to be performed. Such threats often had the wished-for result: the person would immediately rise and beg to be spared such treatment. We shall have to come back to this method in connection with the common eighteenth-century belief that hysterical convulsions were simulated epilepsy. One more test may be mentioned here, because it implies the record of an important diagnostic sign as early as the middle of the eighteenth century. One day a girl suffering from severe deafness was brought before the Viennese clinician De Haen. This complaint having been treated successfully, the girl was brought back by her mother because she was now subject to convulsive attacks. "In order to examine her conveniently," tells De Haen, "I ordered the girl to be kept in the hospital. On the same day I saw her lying in bed in convulsions, and in the middle of her convulsions she shut her thumbs so strongly in her fists that with the greatest effort I could only just release them. She rolled her eyes in a dreadful way. Yet I suspected fraud, first because during the paroxysm the eyes were opened, not blinking, but in a quite healthy manner; secondly, because the pulse was almost normal; thirdly, *because the pupil dilated when the curtains of the bed were closed and, on the other hand, contracted when the curtains were opened*; fourthly, because the pupils contracted very vigorously when a candle was brought near and the girl turned her head as if she felt some harm coming from it."[154] De Haen's suspicions were correct: both the epileptic attacks and the deafness had been simulated.

We have dwelt upon the simulation of epilepsy at some length, because to some extent it illustrates the commiseration felt with the epileptic from the Middle Ages on. The beggar counted on the pity of the public when simulating the disease, and the prisoner condemned to torture speculated on the dispensation that might thus be granted to him. How important this aspect was in the mind of the medieval and Renaissance physician becomes evident from the writings of Paracelsus.

---

[154]De Haen (446), *Ratio medendi*, p. 130 ff.: "Adducebatur mihi puella gravi auditu laborans. Quo revellentibus, et factis in aurem injectionibus, restituto, Convulsiones suboriebantur, quas hoc ordine contingere Mater narrabat. . . . Commodo meo morbum examinaturus, puellam jussi in Nosocomio servari. Vidi illam, eadem die, in lecto decumbentem, convulsam, mediisque in Convulsionibus pollices adeo fortiter intra pugnos firmare, ut maxima vi vix solvere valerem. Oculos horrende agitabat. Attamen dolum subesse suspicabar. 1$^{mo}$, quod oculi durante Paroxysmo non connivendo, sed sano prorsum modo, aperirentur. 2$^{do}$ Quod pulsus fere naturalis esset. 3$^{tio}$ Quod cortinis lecti clausis pupilla dilataretur, vicissimque apertis iisdem contraheretur. 4$^{to}$ Quod pupillae admota candela vividissime se contraherent, et puella quasi nocumentum inde percipiens, caput rotaret."

## 4. PARACELSUS AND HERMETIC MEDICINE

### a. Paracelsus

The feeling that traditional methods were not successful in effecting a cure of chronic epilepsy explains the significance of this disease for the great reformatory attempt of Paracelsus. As early as around 1520 this physician included a chapter on the falling sickness in a collection of pathological essays.[155] About five years later Paracelsus wrote on the pathology and treatment of epilepsy in a psychiatric context.[156] Then, in 1530, he devoted two books to the Falling Evil, the first dealing with the disease in general,[157] the second with the disease from the uterus.[158] In all these works the approach to epilepsy, though similar, is by no means uniform.[159] Since the first book of the treatise of 1530 is the latest of the three and represents the most elaborate presentation, it may serve as a basis for an interpretation of Paracelsus' ideas.

Paracelsus does not begin with an explanation of the name, symptoms, and causes of epilepsy, as might be expected. Instead, the first paragraph deals with compassion as a necessary virtue of the physician. The doctors are accused of lacking compassion for their patients, and yet compassion is the very basis of medicine. For it is the mission of medicine to make sick people recognize God's love. If the doctor is not willing to transmit compassion and love, he will be deprived of his necessary knowledge and will fail in his duty.[160] The heathen think that it is nature's law which effects cures, while the Christians realize that they cannot command nature. Just as man has no innate right to his daily bread but must pray for it, so he has no right to the knowledge of

---

[155] *Elf Traktat von Ursprung, Ursachen, Zeichen und Kur einzelner Krankheiten.* Paracelsus (770), vol. 1, pp. 142-52: "Vom fallend."

[156] *Von den Krankheiten die der Vernunft berauben.* Paracelsus (770), vol. 2, pp. 393-99: "Vom fallenden siechtagen," pp. 427-34: "De cura caduci." In Paracelsus (769), p. 129 ff., Zilboorg has offered an English translation of this treatise.

[157] Paracelsus (770), vol. 8, p. 263: *Von den hinfallenden siechtagen.*

[158] *Ibid.,* p. 319: *De caducis liber secundus, nemlich de caduco matricis das ist, vom hinfallenden siechtagen der mutter, so allein den frauen anhangt.*

[159] The parts dealing with epilepsy in the first two works (see above footnotes 155 and 156) have been analyzed by Pagel (762), p. 167 ff., who has drawn attention to similarities between Paracelsus' chemical imagery and the older theory of catarrh. Particularly, in the *Elf Traktat,* Paracelsus (770), vol. 1, p. 143, ascribes the epileptic attack to an odor reaching the brain, which is at the same time stupefying (like henbane and poppy), inebriating, and mordent, qualities possessed by sulfur of vitriol. If the sulfur in man's body is kindled, the ascending fume is the disease (p. 145). The sulfur will be ignited by the bodily counterpart of a cosmic force. Cf. Pagel (762), p. 167, and (763), p. 114 f. In *Von den Krankheiten die der Vernunft berauben* it is the spirit of life which, when converted into a dynamic agent, can cause epilepsy; cf. Pagel (762), p. 168.

[160] Paracelsus (770), *Von den hinfallenden siechtagen;* vol. 8, p. 264: "dan die arznei und der arzt seind allein darumb, das durch sie der krank entpfintlich sehe und merk die liebe und barmherzikeit gottes, wo nun der arzt in solcher lieb und barmherzikeit nicht geneigt ist, so wird er beraubt des jenigen so im zu wissen zustehet."

medicine but must ask for it. It is true that remedies grow without prayer, but they would be of little avail if we did not know them or how to use them. If we do not pray for this knowledge, we shall never acquire it.[161] Now it is the physician's office to know everything about diseases and in particular about such severe afflictions as epilepsy. Doctors who thrive on slight diseases which cure themselves, but pretend that epilepsy is incurable, are frauds.[162] If the physician loves his patients, then he will obtain the necessary knowledge for his cures, for God has provided remedies for all diseases, including epilepsy.[163] To doubt the curability of this disease means to belie God, our creator, as well as the forces of man.[164] God wants to be glorified in the great diseases; He has created remedies for them so that His great works may be recognized! Therefore, the physician ought not to despair, but should learn and search and should not put his trust in imperfect books.[165]

Paracelsus was not the first to ask for divine help in the treatment of epilepsy or to be moved by love for the sick. Arnald of Villanova too had appealed to Jesus Christ and his compassion for the sufferers from this "unfortunate disease."[166] If He Who on His wanderings had cured the lunatic without compensation did not assist, the experience of the physicians would be idle.[167] Deeming that there existed no greater misfortune than this disease, Arnald was moved to write his work and sought the guidance of the Holy Spirit.[168] But Paracelsus expresses more than the religious sentiment that might be expected from a medieval physician. His denial of the incurability of epilepsy shakes the pious resignation which made Bernard of Gordon exclaim: "I am ignorant, but God has knowledge."[169] Instead, he declares it the physician's duty to search for an effective cure. And whereas Arnald of Villanova remained in the framework of traditional medical doctrine, Paracelsus

---

[161] *Ibid.*, pp. 264–65.

[162] *Ibid.*, p. 266.

[163] *Ibid.*, pp. 266–67.

[164] *Ibid.*, p. 268.

[165] *Ibid.*, p. 269; cf. below, footnote 170.

[166] Arnald of Villanova (58), *De epilepsia*, c. 21; col. 1624: "Medicum supremum, Iesum Christum, obsecro, compatiens toti generi humano ab hoc languore infelici obsesso, et potissime populo Christiano, ut per suam dignam misericordiam tenebras meae ignorantiae dignetur lumine suae gratiae illustrare, ut valeam doctrinam componere, per quam haec species lugubra morbi lunatici curetur faciliter, et resistatur eidem, quam confidens gratis in munere accipere."

[167] *Ibid.*, c. 11, col. 1617: "Eo autem redactus est, ut languori infelici eius, nullo modo Medicorum peritia subvenire possit, nisi summo Medico Iesu Christo opitulante, qui peregre proficiscens, morbum lunaticum gratis curavit."

[168] *Ibid.*, c. 9; col. 1610: ". . . ideo compatiens, ut omnibus eiusmodi morbo infelici obsessis succurrere anxius valeam, et opitulari utilius spiritu sancto duce. . . ."

[169] Cf. above, p. 165.

condemns the books of the authorities. Since they do not help to restore the patient, they are of the Devil.[170] A new way has to be found to explain and to treat the disease, a way which Paracelsus outlined in the subsequent paragraphs of his work, the way of hermetic medicine.

In some respects Paracelsus' attitude is similar to the teachings of the religious and ethical reformers of his century. The interpretation which he gives of the physician's piety puts main emphasis on the fulfilment of the duty to which God has ordained him. To do his duty the physician must be willing to tread new paths and glorify God by new discoveries. Thus, it is not by mere chance that the work on epilepsy gives Paracelsus occasion to expound his ethical ideas. He was well aware that his refusal to admit the existence of incurable diseases must rouse the opposition of his contemporaries, and he points to this objection in his *Seven Defensiones*, a little book in which he tried to defend himself against the accusations made against him. In the very first of these defenses, he deals with the argument that his work is concerned with such incurable diseases as the falling evil, St. Vitus' dance, and gout. Here again his defense ends with an exhortation to further research. "So take heed what is told thee; the rest shall be sought after until the art is found from which good works proceed. For if Christ says: *Perscrutamini Scripturas*, why should I not say of this: *Perscrutamini Naturas Rerum?*"[171]

For both friends and foes of Paracelsus his ideas about epilepsy assumed particular importance. Among his followers, the iatrochemists of the sixteenth and part of the seventeenth century, the cure of epilepsy was a favorite topic. This is understandable if we realize that they liked to proclaim the efficacy of their new remedies for diseases where the old remedies had failed. The adversaries of Paracelsus and of the iatrochemists, on the other hand, were aware of the necessity for a counterattack. Of the four "disputations" which Thomas Erastus (1523–83) directed against Paracelsus, the last was largely devoted to epilepsy.[172] Others returned Paracelsus' accusation by saying that a man who promised to cure leprosy, epilepsy, and possession must be mad.[173] They even blamed him for his alleged willingness to learn from the devils and demons.[174] Thus it was that in the sixteenth century

---

[170]Paracelsus (770), *l.c.*, p. 269: "verlass sich keiner in die geschrift, dan sie ist nit volkomen sonder nichts als ein anweisung aller verzagnus und verzweiflung, nemlich vom teufel und nit von got erdacht."

[171]Paracelsus (769), *Seven Defensiones*, p. 15 (C. Lilian Temkin's translation; cf. also her introduction). The relationship between Paracelsus and Protestant ethics has been elucidated by von Waltershausen (1064).

[172]I have, unfortunately, not been able to obtain a copy of this particular disputation in this country. Cf. Thorndike (1021), vol. 5, p. 652 ff., and Pagel (762), p. 327 f.

[173]Cf. Temkin (1001), p. 258.

[174]*Ibid.*

epilepsy became an important topic in the arguments about medical progress which, in accordance with the character of the time, were of a religious nature.[175]

Paracelsus' work on the falling evil offers great difficulties to the understanding of the modern reader. There is first of all his archaic style and his use of a language not yet adapted to clear scientific reasoning. More important, however, is the difficulty presented by the form of reasoning he employs. His doctrine of epilepsy is not based upon an analysis of direct causes and effects, but upon an interpretation by cosmic analogies.

Paracelsus starts out with the fundamental analogy between microcosm and macrocosm. Man, the microcosm, has in himself everything that exists in the outer world, the macrocosm. The latter is man's "mirror." The theory of what man is in his healthy and diseased state and the anatomy of man have to be discovered by the study of the macrocosm. For the microcosm cannot be understood by itself. Even human diseases correspond to diseases in the outer world. They must first be traced and understood in the outer world, and this will then enable the physician to understand them in the human being too. The pathology of epilepsy must, therefore, not proceed from human anatomy or physiology. The cosmic phenomenon which corresponds to the falling sickness has to be perceived and interpreted, and this will yield an explanation of epilepsy in man.[176] The macrocosm is divided into two parts, Heaven and Earth, and each of these comprises two elements. Fire and air are the elements of Heaven, earth and water are the elements of the Earth. By "elements" Paracelsus does not, however, mean the traditional elements of ancient science.[177] Elements for him are the strata of the cosmos, the "mothers" of things, which bear various fruits. Thus the plants are the fruits of earth, metals and stones those of water, dew is born of air, rain of fire. But apart from their fruits, the elements also show "impressions." Whereas the fruit of fire is rain, its impression is the thunderstorm. These impressions correspond to disease, and in the element of fire, thunderstorm corresponds to epilepsy.[178]

The material from which a thunderstorm is born is mercury, sulphur, and salt. They form its *corpora* just as the body of man is composed of the same chemical principles. For a while the body of a thunderstorm is surrounded by a shell or skin, and as long as this body remains whole

---

[175] Cf. Pagel (766), for the influence of religious thought on scientific progress. Pagel's two books (761, 762) should be consulted for Paracelsus' doctrines in general and for the intellectual background of his work.

[176] Paracelsus (770), *Von den hinfallenden siechtagen*; vol. 8, pp. 273-74.

[177] At least not in the work under discussion.

[178] *L.c.*, pp. 274-75.

the effect of mercury, sulphur, and salt remains enclosed in it. But when the time comes, thunder disrupts its shell and breaks forth.[179]

The genesis of thunder is one form of the genesis of epilepsy in man. There are three more forms corresponding to the fruits and impressions of the other three elements. As fire gives birth to a thunderstorm, earth engenders the earthquake, water the storm, and air a milder form of thunderstorm without rain, hail, and real lightning. Altogether, therefore, the macrocosm reveals four kinds of epilepsy.[180]

Out of mercury, sulphur, and salt, thunder and its analogues in the four elements grow like embryos, enveloped in their skins, which they finally burst. There is a principle of time involved which regulates the growth and birth of these cosmic phenomena. Each element has its *astrum*, its stars which form certain conjunctions and by their course regulate the event of things. Just as seasons follow the revolutions of the heavenly bodies, so every element has its own stars, though they be invisible to the eye. And just as the astronomer predicts future events from the stars, so one must study the stars of all elements to foresee what is to come. For the physician, it is imperative to be skilled in these sciences if he is to understand and to predict the course of the disease. He must be able to read the signs of fire, air, earth, and water; he must be an astronomer of the four elements. "Thus man is nothing but mercury, sulphur, and salt. Now where these three are, there is an astrum and each if fourfold. And thus there is *one* body in the great and in the small world, and it is different only for the eyes."[181]

Having thus outlined the macrocosmic pattern of the paroxysm, Paracelsus compares it step by step with the microcosmic fit. When a thunderstorm is on its way, the weather changes, the animals notice it and become restless. So man too becomes terrified when he feels an epileptic attack approaching. Then clouds gather in the sky, while man's eyesight becomes weakened and he feels sleepy. Next comes the wind, sweeping everything away; in the epileptic, the inner wind makes his abdomen and neck swell. Now the thunder breaks forth, shaking heaven and earth; now the epileptic is convulsed in all his limbs. The thunder sends forth lightning and the epileptic has sheer fire before his eyes. The thunder sheds its rain; the epileptic emits froth. Hail and a stroke of lightning break walls and disrupt everything—so the epileptic's limbs are bent and even broken by the force of the invisible storm and lightning in his body. When the thunderstorm is over the sun begins to shine, but it takes time until it has dried the wetness of the rain and the

---

[179] *Ibid.*, pp. 275-76.

[180] *Ibid.*, pp. 276-79.

[181] *Ibid.*, p. 280: "also ist der mensch nichts als allein ein mercurius, sulphur und sal. wo nun dise drei sind, do ist das astrum und ein ietlichs ist vierfach und also ist ein corpus in der grossen und kleinen welt als allein vor den augen underscheiden."

muddy ways. Likewise, the reason, body, and senses of the epileptic rest until the sun of the microcosm has restored them and he comes back to his former normal state.[182]

Paracelsus assigns the severest epileptic paroxysms to the stars of fire, then follow earth and water, and finally air, whose stars can be recognized in the weakest fits. He emphasizes that the paroxysm can change from one element to another or can even present a mixture of them all. The physician must be able to diagnose the kind of stars under which the patient suffers—but this as well as the knowledge of the manifold symptoms of epileptic attacks Paracelsus leaves to the experience of the medical reader.[183] He now turns to the therapy, which forms the main subject of the following paragraphs.

*Corpora* and stars both act together to form the disease. The only possibility of treatment is to take away the *corpora* from the influence of the stars, since the stars and their operations cannot be changed by man. Such separation can be effected either before the *corpora* are formed and the stars have got a hold over them, or when the time of the "harvest" has come.[184] Paracelsus elucidates this idea by the analogy of conception and the growth of seed. The stars must have their right constellation for seed to be conceived and grow well. If seed and stars do not correspond, something will be wrong; disease will grow with the seed. As far as the generation of man is concerned, God has not given us the knowledge of the right constellations, and we cannot escape disease. All we can do is to cure it by separating the *corpora* and submitting every *corpus* to its proper stars. How this is to be understood Paracelsus explains by the following example. Water and oil are useful and necessary, each of itself. But if mixed together in fire, they are dangerous. They can only be separated in the athanar, the chemical oven, not by mere handicraft. Similarly, in epilepsy the *corpora* correspond to water and oil, the stars to the fire, and the separation of the *corpora* can only be effected by "spagiric arcana," i.e., healing potencies which act analogously to a chemical process. These will separate the *corpora*, break the fatal conjunctions, and put the right *corpus* under its proper star without destroying anything.[185]

But Paracelsus does not immediately proceed to name appropriate remedies. Instead he turns to a consideration of the art of healing. Art, he thinks, was not given man when he was created in Paradise. When Adam was driven out of Paradise and when God told him: "In the sweat of thy face shalt thou eat bread," the second creation took place

---

[182] *Ibid.*, pp. 281–84.

[183] *Ibid.*, pp. 284–85.

[184] *Ibid.*, p. 286.

[185] *Ibid.*, pp. 287–90.

and "the light of nature" was given to him.[186] Now it was that he acquired knowledge, but not all at once; in the light of nature he and his descendents began to learn arts and crafts. Since the light of nature is in every man, knowledge develops from it, just as plants grow forth from the earth. But such potential knowledge must be revealed to the mind of man, therapeutic knowledge in particular, and there are various ways in which this takes place. Spirits, especially angels, have revealed to man the knowledge hidden in him, a chance experience has shown a cure, the similarity of forms between disease and remedy may have indicated the right way. Paracelsus specifies seven ways in which art may be acquired, and he hints at many more.[187] Only then does he return to the treatment of epilepsy, which he arranges in the order of these ways of acquiring art and of which we shall give but a few examples.

There is first of all the revelation by spirits, good or evil,[188] and here Paracelsus mentions three remedies: mistletoe, blood from a decapitated man, and pieces of the human skull. All three of them were known and used before him, but he adds characteristic touches. Mistletoe is good for epilepsy from the element of water and will separate the "epileptic conjunctions" of Venus and Moon, Moon and Saturn, or Saturn and Venus. It must, therefore, be prepared when these planets are in the ascendant; otherwise mistletoe would be of no avail. Similarly, in the administration of human blood certain astrological rules must be heeded, and so generally in all remedies. Regarding the use of the human skull, Paracelsus disapproves of the physicians who use just any of its bones. "There is one bone in the head and it is at its very center: when this bone is drunk, man recovers. . . . The bone is not broader than a penny, somewhat angular, split at the rear, and is not found in all skulls but in some."[189]

As is to be expected, chemical remedies play a great role in Paracelsus' therapy of epilepsy, among them preparations of gold and coral, remedies which he believes to have been discovered by black art.[190] On the other hand, he rejects ordinary oil of vitriol because it does not

---

[186] *Ibid.*, pp. 290–91.

[187] *Ibid.*, pp. 291–94.

[188] *Ibid.*, pp. 296–99.

[189] *Ibid.*, p. 298 f.: "ein bein ist am haupt und nemlich es ist gerad und gleich der centrum, so dasselbig getrunken wird, so geniest der mensch. nun ist aber sein process also und nit wie in die gemeinen arzt getan haben. dieselbigen haben al hirnschalen gefeilet und zu trinken geben; dieselbigen haben getan, wie sie dan in allen dingen nichts sollen. das bein ist nicht uber ein kreuzer breit, etwas ecklet und spalt sich selbs hinden und wirt nit in allen schalen gefunden sonder in etlichen; dan die astra spalten und nit die corpora, auch nit die geburt." The existence of sutural bones here described by Paracelsus was denied by Erastus but reaffirmed by Doringius, Fabricius Hildanus, and others; cf. Sennert (913), *Pract. med.*, I, pars 2, c. 31; vol. 2, p. 240.

[190] Cf. *l.c.*, p. 301.

contain the arcana, i.e., the curative potencies. To be of help in epilepsy vitriol must be made volatile, since it is volatility which commands the stars.[191]

Elsewhere, Paracelsus had given prescriptions how to prepare the spirit of vitriol[192] which, modern chemists suggest, contained ether.[193] He stated that chickens would fall asleep after consuming it, and it may well be that they served him as experimental animals.[194] Paracelsus set great store by the virtue of vitriol. "Regarding what I wrote to you about the vitriol, I strongly beseech you to look at the miserably ill in the falling sickness. May every physician consider his own conscience, God his creator, and [the] love of his neighbor, and may he not reject, refuse, and despise God's gift in the vitriol! Rather, for love's sake, work day and night in these matters, that none may be found idle and all engaged in the work that goes to the profit of your neighbor."[195]

### b. Allegories

The great self-assurance of Paracelsus finds expression in his attacks upon other medical and scientific doctrines. Yet there is a difference between the vehemence with which he opposes the traditional Aristotelian and Galenic teaching and his refutation of older astrological, alchemistic, and magic beliefs. He rejects the former but tries to reform the latter and to give them a broader basis and a wider purpose. Astrology becomes the science of the laws which govern the world and man; alchemy is the art which transforms raw materials into useful things; necromancy, geomancy, cheiromancy, etc., are methods of finding the corresponding properties between diseases and remedies. But however modern the aims of these Paracelsian doctrines may at times appear, they remain bound to their magic, alchemistic, and astrological inheritance. Although Paracelsus initiated a new scientific movement which became important not least for the pathology of epilepsy, he also imparted to it a bias for uncritical and credulous empiricism. On the whole, the iatrochemists of the sixteenth and seventeenth centuries were more superstitious in their therapy than other medical schools.

---

[191] Cf. *ibid.*, pp. 306-7.

[192] Paracelsus (770), *Von den natürlichen Dingen*, ch. 8; vol. 2, p. 146 ff., especially pp. 149-65.

[193] Cf. Pagel (761), pp. 22-24 and (763), pp. 113 and 114. It has to be noted that Paracelsus describes various ways of preparing vitriol for epilepsy, and he particularly praises the spirit of the green oil of vitriol. When, for its preparation, Paracelsus (770), vol. 2, p. 161, advises the use of the mixture suggested for preparing the *spiritus vitrioli*, he may be referring to the alcohol mentioned *ibid.*, p. 154.

[194] Pagel (761), p. 23, and in detail, Pagel (763, 764, 765), where the findings of Eis (317), pp. 1-10, are considered. The reference to the effect on chicken of sulfur obtained from vitriol occurs in Paracelsus (770), *Von den natürlichen Dingen*, ch. 7; vol. 2, p. 133: "das in die hüner all essen und aber entschlafen auf ein zeit, on schaden wider aufstont."

[195] Paracelsus (770), vol. 2, p. 165.

Even such physicians as Sennert or Ettmüller, who would not easily have recognized Paracelsus for their master, abound in antiepileptic remedies of the crudest kind.

In Paracelsus and his followers various mystic ideas about epilepsy are concentrated, ideas stemming from former centuries as well as from their own time. These mystic trends can be recognized in the unchecked use of analogies and in symbolic and allegorical interpretations.

A great many ancient and popular superstitious remedies for epilepsy were probably suggested by some vague analogy to certain symptoms of the disease. Usually the analogy is not expressly stated, but under the influence of the belief in cosmic sympathies and the doctrine of signatures it sometimes finds a rather naïve expression. Pierre Borel, for instance, an iatrochemist of the later seventeenth century, relates the beneficial effect of powdered soap-wort seed, offered for three months at the time of the new moon. He points out that the plant has a "signature" of its property, for if rubbed in water it emits a soap-like foam and is therefore profitable to the frothing epileptics.[196] Long before Paracelsus, however, St. Hildegard had explained the use of a peculiar remedy by various analogies. She recommends a prescription in which the blood of a mole, the beak of a duck, and the nails of a goose are principal ingredients. "For because the mole sometimes shows itself, sometimes keeps out of sight, and because it is wont to dig the earth, its blood resists this disease which at times is felt, but at others hidden." The beak of the duck and the nails of the goose are credited with similar strange properties. Besides, both birds should be of the female sex, "because a woman is more silent than a man, just as this disease is silent until the hour when it has thrown man down."[197]

The symbolic analogies on which St. Hildegard bases her therapy are somehow related to the custom of the alchemists to imply a second and deeper meaning to purely chemical processes. This peculiarity of hermetic philosophy was so well known that it even helped to defend some of the absurdities of the system. Aldrovandi, the famous zoologist of the sixteenth century, quotes some epileptic cures which he had found under the name of one Artephius. He emphasizes that these "experiments . . . contain a parabolic meaning, since they refer to the chemical

---

[196]Petrus Borellus (137), *Historiarum et observationum . . . centuriae*, Observatio 18; p. 27: "Pulvere seminis saponariae ante paroxismos sumpto, semel in mense per tria novilunia ad drag. I. observavi paroxismos valde minui, tum numero, tum violentia. Idque in filia 25. annos nata tentavi, cum felici successu. Nota etiam hanc herbam signaturam hujus proprietatis habere, spumam enim, si in aqua fricetur, saponis instar emittit (unde ei nomen inditum) sicque spumantibus Epilepticis confert." This way of reasoning may have existed in Antiquity regarding frothy poppy; cf. above, II-3c.

[197]St. Hildegard (883), *Causae et curae*, IV; pp. 206–7. A German interpretation of St. Hildegard's work has been offered by Schipperges (884).

art. Therefore they should not be explained literally, for if understood in this way one would be obliged to call them not only incredible but even ridiculous."[198]

The symbolism of alchemy was only one aspect of the allegorical interpretation of the world so popular among philosophers and theologians of the Middle Ages and the Renaissance. It found its source in hermetic traditions, in Neoplatonic mysticism, and, above all, in the allegorical interpretation of the Bible. Origen had already applied this method to the interpretation of the New Testament. The lunatic boy and his father represented the erring soul and its guardian angel.[199] This method transformed an isolated event narrated in the Gospel into general moral and religious sentiments and was extremely popular among theological writers. Thomas Aquinas' exposition of the New Testament, in which he presented a running commentary from various Church Fathers, contains ample material for the mystic interpretation of epilepsy. With reference to St. Mark ix, Theophilus, for instance, says: "This demon is deaf and dumb, deaf in as far as he does not want to hear the speech of God, and truly dumb in as far as he does not want to teach others as it is fitting."[200] St. Bede speculates on the words of St. Matthew, where the boy is called lunatic, and on those of St. Mark, where he is described as deaf and dumb. He thinks that this refers to those who change like the moon, waxing and waning in various vices, who are dumb in not confessing faith, and who are deaf in not listening to the sermon of faith.[201]

The educated of that theological age must have been imbued with similar ideas. Aldrovandi's curious work on monsters contains a whole chapter dealing with the "moral" interpretation of diseases, and the passage on epilepsy almost sounds like a continuation of the words of the Church Fathers. Epilepsy is compared to pride, and the pathology of the disease is brought into close parallel with the features of this vice.

---

[198] Aldrovandi (20), *Monstrorum historia*; p. 117: "Caeterum hic est advertendum, quod haec experimenta Artephii in Scholiis Paracelsi recitata parabolicam sententiam continent, quoniam ad artem chymicam spectant, et diriguntur, ideoque iuxta litteralem sensum, non sunt exponenda; hac enim ratione, non solum incredibilia, sed etiam tanquam ridicula essent celebranda."

[199] Origenes (756), *Coment. in Matth.*, t. 13; col. 1102 f.

[200] Thomas Aquinas (1013), *Expositio continua* [re St. Mark IX]; vol. 4, p. 235: "THEOPH. Daemon autem iste surdus et mutus est: surdus, inquantum non vult Dei sermones audire; mutus vero, inquantum non vult alios, quod condecens est, docere."

[201] *Ibid.* [re St. Luke IX]; vol. 5, p. 435: "BEDA. Mystice autem pro qualitate. . . . Hunc autem daemoniacum Matthaeus lunaticum (cap. 17), Marcus surdum et mutum (cap. 9) describit. Significat enim illos qui ut luna mutantur (Eccl., 27, v. 12) per diversa vitia crescentes et decrescentes; qui muti sunt, non confitendo fidem; et surdi nec ipsum fidei audiendo sermonem."

This affliction [i.e., epilepsy] must beyond doubt be likened to the disease of pride, which in truth can be called a sacred disease, since it triumphs over saintly and perfect men. Likewise, epilepsy is called a damage, so to say, of the upper regions, and not without reason since it has cast down the highest angels. For we read in Holy Script: The Lord has destroyed the seats of proud princes. Thus this affliction of pride is generated when the bad humors of an empty little glory are carried to the ventricles of the mind. This is truly the case when man contemplates the nobility of his birth, the strength of his body, and the amount of his riches, or when he flatters himself extraordinarily over some mediocre literary fame. For then every process of correct function is impeded and the soul falls headlong from the state of grace; and so the tremor of despair, the stridor of wrath and perturbation, the froth of malediction, and the distortion of the face, namely the ugliness of a bad habit, are brought about.[202]

With these ideas in mind we can now understand the following from *The Ancren Riwle*, a treatise on the rules and duties of monastic life, written in the thirteenth century:

The sparrow hath yet another property which is very good for an anchoress, although it is hated; that is, the falling sickness. For it is very necessary that an anchoress of holy and highly pious life have the falling sickness. I do not mean the sickness which is commonly so called; but that which I call falling sickness is an infirmity of the body, or temptation of carnal frailty, by which she seems to herself to fall down from her holy and exalted piety. She would otherwise grow presumptuous, or have too good an opinion of herself, and so come to nothing. The flesh would rebel and become too insubordinate towards its mistress, if it were not beaten, and would make the soul sick, if sickness did not subdue the body with disease, nor the spirit with sin. If neither of these were sick—which is seldom the case—pride would awaken, which is the most dangerous of all sicknesses. If God try an anchoress with any external evil; or, the enemy within, with spiritual disorders, as pride, wrath, envy, or with the lusts of the flesh, she hath the falling sickness, which is said to be the sparrows' infirmity. God so wills it, in order that she may be always

---

[202] Aldrovandi (20), *Monstrorum historia*, p. 256: "Succedit Epilepsia consideranda, morbus capitis praecipuus, ita a Grecis nuncupatus, quia partes superiores comprehendantur, alioquin inter varia nomina, quibus insignitur, morbus sacer cognominatur. Oritur hic affectus, quando humoribus ventriculos cerebri occupantibus, transitus spirituum animalium intercipitur; tuncque patiens convulsus cadit, et cum spuma circa os, stridore dentium, et tortura faciei, toto corpore contremiscere videtur. Haec affectio procul dubio aegritudini superbiae assimilanda est, quae re vera sacer morbus nuncupari potest, cum de viris sanctis, et perfectis triumphum egerit. Item Epilepsia vocatur quasi noxa partium superiorum, nec praeter rationem, cum supernos Angelos prostraverit: legitur enim in sacris paginis. [In Ecclesiast. ca. 10]. *Sedes ducum superborum destruxit Dominus.* Generatur ergo hic affectus superbiae, quando pravi humores inanis gloriolae ad ventriculos mentis feruntur; nimirum quando homo nobilitatem generis, robur corporis, et copiam divitiarum contemplatur, vel quando nomine mediocris cuiusdam litterationis sibi mirifice ablanditur; tunc enim omnis motus rectae operationis impeditur, et anima de statu gratiae praeceps cadit; sicque tremor desperationis, stridor irae, et perturbationis, spuma maledictionis, et tortura vultus, nempe turpitudo malae consuetudinis introducitur."

humble; and, with low estimation of herself, fall to the earth, lest she become proud.[203]

This paragraph summarizes medieval ideas on the falling evil, ideas which, as we have seen, extended far into the Renaissance. The sparrow was popularly believed to be subject to the disease,[204] and Valescus de Tharanta had even dissected the brain of an epileptic sparrow. *The Ancren Riwle*, moreover, uses the vague term "the falling sickness." It does not mean the disease that is usually called so, i.e., epilepsy; rather it means any infirmity which is followed by humiliation and contrition.

### c. Van Helmont

To men brought up in such traditions Paracelsus' way of thinking was much more understandable than to later generations. However great the unwillingness on the part of the majority of physicians to follow his ways, even very sober minds did not escape occasional turns in the same direction. When Georg Agricola, the younger contemporary of Paracelsus, acknowledged the ability of the emerald to avert epilepsy if worn as an amulet or in a ring, he repeated a very old belief. But his explanation of this phenomenon represents more than mere credulity. He states that the emerald fights with epilepsy as with a deadly enemy. If the stone is stronger than the disease, it remains whole; if, however, it is conquered by the disease, it is broken into several parts.[205] Besides, an essential part of Paracelsian doctrines, the chemical explanation of disease, survived even if separated from the theological and philosophical aspects of his work. With the end of the sixteenth century the tendency began to grow to combine iatrochemical with more orthodox views, and various chemists of the seventeenth century opposed the arbitrary symbolism of the earlier alchemists. It is true that at the same time the Rosicrucians tended to combine chemistry with religious mysticism, but this movement became esoteric and lost its connection with the development of medicine.[206] The more concrete attitude can

---

[203] *The Ancren Riwle* (31), p. 177 (Morton's translation).

[204] This idea possibly goes back to St. Matthew X: 29: "Are not two sparrows sold for a farthing? and one of them shall not fall on the ground without your Father." Konrad of Megenberg (591), *Das Buch der Natur*, III, 61; p. 220, 20-22, gives a more rationalistic explanation: "si leident auch in etleichen landen daz vallend leit. daz geschiht allermaist dâ von, daz si ezzent den sâmen iusquiami, daz haizt pilsensâm." For epilepsy in birds cf. Mingazzini (703).

[205] Agricola (13), *De natura fossilium*, VI; p. 622: "at cum comitiali morbo, tamquam cum hoste capitali ita pugnat, ut vel ipse vincat vim morbi minorem, vel a majore vincatur: illo modo manet integer et solidus, hoc in aliquot frangitur partes: itaque reges et divites eum de collo puerorum suspendentes, et gestantes in annulo, saepius periclitantur, si possint illius viribus pellere horrendum istum morbum."

[206] On the fate of hermetic, mystic, and rosicrucian ideas in the seventeenth century cf. Pagel (766). On the influence of Paracelsus and van Helmont on medicine in seventeenth

even be recognized in the scattered passages of van Helmont (1577-1644) where this last of the great hermetic philosophers deals with epilepsy.

According to van Helmont, the sensitive soul, the very principle of life, is situated in the folds of the stomach, especially its orifice. Here it is that the duumvirate of stomach and spleen regulates the functions of life, and here it is that epilepsy is engendered.[207] When the duumvirate "withdraws its government," epilepsies or other diseases result.[208] When the "sharpness of the Stomach doth degenerate, and associate it self with an opiate or drowsie poyson, with a piercing toward the seat of the Soul, the falling evil is straightway present."[209] This is one very important departure from the established theory. Van Helmont concedes that the "occasional nest" of epilepsy may be in the head or feet, "yet the Epileptical fit doth never depart, the which leaves not Thirst behind it, and by that Sign it bewrays that it had pitched its Fold in the Stomack, and that the sensitive Soul was smitten in that part especially, where in it planted the thirsting Power." The phenomenon of epilepsy even serves to prove the location of the sensitive soul in the stomach. "Therefore the Epilepsy painfully and at unawares invading all the Superiority of the sensitive Soul, sitting in the Stomack, doth argue the very seat of the Soul to be there."[210]

The other departure from contemporary theory is van Helmont's denial that epileptic attacks arise from any retained matter or superfluities in the body,[211] or that vapors or fumes are lifted upward.[212] His explanation of epilepsy as a chronic disease is quite different. In the stomach, which is primarily affected, hurtful images are stamped,[213] and the idea of the disease is imprinted into the "Spirit of Life"[214] and acts as a perpetual source of contagion. But although the disease thus originates in the stomach and can be provoked by strong emotions affecting the sensitive soul, it takes on its full character in the head,

---

century England and especially on the relationship of physicians and apothecaries cf. Debus (258), Rattansi (837a), and Thomas (1014a).

[207] Cf. Van Helmont (479), *The Seat of Diseases in the Sensitive Soul, Is Confirmed*, p. 561-63; *The Seat of the Soul*, p. 284; *The Authority of the Duumvirate*, p. 306. All the following quotations of van Helmont are taken from John Chandler's English translation.

[208] *The Authority of the Duumvirate, ibid.*

[209] *From the Seat of the Soul unto Diseases*, p. 292.

[210] *The Seat of Diseases in the Sensitive Soul, is Confirmed*, pp. 561-62. The primary role of the brain in epilepsy had also been denied by other iatrochemists before Helmont, for instance Quercetanus (833), *Tetras*, p. 74 ff.

[211] *Of Archeal Diseases*, p. 550.

[212] *The Seat of Diseases in the Sensitive Soul, is Confirmed*, pp. 561-62.

[213] *Ibid.*, p. 563.

[214] *Of Archeal Diseases*, p. 550.

where its Archeus, i.e., the local ruler, becomes perturbed by the poison-ous images.[215] It is for this reason that amulets may be helpful. "Likewise some external Medicines bound about the head, do preserve from an Epileptical fall and fit, which is for a signe, that either the fruit of the Character is hindered, or the applying of the occasion to the *Archeus*: Indeed in either manner the hurtfull matter is to be letted or prevented, to be extinguished or annihilated, that it be not co-mingled with the *Archeus*."[216]

There is another disease which van Helmont thinks related to epi-lepsy, viz., asthma. It has its original seat in the duumvirate, affects and shakes the whole body, but then concentrates upon the lungs—while epilepsy makes itself felt in the head. Van Helmont is so impressed by the apparent analogy between the two diseases that he says: "We may lawfully therefore, by a Phylosophical Liberty, name an Asthma the falling-Sickness of the Lungs."[217]

Van Helmont's ideas had a peculiar fate as far as the history of epilepsy is concerned. Where he sounds modern, his influence was negli-gible, and it was greatest where he seems to indulge in mysticism. He opposed the old doctrine of catarrhs from the brain;[218] but even during his lifetime this doctrine was not commonly applied to the pathology of epilepsy. He denied the ascension of vapors to the brain; but here his influence was anticipated by Charles Le Pois. Yet van Helmont was not forgotten. When a later generation of physicians turned to a mechanistic interpretation of epilepsy, the vitalistic traditionalists were able to utilize van Helmont's idea of the Archeus. But both Paracelsus and van Helmont were outsiders, and we have now to turn from hermetic medicine to the main development during the Renais-sance.

---

[215] *Ibid.*

[216] *From the Seat of the Soul unto Diseases*, p. 292.

[217] *The Asthma or Stoppage of Breathing, and Cough*, p. 361. Cf. Pagel (759), p. 112, who also gives a German translation of this part.

[218] Pagel and Winder (768) contrast the old theory of catarrh with the modern concepts of Paracelsus and van Helmont and quote additional literature on the topic.

# VI
# Broadening Experience and Changing Theory

## 1. NEW OBSERVATIONS

During the sixteenth century observations were made and published which considerably broadened the clinical knowledge of epilepsy. At the same time a theory was established which, in spite of many errors and imperfections, was preserved in its essential features for a long time. Yet there is nothing very spectacular about this work; it does not reveal any fundamentally new discovery. All the factors which characterize Renaissance medicine combined to advance the clinical as well as theoretical knowledge of the disease. Return to ancient sources served to purify the terminology and led to a clearer statement of the basic ideas. The work of the medieval doctors was not dismissed; some of their arguments were developed more logically and together with a few, but significant, anatomical observations helped to formulate a new theory. A renewed interest in individual cases kept the physicians in touch with reality. The movement which thus started during the Renaissance proper was merely accentuated during the seventeenth century, and only from the middle of the seventeenth century can further chapters be dated.

The humanist aspect of the Renaissance was the first to manifest itself. The absurd linguistic inventions and creations of the Middle Ages were now abolished. Even an Italian of the fifteenth century, Antonius Guainerius, had still derived the word *epilepsia* from " 'epi,' which is 'above' and 'lesis,' which is 'lesion'; a lesion of the upper part, so to say, namely of the head."[219] This kind of etymology now disappeared to-

---

[219] Antonius Guainerius (438), *Tractatus de egritudinibus capitis*, VII, 1; fol. 11$^r$: "Sed dicitur epilepsia ab epi quod est supra: et lesis lesio.

gether with the medieval terms for the three Galenic types. Philip Schopff, for instance, the editor of the 1595 edition of John of Gaddesden's *Rosa anglica*, added a marginal note to his author's statement that the three species of epilepsy were epilepsy, catalepsy, and analepsy. "Neither Galen nor anyone among the Greeks," remarked Dr. Schopff, "has recorded these species of epilepsy."[220] When this terminology was still remembered in the seventeenth century, it was quoted only to be rejected together with the underlying ideas.

The abolition of a traditional terminology was but the outward sign of increased spiritual freedom which expressed itself notably in the attention paid to individual observations. The publication of case histories had not completely stopped during the Middle Ages. Rhazes' clinical observations, for example, which had been translated into Latin and printed together with his *Continens* in 1509, included three cases of epilepsy.[221] The Arabic physician Abulqasim, who claimed the existence of demoniac epilepsy,[222] recorded two cases of epileptics who presented a hallucinatory aura, one of a sexual character, whereas in the other case the patient saw a black woman approaching him, and when she had come near him, he fell down.[223] During the Renaissance such publications became more and more frequent, and by the end of the sixteenth century Schenck of Grafenberg edited a collection of medical observations, chiefly gathered from authors of this period and reflecting a considerable broadening of clinical experience.

Many of the observations made during the sixteenth and seventeenth centuries refer to the various factors which preceded the onset of epileptic attacks. The belief that sudden fear and excitement could cause epilepsy was very widespread,[224] and Mercurialis held it good for

---

quasi superioris partis lesio: quia capitis." Similarly Savonarola (891), *Practica maior*, fol. 71$^V$: "Epilepsia itaque dicitur ab epi quod est sursum, et lesis quod est lesio."

[220] Ioannes Anglicus (535), *Rosa anglica*, p. 34, where the text reads: ". . . cuius tres sunt species, Epilepsia, Catalepsia, Analepsia" and where the editor remarks: "Has species Epilepsiae neque Galenus neque quisquam Graecorum ponit."

[221] These case histories have been translated from the Arabic by Meyerhof (694), where they appear as nos. 17-19 on pp. 341-42. For the Latin translation see Temkin (1002), p. 114 f

[222] Cf. above p. 106. It is a remarkable coincidence that the same author as observed these cases of psychic aura also became convinced of the existence of demoniac epilepsy. Although Abulqasim does not claim any relation, it is not at all impossible that this clinical observation confirmed him in his belief.

[223] Abulqasim (4), *Liber theoricae nec non practicae*, fol. 34$^r$: Alius vero est cui videtur quasi mulier ipsum quaerens ad coitum et festinanter furit ad eam et agit cum ea et post emissionem seminis cessat eius paroxismus et surgit, et ego quidem iam vidi cui hoc accidit . . . et ego quidem iam vidi quendam puerum meum patientem hanc aegritudinem qui dixit mihi quod videbatur ei mulier nigra accedens ad eum habens super ipsam corium quod dicitur parva et quando accedebat ad ipsum mox cadebat et studui ego erga sui curationem, et cessavit illud fantasma ab eo et alleviata est eius aegritudo." Brierre de Boismont (152), *Des hallucinations*, pp. 209-11, reported similar cases from the literature as well as from his own practice.

[224] Cf. Schenck a Grafenberg (892), *Observat. med.*, p. 102.–Io. Baptista Montanus (707), *Consultat. medicin.*, p. 66: "Novi ego duos, qui tantum ex animi affectibus inciderunt in hunc

mothers not to frighten children with fictions and tales.[225] Even the sight of an epileptic attack was reported to have provoked the same disease in some terrified bystanders.[226] The belief in the possible psychogenic origin went so far that Fabricius Hildanus attributed two cases of epilepsy in infants to the imagination of their mothers, who had seen epileptics while pregnant.[227] All this, of course, was not new. The significance of these reports lies rather in the fact that the belief in sudden fright and emotions as causative factors became deeply rooted, not only during this period but also in the centuries to come.

Equal, if not greater, attention was paid to injuries of the head preceding the outbreak of epilepsy. In the fourteenth century, Valescus de Tharanta had described the case of a man with a head-wound penetrating to the pia mater. A fetid ichor had reached the brain and had caused epileptic attacks seven or eight times a day, until the patient died.[228] Some 150 years later, Berengarius da Carpi treated a severe wound of the head where the epileptic paroxysm had supervened about sixty days after the injury, "because of the matter contained in the brain." Berengarius had the man placed feet up and head down; he opened the wound and evacuated a large quantity of watery substance of the color of milk, whereupon the epilepsy ceased immediately.[229] It was, moreover, realized that epileptic seizures might appear many years after the injury to the head. This is proved by the following observation related by Duretus (1527–86). "A bone of the skull of a twelve-year old youth had been broken and depressed by a fall and had by negligence not been restored. The brain was therefore hindered in its growth, since the injured bone itself could not grow so as to become able to hold a larger brain. Consequently, in his eighteenth year, the youth suffered from epilepsy because of the oppression of the brain. He

---

morbum: unus enim fuit quidam Laurentius Brachadenus, et Marcus Antonius Contarenus. Isti tamen in victu erant parcissimi, non erant excrementosi, tantum ex animi affectibus venere in talem aegritudinem: et ita dico quod potuit ista causa concurrere."

[225]Mercurialis, *De morb. puerorum*, II, c. 3; quoted from Schenck a Grafenberg, *l.c.*, p. 102: "Hac in parte laudandus *Plato*, qui monet *in 2. de Republica*, ne matres figmentis, et fabellis filios terreant; et his diebus scriptum ad me, e Germania, de puella quadam, quae tantum ex terroribus facta est epileptica."

[226]Plater (799), *De mentis consternatione*, t. I, p. 14: "Et cum repentinus illorum casus, horrendaque symptomata, maximum torrorem [terrorem?] soleant incutere, adeo ut aliqui ex apprehensione sola mox in eundem affectum inciderint, . . ."

[227]Cf. Fabricius Hildanus (338), *Observ. chirurg. centuria* III, 8, p. 191.

[228]Valescus de Tharanta (1039), *Philonium*, I, 18; fol. 16ʳ: "Inveni etiam hominem in capite vulneratum: cuius vulnus usque ad piam matrem penetrabat: et sanies seu fetida humiditas penetrans usque ad cerebrum faciebat epilepsiam septies vel octies in die: sic mortuus est."

[229]Berengarius a Carpi (104), *Tractatus de fractura calve*, fol. 31ᵛ: "Et sic circa sexagesimum diem ob materiam in cerebro contentam supervenit maximus paroxismus epilepsiae cum maximo omnium membrorum tremore et rigore. Hoc ego videns iussi ipsum pedibus elevari et capite deprimi. et cum stilo paulatim aperui foramen illud praedictum sub craneo in quo inveni magnam quantitatem materiae aquosae colore lacteo coloratae qua evacuata statim cessavit epilepsia et rediit in bonum intellectum."

was, however, cured by the perforation of the depressed bone, for thus the oppression of the brain was removed."[230] This observation is classical in its brevity and clarity and sounds so rational and modern in the treatment reported. Yet it will be seen that trephining was not an unusual practice;[231] besides, some physicians of the period, when confronted with a case of epilepsy of unclear etiology, asked the patient whether he had met with an accident, such as a fall or a blow.[232] They were wont to take any unusual feature into consideration and often arrived at a correct connection of two phenomena. The fact, for instance, that a patient had not passed urine for fully two days was correlated with the ensuing epileptic attacks by Heurnius, who apparently had witnessed a case of uremia.[233]

More difficult to decide was the relation between epilepsy and the newly studied disease, syphilis. It did not escape the attention of the Renaissance physicians that many syphilitics developed epileptic convulsions, and some of the cases show interesting features. A lady who had been afflicted with the *morbus gallicus* suffered for a long time toward the end of her life from most vehement epileptic attacks. Finally, she discharged the processus mamillaris together with a considerable part of the brain through the right nostril(!). The author of this story attributes the latter phenomenon to the "severity of the horrible disease."[234] At another time a "complication" of syphilis with epilepsy and melancholy was observed. While the patient, who had previously been treated with guaiacum, exhibited epileptic fits, pustules broke out on his head. He suffered a series of nervous as well as cutan-

---

[230]Duretus in Hollerius (506), p. 101: "Cum adolescenti cuidam annorum 12. ex casu, os calvariae collapsum atque depressum per incuriam restitutum non fuisset, indeque cerebrum incremento prohiberetur, quia os ipsum quod vitium conceperat, non poterat augeri ut amplioris cerebri capax fieret, anno aetatis 18. epilepsia laboravit ob cerebri oppressionem: sed curationem recepit per ossis depressi terebrationem. Sic enim est sublata cerebri oppressio."

[231]Cf. below, VIII-1c.

[232]Donatus (290), *De historia medica mirabili*, II, 4; p. 147, quotes an illustrative example: "Sic et ex tumore in femore Epilepsiam ortam aliquando testatur *Marcus Cattinaria in sua praxi c. de epilepsia*, ubi meminit cuiusdam, cui saepe adveniebat paroxysmus Epilepsiae, quem cum interrogasset, an ei aliquid accidisset, ut pote casus, vel percussio, ac respondisset, quod non, fecit eum exuere, et invenit unam coxam tumidam, sed nullum percipiebat dolorem, et interrogavit, quod illorum prius ipsi accidisset, scilicet tumor, vel epilepsia, ille nescivit respondere, unde existimavit causam epilepsiae esse illum tumorem, et fecit aperire locum cum cauterio, et inventa est in illo loco humiditas multa putrefacta, et ita dimisso loco aperto, sanatus est."

[233]Heurnius, *De morb. capitis*, c. 22, quoted from Schenck a Grafenberg (892), *Observat. med.*, p. 101 f.: "Non admodum est, quod accersitus fui ad aegrum: vir erat robustissimus, militiae deditus. Hic toto biduo urinam non reddiderat tremulus decumbebat, mens aegre constabat, ac lingua titubabat. A meridie in Epilepsiam incidit nec rediit, sed validis convulsionibus, vitam cum morte sequenti die commutavit: et Avicenna dicit hoc, cum ait, ab humiditate malae substantiae et foetidae Epilepsiam nasci."

[234]Heers (471), *Observationes medicae*, obs. 24; p. 211: "Alia Matrona patricia, gallico morbo olim conflictata, sub finem vitae saevissimis epilepsiae insultibus diu torta; tandem processum mamillarem cum cerebri notabili portiuncula, per narem dextram immani mali saevitia excrevit." Whether "the horrible disease" refers to epilepsy or syphilis remains uncertain.

eous manifestations, until he finally died. When his head was opened
after death, "the left ventricle of the brain was quite full of water and
part of the brain was destroyed, as if it had suffered from gangrene. In
the midst of this destruction were three small bodies like fresh
gummata."[235]

Although in many cases of this kind the authors did not fail to
mention the syphilitic infection, they were by no means certain in
considering it a causal factor, even where the epileptic attacks disappeared under the antisyphilitic treatment. "For more than six years,"
said Thierry de Héry, the friend of Ambroise Paré, "I treated a man
who together with this disease [i.e., syphilis] was tormented by an
epilepsy. And being treated exclusively with remedies proper for the
pox, he was cured of the one as well as of the other disease, so that he
has not noticed them since."[236] Héry was a surgeon, and the remedy
for syphilis used by the surgeons and barbers was mercury, while the
physicians preferred decoctions of guaiacum. The latter often blamed
the mercurial unctions for the resulting epilepsy,[237] for it was believed
that mercury destroyed the "spirits," especially the animal spirit, and
hence caused epilepsy, paralysis, and similar afflictions. "And mercury
causes all this not from some manifest quality, but because by its whole
substance it is hostile to human nature."[238]

When scurvy was studied more closely toward the end of the sixteenth century, epilepsy was numbered among its manifestations.[239]
Fully developed epileptic fits were also observed in the more advanced
stages of the disease which is now called ergotism, and which used to
reign epidemically in former countries.[240] Smallpox, measles, "and
other fevers" likewise entered into this category, especially with regard

---

[235]Quoted (from Crist. Guarinoni) by Bonetus (134), *Sepulchretum* IV, sect. 9, addit.; vol.
3, p. 454. Cf. also Proksch (826), p. 366.

[236]Proksch (826), p. 118: "Héry erzählt auch einen Fall von syphilitischer Epilepsie: 'J'ai
pansé homme plus de six ans, qui, avec cette maladie, estoit tourmenté d'une épilepsie, et estant
traitté seulement avec les remèdes propres pour la vérolle, fut guary de l'une et de l'autre
maladie, de sorte que depuis il ne s'en est senty.'"

[237]Cf. Proksch, *l.c.*, p. 175.

[238]Falloppius (342), *De metal. seu fossilib.*, c. 37; p. 349 f.: ". . . nam hydrargyron destruit
spiritus, ad destructionem autem spirituum sequitur epilepsia, apoplexia, vel alii similes morbi;
et quia spiritus animales sunt magis corruptibiles, quam vitales, et naturales, hinc est, quod
sequuntur potius epilepsia, paralysis, et huiusmodi affectus, quam alii; et haec omnia parit
hydrargyron, non a qualitate aliqua manifesta, sed quia a tota substantia est inimicum humanae
naturae;" etc.

[239]Cf. Eugalenus (332), *De morbo scorbuto liber*, c. 27.

[240]Horstius (515), *Observat. medic.*, VIII, observ. 22, c. 2; p. 423: "Quod si vero morbo
huic incipienti debitis et appropriatis remediis non obviam eatur, ad caput etiam pergit, atque
post multas vellicationes, tensionesque, Epilepsiam cum vehementi artuum jactatione, conquas-
satione et inquietudine parit, qua praesente, aegrotantes nihil amplius sentiunt, aut percipiunt,
neque eorum, quae ipsis interea acciderunt, recordantur, quemadmodum nonnulli in tali exacer-
batione, in obvium ignem praecipitati, misere ambusti sunt, de quo tamen, post paroxysmum ad
se redeuntes, ne minimum quidem sciverunt, aut persenserunt."

to epilepsy in children.[241] The realization of such possibilities led to the concept of *symptomatic* epilepsy, as expressed by Steeghius (c. 1600) in the following words: "Epilepsy is also a symptom of other diseases like smallpox and poisonous bites and ceases together with their cure...,"[242] where "symptom" meant complication rather than a sign.

All this goes to prove that during the period from 1500 to the middle of the seventeenth century, epilepsy was studied under a broadening aspect as far as its *evident* causes were concerned. Even greater attention was paid to the varying symptoms of the disease itself, especially to its unusual forms. While observations of this kind had not been lacking during the Middle Ages, they had been relatively rare and had been pressed into the traditional schemes of "minor" epilepsy or epilepsy without convulsions. This began to change now; the traditional schemata were abandoned more and more; physicians began even to doubt their justification.[243]

The affinity between vertigo and epilepsy was stressed anew; sometimes the physicians did not know whether to classify the case as the one or the other.[244] But then instances of epileptic attacks were related where the patients had neither fallen to the ground nor suffered from convulsions or vertigo. Benivieni was one of the first to describe such a

---

[241] E.g., Sennert (913), *De infantium curatione*, II, c. 10; vol. 3, p. 706: "Epilepsia et motus convulsivi, qui infantes non raro in variolarum et morbillorum principio invadunt, ex se quidem nihil periculi habent, et modo variolae ac morbilli erumpant, nunquam amplius nec adultos epilepsia infestat. Si tamen natura in expellendo succumbat, saepe infantes moriuntur, non epilepsiae, primarii morbi caussa." The same, *Pract. medic.*, I, pars II, c. 31; vol. 2, p. 231: "Massa sanguinea, ut in variolis, aliisque malignis febribus, inter quarum initia Epilepsia excitari solet."

[242] Steeghius (953), *Medicina practica*, VII, c. 3; p. 323: "Est et Epilepsia symptoma aliorum morborum, ut variolarum, et morsuum venenatorum, ad quorum etiam curationem cessat, ..."

[243] E.g., Culpeper's paraphrase of Riverius (853), I, ch. 7; p. 30: "Some of the Ancients make three kinds of Epilepsies: One which is like a deep sleep; another which doth shake the body after divers motions; a third which is made of both the former. The late Physitians deny the first kind, saying, That it is more like a Coma, or a Carus than an Epilepsy; and these two Diseases cannot be otherwise distinguished, but that in a Coma is a deep sleep without a Convulsion, and a Convulsion is a certain sign of an Epilepsie. But *Avicen* saith otherwise, namely, That an Epilepsy comes many times without an apparent Convulsion. And experience teacheth us, That many men in Epilepsies have fits like Coma; and it's known to be an Epilepsie, not a Coma, or a Carus by this; The sleep in an Epilepsie cometh and goeth by fits, when in a Coma it comes all at once."

[244] Erastus, Part. 4, disput. contra Paracel., quoted by Schenck a Grafenberg (892), *Observat. med.*, p. 102: "Vix quispiam fuit doctus, qui non finitimos affectus crederet vertiginem et epilepsiam. Equidem complures ausi sunt asserere vehementiorem vertiginem esse parvam epilepsiam: ut Coel. Aurel. Theod. item Prisc. et reliqui testati sunt. Non in omni epilepsia cadunt aegrotantes, sed aliquando solum caput nonnihil movetur (quod in duabus nobilibus virginibus, cum iam ferme sanatae fuissent, observavi) interdum pedes duntaxat vacillant; ut tamen nondum cadant. Vidi nonnunquam vertigines, inquit Montanus, in quibus accidentia adeo erant similia epilepticis symptomatibus, ut vix dignoscerentur: et a peritis medicis plurimum dubitaretur, utrum vertigines potius censendae, an epilepsiae nominari deberent, propterea quod in finibus utriusque morbi consistere viderentur." Sennert (913), *Institut. medic.*, II, pars 3, sec. 1, c. 9; vol. 1, p. 374: "Et ab aliis pluribus atque a me quoque observatum est, non in omni

case. The patient entered his bedroom, where his wife was lying, and stood still, his eyes wide open, and without reacting to his wife's questions. He was put upon the bed, where he finally recovered, but could not remember what he had been doing. The physicians, though at first uncertain, decided that he could not have been asleep but must have been in a pathological condition. The diagnosis was later on confirmed when he began to suffer from epileptic attacks.[245] While this case of automatism was not recognized as a direct form of epilepsy, another case described by the same author had been recognized as such,[246] and the same is true of the following description given by the Paracelsist, Toxites. It concerned a woman who was able to foresee her attacks and to take appropriate measures. The fit began by involuntary urination; then, with her eyes open, she would look around as if stunned. She would either stand, or go to her spinning wheel, or move a thing from one place to another, or sit down, without saying anything and plainly ignorant of her doings. Only rarely would she fall down, and upon recovering her senses she would ask what she had been doing.[247] Apparently physicians sometimes tried to analyze the state of consciousness during such attacks. Erastus examined a girl who for half an hour used to run up and down in the room while the persons present talked to her and tried to stop her. When afterward asked whether she had seen or heard anybody, she denied it. "But it is a fact," remarks Erastus, "that she saw the walls, and when she came near them she did not proceed further, but turned back."[248]

Such observations, where psychic symptoms prevailed, were supplemented by others where the mind of the patient seemed not to be

---

epilepsia cadere aegrotos, sed aliquando caput, aliquando pedes tantum moveri; vertiginesque etiam visae sunt, in quibus accidentia erant adeo similia epilepticis symptomatibus, ut vix dignoscerentur, et a Medicis dubitaretur, utrum vertigines, an potius epilepsiae nominari deberent."

[245] Benivenius (101), *De abditis morb. causis*, no. 46. For English translations of this case and of the one referred to in footnote 246 cf. Benivieni (102), pp. 99 f. and 181 f.

[246] Benivenius (101), l.c., no. 97. A girl showed no symptoms other than rotations of the neck and head together with complete absent-mindedness and amnesia. The attacks ceased with the menarche.

[247] Toxites, Explicat. 3, par. 3, lib. 3, Paragraphorum Theoph. Paracelsi, quoted from Schenck a Grafenberg (892), *Observat. med.*, p. 104: "Est mihi mulier quaedam nota, quae paroxysmum epilepticum praevidet: itaque cum vel ad aquas lavat, discedit, vel si domi est, aut in eo loco manet, in quo est: aut in alium abit: mox urinam reddit ubicunque est, deinde oculis apertis quasi stupida hinc inde circumspicit, et vel stat, vel ad colum accedit, vel aliquid huc illuc defert, vel sedet, nihilque loquitur, et quid agat, plane ignorat. Raro autem cadit: ubi ad se revertitur, quaerit quid egerit."

[248] Erastus (324), *Comitis Montani*, etc., p. 195 f.: "Et nuper etiam puellam allocutus sum, quae, cum antea gravissime laborasset, ac proxime tanquam mali nihil pateretur, in conclavi per dimidiam horam sursum deorsum cursitasset, atque a me interrogaretur, utrum aliquem vidisset vel audisset (nam allocuti eam sunt, qui aderant, et inhibere motum tentarunt) negavit se quenquam aut vidisse aut audisse. Constat tamen eam parietes vidisse, quos cum ad eos accessisset, protinus cavebat, ac se rursus convertebat. Huiusmodi, inquam, exempla possem alia plurima adferre, si opus esset, quibus manifeste probatur, non ideo non imaginari Epilepticos, quia a paroxismo non recordantur."

affected at all. Ferdinandus (1569–1638) gave an example of a "slight epilepsy," where a girl, under the conjunction of the moon, used to fall down for the time of an Ave Maria, frothing, but without convulsions and in full possession of all her senses.[249]

But the majority of cases deviating from the typical (i.e., the grand mal) referred to attacks where some particular parts of the body were convulsed, with or without fall or loss of consciousness. Many instances were cited of paroxysms starting from the toes, fingers, etc. However, these do not need amplification since they do not represent new experiences, with the one notable exception that the *necessity* of a "breeze" ascending to the head was now denied. It was again Erastus, the bitter enemy of Paracelsus, who said: "Likewise it has been observed by the physicians that this disease in some people often makes its attack from the convulsion of some particular member (forearms, feet, fingers, humerus, shoulder blades), although they do not feel anything ascending to the brain from these members."[250] This remark characterizes the gradual emancipation from traditional views.

It was no longer deemed necessary for the whole body to be convulsed nor even for the patient to fall to the ground. Slight movements of the head or the feet, or perhaps a scarcely noticeable contraction of the lips together with a short state of confusion, might be the only symptoms.[251] Or the convulsions might be pronounced on one half of the body only, as in a case described by Rulandus, where a ten-year-old boy showed convulsions of the mouth, the left eye, and the left hand, while his left arm became stiff and his speech lost. Though frequent, the fits passed off quickly and he did not fall down.[252] Such partial convulsions could be combined with psychic abnormalities. In one of Erastus' patients, a girl, the right lower leg and the forearm of the same side twisted from time to time. If asked questions during the paroxysm, the girl gave appropriate answers, but if left to herself, she laughed,

---

[249] Ferdinandus (350), *Centum historiae*, hist. 24; p. 74: "Respondeo, quod est quaedam epilepsia levis, et incipiens, quae non requirit tantam manifestam convulsionem, et dum haec scribebam habeo prae manibus quandam meam vicinam puellam 13. annorum, filiam Angeli Simeonis dictam Donatam, quae in lunae coniunctione, sive sedens, sive ambulans cadebat in terram sine convulsione, cum admissione sensuum omnium, et cum spuma, et permanebat per spatium unius Ave Maria."

[250] Erastus, Part. 4, disput. contra Paracel., quoted by Schenck a Grafenberg, *l.c.*, p. 103: "Observatum hoc etiam est a medicis, morbum hunc in aliquibus a particularis cuiusdam membri (brachiorum, pedum, digitorum, humeri, spatularum) convulsione saepe incidere, tametsi nihil ex iis ad cerebrum ascendere percipiebatur."

[251] Erastus, *ibid.*, as quoted by Schenck a Grafenberg, *l.c.*, p. 103: "Vidi ego qui facili et brevi delirio cum labiorum vix sensibili contractione tentati statim sibi restituerentur." Cf. also below, footnote 256.

[252] Rulandus (880), *Curationum*, etc., centuria 9, curatio 99; p. 157 f.: "Optime experta et probata in Oberbechinga, ubi Burgl Mairin filius decennis persaepe correptus fuit dies noctesque horribili morbo comitiali, et in paroxysmo oculus sinister, os et manus sinistra convulsa est, loquela amissa, brachium sinistrum, torpuit, sed paroxysmus citissime remisit, et ad se rediit, nec lapsus est, ut fit in graviore epilepsia."

talked strange things, and after the paroxysm had no memory of what she had perceived and done. Sometimes the laughter, change of expression, and silly talk might even be the sole manifestations of the disease.[253] Donatus observed an incomplete form of epileptic attack in an actor who had but a short time before suffered from syphilitic ulcerations. The fits began with a feeling of repletion in the whole head, immediately followed by jerking, contractions of the hands and feet, and an upward twisting of the eyes. He never fell to the ground but had the impression of walking over large balls filled with air and was not quite himself.[254]

These various observations, of which we have cited only some of the more impressive examples, were not always consistent with the traditional definition of epilepsy, for, according to the latter, epilepsy involved both loss of consciousness and convulsions of the whole body.

Marcus Marci (1595–1667) felt justified in broadening the definition of epilepsy "to any affection of the body where the victims are disordered in their minds, while the members [of the body], be it all, or some, or only one, are moved against their will." This broadened definition was to make possible the inclusion of all species of epilepsy. "For he in whom the lips only were convulsed together with a slight delirium, and he who constantly turned around in a circle after the fashion of a whirl or a trundling hoop, and the girl who for the space of half an hour ran forward and backward, must [all] be listed among the epileptics; yes, and he too who was lifted high up by the force of the disease and remained hanging in the air. . . ."[255] Others spoke of a perfect or simple form of epilepsy, which corresponded to the classical definition

---

[253] Erastus (324), *Comitis Montani*, etc., p. 195: "Curavi eodem fere tempore nobilem virginem, et puerum. Illi ex intervallis crus dextrum una cum brachio distorquebantur, ut non concideret tamen. Quae tametsi in paroxismo ad interrogata satis apte responderet, sibi tamen relicta ridebat, alienaque loquebatur: et post paroxismum interrogata nihil prorsus sciebat aut recordabatur eorum, quae vidisset, egisset, dixisset. Quinimo interdum erecta stans ita, ut dixi, risu, vultus mutatione, et deliris sermonibus morbum testabatur, nec gravius aliquid patiebatur. Et tametsi brevi tempore sic afficeretur, nullius tamen rei ad se reversa meminerat. Quod eorum non meminisset, quae in gravioribus paroxismis, quibus aliquando corripiebatur, perpessa fuisset, non admodum mirabar."

[254] Donatus (290), *De historia medica mirabili*, II, c. 4; p. 145.

[255] Marcus Marci (668), *Liturgia mentis*, p. 2: "Nam et is cui sola labia, cum levi delirio convellebantur; et qui in gyrum assidue more turbinis aut trochi se versabat; et ea puella, quae spatio semihorae prorsum et retrorsum cursitabat, inter Epilepticos habendi. Quin et is, qui vi morbi in sublime elatus, in aere pendulus detinebatur: quies enim illa tonica virtute motui aequipollet." I cannot place the last observation. Marcus Marci's contributions to the history of epilepsy have been discussed by Servit (917 and 918). The *Liturgia mentis*, which was written about 1638, was published posthumously in what seems to me an incomplete form. At the end of chapter 9, Marci declares his intention to deal extensively "with the nature of imagination, its powers and various modes of operating. For we cannot know what a disease is and what is abnormal, if we do not know health and disease" (p. 28). The following chapter, "The fundaments of the real cause of epilepsy are laid by investigating the manner in which the sensible pictures are imparted to the external senses and from these to the internal ones," opens a broad and very original discussion of perception, memory, and imagination. But neither here nor in

in contrast to the "imperfect" form which showed certain deviations.[256] This simplified clinical classification represented a real advance
over the elaborate and often artificial divisions of the preceding period.
On the other hand, it introduced an element of uncertainty into the
concept of epilepsy.

It has been noted that unusual cases of epilepsy were open to the
suspicion of witchcraft or possession. Without committing themselves
to a supernatural explanation, some writers believed that imperfect
forms were related to some species of disease different from epilepsy.[257] The main difficulties, however, arose from attempts to coor-
dinate epilepsy and other forms of convulsive disorders.

Since the times of Hippocrates, physicians had been talking about
"convulsions," particularly with reference to children, without clearly
defining the meaning of the term and its relation to epilepsy. From the
end of the fifteenth century on, when pediatric literature increased
considerably, special attention was paid to epilepsy in infancy, and
some attempts were made to draw a line between convulsions and
epilepsy in children. Sennert, for example, believed that in the former
the *materia peccans* aggregated around the spinal cord and the origins
of the muscles, and that, therefore, the general commotion was slighter
and disturbances of psychic functions absent.[258] But, on the whole,
such attempts remained without great consequence. Physicians had long
known that convulsions in early childhood had a different prognostic
significance from epileptic seizures of older persons. But for a very long
time the terminology remained confused. Thomas Sydenham, for example, in discussing convulsions in children preceding the outbreak of

---

the rest of the book does Marci come back to epilepsy. Nor does he take up the promised
discussion of the names of epilepsy "after the nature of the disease has been brought to light"
(ch. 1). Marci's embryological ideas have been analyzed in detail by Pagel (767a), pp. 285-323.

[256] Erastus (324), *Comitis Montani*, etc., p. 195, gives the following case of an *epilepsia
rotatoria et procursiva*: "Superiore anno adolescentem curavi egregium, qui ex alto loco decidit,
et tempus sinistrum laesit, ex quo in epilepsiam incidit, qui paroxismi tempore ter, quater,
saepius in gyrum se vertebat, impetuque facto, si non prohiberetur, versus locum aliquem
procurrebat, priusquam prorsus caderet, (plerunque non cadebat, sed manibus magna vi faciem
confricabat) nec ad se reversus quicquam eorum, quae evenissent, sciebat." All such forms now
entered into the category of imperfect epilepsy: Nymmanus (745), *De epilepsia disputatio*
§ 17: "... alia imperfecta quaedam epilepsia, in qua actiones omnes animales non laeduntur,
ita ut aegri vel non concidant, vel saltem aliquae partes convellantur, et aut caput tantum
concutiatur, aut oculi contorqueantur, aut manus pedesve hinc inde jactentur, aut manus
clausae teneantur, aut aeger se in gyrum convertat, aut hinc inde discurrat, nihil interim loqua-
tur, audiat, sentiat, et paroxysmo finito omnium quae acciderunt ignarus sit; vel a paroxysmo
liberatus eorum, quae acciderunt, recordetur. Quas imperfectas epilepsias cognitas habere utile
est." The term *epilepsia procursiva* is used by Arnoldus Bootius (135), *Observationes medicae
de affectibus omissis*, c. 6; p. 24. Cf. also Gowers (420), p. 39.

[257] Nymmanus, *l.c.*: "Quas imperfectas epilepsias cognitas habere utile est. Etsi enim aliam
potius, quam epilepsiae speciem prae se ferre videantur: tamen cum eandem cum epilepsia
causam habeant, saltem minus vehementem," etc.

[258] Sennert (913), *De infantium curatione*, II, c. 10; vol. 3, p. 707: "In convulsione [i.e., of
children] vero cum materia circa spinalem medullam et in musculorum exortu consistat, omnes
partes ita non concutiuntur [i.e., as in epilepsy], neque animales actiones caeterae laeduntur."

smallpox, scarlet fever, or measles, referred to them as "spasm," "convulsion,"[259] "epileptic paroxysm," and "epileptic insult."[260]

Equal difficulties were presented by the similarity of hysterical and epileptic attacks. Ancient and medieval physicians had tried to establish the differential signs between the two. Guainerius stated that in hysteria the head would usually be inclined toward the knees, and that everything that happened during the fit would be understood and remembered.[261] When hysterical paroxysms had to be distinguished from "idiopathic" epilepsy, the matter was comparatively simple; but the task became extremely difficult in cases where epilepsy was supposed to originate from the uterus. Paracelsus solved this difficulty by denying the existence of any such differences. Epilepsy of the womb for him meant all convulsions which had their cause in the uterus and was identical with hysterical suffocation.[262] Others talked about uterine suffocation as well as epilepsy from the uterus, but neither the clinical nor the pathological differences were clear. Since the Middle Ages a vapor arising from the uterus was believed to induce epileptic attacks.[263] But many physicians of the Renaissance also explained all kinds of hysterical manifestations by vapors from the uterus.[264] Vapors reaching the brain would therefore account for both epilepsy from the uterus and hysteria resulting in epileptic convulsions.[265]

The increase in clinical knowledge gradually made the older classification of convulsive disorders inadequate. Traditionally, epilepsy with

---

[259]Sydenham (983), *Dissertatio epistolaris ad . . . Gulielmum Cole*; pp. 345 and 346.

[260]Sydenham (983), *Observat. med.*, sec. 3, c. 2; p. 120.

[261]Antonius Guainerius (438), *Tractatus de egritudinibus capitis*, VII, 2; fol. 11ᵛ: "A praefocatione cognoscitur [i.e., epilepsy] quia praefocata ut plurimum versus genua caput inclinat: epilepticus non. praefocata item et si respondere nequit: tamen intelligit: et omnium quae in paroxismo facta sunt post paroxismum recordatur." Jacobus Sylvius (985), *De mensibus mulierum*, p. 177, gives the following list of differential symptoms: "Suffocatio ab utero similis epilepsiae, et apoplexiae, et lethargo: quia hi quatuor affectus repente prehendunt: sed epileptica mulier raro recordatur eorum quae illi acciderunt, non audit, non intelligit, habet fere, praesertim cum valens est epilepsia, spumam in ore: menses non habet suppressos, et coitu crebro offenditur: nihil ab utero ad os ventriculi tolli praesentit, sed indidem, vel aliis partibus ad cerebrum, si ex consensum est, et alia habet signa epilepsiae propria," etc.

[262]Paracelsus (770), *De caducis liber secundus*, etc; vol. 8, p. 367: "Also ist auch geent das buch suffocationis oder praecipitationis matricis, das ich caducum matricis nenne; dan der caducus und die krankheit matricis mügen mit ursachen, ursprung und wesen nicht geschiden werden sondern ein ding begreift sich in eim ding."

[263]Albertus Magnus (19), *De animalibus*, IX, 48; vol. 1, p. 692, 26–31, combined this theory with the explanation of imaginary pregnancy. If the male seed were not united with female seed, it would evaporate and raise the uterus, thus deceiving the women into the belief of pregnancy. Besides, the vapor might ascend to the head and cause vertigo or even epilepsy.

[264]Ambroise Paré (772), *Oeuvres*, vol. 2, p. 753: "Et pour conclusion, en la suffocation de la matrice, les vapeurs putredineuses montent quelquesfois iusqu'au diaphragme, aux poulmons et au coeur, qui fait que la femme ne peut respirer ny expirer: lesquelles vapeurs ne sont seulement portées par les veines et arteres, mais aussi par les spiracles occultes qui sont au corps. Et si lesdites vapeurs montent iusqu'au cerueau, causent epilepsie, . . ."

[265]Sennert (913), *Pract. med.*, IV, pars 2, sec. 3, c. 7; vol. 3, p. 582: "Est enim Epilepsiae ex utero causa ille idem vapor et spiritus malignus, qui suffocationem uterinam excitare solet."

its clonic spasms and mental manifestations had been contrasted with the various forms of tetanus, which latter were often called by the simple name "convulsion" or "spasm." Now it was more and more felt that certain cases did not fit into either category. Salius in the latter half of the sixteenth century was one of the first to make this point clear. He described a kind of pathological movement in which the limbs were neither extremely extended nor bent. The movement had a vibrating character and was constant in some patients, while in others it occurred periodically as in epilepsy. Sometimes it was painful, sometimes not; it only rarely affected the whole body, usually only the right or left side, very seldom a single limb. The movement could be more violent and would then cause vehement and very painful distortions of the limbs. If these distortions increased in power and were communicated to the upper parts of the body, and more particularly to the brain, something similar to epilepsy would result. Yet in contrast to real epilepsy, the patients would not froth and would sometimes even preserve their sense of hearing during the paroxysm.[266] Salius' description probably comprises quite a number of different neurological conditions, among others perhaps such forms of epilepsy as had begun with partial convulsions and ended in generalized attacks. But the main point is that his description represents a conscious attempt to introduce a new category of convulsive disorders.

In the seventeenth century these difficulties found their solution in a new phraseology adopted by many physicians. "Convulsion," i.e., tetanus, was now distinguished from "convulsive movements." The latter formed a wide class comprising various diseases ranging from epilepsy to hysteria. Willis gave this concept systematic form,[267] and by this arrangement it was made possible to preserve epilepsy as a well-characterized disease, for the more atypical forms could now be separated as different species of "convulsive movements." The time had not yet come in which the very existence of a definite disease, "epilepsy," was seriously doubted.[268]

## 2. NEW THEORIES

The return to the ancient medical authors was accompanied by a revival of the classical Galenic pathology of epilepsy, including the belief that idiopathic epilepsy was caused by a humoral obstruction of the ventricles of the brain.[269] Nor did this opinion disappear very soon; for a long

---

[266] Salius, De affect. partic., c. 20, quoted by Schenck a Grafenberg (892), *Observat. med.*, p. 114 ff.

[267] Cf. below.

[268] On the scholastic discussions of epilepsy as symptom or disease cf. above, IV-2.

[269] Fuchs (382), *De medendis*, etc., I, c. 18; p. 42: "Gignitur haec passio trifariam. Primum, ubi cerebrum primogenia passione patitur. id quod fit, ubi crassus viscosusque pituitae vel atrae

time it was repeated[270] and even defended against the modernists.[271] In particular, this view could be combined with the theory of catarrhs, i.e., fluxes, from the head. It was suggested that narrowness of the passages from the brain to the spine, or to the palate, or the nose, might lead to accumulation of the "excrements" of the brain in its ventricles. These passages were, furthermore, considered the way by which the brain freed itself from the peccant humors which, in the opinion of a few, formed the froth of the epileptic.[272]

Retaining many features of the old theory of fluxes, Charles Le Pois (1563–1636) worked out a modification which did away with the entire time-honored concept of idiopathic and sympathetic epilepsy. Chapter seven of his work on selected observations and consilia deals with hysteria and epilepsy, and the short argument following the title summarizes his views very clearly. It reads as follows: "Chapter seven. Consilium on epilepsy. In this the symptoms which are commonly called hysterical are referred to epilepsy. Epilepsy itself, however, is proved to be an idiopathic disease of the head, not [brought about] by sympathy of the uterus or the intestines. Furthermore, the conjoint cause of epilepsy is disclosed, viz. a serous flood which, when brought into a state of fervor, attacks and violently distends the origin of the nerves, particularly of the spinal cord and of the sixth and seventh pairs. Finally, the methodical way of its cure is revealed."[273] Le Pois starts out from the case of a woman exhibiting various "hysterical" symptoms. He arrives at the conclusion that the cause of this disease cannot be in the uterus, as usually assumed. The uterus and its blood vessels contain such a small amount of blood that it could not possibly produce a sufficient quantity of vapors to distend the nervous

---

bilis humor spiritus meatum in cerebri ventriculis obstruit, nervorum principio seipsum quatiente, quo excutiat id quod noxium est. A crasso autem humore hanc passionem induci, argumento est, quod et subito fit, et solvitur confestim." Similarly Jacobus Sylvius (985), *De signis*, p. 268.

[270]Riolanus, jr. (852), *Encheiridium anatomicum et pathologicum*, IV, c. 2; p. 270: "Epilepsia est periodica Convulsio totius corporis, cum mentis et sensuum laesione, quae fit obstructis anterioribus Cerebri Ventriculis, ab humore acri, multo, bilioso, vel pituitoso."

[271]Cf. further below.

[272]Hollerius (506), *De morbis internis*, I, 15, scholia; p. 95: "Addunt nonnulli, non sine probabili ratione, quandoque id contingere ob angustiam meatus a posteriore cerebro ad spinam, vel imperforatam, aut strictiorem lacunam ad palatum, aut ad nares. Et certe Galenus de usu partium scribit optime comparatum esse a natura, ut per declives cerebri meatus: tum per palatum in os, tum per corpus narium, orificiis perspicuis ac magnis, pituita, aut alia cerebri excrementa excernantur, ne animal frequenter corripiatur epilepsia: videmusque per illam viam expurgari materiam, quae epilepsiam excitavit, ac spumam ex ore educi." Similarly Valleriola (1042), *Observ. medicinal.*, III, observ. 7; p. 307 f.

[273]Le Pois (633), *Selectiorum observationum . . . liber*, p. 115: Caput VII. de Epilepsia, Consilium. Quo Symptomata hysterica quidem vulgo dicta ad Epilepsiam referuntur: Epilepsia autem ipsa capiti idiopathica esse demonstratur, non per sympathiam uteri, aut viscerum; eiusque porro causa continens detegitur, serosa scilicet colluvies fervore quodam concepto impetens violenterque distendens principia nervorum praesertimque spinalis medullae et sexti septimique parium: denique methodica curandae eius ratio aperitur."

system.[274] Nor are there any ducts through which such a quantity of vapors could reach the head from the uterus.[275] Similar reflections hold true also where parts distant from the brain are believed to cause epilepsy by sympathy.[276] Le Pois thus extends his argument from hysteria to epilepsy. He denies that epileptic paroxysms which start from a finger, or another part, really have their primary seat in that member. Instead, he believes that in such cases the attack, having started in the head, manifests itself and is first felt in the distant part before the fit becomes generalized and the senses lost.[277] Similarly, the ascending "breeze" does not represent the ascent of the morbific agent but is merely a feeling of the affected nerve.[278] Hence, the conclusion is unavoidable that all hysterical symptoms (and the same is true of epilepsy) originate in the brain and are idiopathic.[279]

Having thus refuted the traditional theory, Le Pois now has to elucidate his own. His main points are as follows: The blood vessels of the head carry blood rich in serum (a watery substance manufactured in the digestive organs). This serum passes through the walls of the blood vessels into the empty spaces of the membranes, collects around the base of the head, and from here flows down into the nose and palate, in accordance with the old anatomical and physiological doctrines. But under pathological conditions, especially if the blood is abnormally imbued with serum, there may be a superfluity of the latter in the head. Owing to its watery nature, it can then easily move about; it can effervesce and be dispersed in a very short time; it can flow into the roots of the nerves, fill them, and distend them so that they contract and cause various motions of the body, or affect the senses. If the origin of the entire nervous system is thus attacked, then the whole organism is agitated; if, however, a limited area only is attacked, the symptoms too will be more or less localized.[280]

Le Pois bases his arguments partly on reasoning, partly on clinical observations, and partly on anatomical findings. He cites the case of an epileptic where the entire hind part of the head was found turgid with water and the origin of the nerves, as well as the membranes, drenched with it.[281] Cases like this were to play a great role in the seventeenth

---

[274]*Ibid.*, p. 131 f.

[275]*Ibid.*, p. 132.

[276]*Ibid.*, p. 139 f.

[277]*Ibid.*, p. 140: "... cur ab iis partibus integris et sanis laedi caput censebimus? ac non potius contra capitis contractioni incipienti aliquod membrum v.g. digitum prius compati, quam totum in consensum trahi; eamque particularem contractionem sentiri ante universalem ab ipsis aegris, quia sensus in iis nondum sunt sepulti?"

[278]*Ibid.*, p. 141: "Est igitur aurae frigidae sensus potius nervi ipsius concussi sensus?"

[279]*Ibid.*, p. 144.

[280]*Ibid.*, pp. 144 and 147 f.

[281]*Ibid.*, p. 158 f.

and eighteenth centuries, as can be seen from Morgagni—who discussed the question how far accumulations of fluid could be considered the cause of epilepsy.[282] The main feature, however, of Le Pois' doctrine was his denial of the existence of sympathetic epilepsy and his attributing all premonitory symptoms, including the feeling of the "breeze," to an affection of the central nervous system. But the influence of his ideas made itself felt only later, while his immediate contemporaries adhered to different views.

It was the medieval hypothesis of poisonous vapors affecting the brain which was elaborated by Fernelius and was widely accepted by Renaissance physicians. Fernelius did not confine himself to dialectic arguments but supported his view by new observations. He dissected the brains of two epileptics. One of them had been suffering from an almost continuous headache over a small area of the forehead. He found the cerebral membrane at this spot thickened and adhering to the bone, with a little putrid humor lying in between. The substance of the other brain contained a quantity of very fetid humor. But in both cases the ventricles, as well as the ducts of the brain, were free from any humor or any obstruction. These findings he correlated with the observation of syphilitics who had become epileptic because, as he thought, some of the mercurial ointment used for their treatment had penetrated into the ear and brain. In these cases he attributed the epilepsy to an irritation of the brain by spoiled mercury. This suggested to him that epilepsy was always due to a poisonous vapor which, upon being carried to the brain, violently affected the brain as well as the meninges by the "enmity" of its whole substance.[283]

The anatomical observations of Fernelius were soon supplemented by other writers. Coiter (1534–1600) stated that he had been unable to find anything in the ventricles of the brain besides a watery humor

---

[282] Morgagni (714), *De sedibus et causis morborum*, I, epist. 9.

[283] Fernelius (351), *De abditis rerum causis*, II, c. 15; p. 87: "Ut enim aliquando observavimus e summo capitis vertice, in quo sub pericranio vitiatus venenatusque humor coërcebatur, vaporem manifesto sensu intro subire, qui epilepsiam concitaret, hancque postea caustico persanatam medicamento, ita proculdubio existimari debet intus, vel circum meninges, vel circum cerebri substantiam vitium contineri veneni aemulum, cuius ex intervallis impetu facto, epilepsia suscitetur. Aperto epileptici philosophi qui decesserat capite, qui vehementissimo eoque fere perpetuo dolore, vix digitum lato circa sinciput torquebatur, deprehendimus crassiorem meningem ea sede, calvae ossi adhaerescere, pauculo humore putri interiecto. In altero cerebri substantia humorem foetidissimum, eumque exiguum contineri: utriusque tamen ventriculos et meatus omnis humoris, omnisque obstructionis expertes. Multos ipse (scio) vidisti inde epilepticos evasisse, quod in curanda lue venerea, dum unguentis ex hydrargyro illinerentur, nonnihil in aurem et in cerebrum penetrasset. Hisne quaeso dicas cerebri ventriculos humore multo impleri et obstrui? BR. Minime quidem, sed ipsum corrupti hydrargyri pernicie lacessiri. EV. Talem igitur et in omni alia epilepsia causam existimato: atque si quid aliquando putridi humoris inesse deprehenditur, non ex ea ipsa putredine, sed ex venenata quam concepit qualitate, hoc mali suscitari. Itaque quocunque corporis in loco is fuerit, venenatus illinc vapor in cerebrum sublatus idipsum meningesque totius substantiae inimicitia acriter ferit."

permeating its substance.[284] Erastus, likewise, denied the existence of any obstruction and added that the cerebral ventricles had sometimes been found full of a watery or even bloody humor in people who had never suffered from any epileptic symptoms.[285] Taxil had ordered post-mortem dissections of several children who had died of epilepsy and had never been able to find any considerable quantity of moisture in the ventricles. In one particular case he had noticed a small black spot on the dura mater. He formed the opinion that this spot had been caused by some "malign and biting humors," whence epilepsy had been incited.[286]

These observations confirmed the opinion that epilepsy must be due to an irritation of the brain by some poisonous substance. It is true that some opposition was encountered.[287] In particular it was denied that a poisonous quality had to be involved in all cases of epilepsy.[288] Mercurialis even complained that Fernelius' views would destroy all the fundamentals of medicine.[289] But the idea of an irritation as the fundamental cause remained victorious and stood definitely in the foreground after the beginning of the seventeenth century.

Nevertheless, it was not enough to attribute the epileptic seizure to an irritation of the brain and its membranes and to point to analogies with hiccups and sneezing.[290] The physiological and anatomical basis for such an opinion had to be explained. It was necessary to show which part could be irritated, and how it could be expected to react to

---

[284] Schenck a Grafenberg (892), *Observat. med.*, p. 100. Marcus Marci (668), *Liturgia mentis*, c. 3; p. 6 f., lists Volcher Coiter's observations among the evidence against the traditional pathology of epilepsy, and so does Erastus according to Pagel (762), p. 327.

[285] Erastus, Part. 4, disput. contra Paracel., quoted by Schenck a Grafenberg, *l.c.*, p. 100: "Complurium Epilepticorum cerebrum dissectum nihil habuit, ex quo obstructio colligi posset. Dissecti enim alii sunt, in quibus ventriculi aqueo humore, aliquando etiam cruento pleni apparuerunt, quamvis epileptici nihil fuissent passi." Erastus' theory of epilepsy has been set forth by Pagel (762), pp. 327–29.

[286] Taxil (994), *Traicté de l'épilepsie*, p. 22 f.

[287] E.g., Le Pois, *l.c.*, p. 132.

[288] Duretus in Hollerius (506), *De morbis internis*, I, 15; p. 99 f.: "Et quidem satis mirari non possum doctissimos nostrae aetatis Medicos, qui negant ullam epilepsiam fieri absque venenata qualitate. Quorum opinionem satis refellit puerorum epilepsia, et Galenus ipse qui comm. ad aphor. 45. lib 2. scribit eandem esse epilepsiae et apoplexiae causam, non quidem venenatam qualitatem, sed humorem frigidum et crassum." Similarly Riolanus (851), *De abditis rerum causis comment.* c. 11; p. 150: "De Epilepsia paradoxon est Fernelii, eam semper esse venenatam. Caeteri medici ab aura quidem summe putri et venenata delata ad cerebrum oriri aliquando epilepticos insultus confitentur, quemadmodum a vermibus, et ab ulcere valde putri: Omnem Epilepsiam esse venenatam pernegant," etc.

[289] Mercurialis (684), *Medicina practica*, I, 26; p. 141: "Tertio, destruerentur fundamenta Hip. et totius medicinae, scil. quod non fieret unquam epilepsia repletione, quod tamen falsissimum est. Quapropter sinamus Fernelium cum sua opinione."

[290] For the analogy with sneezing cf. Beverwyck (108), *D. Schatzes d. Ungesundheit* zweiter Teil, d. 12. Hauptstükke, 6; p. 169, and, before him, Erastus: "Sternutatio magna est parva epilepsia" [quoted from Pagel (762), p. 328, footnote 404].

the irritation. Questions of this kind were intimately connected with
the views held about movement and sensibility of the brain and of the
meninges. All these problems, which had their roots in Antiquity, were
now formulated more clearly, though the answers varied for centuries
to come.

Fernelius himself believed that the brain was in constant motion,
while lacking any sense of touch. The meninges, on the other hand,
were immobile but very sensitive to touch, as he had experienced in the
opened skulls of people suffering from wounds of the head.[291] How
this could be coordinated with his view of the origin of epilepsy is not
quite clear. Taxil thought that as a result of its being irritated the brain
contracted like a sea-sponge.[292] While this might pass as a loose way of
expression, it had to be qualified in order to correspond to the more
advanced physiological ideas of the time.

One of the most detailed explanations was offered by Rudius
(†1611). He argued that the brain itself, being void of any sense of
touch, very soft, and lacking fibers, could hardly be expected to contract. It was different in such organs as the stomach, womb, bladder,
and intestines, which were richly endowed with nerves. According to
the current (Galenic) physiology, these parts could "feel" the stimulus,
their expulsive faculty (one of the "natural faculties" common to all
vegetative organs) would be irritated and would respond by contraction. Now, for the reasons stated, this could not be the case with regard
to the substance of the brain proper. It could, however, as Rudius
concluded, be true with regard to the cerebral membranes, which possessed an exquisite sense of touch.[293] Thus "the moderns" came to

---

[291] Fernelius (351), *Physiologia*, lib. V, c. 10; p. 73 f.: "Cerebri corpus motu agitatur
assiduo, nullo tamen tangendi sensu praeditum: contra vero quae idipsum ambiunt meninges,
immobiles per se sunt, praesertimque crassior: tactu autem eae valent exquisitissimo, quae
singula ut Galeni fide confirmata sunt, ita etiam vulnerata, apertaque calva contrectantibus
nobis sunt deprehensa."

[292] Taxil (994), *Traicté de l'épilepsie*, p. 18: ". . . mais c'est à cause que ceste contagieuse
malignité, irritant le cerueau par toute sa forme, faict que le cerueau se comprime et reserre en
soy comme une esponge, et par consequant la pituite decoule en bas. . . ."

[293] Rudius (877), *De humani corporis affectibus*, I, 9; fol. 38ʳ: "Verum hoc in loco perpul-
chra oritur dubitatio, quo nam modo cerebri expultrix possit adeo stimulari, ut cerebrum se
ipsum concutiat, et moveatur: non enim quemadmodum ventriculus dum a prava materia
irritatur in singultu, et aliae quoque nervosae partes ratione stimuli, ut noxium expellant,
contrahuntur; ita videtur cerebrum contrahi, et moveri posse: nam vetriculus, uterus, vesica,
intestina stimulum facillime sentiunt, cum hae partes nervosissimae sint, et iisdem de causis
facillime, irritata expultrice, contrahuntur. sed cerebrum ipsum cum sensu tactus, ut ait
Galenus, sit destitutum, et mollissimum sit, et sine fibris; non videtur rationi consonum, ut se
ipsum, propter irritatam expultricem, concutiat. neque credendum est, ad motum hunc producendum, eius vim expulsivam simpliciter naturalem, et nulla tactiva sensatione concurrente,
sufficientem esse, quoniam expultrix penitus naturalis, ut in sermone de virt. cordis ostensum a
nobis est, sine partis expellentis contractione, et aperto motu fit. quod autem cerebri substantia
penitus non sentiat ne dum in magnis capitis vulneribus, saepius experientia comprobavimus,
verum etiam validis rationibus probari potest. Namque, ut dictum est, cerebrum est mollissimum sine fibris, et omnino exangue. quae autem omnino exanguia sunt, ut docet experientia,
tactiva functione carent, quia, ut recte inquit Aphrodiseus, sine tenui sanguine, in quo spiritus,

consider irritation of the cerebral membranes the proximate cause of the epileptic attack.[294]

It is scarcely necessary to point out the shortcomings of this form of the irritation theory. Of course, neither the brain nor the meninges contract.[295] These mistakes were corrected only later. But judged on the basis of contemporary physiological and clinical knowledge, this theory offered an explanation of a variety of phenomena. Above all, it accounted for epileptic attacks following wounds or syphilitic affections of the skull, ulcerations of the cerebral membranes, and subcranial bleeding.[296]

Perpetuating older hypotheses, it was believed that any part of the body could be a source of irritation for the meninges and the brain. Paré maintained that the dura mater covered not only the brain and the spinal cord, but every nerve and membrane of the body as well. An ulceration of any part, e.g., of the foot, could affect the local membranes, whereupon the patient might feel something creep upward until it reached his brain and an epileptic attack ensued.[297] Usually, however,

---

et calor residet tactus fieri non potest. Cui difficultati satisfacientes dicimus cerebrum secundum expultricem irritari, ut fiat ille motus seu concussio, non quidem in virtute propriae substantiae cerebri, sed merito membranarum, quae quidem eximio, et exquisitissimo sensu praeditae sunt, et praesertim tenuioris, quae per cerebri substantiam pluribus in locis disseminatur." Similarly Sennert (913), *Pract. med.*, I, pars 2, c. 31; vol. 2, p. 237: ". . . recte etiam hic statuimus, cerebrum in Epilepsia affici, quatenus ob membranas suas sensu praeditum est. Etsi enim cerebri substantia non sentiat: tamen in membranis cerebri, et quae illud continent, et in tenuissima illa membrana, quae ventriculos cerebri intus investit, sensus inest. Et hinc fit, ut malignitate et acrimonia materiae Epilepticae vellicatum cerebrum sese cum nervoso genere concutiat, atque id, quod molestum est, excutere conetur."

[294] Bruno (177), *Theses inaugurales medicae de epilepsia*, IV: "Causa epilepsiae continens seu proxima diversa itidem a diversis statuitur: neoterici ut plurimum eam statuunt irritationem sue vellicationem cerebri meningum ab allisione spiritus acris aut maligni, cerebri meningas, quae exquisiti admodum sensus sunt ferientis et tristi quodam sensu afficientis: quamvis etiam sententia Galeni non incommodo defendi possit." A subtle argument arose over the question whether the natural faculty (Comes Montanus) or the animal faculty (Erastus) or both together (Sennert) would account for the convulsive motions; cf. Sennert, *l.c.*, vol. 2, p. 237 f.

[295] Coiter denied movement to the brain: "Agnorum, hoedorum et canuum viventium, quo certo, num cerebrum movetur, deprehenderem, aperui capita at nullum cernere quivi in iis motum" [Quoted from Neuburger (731), p. xxvi]. According to Neuburger (*l.c.* and p. 72) Coiter denied the phenomenon of cerebral motion altogether, whereas according to Pagel (760), p. 111, Coiter saw the pulsating motion of the brain but referred it to the arteries, thus denying to the brain any autonomous movement.

[296] Cf. Steeghius (953), *Medicina practica*, VII, 3; p. 320. "Irritation" of single nerves and muscles by humors and vapors was also conceived as an explanation of convulsive phenomena. The fact, for example, that some epileptic seizures began with convulsions of the eyebrows, the eyes, or the whole face was explained by Spigelius as an irritation of the third pair of cerebral nerves; Spigelius (944), *De humani corporis fabrica*, VII, 2; p. 206 f.: "Solet quoque in nonnullis Epilepsiae praeludium in palpebris, facie tota, ac oculis, eodem nomine oboriri, cum tertium hoc par [i.e., of cranial nerves] ab humoribus epilepsiam generantibus vellicetur, sicque convulsio oculorum et faciei nascatur." Sennert attributed partial convulsions in scurvy to the evil vapor penetrating and nipping a particular muscle or nerve; Sennert (913), *Pract. med.*, III, pars 5, sect. 2, c. 4; vol. 3, p. 264: "Nonnunquam tamen particulares convulsiones excitantur [i.e., in scurvy], vapore isto pravo peculiarem aliquem musculum, vel nervum occupante, eumque vel acrimonia, vel peculiari proprietate vellicante."

[297] Paré (772), *Oeuvres*, vol. I, p. 211.

an ascending vapor was held responsible for the irritation of the brain evoked from a distant part. At the same time it was considered theoretically unimportant which part had been afflicted, whether the stomach, uterus, legs, or arms, since the mechanism would always be the same. This led to a simplification of the traditional scheme. From now on, most authors recognized but two types of epilepsy: idiopathic epilepsy originating in the brain itself, and sympathetic epilepsy arising from some other organ. The distinction between epilepsy from the stomach and from other parts was abandoned as being unessential, and the three Galenic types were now put aside.[298]

The irritation theory of epilepsy, included in Galen's pathology and generalized during the Renaissance, is not without interest for the history of physiology. It shows that long before Glisson and Willis, physicians were acquainted with the term as well as concept of irritation. Although not backed by experimental evidence, the opinion that a strong stimulant would lead to a contraction of the irritated parts was familiar enough.[299] For most of the older physiologists and pathologists an epileptic seizure was a purposeful act by which nature through her expulsive faculty tried to rid the organism of a harmful agent. Only after Harvey's discovery of the circulation of the blood and Descartes' mechanistic philosophy had defeated the old physiology did some physicians begin to view the epileptic fit not as a beneficial reaction but as a mere necessary consequence of pathological forces.

---

[298] Culpeper's paraphrase of Riverius (853), p. 29: "There is in Galen, and almost all Authors, a threefold Epilepsy. The first is that which hurts the Brain, in which the Disease is: The second is that which hurts the Brain by consent from the Stomach: The third is when the disease is sent from other parts of the Body to the head: And these have their proper names; The first, as being chief, is called Epilepsia; the second Analepsia; the third, Catalepsia: But (by Galens leave) that division is superfluous, and in vain is that Epilepsy which comes from the Stomach separated from those which comes by sympathy from other parts; when all ought to be called Sympathicae, or Epilepsies by consent. Neither is it sufficient to say that an Epilepsy from the Stomach is distinct from others, because it is most frequent since that which comes from the Stomach and Spleen, is as usual and as frequent, if not more. Therefore we divide an Epilepsy into a Proper one, and one by Consent. Again, we subdivide that which is by consent according to the divers parts from whence these sharp and malignant vapors are sent to the Brain, for there is almost no part in the Body from which a malignant vapor cannot be sent."

[299] Cf. Temkin (998).

# PART FOUR

# THE GREAT SYSTEMS AND THE PERIOD OF ENLIGHTENMENT

# VII
# The Great Systems

## 1. IATROCHEMISTS AND IATROPHYSICISTS

The latter part of the seventeenth century developed some theories of epilepsy which took into account the new discoveries in the fields of chemistry and physics. The trend had already started among some iatro-chemists of the Renaissance, when an attempt was made to give the vague notion of poisonous vapors a more concrete chemical meaning. Quercetanus (1521–1609) put the blame on a vitriolic vapor of mercury, and his theory, although rejected by the more ortho-dox, nevertheless must have made a great impression since it was quoted by so many authorities from the beginning of the seventeenth century on.[1]

Such early attempts were, however, not much more than chemical interpretations of current theories. A real break with tradition set in with the development of the great chemical systems of Sylvius and Willis on the one hand, and with the iatrophysicists on the other.

Sylvius (1614–72) places the cause of epilepsy in the animal spirits themselves, which are necessary for the functioning of both movement and sense percep-tions. If the animal spirits become ill-disposed, move-ment and sense perceptions will be affected. Sylvius finds the proximate cause of epilepsy in a deviation and inordinate motion of the animal spirits; this, he thinks, accounts for the various symptoms of the epi-

---

[1] Cf. Quercetanus (833), *Tetras*, p. 114 ff. Horstius (515), *Centuriae problemat.*, decas 2, quaestio 9; t. 3, p. 33, and particularly Sennert (913), *Pract. med.*, I, pars 2, c. 31, quaest. 3; vol. 2, p. 237, who discusses the theories of various Paracelsists.

leptic attack.[2]  But what affects the animal spirits in such a way?
Sylvius answers: an acid volatile spirit; this spirit is the remote cause of
epilepsy,[3] and if it mixes with the animal spirits, it disturbs them violently.[4] From this chemical explanation Sylvius deduces the principle
of his chemical therapy: antiepileptic remedies are those which contain
a basic or other salt of a fixing quality.[5]

In the chapter on epileptic seizures in children Sylvius develops his
theory of the various causes of epilepsy and of their interaction more
systematically. Here again he assumes acid spirits or vapors to be the
main factor, irritating the spinal cord and brain and mingling fatally
with the animal spirits. The former action explains the convulsive
motions, the latter the mental symptoms of epilepsy.[6] In addition,
Sylvius follows the development of this harmful agent step by step and
distinguishes at least five causes. Bile and pancreatic juice form the
*antecedent* cause of epilepsy. As such, they are not yet pathogenetic,
but become so under the influence of some *irritative* cause (*causa irri-
tans* or *causa procatarctica*). The air, a wrong diet, fright, or something similar, make the acid pancreatic juice and the bile effervesce in
the intestines, thus creating the harmful *remote* cause, i.e., the acid
evaporations. These vapors pass from the lacteal vessels into the blood
and are carried to the brain, where they now constitute the *conjoint*
(*causa continens*) as well as *proximate* cause. They act as a proximate
cause since they account for the symptoms of the attack, and as the
conjoint cause since the symptoms last as long as the vapors are
present.[7]

Sylvius was one among many physicians of the sixteenth and seventeenth centuries who put even greater emphasis on the formal distinction of the causes of epilepsy than had the medieval doctors.[8] He and
his contemporaries were not always unanimous in their definitions of
the various causes and did not always distinguish the same number. Yet

---

[2] Sylvius (984), *Prax. med.*, II, c. 20, 83; p. 319: "Adeo ut proxima laesarum primario in
Epilepsia functionum causa sit Animalium Spirituum a sensoriis aversio, sive amandationis
naturalis ad ipsa defectus; atque ad motus organa interruptus, inordinatus, conturbatusque ac
vehemens motus."

[3] *Ibid.*, c. 20, 89; p. 320: "Ex quibus omnibus et similibus ex praxi desumendis concludo,
Causam Epilepsiae remotiorem, et animales spiritus ad paroxysmum producendum disponentem
esse Spiritum acidum volatilem."

[4] *Ibid.*, c. 20, 92; p. 320.

[5] *Ibid.*, c. 20, 125; p. 321: "Remedium autem ipsi futurum salem lixiviosum vel fixum, vel
volatilem quidem, ast simul fixantem; atque, alterutrum observari in plerisque Antepilepticis
medicamentis."

[6] Sylvius (984), *Prax. med. appendix*, tract. 1, c. 6, 27; p. 459.

[7] *Ibid.*, p. 459 f. This complicated system of causes goes back to ancient sources; for the
latter cf. Wellmann (1079), p. 154 ff., and Senn (912), p. 234 ff.

[8] Cf. above, p. 130 f.

it was more than a mere logical exercise. Particularly in a disease like epilepsy was it felt necessary to account for the various factors which cause the disease and to explain the sudden occurrence of its attacks. Every pathology of epilepsy considers these points, and it is only a question of logical neatness whether the various causes are differentiated implicitly, as in *On the Sacred Disease*, or numbered and named, as they were by physicians from the sixteenth to eighteenth centuries. Even in the eighteenth century, when scholastic niceties counted for little, these causes were still separated, and it was only in the later nineteenth century that the feeling for an orderly logical arrangement was lost.

For Willis (1622–75), ordinary muscular motion is brought about by an explosion. He acknowledged Gassendi as a sponsor of this idea,[9] but as *explosio Willisiana* it remained connected with his name.[10] The spirits in the muscular fibers contain spirituosaline particles, while the arterial blood supplies the muscles with nitrosulphurous particles, and these two kinds of particles are mixed like the nitre and sulphur in gunpowder. The action of the nerves ignites these particles and makes them explode, whereupon the muscles become inflated and shortened.[11]

Before applying his new theory to convulsive disorders, Willis reviewed some of the older opinions, in particular that of irritation. Well acquainted with the experimental work of his time, he knew that stimulation of the spinal nerves with a knife will bring about a response in the muscles. He also admitted that irritation of the nerves might cause slight and transient convulsions, but he thought that the conjoint and procatarctic causes of severe and repeated paroxysms had to be sought elsewhere.[12] To explain convulsions of this kind Willis assumed the existence of a "spasmodic explosive copula." In contrast to normal movements, this copula did not affect the muscles directly;[13] instead, "The Convulsive Disease . . . for the most part, takes its Original from the head: to wit, as often as the heterogeneous and explosive particles, being diffused from the Blood into the Brain, or its medullarie Appendix, are afterwards derived to the Nervous stock, and there grow together with the spirits."[14] As long as the particles were not too numer-

---

[9] Willis (1108), *De morbis convulsivis*, I, c. 1; p. 3; cf. Meyer and Hierons (688), p. 6, and Isler (537), p. 97.

[10] Wepfer (1085), *Observationes medico-practicae de affectibus capitis*, Observ. 133; p. 629: *"Explosioni Willisianae* hactenus assentire nequii . . ."

[11] Willis (1108), *De morbis convulsivis*, c. 1; p. 2.

[12] *Ibid.*, pp. 3–4.

[13] Although in some cases of partial convulsions this may be the case, cf. *ibid.*, p. 5.

[14] Willis (1107), *Of Convulsive Diseases*, ch. 1; p. 5 (Pordage's translation).

ous, they could mix with the spirit without any explosion taking place. A steady influx of particles could be assumed to remain unnoticed until a certain amount had been accumulated, or until some evident cause started off the process.[15] Willis knew quite a number of such evident causes, including one class where the convulsions were incited by reflex action.[16] Intestinal worms, drugs, and acrid humors might have this effect when they irritated some part of the nervous system, an irritation which was then communicated to the brain.[17]

After these general remarks about the nature of convulsive diseases, Willis approached the most important of all of them, epilepsy. The symptoms of the disease made it clear to him that it must have its seat in the brain.[18] But he disagreed with those of his predecessors who placed the origin either in the middle of the brain itself or in its meninges. He rejected the former opinion on the ground that the soft substance of the brain is not capable of contraction, and he dismissed the latter view because the meninges are so strongly fixed to the skull or tied up by blood vessels that they cannot possibly contract to any great degree.[19] Instead, he proposed the following hypothesis: the brain being of a weak constitution, and a strong spasmodic copula being distilled from the blood into the brain, the animal spirits which lie in the middle of the brain will be affected and will explode.[20] This will cause all the mental symptoms of the epileptic attack, and a series of similar explosions occurring along the rest of the nervous system will bring about the convulsions of the body.[21]

Willis accepted the division of epilepsy into idiopathic and sympathetic and was well aware of the various premonitory symptoms, including the ascending "breeze" which the patients may feel. Here he made a very important remark. Whereas physicians before him, with the exception of Le Pois, had assumed that such premonitory or initial symptoms corresponded to some lesion or corruption in the particular part of the body, Willis now pointed out that very often the cause lay in the brain. When the animal spirits in the brain and the spinal cord were all ready to explode, a more distant part deprived of the normal influx of animal spirits would sometimes begin to show spasms; this

---

[15] Willis (1108), *De morbis convulsivis*, c. 1; p. 8.

[16] *Ibid.*: "Quoad alterum causae evidentis genus, quo scilicet Spasmi actu reflexo incitantur." On Willis' concept of the reflex cf. Canguilhem (199), ch. 3. For more details of Willis' theory of epilepsy cf. Isler (537), pp. 96–105.

[17] Willis, *ibid.*

[18] *Ibid.*, c. 2; p. 12.

[19] *Ibid.*, pp. 12–13.

[20] *Ibid.*, p. 13.

[21] *Ibid.*, pp. 13–14. Brain (146), p. 323: "This is precisely the modern view of the nature of constitutional epilepsy, if we substitute the idea of an electric discharge for a discharge of animal spirits." Cf. Also Canguilhem (199), p. 76, and Isler (537), pp. 98 and 101.

process would spread backward along the nerves till it reached the central nervous system, where now the explosion would take place.[22]

The theories of Sylvius and Willis are two outstanding examples of the new way of explaining epilepsy. Other physicians near to the iatro-chemical school proposed hypotheses of their own with more or less far-reaching modifications. Resemblance to Willis can be found in the views of Blankaart (1650-1702),[23] who repeats the idea of an explosion of the animal spirits in the brain. Others are more inclined toward Sylvius or hold opinions which are mainly their own. Many, like Ett-müller (1644-1683) and Barbette (d. 1666), reject the idea of ascending vapors, the former calling it "a false imagination" and "a vulgar error."[24] Barbette finds that "the nearest Cause is the Lympha vitiated in the Brain, and irritating the nerves by it's Sharpness. The remote Causes are to be sought for in the milky glandules, the womb, and in other parts." It "is the Brain, and consequently the Nerves, but in no wise the Membranes" which are primarily affected.[25] The desire to connect the pathology of the disease with the most recent physio-logical discoveries is perhaps best illustrated by Mayow (1645-79). Having inferred the existence of "nitro-aërial particles," which have some of the properties of what we call oxygen, Mayow identifies them with the animal spirits, which are of necessity sent to the brain. Saline-sulphurous particles, on the other hand, must be prevented from reaching the brain since their action on the animal spirits would cause disturbed movements, epilepsy, and similar conditions.[26]

Manifold as these chemical theories of epilepsy are, they have one common tendency: to make the epileptic attack appear, as far as possible, a necessary result of chemical forces. This is obvious in Willis' views, where irritation is relegated to a secondary place, and where all the phenomena are explained by the explosion of the animal spirits. The epileptic fit is not seen as a purposeful act, but as a physical consequence. Nevertheless, the idea of irritation in the traditional sense was not banished altogether, as is shown by a few short remarks of Borelli's (1608-79) on normal and pathological motions. Under normal conditions and under the influence of the will, the animal spirits twitch the beginning of the nerves in the brain and cause the excretion of a few drops of nervous juice from the nerves into the blood of the

---

[22] Willis, *ibid.*, c. 13; p. 15.

[23] Blancard (120), *The Physical Dictionary*, s.v. *Epilepsia*, p. 85 f.

[24] *Ettmullerus Abridg'd* (331), p. 494-95.

[25] Barbette (78), *The Practice* etc., p. 2 (contemporary translation).

[26] Mayow (675), *On Muscular Motion and Animal Spirits*, p. 279. Mayow's views on epilepsy, since expressed parenthetically, are not quite clear. In another passage of the same treatise (p. 261 f.) he thinks that epilepsy may sometimes arise from a convulsion of the dura mater.

muscles. Hence, an explosion occurs which causes inflation of the muscles. Under pathological conditions, a morbific agent takes the place of the normal action of the animal spirits. Borelli reaches the conclusion that a sharp and saline humor, when acting upon the nerves, may thus produce convulsive motions. Yet the nerves do not react mechanically. After death the distortions of the body cease, because now "the sensitive faculty" in the nerves is dead, and with it the sense of being molested, which made the nerves twitch. Forthwith, they no longer pour out the spirituous juice.[27]

It is remarkable how near this view of Borelli's, one of the main iatrophysicists, comes to the ideas of the iatrochemists. This goes to show that the differences between the two schools, though striking in many instances, were not of a fundamental nature.

Borelli's erstwhile friend Malpighi (1628-94) is famous for his anatomical and physiological rather than for his pathological investigations. Yet some of his medical consultations which deal with epilepsy show that he was ready enough to draw medical consequences from his scientific research. One of the less fortunate conclusions at which Malpighi arrived was his idea concerning the structure and function of the brain. He pictured the cerebral cortex as a conglomeration of glands which, under the influence of a constant contraction of the brain, excreted nervous spirits or juice, first into the fibers of the brain, and hence into the nerves, muscles, and membranes. The result was a moderate tension of the fibers of the brain, so that the waves arriving from external objects and communicated by the sense organs were presented to the soul. At the same time clefts were held open in the muscles, into which humors could flow and effect the tension of the muscular fibers. In epilepsy, however, vitriolic and arsenical particles reached the brain, affected the nervous juice, and irritated the cerebral fibers, so that their normal tension was changed into a spasm. Consequently, the nerves drew back, the clefts in the muscles stayed open, the soul lost its power, and both senses and movements were impaired.[28]

---

[27] Borellus (136), *De motu animalium*, propos. 213; p. 433 ff.

[28] Malpighi (662), *Consultat. medic.*, consil. 10; p. 33: "Morbus hic ignotissimus est, cum adhuc circa ipsius causas, et generationem famigeratissimi etiam Medici insudent. Ex emergentibus tamen productis probabiliter philosophari licet, convulsionem esse totius cum sensuum internorum, et externorum motusque laesione. Ut autem haec magis pateant, praesciendum, in naturae statu perpetuo in corticalibus glandulis cerebri separari volatiles, mitesque spiritus, sive succum nerveum, qui in determinata quantitate ex perenni, blanda cerebri contractione in productas ejusdem fibras, et ex his in continuatos nervos exprimitur, et postremo in musculos, et membranas imperio etiam voluntatis propellitur; ita ut sensus externi, et interni motusque naturales peragantur, quatenus inducta mediocri tensione in cerebri fibris undulationes ab externis objectis mediis sensoriis communicatae recipiuntur, et animae objiciuntur, et in musculis hiatus patent humoribus, a quibus fibrarum in musculis subita succedit tensio. In hoc autem morboso statu immutata nervei succi natura, nativa fibrarum cerebri tensio ex irritatione in spasmum, et convulsionem interpolatam immutatur; et retractis singulis nervis tumultuarie, et absque imperio animae patentibus fibrarum carnearum meatibus, musculi in motu detinentur,

Malpighi's errors were destined to influence the pathology of epilepsy of generations of later physicians. They were partly taken over and elaborated, with certain modifications, by Baglivi (d. 1707), who is usually considered the most radical representative of the iatrophysical school. On the basis of anatomical and clinical observations, physiological experiments, and physical speculations, Baglivi worked out a neurological theory which was modern for its time and wrong from the present point of view. Shortly before Baglivi, Vieussens had described the fibrous texture of the dura mater, and his results were confirmed by Baglivi and Pacchioni.[29] Baglivi proceeded to distinguish two types of fibers: membranous fibers, which had their origin in the membranes of the brain, and fleshy fibers, which were chiefly represented by the muscles.[30] But he did not restrict contraction to muscular fibers; on the contrary, he believed that the fibers of the dura mater participated in this activity to an even higher degree. The heart, by its regular motions, kept the blood circulating in the body, and the dura mater, according to Baglivi, was the heart of the brain, moving in regular systole and diastole.[31] This movement was not dependent on the pulsation of the arteries of the dura mater[32] but must be considered autonomous. Its function was to distribute the nervous fluid over all parts of the body. For the cortex of the brain was but a conglomeration of glands where the nervous fluid was separated from the arterial blood. The excretory ducts of these glands formed the medullary part of the brain and of the spinal cord, and the nerves were the canals through which the nervous fluid passed to the various organs. The dura mater pressed the nervous fluid from the cortical glands into the excretory ducts and canals, and upon its activity depended the regulation of bodily movements by the soul.[33] Besides, the membranes, not the medullary substance of the nerves, were the seat of sensation[34] and became thus the main instrument of the soul. The regular movement of the dura mater could be explained on purely mechanical grounds. The arrangement of the fibers gave it a high degree of elasticity, and under normal circumstances the dura mater moved under the same influence of elastic forces, like a clock. The nervous fluids, moreover, when propelled to the parts, sup-

---

et ita sensus interni, et externi motusque labefactantur vitiato organo. Excitatur igitur probabiliter haec convulsiva contractio in cerebro, et appensis nervis a particulis vitriolatis, et arsenicalibus, quibus veluti ab aqua stygia alte penetrante, et erodente tenella fibrarum cerebri structura lacessitur."

[29] Cf. Baglivi (73), *De fibra motrice*, c. 5, p. 272 f.

[30] *Ibid.*, c. 3. On the doctrine of fibres cf. Berg (105) and Bastholm (84).

[31] Baglivi, *l.c.*, c. 5, p. 273.

[32] *Ibid.*, p. 280.

[33] *Ibid.*, p. 282 f.

[34] *Ibid.*, p. 287: "Solum systema membranarum sentit, ipsique nervi sunt adeo acuti sensus, non ob medullarem sui substantiam, sed ob membranas, quibus involvuntur."

plied the latter with tonus and a kind of oscillating movement which was reflected toward the dura mater, so that the whole organism was in a state of elastic equilibrium.[35]

Many physicians of the eighteenth century accepted this physiological theory as a basis for the understanding of epilepsy. Baglivi himself made some contributions in this direction. Under the influence of some violent agent the normal action of the dura mater would be changed into a pathological, i.e., vehement and irregular, movement; the course of the nervous fluid would also become irregular and disturbed, and all kinds of nervous diseases, including epilepsy, would follow.[36] If, on the other hand, the equilibrium between the various parts of the body were disturbed, then convulsive movements, excited in some part, might be reflected to the head. In this way Baglivi explained Galen's case of the epileptic boy whose fit had started from the toe.[37]

Baglivi thought that observation and experiments supported his views. If the medullary part of the brain were touched in a patient suffering from a wound of the head, he would remain quiet; whereas touching the dura or pia mater would produce convulsions in the whole body.[38] New-born lambs would show convulsive movements, particularly on the side on which the dura mater was pricked either with a fine needle or acrid fluids.[39] Similar results were obtained when the vertebrae of various animals were trephined and acids injected: convulsions and other symptoms were present.[40]

The influence of Baglivi is evident in Fr. Hoffmann,[41] who, however, modified his basic concepts in some respects. Hoffmann knew that there were many remote causes which could be responsible for epilepsy. But there was one proximate cause that explained the various features of the seizure, viz., a stricture of the dura mater.[42] Such a stricture arose from a stagnation of the blood in the sinuses of the dura mater. The circulation of the blood in the brain was now impeded, and coarse particles (instead of the usual fine ethereal substance) entered from the cerebral arteries into the brain. At the same time, the blood vessels were dilated, and this led to the spastic stricture of the cerebral membranes. The brain was compressed; more nervous fluid than was normal flowed

---

[35]*Ibid.*, p. 281.

[36]*Ibid.*, p. 276.

[37]*Ibid.*, p. 281 f.

[38]*Ibid.*, c. 8, p. 322.

[39]*Ibid.*, c. 5, p. 274 f.

[40]*Ibid.*, p. 277 f.

[41]Cf. Hoffmann (503), *Medicina rationalis systematica*, tom. IV, pars 3, sec. 1, c. 1, § 10; vol. 2, p. 11, where Baglivi is quoted.

[42]*Ibid.*, § 12: "Ex his adparebit, in omni epilepsia praesto esse membranae cerebrum, medullam spinalem, ac nervos investientis structuram, ceu caussam illius proximam."

into the nerves and caused convulsion in the motor organs, particularly the muscles. The nerves which communicated with the sense organs were, on the other hand, constricted, which resulted in a temporary loss of the external as well as internal senses.[43] The process which in the brain produced the epileptic fit accounted for other convulsive motions without the stigmata of epilepsy, if it took place in the membranes of the spinal cord[44] or of the joints.[45] And, since the membranes of the brain, of the spinal cord, and of the articulations were intimately connected, it was obvious why convulsive motions so often passed into epileptic seizures.[46]

## 2. ANIMISM AND ECLECTICISM

With Baglivi and those influenced by him, the mechanical theory of epilepsy had reached its extreme. Epilepsy was now explained by disturbed elastic equilibrium of fibers, pressure in blood vessels, etc. The great number of different theories of this kind suggests of course that none of them proved satisfactory. There were too many factors of a purely speculative nature involved, and everyone speculated differently. Very little was known about the structure and physiology of the brain, meninges, nerves, and muscles; and the chemical knowledge was equally unsatisfactory. Various kinds of fibers, glands of the brain, vitriolic, arsenical, and other particles were chiefly products of the imagination. Complicated as many of these theories of epilepsy were, they still failed to explain all the details.

Toward the end of the seventeenth century opposition to a purely mechanical physiology and pathology gained strength. The movement, which became very strong during the eighteenth century, was characterized by the renewed emphasis upon a teleological principle in the explanation of biological processes. It reached a climax with the animism of Stahl, but many later physicians, though opposed to Stahl, belonged to it because of their opposition to mere mechanism. This movement, for which a common name is lacking, was not at all uniform. But, at least as far as the theory of epilepsy is concerned, it showed a uniform tendency to view the epileptic attack as a purposeful and essentially beneficial reaction of the soul or of "nature."

The new point of view and its connection with earlier pathologists can perhaps be best understood from an analysis of some principles laid down by the Swiss physician Wepfer (1620–95). In a work on hemlock Wepfer investigated the action of poisons, particularly their

---

[43] *Ibid.*, § 11.
[44] *Ibid.*, c. 2, § 2; p. 24.
[45] *Ibid.*, c. 3, § 2; p. 34.
[46] *Ibid.*, c. 2, § 8; p. 25 and c. 3, § 2; p. 34.

irritative effects. Wepfer is one of the scientists of the later seventeenth century to whom the experimental study of irritability owes a great deal. Having observed spasms and convulsions in various cases, Wepfer put the question whether epilepsy could be explained by the action of irritative agents alone. His answer was a negative one, and his reasons were the following: there are many diseases, like syphilis and cancer, which (in the opinion of the time) are accompanied by corruption of the humors and where acrimonious irritants are certainly present in the body. One would, therefore, expect these diseases to be frequently complicated by epilepsy, yet Wepfer says that this is rarely—if ever—the case.[47] Again, if in other diseases where convulsions occasionally occur the irritating humors alone were responsible, all or most cases should show convulsive attacks—whereas in reality this is not so.[48] Epilepsy can, therefore, not be explained as the necessary result of an irritating agent. One has to assume the existence of a higher selective principle, which Wepfer calls the "president" of the nervous system,[49] and which he compares with the *archeus* of van Helmont and the *appetitus sensitivus* of Glisson.[50] Under the command of the "president" the body tries to rid itself of harmful irritants, a response which is both purposeful and beneficial. But the "president" is not endowed with any clear judgment and does not know whether the forces at his command suffice to expel the irritant. If the latter is very strong, the "president" may be provoked to a wild and unreasonable reaction, and thus it happens that convulsions very often are a sign of death.[51]

It may seem surprising that Wepfer connects his own views and those of van Helmont with Glisson, since we are accustomed to consider Glisson (1597–1677) as the forerunner of the *modern* theory of irritability. But Glisson himself refers to the *archeus*,[52] and his principle of irritability presumes the existence of some kind of perception in the organs. While it is true that he used the term "irritability" for a general property of the fibers, he neither gave it a mechanical interpretation nor did he accept it as a basic physiological phenomenon independent of all sensibility. The clear distinction between sensibility and irritability was the work of Albrecht von Haller.[53]

From Wepfer we learn how the new theory of epilepsy was connected with earlier scientists. On the other hand, Wepfer's ideas antici-

---

[47]Wepfer (1084), *Cicutae aquaticae historia*, p. 99: "Denique saepe pessimae notae particulae illaeque acerrimae sanguini confunduntur, a quibus nunquam vel rarissime Epilepsia excitatur."

[48]*Ibid.*, p. 103.

[49]*Ibid.*, p. 100: "Ad rem hanc obscurissimam explicandam aliquo modo necessario statuendus videtur *Praeses* aliquis *toti Systemati nervoso praefixus*," etc.

[50]Cf. *ibid.* The connection of these concepts has been brought out by Pagel (758), p. 53 ff.

[51]Wepfer, *l.c.*, p. 107.

[52]Glisson (415), *Tractatus de ventriculo et intestinis*, c. 8, 6; p. 161.

[53]For details on Glisson's ideas of irritation and irritability cf. Temkin (998).

pate Stahl's doctrine of convulsions and epilepsy. According to Stahl (1660-1734) it is the soul which rules the living body, watches over the vital tonus, and regulates the movements of the organism. Convulsions[54] and epilepsy[55] cannot be explained as mechanical processes. All kinds of stimuli, even foreign bodies in the ear,[56] or worms,[57] can provoke epileptic convulsions. But they do not cause the convulsions *in* the parts (i.e., by some kind of mechanical action); rather they provoke the organism to carry out these movements *by* the parts, i.e., as a purposeful reaction.[58] Some idea arising from wrath or anxiety expresses itself through the disturbed motions and lies at the bottom of the disease.[59] The causes of the epileptic seizure do not come from outside but lie inside the human organism; its true architects are sufferings of the soul brought about by anxious and terrifying "prefigurations."[60] The fact that convulsions so often are seen in psychic disturbances is one of the main arguments for their moral rather than mechanical origin.[61]

In his classification of convulsions Stahl makes a suggestion which foreshadows a later development. Epileptic and other convulsive movements cannot be distinguished by the more or less severe character of the symptoms. The only logical distinction according to Stahl would be to consider as symptomatic convulsive movements all those convulsions which appear as complications of some disease, and to recognize as epileptic convulsions only those whose vehemence has no relation to other diseases.[62]

Stahl's theory, the very opposite of the contemporary iatrochemical and iatrophysical explanations, exerted a great influence upon a number of physicians, particularly in England, who, though averse to mysti-

---

[54] Stahl (948), *Theoria medica vera*, Pathologia, pars 2, sec. 3, membr. 3; vol. 2, p. 264, where Stahl uses the same arguments as Wepfer.

[55] *Ibid.*, pars 3, sec. 2, membr. 4, art. 2; vol. 3, p. 320.

[56] *Ibid.*, vol. 3, p. 323 f., where Stahl refers to an observation by Fabricius Hildanus.

[57] *Ibid.*, p. 325 f.

[58] *Ibid.*, p. 322: ". . . sed *incitamenta motuum*, non tam simpliciter *in* partes inducendorum, aut *in* partibus agitandorum, sed vere *per* partes exercendorum, et non aliter, quam alias etiam ad manifestos certos fines solent, instruendorum."

[59] *Ibid.*, p. 320: ". . . non minor certe ex horum comparatione elucescit probabilitas, quod hi motus [edit. has 'modus'] tamquam ideam aliquam seu qualemcunque impressionem, tamquam iracundam aut tamquam anxie trepida intentione subnixam, pro fundamento habeant;" etc. It is, therefore, not surprising to see Stahl stress the emotional cause of epilepsy in children, possibly by the mediation of the nursing mothers; see Stahl (949), pp. 32 and 34, for the German translation of pertinent passages from the *Disputatio inauguralis de passionibus animi corpus humanum varie alterantibus* of J. J. Reich.

[60] Stahl (948), p. 317.

[61] *Ibid.*, pars 2, sec. 3, membr. 3; vol. 2, p. 267: "Quae res ut omnino moralem magis, seu finalem harum rerum efficaciam impulsivam declarat, ita illustrat hanc eo magis notissima illa, et penitus quod aiunt confessa, energia ad producendas convulsiones, tamquam magis simplices et idiopathicas, quam exserunt animi pathemata." For the relationship of Stahl and van Helmont cf. Pagel (758).

[62] Stahl, *l.c.*, p. 263.

cism, yet believed a merely mechanical explanation insufficient. Even from a physiological point of view it helped to simplify matters considerably. Iatrophysicists and iatrochemists alike had found it necessary to uphold the hypothesis of psychic spirits or of a psychic fluid. This hypothesis was not essential for the followers of Stahl. Since the soul itself commanded all vital motions, the assumption of psychic spirits, i.e., special instruments of the soul, could be abandoned. This aspect of Stahl's system recommended itself to men like Cheyne[63] and others, who combined Stahl's animism with the principles of Newtonian physics. Cheyne (1671–1743) compared the relation of soul and body to that of a musician and his instrument.[64] The instrument of course is a physical object and renders sounds according to purely physical laws. But the instrument needs the musician to play it. Similarly, Cheyne explained most nervous functions through the elasticity of the fibers, which conveyed impressions to the sentient principle situated in the brain. Nervous functions had a physical basis but obeyed a psychic principle, and nervous disorders, although caused by disturbances of the nervous system, were not mere mechanical phenomena. Thus, Cheyne could again consider the convulsions accompanying epilepsy as "the Struggle of Nature to throw off the peccant Cause . . . ."[65] This teleological view of epileptic convulsions was also shared by others who did not agree with Stahlian doctrines. The latter made it very difficult to explain those muscular movements which did not depend upon the exertion of the will and might even be provoked a long time after death. Robert Whytt (1714–66) recognized this difficulty: for the explanation of involuntary movements he accepted some kind of sensibility with which the parts of the organism were endowed and a "general sympathy which prevails throughout the whole body."[66] As one of the examples of sympathy he mentioned epileptic fits which resulted from a mechanical irritation of the nerves of the great toe or the calf of the leg.[67] But he confessed ignorance as to the manner in which irritation of the brain or any other part induced convulsions in the body.

> And here we must rest; for to endeavour to explain more particularly, either how the passions, or an irritation of the brain or other sensible parts, bring on alternate convulsions or fixed spasms of the muscles, would be to no purpose, till we are better acquainted with

---

[63] For a refutation of animal spirits, Cheyne (218), *The English Malady*, p. 78, refers to the Stahlian Goelike and to Pemberton.

[64] Cheyne (218), *The English Malady*, p. 69 ff.

[65] *Ibid.*, p. 225.

[66] Whytt (1097), *Observations on the Nature, Causes, and Cure of those Disorders which are commonly called Nervous, Hypochondriac or Hysteric*, p. 494.

[67] *Ibid.*

the structure of these organs, and with that cause which immediately produces their contraction; points which will probably for ever elude our researches. All we know is, that whatever irritates or disagreeably affects the brain, nerves, or any of the more sensible parts, occasions continued spasms or convulsive motions, either in the parts themselves, if muscular, or in those with which they have any considerable sympathy; and that, when the nervous system is delicate, or the irritation great, almost all the muscles will be sometimes agitated with alternate contractions, or affected with a *tetanus* or general rigidity.[68]

The work from which this quotation has been taken was first published in 1764. Its note of resignation evidences the fate of the great medical systems. While the beginning of the eighteenth century marked the height of their development, and epilepsy was explained according to one or a few principles, none of these explanations had received general approval. It is true, theorizing on this line did not stop during the century, and at its end it found a new vehicle in the systems of Cullen and Brown. But at the same time an eclectic clinical attitude became more and more pronounced and expressed itself in Boerhaave (1668-1738) and his pupils. This school did not altogether avoid pathological systems. Boerhaave himself, an academic teacher of great accomplishment, was more open to scholastic traditionalism than is usually recognized. In his *Praelectiones de morbis nervorum*, which was published posthumously in 1761, he still implicitly followed the Galenic classification of epilepsy. He distinguished between *epilepsia idiopathica* and *epilepsiae deuteropathicae*, the latter having their seat either in the stomach or somewhere else outside the brain.[69] The influence of van Helmont, whom he often mentioned in the chapter on epilepsy, is unmistakable, and he went so far as to quote a prescription containing human blood as a specific against *some* kinds of epilepsy.[70] Even in his short and concise *Aphorisms*, one of his most influential works on the diagnosis and therapy of diseases, Boerhaave revealed his systematic tendencies. Having pointed out the great variety of muscular contractions in the epileptic attack, he said: "But all those varieties consist only in changing the motions of the moveable parts, and therefore of the muscular; wherefore they only suppose various contractions of the muscles; hence various influxes of the nervous liquid, and thence the various distribution of it from the common sensory to the nerves; and lastly therefore various causes in the medulla of the brain pro-

---

[68] *Ibid.*, p. 591.

[69] Cf. Boerhaave (130), *Praelectiones*, p. 834, where he refers to Fernelius.

[70] *Ibid.*, p. 849 f.: "Spiritus salis sanguinis humani magno Helmontio dicitur remedium certissimum ad curandam Epilepsiam [follows recipe] . . . Omnia haec remedia valent ad quasdam Epilepsias, non vero ad omnes, uti ex antecedentibus satis patuit."

ducing these distributions, etc. which are best known from the historical account of them."[71] The pathological hypotheses implicit in this
aphorism, such as the existence of a nervous liquid, its distribution into
the nerves from the medullary part of the brain, are reminiscent of the
iatrophysical school. But they play a subordinate role. Boerhaave's
emphasis lies much more on the enumeration of those factors which
can actually be observed either in the living patient or on the dissecting
table. The chapter on epilepsy in the great commentary of Boerhaave's
pupil van Swieten (1700–72) on his teacher's aphorisms is a product of
the tendencies of this school. This chapter is interesting for its omis-
sions as well as its contents. It contains good clinical descriptions of the
disease in its various forms and of the relation to other diseases, such as
apoplexy and hysteria. Van Swieten also tries to explain the various
symptoms, such as the initial cry, the swelling of the veins, frothing, on
the basis of the physiological facts known in his time. He does not try
to trace them all back to one pathological theory. He seems scarcely
interested in the systematic attempts of the preceding generations and
does not discuss them at any length. On the other hand, he is remark-
ably well versed in the literature of the ancients; Hippocrates, Aretaeus,
Galen, Caelius Aurelianus, and a few others are authorities as far as
observations are concerned, whereas the literature of the Middle Ages,
both Arabic and Latin, is nonexistent for him. He gives an almost
exhaustive account of the various causes observed by himself or by
others, and he emphasizes the multiplicity of such causes and the therapeutic consequences. Epilepsy cannot be cured by the same procedure
in all cases, hence, the trust in one specific is ridiculous. The practitioner has to investigate every case carefully, and even though the predisposing cause may be hidden, he can at least find the provoking cause
and eliminate it. He will thus be able to prevent the occurrence of
further attacks, and there is no necessity for exaggerated pessimism.

From this short analysis it is possible to recognize not only a new
approach toward the study and cure of epilepsy but also a new type of
physician. It is the scientifically trained and scientifically interested
practitioner who is an eclectic rather than a dogmatist. A classical
scholar, he is yet conscious of the progress of his times and inclined
toward contempt for the Middle Ages. He is full of optimism in the
exertion of his art and trusts in observation and his power of reasoning.
This new type of physician assumed an important role in the bourgeois
society which gradually established itself from the seventeenth century
on. He was a leader in many branches of civic and cultural life, and
particularly in that movement which is called "Enlightenment." En-

---

[71] Boerhaave, *Aphorisms*, sec. 1074, quoted from the contemporary English translation of
van Swieten's (982) *Commentaries*, vol. 10, p. 343 f.

lightenment had a marked influence upon the history of epilepsy; at the same time the attitude of the physicians toward this disease reflects the progress and intensity of Enlightenment. Many of the medical views of the eighteenth century about epilepsy have been abandoned, but our general attitude toward it was influenced decisively by the "enlightened" physicians of this period. For Enlightenment did not end with the eighteenth century; in many respects the process is still going on. Before returning to the development of medical observations and theories we shall, therefore, discuss the emergence of new views about epilepsy and its relation to supernatural forces, cosmic phenomena, and occult remedies.

# VIII
# The Enlightenment

## 1. THE FIGHT AGAINST THE SUPERNATURAL AND OCCULT

### a. The Rationalistic Interpretation of Possession

The process which we commonly call "Enlightenment" began in England in the late seventeenth century. It slowly spread to other Western countries, until at the end of the eighteenth century it was counterbalanced by increasing romantic tendencies. In every country enlightenment had its own antecedents and its own controversies with customs, beliefs, and practices that were to be declared superstitious.

In England, enlightenment followed the intense religious excitement of the puritan age. Trembling, convulsions, frothing were frequently seen among sectarians and especially among the enthusiasts[72] and came to life again among the Methodists of the eighteenth century. During the Salem witchcraft trials, possession with its classical features played a decisive role. In France, the convulsionists of St. Médard[73] showed by their very designation that they belonged in the same group. These are only some of the historically outstanding examples of "possession," divine or devilish, which formed the religious background against which the Enlightenment viewed epilepsy.

As a whole, physicians during the second half of the seventeenth century and a great many of them in the first half of the eighteenth century did not exclude the infliction of epilepsy by the Devil and by witches. Willis, in commenting upon the name "Sacred Disease" and the belief in demoniacs

---

[72] Rosen (872), p. 207 f., and Rosen (871), p. 414.
[73] See below.

as expressed in the Gospel, said: "In truth, in this Distemper [i.e., epilepsy], no marks at all of the Morbifick matter appears, or are so very obscure, that we may have deservedly suspected it to be an inspiration of an evil spirit; at least it is probably, that as often as the Devil is permitted to afflict miserable Mortals with his delusions, he is not able to draw more cruel Arrows from any other Quiver, or to shew Miracles by any better Witch than by the assaults of this monstrous Disease."[74] Others went beyond this kind of ambiguous admission. Hoffmann proved in a special thesis that the Devil had physical power and could cause epilepsy.[75] The animist Stahl stated dogmatically that witches and magic sometimes caused the disease.[76] The main argument brought forward in defense of such opinions was the appeal to supposedly incontrovertible facts: Christ had cured the lunatic boy who was possessed by an unclean spirit and who had obviously been an epileptic. "But can it be absolutely denied," asked van Swieten, "that this disease was never produced from supernatural causes? Certainly no; for that epileptic boy, who is mentioned in the comment to the preceding section, was cured by our blessed Saviour, by throwing out the devil."[77]

For Bartholinus, the chief medical interpreter of biblical diseases in the latter half of the seventeenth century, the demoniac nature of the biblical case of epilepsy was undoubted.[78] The same is true of the very learned English physician, Dr. Jonathan Harle, who wrote about half a century later. "That there were some actually possess'd by the devil, is a truth as plain as words can make it: 'Tis true, in one place a person is said to have a devil, and be mad, and another to be a demoniack, and yet is call'd a lunatick, or one troubled with the falling sickness. If we take in both texts, we have the full meaning, which is, that the madness and epilepsy these people labour'd under were caus'd by the devil."[79] This is clear enough as far as the Bible is concerned, but Harle's views are much more sceptical and enlightened when he discusses other supernatural beliefs associated with epilepsy. He says that in all ages its strange symptoms have been attributed to God or spirits, and epileptics have been esteemed prophets.[80] "Among us it is called lying in a trance,

---

[74]Willis (1107), *Of Convulsive Diseases*, ch. 2, p. 11 (Pordage's translation).

[75]Hoffmann (503), *De diaboli potentia in corpora*, § 21; vol. 3, p. 100.

[76]Stahl (948), *Theoria medica vera*, Pathologia, pars III, membr. 4, art. 2; vol. 3, p. 317: "Enimvero subesse in hoc talia quaedam phaenomena, quae ortum etiam eius aliquando veluti vere spiritualem innuere possint, nemo plane negaverit, cui exempla nota fuerint; ortus eius aliquando per superstitiones, fascinum, et nefarias magicas artes incussi, seu excitati; imo per nefandas imprecationes velut evocati: quarum utrarumque rerum exempla vulgo notiora sunt, quam ut prolixam assertionem postulent."

[77]Van Swieten (982), *Commentaries*, vol. 10, p. 334 (contemporary translation).

[78]Bartholinus (82), *Histor. anat. cent.*, II, hist. 72; p. 299 f.

[79]Harle (454), *An Historical Essay*, etc., p. 22.

[80]He relates, p. 125, quite an interesting interpretation of the stages of the epileptic fit. According to these beliefs it was assumed "that all those motions were from their [i.e., the

when the fits are long, and seeing strange things, which they relate, and have the good fortune severally to be believed; especially if in the almost infinite variety of rambling thoughts, from a strong and active imagination, they chanced to hit upon some thing that has happened during their state of insensibility, and the retiring of their senses inward. On the other hand, some are said to be bewitched, and grievously tormented of the devil, and no otherwise to be deliver'd but by the help of charms, amulets, exorcisms, or religious conjuration."[81] All this, as can be inferred from the rest of Harle's book, he thinks nothing but old wives' tales.

Obviously then, the Enlightenment represented a different attitude toward matters known to previous generations. The occurrence of natural ecstasies and visionary epileptic states had long been admitted. Nobody, said Casaubon, doubted that "melancholici, maniaci, ecstatici, phrenitici, epileptici, hystericae mulieres" all suffered from natural diseases. "To all these naturall diseases and distempers, enthusiastick divinatory fits are incidentall."[82] The man of the Enlightenment now refused to allow any exceptions short of the Bible, and the final step in the progress of enlightened medicine was the denial of demoniac influence even in the biblical cases. This could be done by complete disbelief in the truthfulness of the account, a course which very few, if any, dared to take. It could also be done without suspicion of atheism by combining a historical interpretation of the cases with the belief in their miraculous nature. Willis already referred to "the conjecture of a certain Divine of our own Country, of no small note, to wit, that many who were taken to be Daemoniacks, or possessed with the Devil in the New Testament, were only Epilepticks; and that they called the cure of this Disease by our Saviour Jesus Christ, an ejection or exorcism of the evil spirit."[83] He possibly had in mind the theologian Joseph Mead (or Mede, †1638) to whom his younger relative Richard Mead credited his own rationalistic views.[84] Whether Joseph Mead really had taught that the demoniacs of the Gospel were simply suffering from a natural disease is doubtful,[85] but such, at any rate, was Richard Mead's opinion. He maintained that the Jews attributed not only madness and epilepsy, but some other diseases as well, to demons,[86] and that this

---

patients'] inability to receive the god or demon, or bear their communications; the following quiet and silence, the season of inspiration and union, and the coming out of the fit, the time of uttering oracles."

[81] *Ibid.*, p. 125.

[82] Casaubon (205), *A Treatise Concerning Enthusiasme*, p. 36 f.

[83] Willis (1107), *Of Convulsive Diseases*, ch. 2, p. 11 (Pordage's translation).

[84] Mead (677), *Medica sacra*, p. ix f.

[85] Cf. *Dictionary of National Biography* (268), s.v. Mead, Joseph.

[86] Mead, *l.c.*, p. 75: "Neque maniam tantum et epilepsin, sed et alios etiam morbos nonnullos ad daemonas pariter illi referebant."

popular belief was reflected in scripture. "Yet the Lunatick . . . whose disease is described in the gospels, was affected with the falling sickness. Wherefore this patient . . . was either mad and epileptick at the same time, which is not uncommon; or he laboured under a periodical epilepsy, returning with the changes of the moon, which is a very common case."[87] The *miracle* consisted in Christ's curing natural diseases immediately by the mere command of his voice and thus superseding the laws of nature. The belief in the demoniac origin of diseases at any place or any time was mere superstition, the very thing which Mead wanted to combat in his book.

The changing interpretation of the biblical story of the epileptic may suffice as an instance of the progress of enlightened medicine in its denial of demoniac powers. It is well known how the spiritual leaders of the "philosophic" century successfully combated the older acceptance of demons and witches. Nor is it necessary to dwell at length upon the more or less mystic movements which formed the counterpart of the struggle for enlightenment. As long as men like Hoffmann and Stahl believed in supernatural forces, it is not remarkable to find laymen and physicians, especially in Germany, who attributed cases of epilepsy to demoniac influence. From the second half of the eighteenth century on, when such notions began to disappear from authoritative literature, they were still alive among rosicrucians, alchemists, and all the uneducated, as well as such educated people as were not satisfied with a sober view of reality. Still later these tendencies passed into the Romantic German medicine of the early nineteenth century, when a few physicians like Justinus Kerner (1786–1862) seriously tried to revive the belief in demoniac possession. Interesting as these mystic movements are in themselves, we can yet pass them over as undercurrents which exerted no lasting influence upon the history of epilepsy. Only in one point do they demand our attention. Enlightened physicians might scoff at the *idea* of divine or demoniac possession, yet they could not disregard the behavior of persons allegedly possessed. In general their answer can be summed up by quoting Cheyne, who wrote: ". . . I hope I have explain'd the Nature and Causes of Nervous Distempers (which have hitherto been reckon'd Witchcraft, Enchantment, Sorcery and Possession, and have been the constant Resource of Ignorance) from Principles easy, natural and intelligible, deduc'd from the best and soundest Natural Philosophy . . . ."[88] In other words, persons deemed possessed were actually suffering from a nervous disease: an answer as old as the book *On the Sacred Disease*.

The reduction of religious experiences to morbid conditions, the hallmark of "medical materialism," to use an expression of William

---

[87]Mead (678), *The Medical Works*, p. 625 (contemporary translation).

[88]Cheyne (218), *The English Malady*, p. x.

James,[89] was one thing; to identify and to explain the particular abnormality was quite another. Phenomena of this kind could be assigned to various classes of diseases. They could be grouped under the broad traditional category of melancholy, of which Burton, in 1621, had given a most comprehensive account; they could be classified as hysterical or hypochondriac, as ecstasies, vapors, or convulsions. There was no lack of names, but there was no consistent or clear definition. Many physicians were inclined to consider the patients epileptic, or at least suffering from a disease closely related to epilepsy, especially if convulsions were present.[90] At the cemetery of St. Médard, in the twenties of the eighteenth century, an increasing number of people, particularly women, began publicly to exhibit convulsions and trance-like states accompanied by religious emotions. These events, which led to public disorders, were hailed by some Jansenist theologians as miracles of divine inspiration. Others, above all the physician Philippe Hecquet (1661–1737), opposed these convulsionists and their theological defenders. Hecquet claimed that the whole thing was a contagious disease, an epidemic, and therefore belonged to the realm of medicine, not of theology.[91] Moreover, he stated that these convulsions were related to the epilepsy peculiar to young women and that several of the victims were truly epileptic.[92]

From Hecquet's remarks it becomes evident that one of the reasons for associating various neurotic phenomena with epilepsy was the theoretical, and even more the practical, inability to differentiate between epilepsy, hysteria, and kindred affections. The growing recognition that hysteria was a nervous disease which need not originate from the uterus helped to make it a competitor of epilepsy in the diagnosis of convulsive neuroses. The practical distinction was often very difficult. Willis, the foremost theoretician of hysteria of the seventeenth century,[93] may have diagnosed cases as hysterical which, in reality, were epilepsies with lesions of the temporal lobe.[94] In the early eighteenth century, epilepsy and hysteria were seen in close proximity. That hysteria might end in

---

[89]James (560), *The Varieties of Religious Experience*, p. 14: "Medical materialism finishes up Saint Paul by calling his vision on the road to Damascus a discharging lesion of the occipital cortex, he being an epileptic." See also Laski (614), p. 254.

[90]Cf. Semelaigne (909), vol. 1, p. 51.

[91]Hecquet (470), *Le naturalisme*, etc. p. 21: "Car c'est une *contagion* ou une *épidémie*, et les maladies contagieuses sont du ressort de la Médecine;" etc.

[92]*Ibid.*, p. 21 f.: "Or que les convulsions soient épidémiques, elles le sont spécialement en ce qu'elles tiennent par elles-mêmes, ou de leur nature de cette *épilepsie* propre, et particulière aux jeunes personnes du sexe, parce qu'elle leur est familière.

Mais cette affinité avec *l'épilepsie* est d'autant plus sensible dans les convulsions régnantes, qu'il est de notorieté que plusieurs des convulsionnaires sont vraiment *épileptiques*, soit par elles-mêmes, soit parce qu'elles sont nées de meres *épileptiques*."

[93]On Willis and hysteria see Veith (1046), p. 132 ff., and Isler (537), p. 105 ff.

[94]Hunter and Macalpine (521), p. 188.

epilepsy was maintained by Boerhaave[95] as well as his pupil van Swieten, who stated that "the hysteric passion has frequently been observed to degenerate into the epilepsy."[96] Cheyne, whom we quoted as attributing all possession to "nervous distempers," said that epilepsy "differs very little, or not at all, or at most, in a few Circumstances only, from Hypochondriacal and Hysterick Fits: which last, when violent, terminate always in these Epileptick Fits, as they, on the other Hand, when they become weak, dwindle into the Hysterick Kind."[97] Similar views were held by John Purcell, who thought that the treatment too should be the same.[98]

There were, of course, others who did not believe in the essential identity of epileptic and hysterical convulsions, and this nosological differentiation gained in the course of the century. Tissot, for instance, denied ever having seen hysteria or "vapors" degenerate into epilepsy.[99] He argued against the establishment of such a group as *epilepsia hysterica*.[100] In cases where epilepsy originated from the uterus, it was one of its many sympathetic forms but had nothing to do with hysteria. Still others, while counting epilepsy and hysteria as two different nosological entities, yet recognized *epilepsia uterina* as a subdivision of the former disease,[101] though they might consider it different from "true epilepsy" and "peculiar to women of the hysteric temperament."[102] Toward the end of the eighteenth century, it is true, the view prevailed that epilepsy and hysteria should not be confused, even if their practical distinction was sometimes very difficult.[103]

However ecstatic convulsive states were diagnosed in the individual, account had to be taken of their frequent occurrence in epidemic form. An explanation was needed of how such phenomena, which were still frequent in the eighteenth century,[104] could spread within small or large groups. An event in the practice of Boerhaave assumed some importance, since it became famous in the medical literature of the century. Speaking of simulated epilepsy, this author remarked in his

---

[95] Boerhaave (130), *Praelectiones*, p. 846: "Uteri affectiones, inprimis genus nervosum spectantes, adeo multiplices observatae fuerunt, ut inde ortae fuerint convulsiones, et cum illis saepe Epilepsia (illam enim a convulsionibus distinguimus)."

[96] Van Swieten (982), *Commentaries*, vol. 10, p. 375 (contemporary translation).

[97] Cheyne (218), *The English Malady*, p. 253.

[98] Purcell (830), *A Treatise of Vapours or, Hysterick Fits*, p. 132; cf. Hunter and Macalpine (521), p. 288.

[99] Tissot (1024), *Traité de l'épilepsie*, p. 176: ". . . mais je n'ai jamais vû l'hysterie ou les vapeurs dégénerer en cette maladie; je suis même convaincu que cela est très rare, et Andrée, Medecin Anglois, qui établit que cela est très fréquent, s'ést assurément trompé."

[100] *Ibid.*, p. 81 f.

[101] Cf. Boissier de Sauvages (890), *Nosologia methodica*, cl. 4, ordo 4, 19; vol. 3, p. 115.

[102] Macbride (654), *A Methodical Introduction*, etc., p. 558.

[103] Cf., e.g., Duncan (304), *Medical Cases*, p. 13.

[104] See Rosen (872), ch. 7.

*Praelectiones* that such cases had frequently been cured by the threat of flogging. And "by menacing to apply a hot iron," so he added, "I once cured the entire orphanage of Haarlem."[105] Cures of this kind, as we have seen, were nothing unusual with regard to simulated epilepsy. But this case, as related in greater detail by Boerhaave's nephew, Abraham Kaau, was of a different nature. A girl belonging to the Haarlem institution had been frightened and was seized by a "convulsive nervous disease." In the course of a few days nearly all boys and girls living there exhibited the same disease. The best anti-epileptic remedies were of no avail. Boerhaave was summoned and noticed how several of the patients were stricken "with a kind of epilepsy" as soon as one had been seized by a fit.[106] Since medicine was of no use and the disease spread by imagination,[107] he hit upon the above-mentioned cure, viz., the threat of painful cauterizations.

In this case the attacks were not simulated in the ordinary sense of the word, nor were they identical with the usual form of chronic epilepsy. It was the power of imagination or imitation which produced them, according to the physicians. Proofs for this contention were not lacking. An epidemic similar to that in the orphanage of Haarlem had started in a church in France in 1780 in connection with religious ceremonies. The epidemic had stopped after the children had been sent home to their parents,[108] i.e., after they could no longer see and imitate one another. The same hypothesis that still hides behind such expressions as *chorea imitativa* seemed adequate to explain the convulsions which occurred during the séances held by Mesmer and his pupils. Mesmer, of course, attributed these convulsions to animal magnetism, whereas the foes of mesmerism regarded them as another example of the power of imitation.[109]

At any rate, so much seemed certain: a convulsive disease which was not clearly, if at all, separated from epilepsy could spread like any other epidemic. To this were added older observations of people who had become epileptic by accidentally witnessing an attack.[110] All this led to the conclusion that epilepsy, by some kind of mental infection, could

---

[105] Boerhaave (130), *Praelectiones*, p. 806 f.: "Tales Epilepsiae virgarum minis in paroxysmis repetitis sanatae fuerunt; sic intentato ferro candenti olim sanavi integrum Orphanotrophium Harlemense," etc.

[106] Kaau Boerhaave (129), *Impetum faciens dictum Hippocrati*, p. 356: ". . . et dum rem examinat, invadente in unum paroxysmo, vidit convelli plures specie epilepsiae."

[107] *Ibid.*: "Datis incassum optimis remediis a Medicis sapientibus, et ad imaginationem ex uno in alterum traducto morbo," etc.

[108] This story appeared in the report of the French commission charged with an investigation of animal magnetism and was reprinted in Falconer (341), *A Dissertation on the Influence of the Passions upon Disorders of the Body*, p. 65 f. footnote.

[109] Cf. *ibid.*

[110] Cf. references given by Kaau Boerhaave (129), *Impetum faciens*, p. 355, and Falconer, *l.c.*, p. 65.

be transmitted from one person to another. Or to quote a contemporary: "But it is well known, that, with very delicate habits, diseases which cannot be said to be infectious, are yet catching, from the principle of imitation."[111]

It was a paradoxical result that the enlightened century, on a different level it is true, revived an idea rooted in the belief in the demoniac contagion of epilepsy. Hecquet even cited the ancient customs regarding epileptics in evidence of his own medical theory about the convulsionists of St. Médard.[112] In its new form this idea had considerable consequences, for it lasted far into the nineteenth century and gave a strong impetus to the demand for the isolation of epileptics.

### b. The Revolt against the Occult

The rejection of all belief in the demoniac nature of epilepsy reflects a changed attitude toward unexplained and obscure phenomena. What general factors caused this changed attitude, which we call Enlightenment, need not be answered here. Confining ourselves to epilepsy we must, however, realize that it was this changed point of view which made demons and witches disappear, rather than any progress in the pathology of the disease, or any fundamentally new clinical observations. The same is true with regard to the acceptance of the imagination of the pregnant mother and of the moon as causative factors of epilepsy. Originally, at least, these beliefs were not disproved by statistics or anything of the sort, but were discarded because they seemed to be irrational and to postulate the impossible.

Influence of the moon upon epilepsy was taken as an established fact until the end of the seventeenth century. Some physicians attributed it to the general interrelation of cosmic phenomena. Bartholinus related the case of an epileptic girl who had spots on her face which changed in color and size according to the phase and mutation of the moon.[113] Stahl was inclined to see something mysterious and inexplicable in the lunar aspect of epilepsy.[114] But the majority of physicians, in continuing the classical tradition, looked for a more physical explanation. Most medieval textbooks had devoted some space to the discussion without, however, necessarily displaying astrological tendencies. In the sixteenth century Ferdinandus imputed a case of epilepsy to the pa-

---

[111] Duncan (304), *Medical Cases*, p. 15.

[112] Hecquet (470), *Le naturalisme*, p. 22: "Mais de plus, l'épilepsie étoit tellement reconnue pour contagieuse parmi les Anciens, que les Epileptiques étoient exclus des Assemblées publiques, d'où est venu à l'*épilepsie* le nom *comitialis morbus*, parce que la presence d'un Epileptique ne se souffroit point dans les Assemblées. Et encore, les Epileptiques étoient, leur sembloit-il, si contagieux pour les personnes de la même famille, qu'il étoit d'usage de les tenir à la campagne pour les éloigner de dessous les yeux de leurs parents."

[113] Bartholinus (82), *Histor. anat. cent.* II, hist. 72; p. 300.

[114] Stahl (948), *Theoria medica vera*, Pathologia, pars 3, membr. 4, art. 2; vol. 3, p. 332.

tient's having spent a summer night under an olive tree while the air was tepid, humid, and filled with a slight warmth from the light of the moon.[115]

The physical influence of celestial bodies upon the earth had been confirmed by Newtonian physics, viz., by the law of gravitation and the lunar explanation of the tides. This seemed to offer a new mechanical basis for the assumed relationship between the moon and epilepsy. Friedrich Hoffmann, who believed implicitly in the influence of stars upon the organism, expected a future explanation of these phenomena from mechanics.[116] Even the more enlightened physicians, like Richard Mead, saw now a possibility for a satisfactory explanation. Richard Mead gave various examples of epileptic attacks occurring regularly at certain constellations of the moon.[117] The moon, he thought, exerted its power above all upon the animal spirits, these being the thinnest and most elastic parts of the body. Hence the lunar effect was greatest in all those diseases which were caused by morbid changes of these spirits.[118] It may partly be due to the authority of Mead's name that belief in the influence of the moon survived so long in British medicine, even among men like John Hunter[119] and Erasmus Darwin.[120]

In contrast, Mesmer in Vienna admitted in his dissertation of 1766 that his attempt "to bring back the influence of the stars" was something of an anachronism "after so many attempts from the pen of the most famous Mead."[121] In France, where the Enlightenment became more radical than in other countries, scepticism as to the alleged powers of the moon was more pronounced. What probably aroused the suspicion of scientists and philosophers was the variety of actions attributed

---

[115] Ferdinandus (350), *Centum historiae*, hist. 24; p. 72 f.: "Quantum ad res non naturales, licet erat aestas, tamen aer in quo per noctem moratus est aeger, erat tepidus, humidus cum pusillo calore, qui a lumine lunae proveniebat, deinde manens sub umbra olivae occasio fuit exhibita generationi istius symptomatis, ab aere igitur opaco, et humido, et ex lunae radiis sumpsit ansam affectus praeter naturam. . . ."

[116] Hoffmann (503), *De astrorum influxu in corpora humana*, § § 15 and 35; vol. 3, pp. 73 and 76.

[117] Mead (676), *De imperio solis*, pp. 35, 36 ff., and 42 f.

[118] *Ibid.*, p. 33 f.: "Et hoc primum mihi satis constare videtur, lunaris hujus potentiae vim majorem necessario esse in illum corporis nostri humorem, qui nervos irrigat, quem *spiritus animales* dicimus; quam in ipsum sanguinem, aut alios quoscunque vitales liquores. Cum enim is sit partium tenuissimarum, et (sicut alias monstravi) elasticarum, virtuti causae cujusvis externae facilius obtemperabit. Idcirco, ad illos praecipue morbos spectabit vis lunae, qui a vitiis subtilissimi hujus spiritus oriuntur."

[119] Cf. Hunter (519), *Works*, vol. 1; p. 346.

[120] Darwin (256), *Zoonomia*, vol. 1, p. 377, cites Mead in connection with the lunar influence upon epilepsy and so does Leake (621), *A Practical Essay*, p. 401. Sceptics were of course not lacking: Macbride (654), *A Methodical Introduction* etc., p. 556, for instance, writes: "It is generally supposed, that the change and full of the moon have some influence in bringing on the fits; this, however, is much to be doubted."

[121] Quoted from Pattie (777), p. 277. Pattie has shown that in his dissertation Mesmer largely depended on Mead's work.

to the moon and their obvious connection with popular beliefs. Already, in 1705, the physicist La Hire, plainly doubtful of all these stories,[122] raised the question whether the moon reflected enough heat to exert any possible influence in this way. His computations showed that the amount was negligible, a result that knocked the bottom out of the ancient astrophysical theory of epilepsy. Still, the innumerable reports of epileptic attacks coinciding with some phase of the moon had to be accounted for. Tissot solved this dilemma by considering such cases as examples of the many curious variations of the disease. "One has seen it [i.e., epilepsy] coming back every month regularly at the same day of the moon, although this does not prove the chimerical influences of the latter."[123]

Tissot's *Treatise on Epilepsy*, published in 1770, is the first book on this subject to show all the characteristics of Enlightenment in medicine. Written in the French vernacular,[124] it is at once learned, scientific, and readable. A friend of Haller and Zimmermann, a propagator of the new theory of sensibility and irritability, progressive in his care for the health of the rural population, Tissot (1728–97) is to be found on the side of those opposing old beliefs for which no adequate reason could be given. His rejection of the chimerical influences of the moon is one example; another one is his refusal to accept the imagination of the pregnant mother as a cause of epilepsy. Here the situation presented itself to Tissot as follows.

In enumerating the causes of epilepsy, Boerhaave had written: "But these are, 1. hereditary, from a family taint of the father, mother, relations, or ancestors; the disease frequently lying dormant in the father, while it is derived from the grandfather to the grandchild. 2. Born with one [i.e., epilepsy], from the imagination of the mother when she was pregnant being shocked at the sight of a person in an epileptic fit."[125] Tissot did not altogether deny the possibility of hereditary epilepsy and thought it the duty of epileptics to remain unmarried.[126] But with regard to the second cause, Tissot was quite incredulous. He was certainly not the first to deny the power of imagination over the fetus, and he quoted the names of those who had rejected such a possibility.[127] Yet it is interesting to compare his attitude with that of

---

[122] La Hire (495), *Sur la chaleur que nous peuvent causer les rayons du soleil reflechis par la lune*, 1705, p. 346: "On sçait qu'un assez grand nombre de personnes attribuënt à la Lune beaucoup de qualités, sans avoir des raisons fondées sur de bonnes experiences."

[123] Tissot (1024), *Traité de l'épilepsie*, p. 182.

[124] Tissot can, therefore, be considered as affiliated with the French sphere of culture, although he was Swiss.

[125] Boerhaave, *Aphorisms*, sec. 1075, quoted from the contemporary English translation of van Swieten's (982), *Commentaries*, vol. 10, p. 351.

[126] Tissot, *l.c.*, p. 29.

[127] *Ibid.*, pp. 31–32, footnote.

van Swieten. The latter, in upholding Boerhaave's view, was well aware "that all those things are denied by some persons, because they cannot conceive, how a change of thought in the mother can so affect the foetus; and they laugh at men of sense as being too credulous, for believing what they have seen themselves, or have read in authors of approved veracity. I own, that I do not understand the connection of the cause acting upon the mother with the effect observed in the foetus; and why that fright should not rather render the mother epileptic, than the foetus; but it must not therefore be denied, that such a thing has really happened."[128] For Tissot, on the other hand, it was enough to point out the anatomical and physiological reasons which made such occurrences highly improbable in order to deny their existence.[129]

A change of mind which leads to the renunciation of old beliefs usually also leads to the creation of new ones, and superstitions are often exchanged rather than abandoned. The same enlightened physicians as moulded our modern concept of "superstition," relegating to it all notions of occult forces, established a new superstitious belief. They claimed that epilepsy could be caused by masturbation, and here again Tissot assumed a leading role. In Antiquity the influence of sexual intercourse upon epilepsy had been widely discussed. During the Middle Ages and Renaissance the opinion prevailed that sexual excesses were harmful for epileptics,[130] while complete continence might also engender attacks of the disease. From the second half of the eighteenth century, this point of view was strongly emphasized. Tissot was positive in his belief "that sexual excesses bring about epilepsy in the most robust persons who have never been attacked by it."[131] On the other hand, he admitted that in some individuals excessive continence could have the same effect.[132] From the point of view of contemporary pathology these opinions were understandable, since overpowering passions, disintegrating humors, etc. were generally admitted as factors in the pathogenesis of epilepsy. At the same time, however, the attention of the physicians began to concentrate not so much on sexual excesses in general as on masturbation. Earlier centuries had condemned this habit on religious grounds; now it was blamed as the source of a multitude of diseases. In his book *On Masturbation*, which became an early classic on the subject, Tissot summarized observations of earlier physicians, of contemporaries, and of his own. He described the dire conse-

---

[128] Van Swieten (982), *Commentaries*, vol. 10, p. 355 (contemporary translation).

[129] Tissot, *l.c.*, pp. 29–33.

[130] E.g., Sennert (913), *Pract. med.*, 1, pars 2, c. 31; vol. 2, p. 230: "Venus in hoc morbo, ut pestis, fugienda."

[131] Tissot, *l.c.*, p. 70.

[132] *Ibid.*, p. 73.

quences of masturbation—among which epilepsy looms large.[133] He makes a point of it that masturbation is much more dangerous than mere sexual debauchery. "Too great a quantity of semen being lost in the natural course produces very direful effects: but they are still more dreadful, when the same quantity has been dissipated in an unnatural manner. The accidents which happen to such as waste themselves, in a natural way, are very terrible: those which are occasioned by masturbation are still more so."[134] Tissot gives many reasons why this should be so, reasons which, however, do not sound very convincing. "We subject ourselves to want without being in want; and such is the case of masturbators. It is imagination, habit, and not nature that importune them. They drain nature both of that which is necessary, and also of that which she herself would have taken care to dispose of."[135] It is not clear why this, one of Tissot's main arguments, should not be true of all sexual excesses.

For more than a century and a half masturbation figured as one of the main causes of epilepsy in medical literature. There were but few authors who did not emphasize or at least mention it as such. Schroeder van der Kolk (1797–1862), who cited abnormal excitability of the medulla oblongata as the cause of epilepsy, named among the irritants "... above all, onanism, which acts so very much on the medulla oblongata, and must be regarded as a very frequent cause of epilepsy."[136] Fournier (1832–1914), one of the leading French physicians, wrote: "One of the nervous affections which onanism occasions most frequently is epilepsy. . . . There are very few physicians who have not observed cases where it has been produced, maintained or aggravated by the practice of this pernicious habit."[137]

These are a few examples which could be multiplied almost indefinitely. The superstition reached its climax in the last third of the nineteenth century, when recourse to clitoridectomy[138] and to castration in extreme cases was considered. At the annual meeting of the British Medical Association at Cambridge in 1880 the following remarks were exchanged:

> Dr. BACON had castrated two male epileptics, with the result, in one case, of great improvement.
> Dr. HACK TUKE asked under what conditions such an operation would be indicated?

---

[133] Tissot (1023), *L'onanisme*, pp. 23, 26, 46.

[134] Tissot (1022), *An Essay on Onanism*, p. 11 (Hume's translation).

[135] *Ibid.*, p. 65 f. (Hume's translation).

[136] Schroeder van der Kolk (902), *On the Minute Structure* etc., p. 250 (Moore's translation).

[137] Fournier (373), *De l'onanisme*, p. 98.

[138] Cf. Duffy (302).

Dr. BACON replied, in cases of confirmed masturbation in incurable cases of epileptic insanity.[139]

Castration had been performed in the same century in cases of supposed sympathetic epilepsy originating from the testicles.[140] Such a view may have been erroneous but could at least be defended on the basis of sober pathological principles current at the time. But here castration was advised to stop masturbation and thereby cure epilepsy. Lest any doubt exist about this interpretation, it is dispelled by Gowers. In 1881, this leading English neurologist stated that castration had proved unsuccessful as a therapy of epilepsy.[141] Then he added: "It [i.e., castration] has been lately revived by Bacon as a means of arresting epilepsy *due to masturbation* in adult insane patients."[142] But even Gowers believed in masturbation as a causal factor and advocated surgical measures, for he continued: "In boys, however, *circumcision*, if effectually performed, is usually successful, and should be adopted in all cases in which there is reason to associate the disease with masturbation."[143] This is all the more surprising, as the suspicion had long before been voiced that excessive masturbation might be one of the abnormalities accompanying certain diseases, rather than a cause.[144] But then, the whole idea had its origin not so much in rational pathology and critical observation as in the peculiar attitude of contemporary society toward matters of sex.

### c. The Purging of Therapy

During the eighteenth century, partly under the direct influence of Enlightenment, the therapy of epilepsy underwent a metamorphosis which affected dietetic, pharmacological, and surgical treatment. A review of the cure of epilepsy since the Middle Ages shows it to be a partial break with tradition.

The medieval physician ordered regimen, drugs, cauterization, and trephining in continuation of ancient traditions. It can perhaps be said

---

[139] *The Journal of Mental Science*, vol. 26, 1881, p. 470.

[140] Cf. below, p. 293. See also Billings (112), p. 339.

[141] Gowers (420), *Epilepsy*, p. 286.

[142] *Ibid.*; italics are mine.

[143] *Ibid.*; italics are in text. Cf. *ibid.*, p. 178.

[144] Cf. Flemming (364), *Über das Causal-Verhaeltnis der Selbstbefleckung zur Geistesverirrung*, who doubts the etiological role of masturbation in insanity. In 1866 West (1086), *Clitoridectomy*, p. 585, clearly stated: ". . . I have not in the whole of my practice seen convulsions, epilepsy, or idiocy *induced* by masturbation in any child of either sex . . ."; cf. Duffy (302). In fairness to Gowers it must be stated that he was not dogmatic as to the causal relationship between masturbation and epilepsy; cf. Gowers, *l.c.*, p. 31 f., where he also says: "I am inclined to think that it is much less frequently a cause of true epilepsy than of untypical attacks, sometimes hysteroid, sometimes of characters intermediate between hysteroid and epileptoid form. I have so frequently in boys met with this form of attack in association with the practice, that I can scarcely doubt their etiological connection." The possibility must not be overlooked that the severe mental stress imposed by parents and educators upon the onanist might sometimes have led to hysterical reactions.

that the regimen was not quite as well reasoned as it had been in the great classical authors. It was more concerned with the choice and rejection of foods, beverages, and daily habits than with the arrangement of a strict daily program. The use of drugs, on the other hand, was strongly emphasized and played a greater part than in Antiquity. Both regimen and drugs were prescribed according to a rational scheme and not in any haphazard fashion. The great pharmacological textbook of the Middle Ages which went under the name of Joannes Mesue stresses the following six points in the treatment of epilepsy: (1) arrangement of a regimen; (2) the morbid matter is made ready for evacuation; (3) it is evacuated; (4) care is taken that the residue of the morbid matter be diverted to other parts of the body; (5) the brain, and any other organ where the disease originated, is restored; (6) the various symptoms incidental to the disease are set right.[145]

Although the remedies used for epilepsy were largely those of the ancients, the medieval physicians were not altogether lacking in ingenuity. During the attack a small wooden knife was inserted between the teeth,[146] and obstacles to free respiration were removed as far as possible.[147] Arnald of Villanova actually proposed a fever treatment for the cure of epilepsy, at least of that form which originated from black bile. First leeches were to be applied over the spleen and then a poultice of pigeon's dung and raven's eggs. This was supposed to draw the morbid matter from the head to the spleen, to generate fever, and thus to cure the epileptic—particularly if done in the autumn.[148]

Of surgical measures cauterization took the first place (cf. Fig. 4). The hot iron was usually applied to several places on the head, specifically the occiput and bregma,[149] sometimes to other regions like the vertebral column,[150] the chest,[151] or even the arm.[152] Cauterization as a therapy or prophylaxis for epilepsy had a strong popular appeal and

---

[145] Joannes Mesue (686), *Grabadin*, lib. II, summa 3, c. 26; fol. 208$^r$: "Cura huius aegritudinis sunt sex res. Prima ponit regimen in vita. Secunda aequat, et coaptat materiam. Tertia abscindit eam. Quarta ponit regimen in conversione residui eius ad partes diversas, et oppositas. Quinta rectificat membrum mandans, si est aliquod mandans, et rectificat cerebrum. Sexta corrigit accidentia." Similarly Arnald of Villanova (58), *De epilepsia*, c. 7; col. 1608.

[146] Cf. Antonius Guainerius (438), *Tractatus de egritudinibus capitis*, VII, 4; fol. 12$^r$.

[147] Cf. Arnald of Villanova (58), *Breviarium*, I, c. 13; col. 1074.

[148] *Ibid.*, col. 1075: "Cum epilepsia fit ex melancholia, accipe stercus colombinum, pista ipsum, et cum ovis corvorum misce, et cataplasma super splenem apponatur, prius appositis sanguisugis: hoc enim cataplasma materiam trahit a capite ad splenem et generat febrem, et sic epilepticum liberat, et maxime si fiat in autumno."

[149] Cf. Abulqasim (3), *De chirurgia* I, sec. 10; vol. 1, p. 31; *Chirurgia Rogeri*, in Sudhoff (968), vol. 2, p. 171; De Renzi (840), vol. 4, pp. 55 and 143; Arnald of Villanova (58), *Breviarium*, I, c. 13; col. 1074.

[150] Cf. Abulqasim, *l.c.*

[151] Cf. Gilbertus Anglicus (412), *Compendium medicinae*, fol. 112$^r$.

[152] Montanus (707), *Consultat. med.* 10; p. 69: "De cauteriis, ego summopere laudarem cauteria in brachiis, imo hoc est familiare remedium. Et vidi anno praeterito unum qui solo cauterio sanatus est. Et erat senex in LII. anno aetatis suae constitutus."

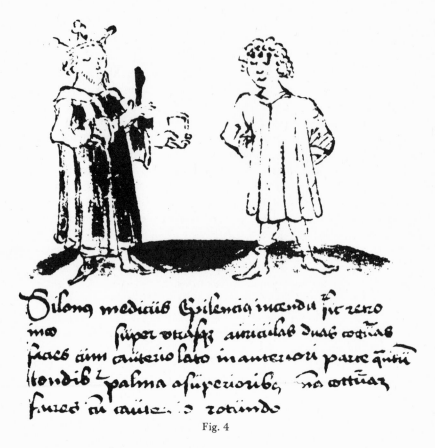

Fig. 4

Cauterization of epileptic. Manuscript of the
fifteenth century. (Sudhoff, *Beiträge zur Gesch.
d. Chirurgie im Mittelalter*, vol. I, Leipzig,
Johann Ambrosius Barth, 1914. Table 36.)

was sometimes performed by laymen without the help of proper surgeons. We are informed that the women of Florence used to cauterize
their children on the back of the head and that peasant women handed
their children over to the priest, who would perform the operation.[153]
The motives behind this practice are obscure. Was it a remnant of the *T
sincipital* of prehistoric times? Unfortunately, our explanation of prehistoric cauterization rests largely upon speculation, and it is by no
means certain that it had a definite therapeutic aim. Or was it simply a

---

[153] Rondeletius (866), *Methodus curandi morbos*, I, c. 36; pl. 175: "Florentinae mulieres
cauterio occiput urunt, idque habent in communi usu, edoctae quotidiana experientia. Rusticae
pueros sacerdotibus deferunt, ut cauterio, vel carbone ignito partem illam posteriorem urant,
quod maxime confert, si epilepsia facta fuerit per idiopathiam."

continuation of ancient therapy, or possibly both? In attempting to answer these questions we are not much helped by the fact that the medieval physicians had a rational theory ready at hand. They claimed that the hot iron counteracted the deficiency of warmth and the superfluity of humors,[154] and it was believed efficacious in idiopathic epilepsy, where the disease was caused in the brain by phlegm.[155]

What has just been said about cauterization is equally true of trephining, also one of the extreme remedies to be tried.[156] The *Quattuor magistri*, a surgical text probably of the thirteenth century, advised opening the skulls of melancholics, epileptics, and others, "that the humors and air may go out and evaporate."[157] Even prophylactic opening of the fontanelles of children was advised from similar considerations.[158] A story related by Donatus became famous in subsequent centuries. A French nobleman suffering from epilepsy travelled to Italy in order to consult the physicians of that country. On his way he was attacked by Spanish mercenaries, robbed, and severely wounded. A friend took him to the next village, where he was treated by a surgeon. One wound in his forehead was, however, so large and had caused such a considerable loss of bone that it took a very long time to heal. But when he arrived in Padua, more than two months after the infliction of this wound, he was free from all epileptic attacks and returned home the next spring.[159]

Trephining was still practiced in the seventeenth century in epilepsy and allied disorders, in order to give an outlet to the materia peccans. "If al means fail," says the English interpreter of Riverius, "the last remedy is, to open the fore part of the Skul with a Trepan, at distance from the Sutures, that the evil air may breath out. By this means many times desperate Epilepsies have been cured, and it may be safely done if the Chyrurgeon be skilful."[160]

In many cases where epilepsy was caused by a malign vapor, trephining was considered an adequate though dangerous treatment by Fienus (one of the teachers of van Helmont) since it would facilitate the escape

[154] Cf. De Renzi (840), vol. 2, p. 659.

[155] Cf. above footnote 149. Abulqasim, *l.c.*, expressly says: "Sit autem Epilepticus cujus Epilepsia ex phlegmate ortum suum trahit."

[156] Gilbertus Anglicus, *l.c.*, fol. 112$^r$: "Ultima cura in his est cauterium in furcula pectoris: et apertio cranei."

[157] De Renzi (840), vol. 2, p. 698.

[158] Ponze Sanct a Cruz (886), *Praelectiones Vallisoletanae*, p. 69: ". . . hoc loco plures confirmant fontanellas aperiendas puerulis, quibus deficiunt expurgationes cerebri, ne incidant in Epilepsiam."

[159] Donatus (290), *De historia medica mirabili*, II, c. 4; p. 149. A somewhat similar case was communicated by Boucher to the Académie Royale des Sciences in 1757 (495), p. 28. An epileptic child had suffered a compound fracture of the occipital and parietal bones. After trephining, the epileptic attacks gradually disappeared.

[160] Riverius (853), *The Practice of Physick*, p. 32 (Culpeper's paraphrase.)

of such vapors; whereas, in cases caused by humors in the brain he thought trephining out of place.[161] As late as 1733 a second edition of Fienus' book appeared, and at about the same time La Motte (1655–1737) published his treatise on surgery, where he told of the relief given an epileptic by trephining. In this case the patient had not reported any old injury of the head. La Motte, nevertheless, proposed trephining as a last resource and thus brought about an abatement of the attacks.[162] In the course of the operation La Motte found the middle of the left parietal bone much thickened and without diploë. Tissot, who showed great interest in this case history, concluded "that the brain at certain times was too much compressed by the skull and that then the compression produced epilepsy"; furthermore, that the slight diminution of this compression by means of trephining had effected the relief.[163] Tissot advised trephining in all cases where the symptoms pointed to a seat of the disease accessible to the trephine, even if there were no conspicuous previous injury. He believed, moreover, that if performed in good air, by a good surgeon, and on a patient with healthy blood, the operation was not very dangerous.[164]

Tissot envisaged a broader indication for trephining and was more optimistic about its success than most of his contemporaries. Gradually the indications for trephining in epileptic patients had been limited to the following two eventualities: (1) a morbid condition of the skull due to contusion, fracture, caries, or other lesion of the bone; or, (2) an accumulation of humors directly under the skull. These were the points stressed by Steeghius in the beginning of the seventeenth century,[165] as well as by van Swieten in the middle of the eighteenth century. Trephining for other reasons was believed of little avail.[166] It can therefore not be said that trephining for epilepsy was unknown in the eighteenth century. Since the times of Antiquity there is an almost unbroken chain of evidence of its existence.[167] What changed was probably the frequency of, and certainly the indication for, its performance.[168] The older notion of giving an outlet to vapors and humors had, by the eighteenth century, yielded to the stricter idea of removing a localized pathological condition affecting the brain and its membranes.

---

[161] Fienus (357), *Libri chirurgici*, pp. 4 and 10.

[162] La Motte (607), *Traité complet de chirurgie*, obs. 172; vol. 1, p. 648 ff.

[163] Tissot (1024), *Traité de l'épilepsie*, p. 263 f.

[164] *Ibid.*, p. 259 f.

[165] Steeghius (953), *Medicina practica*, VII, c. 3; pp. 321 and 323.

[166] Van Swieten (982), *Commentaries*, vol. 10, p. 425.

[167] Severinus (419), *De efficaci medicina*, p. 126, gives a list of ancient and later authors recommending trephining in epilepsy. According to Lopez Piñero and Garcia Ballester (648), p. 20, the Renaissance witnessed an excessive popularity of trephining in general.

[168] Heister (477), *A General System of Surgery*, part 2, sec. 2, ch. 41; p. 356: ". . . but the modern Surgeons never use the Trepan at present for internal Disorders of the Head . . ." (contemporary translation).

From the sixteenth century on, cauterization and trephining were often replaced by the setting of a seton.[169] Warmly recommended by Ambroise Paré,[170] this practice was made popular by Fabricius Hildanus, who reported great success and described the procedure in detail.[171] The effect of this cure was first attributed to a removal of peccant humors,[172] but as a "derivative" treatment it lasted far into the nineteenth century, together with cuppings, scarifications, and the application of leeches.[173]

The change in therapeutics in the eighteenth century manifested itself most strikingly in the rejection and choice of specifics and drugs. Until the end of the seventeenth century, almost all textbooks mention occult "specifics." From the sixteenth century on, but particularly in the seventeenth, the number of old and medieval specifics was largely supplemented by chemical preparations, very often of an equally doubtful character. True, already at that time some physicians objected vigorously to the whole idea of specifics. "I believe," said Gui Patin (1602-72), "that there is no antiepileptic remedy. Those praised as such by Crollius and the nation of the chemists are fictions and pure fables. I do not except the mistletoe, the elk's foot, peony root, nor other similar trifles."[174] Now Gui Patin was a reactionary and his opposition to all these remedies was mainly motivated by his hatred for medical innovations. Nevertheless, he was quoted with approval by Tissot,[175] and it is interesting to note that the reactionary sentiments of one period may sound progressive to another.

To the physicians of the eighteenth century the problem of specifics presented itself approximately as follows: A great many remedies had been recommended by the preceding generations as possessing an occult power over the disease epilepsy. The school of Boerhaave rejected this idea because it did not believe in any single cause of epilepsy. To its analytical way of thinking, epilepsy could be caused in many ways. It was, therefore, nonsensical to assume that certain remedies would remove the disease as such, regardless of the etiology of the case. The enlightened physicians, furthermore, could not let the concept of "occult powers" pass, since this claim largely rested on superstition. There

---

[169] The seton was well known during the Middle Ages; cf. Sudhoff (968), vol. 2, index. It was probably used in epilepsy, though I have not been able to find a definite reference.

[170] Paré (772), *Oeuvres*, vol. 2, p. 80.

[171] Fabricius Hildanus (338), *Opera omnia*, p. 34 ff.

[172] Cf. Riverius (853), *The Practice of Physick*, p. 32.

[173] E.g., cf. Schroeder van der Kolk (902), *On the Minute Structure* etc., p. 259 ff. As a curiosity the intravenous injections of anti-epileptic remedies as practiced in the seventeenth century may be mentioned here. Two cases of this kind are published by Bonet (133), *Medicina septentrionalis*, I, sec. 14, c. 25; vol. 1, p. 118, from "D. Fabri, Medici Gedanensis, in Actis Philos. Angl. Dec. 1667."

[174] Quoted from Tissot (1024), *Traité de l'épilepsie*, p. 230 f.

[175] *Ibid.*

ensued the elimination of such "disgusting" remedies as human blood and bones and animal dung, as superstitious, useless, or even harmful.[176] If, nevertheless, useless specifics occasionally proved effective, their success was attributed to the power of imagination,[177] an explanation which was extended to the cure by relics of saints, etc.[178] If even the physician had sometimes to prescribe such remedies, then only "that they may satisfy the patient and his friends in the mean time, while the physician collects the history of the disease. For they would all imagine the patient to be neglected by the physician, if he was to give them no remedy in so violent a complaint."[179]

In principle at least, if not in practice, this did away with the occult remedies and the *Dreckapotheke* of former times, a pharmacological purge which took place in the period between 1700 and 1750. Obviously, this time was much too short to have proved the actual inefficacy of all such medicaments. Here again the enlightened physicians were guided more by their philosophical views than by experience,[180] as becomes evident if we consider those specifics which were not rejected by the majority. In order to avoid any superstitious connotation, a new definition had to be given of what was meant by a *specific* remedy for epilepsy. Tissot, for instance, said that by this term he merely understood those known remedies which were the most proper to change the epileptic disposition of the brain.[181] But on his own admission this disposition was an unexplained factor. Specifics, therefore, were something that somehow changed something unknown. Strictly speaking, their powers were just as occult as those of human blood and the other "disgusting" remedies and could only be ascertained by their empirical results. And a real empirical basis was still lacking in the eighteenth century, as becomes manifest in the evaluation of those drugs whose superstitious character could not be assumed a priori, e.g., peony root and mistletoe. The efficacy of peony had been disputed for a long time, and many physicians denied its usefulness in epilepsy. Others, however, claimed that the wrong plant had been used or that it had been collected at a wrong time.[182] On the whole, the

---

[176] Cf. van Swieten (982), *Commentaries*, vol. 10, pp. 441–47, and Tissot, *l.c.*, p. 357.

[177] Falconer (341), *A Dissertation on the Influence of the Passions*, p. 65, thinks that if such "hideous remedies could have any efficacy, it must be owing to their absorbing the attention, and of course leaving no room for the apprehension and recollection of the disorder to operate . . ."

[178] Cf. Falconer, *l.c.*, p. 67 f.

[179] Van Swieten, *l.c.*, p. 447 (contemporary translation).

[180] Cf. McKenzie (657), p. 163. I am indebted to Dr. Erwin H. Ackerknecht for having directed my attention to this reference which corroborates my own opinion.

[181] Tissot (1024), *Traité de l'épilepsie*, p. 354 f.: ". . . quand je dis que tels remedes sont spécifiques dans cette maladie, j'entends seulement par-là, que ce sont les remedes connus, les plus propres à changer la disposition épileptique du cerveau . . ."

[182] Cf. Schenck a Grafenberg (892), *Observat. med.*, p. 111.

popularity of the peony was on the decline from the seventeenth century on,[183] and Tissot discarded it altogether, although as great a clinician as De Haen placed it among the main drugs, together with mistletoe and valerian.[184] No definite agreement was reached as to the efficacy of peony, and the evaluation of mistletoe varied from praise to contempt.[185] Valerian, on the other hand, was a drug that steadily gained as a remedy for epilepsy from the sixteenth century on. It had been introduced by the epileptic Fabius Columna, who wished to find an efficacious help for his ailment. According to Fabius Columna's own testimony, the root of the valerian cured him completely.[186] This story was not forgotten during the following century,[187] and at the beginning of the eighteenth century Marchant helped to put the drug in vogue.[188] Apart from the old traditional specifics, the physicians of the eighteenth century discussed a great variety of remedies for epilepsy and even added some new ones, e.g., oxide of zinc, which had been sold by an empiric to Gaubius (1704-80).[189] Cold baths were ordered, and nux vomica was tried;[190] there was a good deal of experimenting by practitioners who followed their own judgment. Advanced men like Home (1719-1813) recognized the uncertainty of their own experiments with antispasmodics and the weakness of unrelated observations by individual physicians.[191]

The mistrust of specifics and the realization that they did not know the predisposing cause of epilepsy did not lead the physicians of the eighteenth century into therapeutic nihilism. On the contrary, few authors have ever been so optimistic as, for instance, Tissot. If they could not rationally attack the predisposing cause, at least they might prevent everything that put the predisposing cause into action. Van Swieten recognized the value of keeping the patient free from attacks for some time at least. "For when the paroxysms can be prevented for a while, the predisponent cause seems gradually to diminish, having not been excited for a great length of time."[192] To keep the patient under the most favorable conditions, under a healthy regimen, and safe from all exciting causes became a strongly emphasized therapeutic principle.

---

[183]Cf., e.g., Sylvius (984), *Prax. med.*, II, c. 20, 129; p. 321.

[184]Cf. Tissot, *l.c.*, pp. 314-18.

[185]For the history of mistletoe and particularly as an anti-epileptic remedy cf. Kanner (572).

[186]Cf. van Swieten (982), *Commentaries*, vol. 10, p. 367.

[187]Cf. Sennert (913), *Pract. med.* I, pars 2, c. 31; vol. 2, p. 226. Riverius (853), *The Practice of Physick*, p. 32 f. Sylvius (984), *Prax. med.*, II, c. 20, 130; p. 321.

[188]Cf. Marchant (667), *Sur les vertus de la racine de la grande Valeriane sauvage.*

[189]Cf. Sprengel (946), vol. 5, 2; p. 696.

[190]Mildner (700), cites instructive examples.

[191]Home (511), *Clinical Experiments*, pp. 153-234.

[192]Van Swieten (982), *Commentaries*, vol. 10, p. 417 (contemporary translation).

The exact steps to be taken were not formulated in an abstract rule but had to be decided according to the individual case. It was a treatment of epileptics rather than of epilepsy.

The tendency toward prevention can be studied in one of its most radical forms in Thomas Beddoes' (1760-1808) *Essay on the Nature and Prevention of some of the Disorders, commonly called Nervous.* In this essay, epilepsy is chosen as the example of nervous maladies[193] and is studied in connection with other seizures which are not epileptic or *not yet* epileptic. For Beddoes believes that the disposition toward epilepsy is widespread. He pays particular attention to the changes which develop before the onset of definite epileptic attacks, and he finds that these pre-epileptic states are similar to the manifestations of hysterical and other nervous complaints. Beddoes' essay is probably one of the most comprehensive early studies of incipient epilepsy. It is largely based on the book of an epileptic who gave a detailed account of the history of his own disease.[194] At the same time Beddoes' work leaves a frightening impression. He finds such great similitude between incipient epilepsy and other nervous disorders that all differences between the various classes of disease begin to disappear. Everybody suffering from the slightest nervous complaint finds himself threatened with future epilepsy and should therefore take steps to root out the disposition to such a horrible disease. "I wish that the following observations may contribute to increase the interest he [i.e., the reader] may have taken in the subject, and put him upon his guard against the causes of those semi-epileptic qualms, with which more, I am afraid, than three out of ten in every genteel circle are not unfrequently overtaken."[195]

For an understanding of Beddoes' exaggerations it is necessary to know that the above-mentioned essay is part of his *Hygeïa,* a work which, according to its subtitle, contains "Essays Moral and Medical, on the Causes Affecting the Personal State of our *Middling and Affluent Classes.*"[196] It is concerned with that stratum of society which indulged in sentimentality, swooning fits, and a yearning for nature. Beddoes gives to all this a medical basis. He takes the complaints of nervous persons seriously—just as seriously as a neurotic patient would like to have them taken. He warns his "genteel" readers against the "vulture of fashion,"[197] against too much reading (especially of novels),[198] he

---

[193] Beddoes (93), *Hygeïa,* vol. 3, p. 16.

[194] Cf. *ibid.,* p. 33. This book was the *Diaetophilus, physische und psychologische Geschichte seiner siebenjährigen Epilepsie* (Zürich, 1798), by K. W. L. von Drais.

[195] Beddoes, *l.c.,* p. 69.

[196] Italics are mine.

[197] *Ibid.,* p. 107.

[198] *Ibid.,* p. 164 ff.

praises the advantages of "a simple and natural life"[199] (particularly gardening), gives most detailed instructions as to when and how to sleep, and thinks that the study of mathematics, experimental sciences, and the law will have a salutary influence upon the nervous system.[200] Beddoes' essay is another example of how people who had freed themselves of the fear of demons and witches now invented new anguishes. Their hypochondria led them to the praise of a simple life, near to nature and devoted to studies, a kind of secularized monastic idyll.

## 2. PATHOLOGY AND NOSOLOGY

### a. Pathology

The dogmatic physicians of the seventeenth and early eighteenth centuries had been intent upon the search for the proximate and conjoint causes of epilepsy. They had tried to find out what morbid change in the epileptic organism might in all cases account for all the symptoms of the disease. Toward the middle of the eighteenth century this dogmatic interest abated; instead, many physicians became pessimistic as to whether such a goal could ever be reached. We have already discussed the manner in which a shift toward a more practical attitude corresponded to the emergence of the enlightened physician. We shall now have to show that the period of Enlightenment also represented a more positive approach toward the pathology of epilepsy.

Irritability, which for centuries had played such an important part in the theories of epilepsy, was given a new experimental definition by Haller (1708-77). Whereas many scientists of the old Galenic as well as the Stahlian school had connected it with some kind of sensibility, he separated these two concepts. According to Haller, sensibility was a response which expressed itself in manifest psychic reactions, like signs of pain, and was bound to the nerves. Irritability, on the other hand, was determined by contraction and was a property of the muscles.

Haller's work did not remain unchallenged. Some of his observations were debatable, e.g., his denial of any sensibility of the dura mater.[201] Besides, his definitions were too restricted; irritability as a phenomenon of organic life is more than contractility. Some necessary corrections were made during the half century between Haller's publication and the work of Bichat. But with all its faults, Haller's research led to one important result: neither the dura mater nor the brain was capable of any active movements.[202] In principle, this put an end to the theories of epilepsy implying a movement of the brain or of the meninges. It

---

[199] *Ibid.*, p. 107.

[200] *Ibid.*, p. 161 f.

[201] Haller (451), *A Dissertation on the Sensible and Irritable Parts of Animals*, p. 17 ff.

[202] *Ibid.*, pp. 19 and 30.

was, however, much more difficult to give an adequate explanation on the basis of the new findings. Haller knew, of course, that muscles contracted upon stimulation of the nerves, and it was also clear to him that epilepsy originated from the brain. The question, therefore, was how the impulse to general convulsions could come from the brain. As far as contemporary experiments and clinical observations were concerned, the results were rather confusing.[203] Even before his time it had been denied that irritation of the cerebral cortex would produce convulsions.[204] Haller stated that it was necessary to irritate the medullary part of the brain at a rather deep point.[205] This was the part of the brain where he located the seat of sensation and the origin of movement,[206] and it seems that he referred epilepsy to pressure exerted upon the white matter of the brain.[207] It is, however, difficult to explain how this irritation or pressure could obtain in cases where the membranes or only the surface of the brain appeared to be affected.[208]

Since Haller was chiefly a physiologist, the lack of a clear theory of epilepsy in his works is excusable. Most of the authors who wrote more effusively on the subject either adhered to some older theory or implied some rather vague notions of increased irritability. Tissot, for instance, whose views agreed to a certain extent with those of Haller, thought that the cause of epilepsy was in the brain, which, when compressed or contracting, sent the animal spirits into the motor nerves and prevented their reception by the sensitive nerves. A convulsion of the brain might produce this effect[209]—but one may well ask how a contraction or convulsion of the brain could be maintained in the light of Haller's findings. Tissot himself was quite frank about it. He said that we could understand the convulsions of the muscles as caused by the animal spirits sent there by the irregular action of the brain. "But," he added, "we do not understand at all the convulsion of the brain, and the conjectures one may make about it seem to me so uncertain that I deem it useless to venture upon them."[210] This was practically the

---

[203]The history of these experiments has been given by Neuburger (731). Since they have only an indirect bearing upon epilepsy, I refer to this book as well as to Soury (939).

[204]Cf. Kaau Boerhaave (129), *Impetum faciens dictum Hippocrati*, p. 257.

[205]Haller (452), *Elementa physiologiae*, X, sec. 7, § 27; vol. 4, p. 327, and sec. 8, § 23, p. 392.

[206]*Ibid.*, sec. 8, § 23, p. 392 f.

[207]Cf. *ibid.*, sec. 7, § 27, p. 328 f.

[208]Cf. *ibid.* Haller probably agreed with Boretius, whose disputation he incorporated into one of his collections. Explaining the pathology of epilepsy due to depression of the skull, Boretius (138), *Disputatio inaug. de epilepsia ex depresso cranio*, p. 69, wrote: "Cranio intropresso, premitur dura et pia mater, cortex cerebri, ejusque medulla, nervorum origo. Hinc praecise in hac parte cerebri, in qua premitur, fomes semper haeret; qui a causa quadam physica, eaque minima, in actum deductus, nervos afficiendo suum sortitur effectum."

[209]Tissot (1024), *Traité de l'épilepsie*, p. 25 f.

[210]*Ibid.*, p. 44.

conclusion to which Whytt had resigned himself some years before.[211] Zimmerman, himself one of Haller's main collaborators in the experiments on irritability, pointed to a concretion in the brain which, allegedly, had caused epilepsy through irritation of the dura mater.[212] Cullen (1712-90) admitted lack of exact knowledge of the proximate cause of epilepsy and hinted at some abnormality in the energy of the brain.[213] Many authors evaded the question altogether.

In the main, interest shifted from speculation about the proximate cause to a discussion of predisposing factors and provoking causes. It was recognized that the nervous system of epileptics must differ in some way from that of healthy people, since the same causes provoked an epileptic attack in the former but not in the latter. The predisposing cause might be inherited or acquired later on in life, constitutional factors might play a role, or a strong emotion might engender the first attack and hence the disposition to the disease.[214] Tissot did not dare to decide what change occurred in the brain when it became disposed to epileptic attacks.[215] Cullen thought that the predisposing cause was connected with "a mobility of constitution,"[216] and that this in turn "consists in a greater degree either of sensibility or irritability."[217] The rather unsuccessful quest for the predisposing cause did not lead much further than the recognition of its existence. Anatomical and physiological investigations contributed little. However, both came into full play in the search after the *provoking* causes of epilepsy. The provoking, occasional, exciting, procatarctic, or determining causes, as they were variously called, were those which determined the manifestation of the disease once the disposition toward epilepsy was given. These were the causes to which most attention was paid by the physicians from Boerhaave on. According to a customary division, they were classified as either moral or physical.[218] The moral causes were those which nowadays are called psychic causes; chief among them were strong passions, shock, mental overwork, and, above all, sudden fright. Apart from eliminating the belief in witchcraft and possession, the eighteenth century here followed traditional lines. But in the class of physical causes an impressive amount of anatomical material was accumulated.

---

[211]Cf. above, VII-2.

[212]Zimmermann (1118), *Dissertatio physiologica de irritabilitate*, pp. 6-8. However, Zimmermann argued, the brain was as likely to have been irritated as the dura mater.

[213]Cullen (247), *First Lines of the Practice of Physic*, vol. 3, p. 180 f.

[214]Cf. Tissot, *l.c.*, p. 43.

[215]Cf. *ibid.*

[216]Cullen, *l.c.*, p. 201.

[217]*Ibid.*, p. 202.

[218]Cf. Tissot, *l.c.*, p. 44.

During the preoccupation with iatrochemical and iatrophysical systems the theory and pathological anatomy of epilepsy were badly coordinated. The large number of dissections recorded in the literature of the seventeenth century found a much greater appreciation in the next period, when manifold new findings of pathologists and surgeons were added. Bonet's *Sepulchretum*, in the enlarged edition of 1700 by Manget, shows what observations had been made concerning morbid changes in the brains of epileptics by the beginning of the eighteenth century. Among the more remarkable cases, we may mention that of Rhodius, who had found a fleshy tumor in the ventricle of the brain of an epileptic. By compressing the brain this tumor had rendered the disease incurable.[219] Another case of brain tumor had been observed by Plater in a young man, where the malady had started with headache, stubborn insomnia, and deterioration of his faculties and had ended with frequent convulsive attacks and emaciation. The post-mortem dissection revealed a tumor in the anterior part of the brain.[220] Again, a soldier often fell from his horse in a state of unconsciousness, complaining afterward of headache and ringing in the ears. Six years later he became epileptic and died. When the skull was opened, the dura mater was found gangrenous in the region from the coronary suture to the forehead, and in the middle of the brain a rather big bone was concealed which, with its sharp point, had caused inflammation and rotting of the membrane. No sign of former fracture of the skull or of an old scar was found.[221] Bony concrescences were frequently reported in the eighteenth century. The surgeon La Motte gave the history of a young man who, as a boy of nine, had suddenly been seized with a violent headache, vomiting, fever, and loss of consciousness. On recovering from this, he had suffered complete amnesia and had even had to be taught to speak again. During the following six or seven years he had had very slight epileptic attacks which had become more considerable at the age of sixteen to seventeen and, at twenty-four, had reached a frequency of two or three a week. All exercise caused severe headache and epileptic attacks. The patient died, when twenty-seven years old, of a pulmonary abscess. In the duplicature of the falx cerebri a number of very small bones was found "which seemed to originate from the internal surface of the dura mater and turned their very sharp points toward the pia mater, as if to prick it. They pricked it effectively on the slightest stir, and, since it is extremely sensitive, this gave rise to the great headaches and the epileptic attacks."[222] La Motte's observation

---

[219] Rhodius (844), *Observat. medic.* cent. I, obs. 55, p. 33 f.: "in cerebri ventriculo tumor carnosus fuit inventus, qui cerebro compresso inanem huic morbo medicinam docuit."

[220] Cf. Tissot, *l.c.*, p. 117.

[221] Cf. Bonetus (134), *Sepulchretum*, I, sect. 1, obs 49; vol. 1, p. 32.

[222] *Histoire de l'Acad. Roy. d. Sciences*, année 1711 (495), p. 28.

was supplemented by that of Hunauld, who in one of the lateral walls of the sinus longitudinalis superior found small pointed bones which became entangled in the brain and must have "pricked" it.[223] And Lieutaud described a bony formation embedded in the cerebellum but also connected with the dura mater.[224] These observations of French surgeons made quite an impression upon the pathologists of the eighteenth century. In 1781 Vicq-d'Azyr considered it necessary to dwell on the inconclusiveness of such concretions. He had found them on the dura mater, on the falx, and on the pia mater of persons without epileptic symptoms, and he had, on the other hand, dissected the heads of several epileptics without finding any bony concretions.[225]

Cases where some former injury of the skull could be traced were, of course, frequently observed during the seventeenth as well as the eighteenth century. Clossy reported a case which is interesting because the operative treatment is mentioned, although it led to the death of the patient. In this instance epileptic attacks had occurred several times a day for three years. "On examining the Head, there appeared a fulness on the left Parietal bone, which had remained from a stroke of a saplin about the time of the commencement of the fits." Trephining was then performed, and "in the operation the Bone was found cellulous and spungy with Pus in the midst; to the Bone the Dura Mater firmly adhered." A short time afterward the patient died, and a post-mortem examination was made. "The Cranium with the Dura Mater being removed, there was a circular asperity on the inside the Bone, about the size of a crown, and several abscesses in the Membrane about the size of peas adjacent to the hole."[226] Although interesting and instructive in detail, these observations merely amplified those of earlier times and need not be repeated here. The same is true of syphilitic epilepsy. It is, however, worth mentioning that injuries suffered at birth were now seriously considered as a possible cause of epilepsy. Boerhaave accused the midwives who, in their endeavors to extract the child, "move its head, press, draw, and twist it and thus cause the predisposition to

[223] *Ibid.*, année 1734, p. 44: "Quand il fut mort, on lui trouva dans une des parois latérales du Sinus longitudinal supérieur de petits Os hérissés de pointes qui s'engageoient dans le Cerveau, et devoient le picoter."

[224] *Ibid.*, année 1737, p. 51.

[225] Vicq-d'Azyr (1048), *Recherches sur la structure du cerveau*, p. 498 f.: "Je dois ajouter que j'ai vu plusieurs fois des concrétions sur la dure-mère, sur la faulx et sur la pie-mère, sans que les malades eussent éprouvé le moindre symptôme épileptique, ni même des maux de tête bien marqués; ce qui doit jeter quelque doute sur l'importance que l'on a attachée à ces sortes de concrétions, lorsqu'on les a observées dans les corps des personnes sujettes à ces différentes maladies: Morgagni avoit déjà fait cette remarque qui paroîtra plus vraisemblable encore, en ajoutant que j'ai ouvert le crâne de plusieurs personnes sujettes à des accès fréquens d'épilepsie, et que je n'y ai point trouvé de concrétions osseuses."

[226] Clossy (228), *Observations on Some of the Diseases of the Parts of the Human Body*, p. 17 ff. On Clossy cf. Stookey (963).

epilepsy, which will not only soon come into existence, but will last throughout the entire life."[227] To this van Swieten added in affirmation: "I remember to have seen several, in the hospitals for incurable epileptic persons, and ideots, in whom the shape of the skull could plainly be observed to be faulty."[228]

Various other observations were published of destruction of the corpus striatum,[229] hardening of the cerebral hemispheres, and other gross changes. Rhaetus, for instance, described the case of a thirty-five-year-old man who had begun suffering from dull pains in the head two years before and had later developed epileptic attacks and died. The anterior part of the right hemisphere toward the dura mater and in the region of the crista galli was found hard, callous, and adhering to the dura mater. On the left side a small quantity of bloody extravasate was found in the anterior part of the brain.[230] In addition to observable changes in the solid parts of the brain, humoral processes were believed of equal importance. Acrid humors were much talked about, and to them Boerhaave attributed "epilepsy" after prolonged retention of urine.[231] Plethora, over-extension of cerebral blood vessels, as well as hemorrhages producing collapse of the brain, were also counted among the causes of epilepsy.[232] However, doubts were voiced as to how far an accumulation of serous fluid in or around the brain should be considered a cause. Le Pois, Wepfer, and others believed it to be so; Morgagni was undecided; Tissot doubted it.[233] This doubt was expressed in spite of the many examples of edema of the brain or a fluid between the brain and its membranes.[234] The facts were not denied as such, but, like some other morbid changes, they were declared effects rather than causes of the epileptic attacks.[235] It had become clear in the eighteenth century that the attacks were accompanied by changes in the body, that these changes might then persist and be mistaken for causes of the disease.[236]

---

[227]Boerhaave (130), *Praelectiones*, p. 794: "Huc refertur vitium obstetricum, quae saepe infantem jam pariendum, et stantem inter angustias ossium pubis et coccygis, et conniventias ossium Ischii, educunt, tumque caput movent, premunt, trahunt, torquent, et hoc modo non tantum Epilepsiae mox futurae sed per totam vitam duraturae, faciunt praedispositionem insanabilem."

[228]Van Swieten (982), *Commentaries*, vol. 10, p. 410 (contemporary translation).

[229]Cf. Haller (452), *Elementa physiologiae*, X, sec. 7, § 33; vol. 4, p. 343.

[230]Cf. Mihles (699), *Medical Essays... Abridg'd from the Philosophical Transactions*, p. 163 f.

[231]Boerhaave (130), *Praelectiones*, p. 797: "Videtis hic, quod humor acerrimus et tenuis ortum dederit Epilepsiae; et simul patet, quare illi, qui vera Ischuria laborant, semper ante mortem aliquid Epileptici patiantur."

[232]Cf. Cullen (247), *First Lines*, vol. 3, pp. 187 ff. and 193 f.

[233]Cf. Tissot (1024), *Traité de l'épilepsie*, p. 149 ff. Cf. also above, p. 197 f.

[234]Cf. Mihles, *l.c.*

[235]Cf. Tissot, *l.c.*, p. 148 ff.

[236]Van Swieten (982), *Commentaries*, vol. 10, p. 388: "It will appear in the comment to the following section, what wonderful changes happen both in the fluid and solid parts of the

The observations which we have discussed in some detail by no means exhaust the catalogue of occasional causes of epilepsy as they were known or assumed at the close of the century. The following list may give an idea of their great and ill-assorted variety. "The occasional or exciting causes are, tumours pressing upon the brain, irregularity in the arrangement of the bones of the cranium, mal-conformation of the cranium, sharp-pointed ossifications within the cranium, splinters, or depression of the bones of the cranium from fracture, serous or other effusions into the ventricles, or upon the membranes of the brain, an abscess formed in the tuberculum annulare, or its neighbourhood, violent joy and anger, pressure upon the medulla oblongata and medulla spinalis, worms, dentition, derangement of the primae viae, suppression of any habitual haemorrhage or accustomed evacuation, syphilis, over-distension of the blood-vessels of the brain, the eruptive fever in certain exanthemata, as the variola and scarlatina, nervous sympathy, profuse haemorrhages, terror, horror, pungent odours, certain poisons, difficult parturition, a diseased state of the liver, the aura epileptica, and external irritations."[237]

This list shows a few peculiarities of the school of Cullen but is otherwise representative of similar lists. The aura epileptica is here considered a cause, and this had a precedent in the preceding century.[238] Furthermore, its very concept had begun to broaden and was no longer restricted to the "breeze" exclusively.[239] Cullen described the aura as the sensation of something moving in some part of the body and creeping toward the head.[240] Apart from the aura, the list includes many causes which do not affect the brain directly and which belonged to the traditional group of *sympathetic* epilepsy.

### b. Nosology

The division into idiopathic and sympathetic epilepsy prevailed throughout the eighteenth century and far into the nineteenth. It was in agreement with experience as well as with neurological theories of the time, which admitted sympathy of the nervous system, or at least spread of irritation from one nerve to others. The difference between the two was easily defined: idiopathic epilepsy had its cause in the

---

body, during the time of the epileptic paroxysm; wherefore these may likewise be observed after death, but they are sometimes the effects of the epilepsy, and not always the causes." (Contemporary translation).

[237] Clarke (224), *The Modern Practice of Physic*, p. 288.

[238] Ferdinandus (350), *Centum historiae*, hist. 24; p. 72: ". . . Casus Vigesimus quartus, Epilepsiae ab aura."

[239] Herpin (487), *Du pronostic et du traitement curatif de l'épilepsie*, p. 396, claims that Hollier in the sixteenth century had already used the expression *aura* ". . . comme d'un mot générique, car les phénomènes qu'il décrit, tous convulsifs, n'ont aucun rapport avec le vent ou la vapeur froide du malade de Galien."

[240] Cullen (247), *First Lines*, vol. 3, p. 197.

brain, while in sympathetic epilepsy the cause was transmitted to the brain either from some internal or external part of the body.[241] This division, moreover, though inherited from Antiquity, seemed now to rest on a more solid basis. The anatomical changes found in the heads of many epileptics, together with plethora and acridity of humors, were thought by some to be manifest causes of idiopathic epilepsy.[242] But then the question arose, how to classify those cases where no definite cause could be discovered at all. To this kind of epilepsy, which seemed to depend solely on the epileptic disposition of the brain, Tissot reserved the title of *essential* epilepsy.[243] Since, however, Tissot admitted that the nature of the epileptic disposition of the brain was unknown, he implicitly defined essential epilepsy as that group of cases which could not be attributed to any known cause. Contrasting it with the groups which seemed etiologically clear, he came very near the modern distinction between genuine and symptomatic epilepsy.

Neither Tissot nor other physicians of the eighteenth century stressed this point. However, a minority challenged the concepts of sympathetic and symptomatic epilepsy and established a system of classification on different grounds. Preceded by Le Pois and Willis, de Moor at the end of the seventeenth century had categorically asserted that all epilepsies were idiopathic.[244] Boissier de Sauvages (1706-62) did not go quite so far; he rejected the opinion that all convulsions had their origin in the brain but believed that the distinction between idiopathic and sympathetic convulsions met with great difficulties.[245] De Sauvages, who was strongly influenced by Stahl, considered the cause of convulsion to be nature's attempt to free the organism of any morbid agent.[246] This attempt could, of course, be provoked in any part of the body. But de Sauvages also recognized that an irritation of the origin of the nerves in the medullary part of the brain might provoke the same sensations as irritation of the parts where these nerves ended.[247] Hence,

---

[241] Cf. Tissot (1024), *Traité de l'épilepsie*, pp. 44-48.

[242] Cf. *ibid.*, p. 225 f.

[243] Cf. *ibid.*, p. 270. He was not the first to base the diagnosis of "essential" epilepsy on lack of any anatomical changes. Bonet (134), *Sepulchretum*, vol. 1, p. 288, quotes the following observation from Schneider: "Infantium Epilepsia extinctorum cerebra perspexi, saepius nihil in iis unquam notavi. Quos tamen medentes concordi assensu confirmabant Essentiali, ut loquuntur, Epilepsia conflictatos fuisse: multos hic morbus a teneris unguiculis exercuit, nec ulla nota offensi cerebri post mortem eorum in capitibus deprehendi poterat." The term "essential epilepsy" can also be found in Alsarius (25), *De morbis capitis frequentioribus*, p. 234: ". . . si de essentiali Epilepsia loquamur."

[244] Cf. Tissot, *ibid.*, p. 100.

[245] Boissier de Sauvages (890), *Nosologia methodica*, classis IV, Spasmorum theoria, § 63; vol. 3, p. 21.

[246] *Ibid.*, § 55, p. 18.

[247] *Ibid.*, § 63, p. 21: "Notum est, molestatis nervorum principiis in medulla cerebri subsequi imaginationem, seu perceptionem illi similem, quae irritatis organis externis, quibus prospiciunt illae fibrae medullares, subsequi solet;" etc.

it was difficult to decide where the irritation actually had its seat, and it was not justifiable to admit the existence of sympathetic or symptomatic epilepsy as a special group of attacks beginning with symptoms which the patient localized in parts other than the brain.[248]

In his classification of epilepsy de Sauvages followed the general principles of his system, which imitated the classifications of the botanists. The fourth class in the system comprised the convulsions. These were divided into four orders, the fourth order dealing with general clonic convulsions[249] and including epilepsy. De Sauvages tried to give a clear definition of epilepsy which would distinguish it from other diseases. He defined it as a general clonic disease of a chronic and periodic character, with insensibility during the paroxysms and oblivion of previous acts.[250] De Sauvages' definition was not accepted by all nosologists of the time; Cullen, for instance, defined epilepsy "as consisting in convulsions of the greater part of the muscles of voluntary motion, attended with a loss of sense, and ending in a state of insensibility, and seeming sleep."[251] And whereas both Cullen and de Sauvages stressed the generalized character of the convulsions, Tissot allowed the convulsions to be more or less violent and to show in a greater or smaller number of parts.[252] But all agreed in one point, viz., that epileptic attacks were accompanied by insensibility and loss of consciousness, and this was accepted as the distinguishing mark between epilepsy and other convulsions.[253]

Although by definition epilepsy involved unconsciousness, it was, on the other hand, recognized that mere convulsive movements might develop into epilepsy.[254] The same definition facilitated the recognition of the epileptic character of what is now called "absence." Some cases

---

[248] *Ibid.*, classis IV, Spasmi universales clonici, pp. 112 and 117.

[249] The distinction between clonic and tonic convulsions had been well defined by de Gorter (419), *Medicinae compendium*, p. 62: "si alterne contrahuntur musculi, convulsionem Clonicam; si vero contracti manent, convulsionem Tonicam vocant."

[250] Boissier de Sauvages, *l.c.*, p. 109: "Est morbus clonicus universalis, chronicus et periodicus, cum sensuum feriatione in paroxysmo, et anteactorum oblivione."

[251] Cullen (247), *First Lines*, vol. 3, p. 177.

[252] Tissot (1024), *Traité de l'épilepsie*, p. 1: "L'épilepsie, est une maladie convulsive, dont chaque accès fait perdre sur le champ le sentiment et la connoissance, et est accompagné de mouvements convulsifs plus ou moins violents, et dans un plus ou moins grand nombre de parties."

[253] Cf. *ibid.*, p. 16 f.; Beddoes (93), *Hygëia*, vol. 3, p. 20.

[254] Cf. Tissot, *l.c.*, p. 175 f. In 1727 Wepfer's (1085) posthumously published *Observationes medico-practicae de affectibus capitis*, observ. 134, p. 631, carried Camerarius' observation of a young man who, every four to six days, suffered from spasmodic movements of the left middle finger, spreading to the four other fingers and to the palm of the hand. One morning the patient laughingly exhibited the movements to his brother and sisters when, suddenly, the whole arm contracted, which was followed by a violent epileptic attack. The course of these attacks was then carefully described. Herpin (487), *Du pronostic et du traitement curatif de l'épilepsie*, p. 403, translated the story into French.

described in the older literature already suggest this interpretation,[255] and in 1705 Poupart reported an example to the Académie Royale des Sciences. At the approach of an attack the patient would sit down in a chair, her eyes open, and would remain there immobile and would not afterward remember having fallen into this state. "If she has begun to talk and the attack interrupts her, she takes it up again at precisely the point at which she stopped, and she believes she has talked continuously."[256] Tissot himself was consulted concerning a fourteen year old girl whose case illustrates both these points. In good health until the age of seven, she had been much terrified by a storm. "A few days afterwards, one noticed a movement of the eyelids which at first seemed to be a tic, but which was soon recognized as convulsive." Even medical care could not prevent the development of severe and frequent attacks of epilepsy, attacks which went on for several months, and "during part of this time the young patient, in the intervals between the *great* attacks (*grands accès*), frequently had very short, *little* (*petits*) attacks, which were merely marked by an instantaneous loss of consciousness interrupting her speech, together with a very slight movement of the eyes. Often, when recovering, she finished the sentence in the middle of which she had been interrupted; at other times she had forgotten it. During another part of the same period these instantaneous attacks only seized her when she was walking: she stopped, senseless for a few seconds, and there was always a slight convulsive movement in the leg which was in front."[257] This story not only describes the interplay of grand mal and petit mal but also distinguishes them terminologically as *grands accès* and *petits accès*.

By defining epilepsy as a *chronic* disease, Boissier de Sauvages tried to differentiate it from the great group of "acute clonic convulsion with insensibility during the paroxysm," to which he gave the name of eclampsia.[258] This distinction proved of importance later when it became generally accepted and was used to designate epileptiform convulsions accompanying other diseases. Convulsions during pregnancy and convulsions of infants were thus separated terminologically from epilepsy. De Sauvages included both conditions in his nosological genus of eclampsia and used the term *eclampsia parturientium*[259] for the former,

---

[255]Cf. above, pp. 189-92.

[256]*Histoire de l'Acad. Roy. d. Sciences*, année 1705 (495), p. 50: "Si elle avoit commencé un discours que son accès ait interrompu, elle le reprend précisément au même endroit où elle l'avoit quitté, et elle croit avoir parlé tout de suite."

[257]Tissot (1024), *Traité de l'épilepsie*, p. 21 ff. Italics are mine. Lennox (632), vol. 1, p. 69, considers this the first account of "pure" petit mal, essentially identical with pyknolepsy described by Adie (9) in 1924.

[258]Boissier de Sauvages (890), *Nosologia methodica*, vol. 3, p. 97.

[259]*Ibid.*, p. 99.

referring to Moriceau, the great-French obstetrician who had paid particular attention to this syndrome.[260] He also used it of uremic attacks, which he designated as *eclampsia ab ischuria*,[261] and various other epileptiform convulsions which had hitherto been termed epilepsy.

The terminological innovation was not accepted at once. Indeed, it must be acknowledged that hesitation was not wholly unjustified. The distinction between epilepsy and eclampsia was purely clinical and rested on the single feature that the former was chronic, the latter acute. In extreme cases, like *eclampsia parturientium*, on the one hand, and chronic epilepsy with psychic deterioration, on the other, the differentiation was easily made. But it was known to the physicians of the eighteenth century that some cases of epilepsy showed few attacks and were free from the sinister consequences of the inveterate form of the disease. Tissot stated quite clearly "that these fatal consequences need only be feared for those who have frequent or violent attacks; I have seen epileptics in whom the attacks were rare and not severe, and in whom it was rather difficult to discover any noticeable alteration depending on this cause. . . ."[262] In such cases it was difficult to say whether the single attack should be diagnosed as epilepsy or as a kindred convulsive disorder.

In spite of the great difficulties of differential diagnosis, which were frankly admitted, the nosological entity of epilepsy seemed to the physicians of the eighteenth century to be well established. How little justified this assurance was is evidenced not only by the already mentioned confusion with hysteria[263] but also by the general character of the subdivisions of epilepsy made by Boissier de Sauvages and others after him. Epilepsy could be the result of syphilis or of worms, and all such possibilities had to find a place in the system. Since there was no guiding principle in the choice and arrangement of subdivisions, they became a pell-mell of historical data. As far back as the Middle Ages, when the Galenic doctrine had been prevalent, adjectives had been used to designate the organ from which epilepsy had presumably arisen. Idiopathic epilepsy, since it originated directly from the brain, was named "cerebral epilepsy," while the various forms of sympathetic epilepsy were called *stomachica, splenetica*, etc.[264] It is simply an extension of such older usage when later on we find forms like *nephritica*,

---

[260] Cf. Fasbender (346), p. 171.

[261] Boissier de Sauvages, *l.c.*, p. 102. Cullen (249), *Synopsis nosologiae methodicae*, p. 299, footnote, objected to the separation of eclampsia from the genus epilepsy.

[262] Tissot (1024), *Traité de l'épilepsie*, p. 205 f.

[263] Cf. above, VIII-1a.

[264] Jacobus Forliviensis (370), *In Hippocratis aphorismos* etc., fol. 158[r]: "Per proprietatem appelatur epilepsia cerebralis. Per communitatem recipit denominationem a communitate membrorum ut dicatur stomatica (!) splenetica myrachia, et sic de aliis."

*hysterica, verminosa.*[265] Boissier de Sauvages collected all such particular forms of epilepsy from literature and classified them as subdivisions, adding the name of the author from whom the description was taken. If his source had not done so already, and if it seemed convenient to do so, he himself would coin an adjective. Thus we read *"epilepsia syphilitica Bonet*, Sepulchretum," which means that de Sauvages had found this particular form described in Bonet's *Sepulchretum*,[266] and Hecquet's discussion of the convulsionists of St. Médard[267] is referred to as *epilepsia simulata.*[268] The latter example illustrates the lack of real criticism characteristic of this and similar systems. Cullen established two main categories: idiopathic and symptomatic epilepsy. Idiopathic epilepsy included three major subdivisions: (1) *Epilepsia cerebralis*, "suddenly coming on without manifest cause; not preceded by any troublesome sensation, unless perhaps of vertigo and dimness of sight." (2) *Epilepsia sympathica*, also with manifest cause but preceded by an aura. (3) *Epilepsia occasionalis*, "arising from manifest irritation, and ceasing when the irritation is removed." There being many and diverse irritations, the last named subdivision contained the usual multitude of epilepsies: "from injury done to the head," "from poison," "from affection of the mind," and many others. Cullen did not account satisfactorily for the difference between "occasional" and "symptomatic" epilepsy; for instance, exanthematic epilepsy is listed among both.[269]

Though some of their terms survived, these systems did not greatly advance the understanding of the disease and were contradictory in themselves. At least one contemporary of de Sauvages considered them practically useless.[270] Yet the persistence of nosological schemes into the present indicates the need for classification in the interest of clearness as well as mutual communication.

---

[265]Cf. Hoffmann (503), *Medicina rationalis systematica*, t. IV, pars 3, sec. 1, c. 1; vol. 2, p. 12.

[266]Cf. Boissier de Sauvages (890), *Nosologia methodica*, vol. 3, p. 119. Although Bonet described epilepsy in syphilitics (cf. above, VI-1, footnote 235), I have not been able to trace the term *epilepsia syphilitica* in his collections.

[267]Cf. above, VIII-1a.

[268]Boissier de Sauvages, *l.c.*, p. 115.

[269]Cullen (248), *Nosology: or a Systematic Arrangement of Diseases*, pp. 115-17. On the history of neurological classification from Cullen to the twentieth century cf. Riese (848).

[270]Macbride (654), *A Methodical Introduction* etc., p. 558: "It seems of very little practical use to distinguish the epilepsy into different species; although Sauvages makes fourteen, to whom we refer. The *epilepsia uterina*, or hysteric epilepsy, is the only one that requires much notice."

# PART FIVE

# FIVE

# THE NINETEENTH CENTURY: 1800-1861

# First Period: 1800-1833

## 1. THE HOSPITALIZATION OF EPILEPTICS

Once the fetters were taken off the insane, their former prisons began to assume the character of asylums or of hospitals. This change benefited epileptics too, for they had often been confined with the insane. Certain differences had been made between epileptics and alienated persons; in the eighteenth century, for example, epileptics in the Bicêtre were allowed to go to Mass on Sundays.[1] In the same century we occasionally hear of epileptics who were under observation in a hospital or confined in prison-like institutions.[2] But, in general, it was only from the time of Pinel (1745–1826) in France, of Chiarugi (1759–1820) in Italy, and the Tukes in England, that confined epileptics became the object of systematic medical attention. In 1815 Esquirol made a strong plea for the establishment of special divisions for epileptics. Altogether, the care of epileptics, particularly of children, progressed slowly. Only in 1838 were such children, in Paris, transferred from the hospital of the incurably ill to the Bicêtre and some kind of education provided for them.[3]

The reasons given by Esquirol (1772–1840) for separating epileptics and insane persons are somewhat surprising. He was not motivated by solicitude for the epileptics, who might suffer from contact with the insane. This is partly understandable, since the ma-

---

[1] Cf. Bru (176), p. 162.
[2] E.g., Gredings's (423), careful studies at the poorhouse of Waldheim, Germany.
[3] Cf. Bru, *l.c.*, p. 274.

jority of confined epileptics were mentally affected. Rather, Esquirol was anxious for the well-being of the insane. He believed that the sight of one epileptic attack might suffice to make a healthy person epileptic. Now if this held true of healthy people, how much greater was the danger for the mentally deranged, who were so much more impressionable.[4] Such views appear to be a direct consequence of the theory that epilepsy was an infectious disease.[5] In the middle of the century the question was still discussed, whether prolonged imitation of epilepsy would lead to the firm establishment of the disease itself.[6]

In many countries new institutions were built, for instance the county asylums in England, and the confinement of epileptics in separate wards of lunatic asylums became the established procedure around 1850.[7] Then, when segregation had become a fact, the next step was the request for special institutions for epileptics. But, although demanded repeatedly, the scheme was slow to materialize. The National Hospital for the Paralysed and Epileptic, Queen Square, London, was opened in 1860.[8] In Germany the Heil- und Pflegeanstalt für Schwachsinnige und Epileptische, Stetten i. R. goes back to 1849, and Bethel, near Bielefeld, was founded in 1867.[9] Also in 1867, the Epileptic and Paralytic Hospitals were established on Blackwell's Island, New York, but the first separate institution for epileptics in the United States, at Gallipolis, Ohio, dates from 1891.[10] Regarding the most common form of epilepsy among the inmates of asylums, the superintendent of an English county asylum in 1858 described it as "that in which the attack commenced in childhood" and where "the mind has never been developed and we have the idiot whose course is generally cut short in early life," or where "some considerable amount of intelli-

---

[4]Esquirol (329), *Des maladies mentales*, vol. 1, p. 331: "Ils ne doivent pas habiter pêle-mêle avec les aliénés, comme cela se pratique dans presque tous les hospices où l'on reçoit les épileptiques et les aliénés. La vue d'un accès d'épilepsie suffit pour rendre épileptique une personne bien portante. Combien plus grand est le danger pour un aliéné quelquefois si impressionnable!"

[5]Cf. above, VIII-1a.

[6]Cf. Hasse (461), *Die Krankheiten des Nervensystems*, p. 267.

[7]Cf. Hunter (520), p. 167. Meyer (689), *Aus der Krampfkranken-Abtheilung der Charité*, p. 1: "Die Beunruhigung, welche die gesellschaftlichen Verhältnisse durch die Mehrzahl der sogenannten Epileptiker leiden, die Nothwendigkeit, diese Kranken unter eine dauernde Aufsicht zu stellen, die häufigen Complikationen mit Wahnsinn, hat die Unterbringung derartiger Krampfkranken in besonderen Abtheilungen grösserer Irrenanstalten zu einer fast allgemeinen Praxis erhoben."

[8]Cf. Holmes (509), p. 11.

[9]Cf. *Institutions* etc. (533), pp. 105 and 106.

[10]Cf. Shrady (923), *The Medical Register of New York*, p. 75, and Deutsch (267), p. 381. According to Shanahan (921), the Ohio Hospital (Gallipolis) "was opened to patients November 30, 1893."

gence has been developed, but is afterwards destroyed by successive convulsive attacks."[11]

Pinel had made it possible to study epilepsy under more favorable conditions than before, and he was also one of the first to see the importance of such studies, stimulating his pupil Maisonneuve to undertake them at the Salpêtrière.[12] When Maisonneuve's book was published in the year 12 of the French Republic (1804), it gave programmatic expression to this principle of investigation. "And first of all," wrote Maisonneuve, "epilepsy, like all chronic diseases, can be studied well only in the hospitals; there alone is it possible to find all its varieties together, to see it in all its nuances, and to acquire in short time more experience of this disease than in the whole course of ordinary practice."[13] Most of the classical studies of epilepsy which appeared in France and England during the following years came from physicians who were closely connected with hospitals for the insane, with asylums for epileptics, or with the epileptic wards of general hospitals. This fact in itself accounts for some of the new aspects which were developed during the early part of the nineteenth century: establishment of a new terminology, increasing use of statistics, and interest in the psychiatric side of epilepsy.

### a. Terminology

Some terms still used today for designating certain types of epileptic attacks have preserved their French forms. We still speak of "grand mal," "petit mal," and "absence." These terms do not indicate any form of epilepsy unknown before the nineteenth century; they were customary in the hospitals of Paris and hence gradually came into general use in the literature of epilepsy.[14] In 1815 Esquirol stated that "sometimes the attacks alternate in intensity: there are severe and slight attacks; this is what is called *le grand* and *le petit mal* in the hospitals."[15] Esquirol's definition of these two terms is obviously vague. Even if it is understood that *le grand mal* means the fully developed fit with loss of consciousness and general convulsions,[16] it leaves *le petit*

---

[11]Manley (658), *On Epilepsy*, p. 245.

[12]Pinel (797), *Nosographie philosophique*, vol. 3, p. 75. On Pinel's influence on the young Paris school see Ackerknecht (6), p. 47 ff.

[13]Maisonneuve (661), *Recherches et observations sur l'épilepsie*, p. 8.

[14]For the whole history of the Paris hospitals during this period Ackerknecht (6) should be consulted.

[15]Esquirol (329), *Des maladies mentales*, vol. 1, p. 281: " ... quelquefois les accès alternent pour l'intensité: il y en a de forts et de faibles; c'est ce qu'on appelle dans les hospices *le grand et le petit mal.*"

[16]Cf. *ibid.*, p. 288.

*mal* badly defined. This looseness is particularly obvious if the two names are compared with their medieval analogues: *epilepsia maior* and *minor*, which connoted two stereotyped forms of epileptic fits.[17] Esquirol himself did not make things clearer by using, in addition, the term *vertige épileptique* (epileptic vertigo).[18] Here again there is a much older precedent, the ancients already having called vertigo "a little epilepsy."[19] But from Esquirol's descriptions it is not possible to tell whether *vertige épileptique* and *petit mal* were synonymous for him.

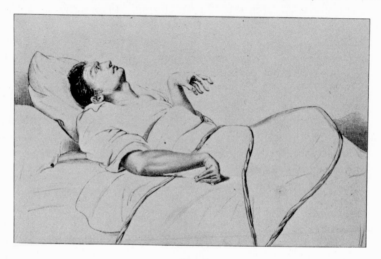

Fig. 5

Epileptic. (Esquirol, *Des maladies mentales*, Atlas, Paris, 1838, plate 1.)

For some time the two expressions rivaled one another,[20] but during the later part of the century "petit mal" began to prevail. The latter term had obvious advantages. It did not emphasize a subjective symptom, vertigo, and it was less apt to lead to confusion with other forms of vertigo, particularly Ménière's disease, which was well described in 1861. But its chief advantage lay in its breadth, particularly since

[17]I am not able to say whether there is any real historical connection between the two sets of names.

[18]Esquirol, *l.c.*, p. 278.

[19]Cf. above, II-1e.

[20]Most authors used the two expressions synonymously. According to Calmeil (197), *De l'épilepsie*, p. 13 f. "Petit mal, vertiges, étourdissemens parmi les malades" (without proper distinction) are the second form of epilepsy in contrast to the grand mal, its first form. Cf. also Foville (374), Article *Épilepsie*, p. 416; Watson (1067), *Lectures* etc., p. 342. Trousseau (1032), *Clinique médicale*, p. 104: " . . . des accès de *petit mal* (c'est le nom qu'on a encore donné aux vertiges épileptiques)." On the conceptual history of petit mal cf. Daly (252).

Calmeil (1798-1895) in 1824[21] had familiarized the medical world with the term "absence." The fully developed fit was distinguished by the name of "grand mal"; those cases characterized by a passing mental confusion without any definite physical symptoms were easily characterized as "absences"; vertigo could be extended to include mental aspects of epilepsy; while "petit mal" remained a convenient term to comprise the great variety of attacks which did not have the character of grand mal. From a logical point of view this terminological looseness might appear unsatisfactory, but from the point of view of a progressive science it proved adequate.

Another term which, if not coined, was at least made familiar in the hospitals, was "status epilepticus" or its French equivalent, état de mal, as used at the Salpêtrière and Bicêtre.[22] Calmeil seems to have been the first author to differentiate between severe fits and état de mal, a series of attacks following one another uninterruptedly and presenting a bad prognosis.[23] The opportunity to observe great numbers of epileptics and the necessity of discussing the cases with fellow physicians, students, and attendants led not only to the adoption of certain terms but also to doubts of the correctness of others. It was particularly the concept of the epileptic "aura" which began to undergo a decisive change. By the end of the eighteenth century its definition as an ascending "cold breeze" had already been broadened to include other ascending feelings. In 1823 Georget (1795-1828), physician at the Salpêtrière, maintained that aura of the classical type must be very rare, that one did not encounter it where many epileptics were united, and that usually the same few examples were carried along in the literature.[24] A year before, Prichard (1786-1848), who could look back upon a hospital experience of ten years,[25] gave the following description of a certain type of prodromal symptom: " . . . the attack seems to

---

[21]Calmeil (197), De l'épilepsie, p. 14: "Troisième nuance.—Absences. . . . Je serais porté à croire que l'absence n'est qu'un vertige avorté, de même que les vertiges pourraient bien être des accès incomplets de grand mal."

[22]Cf. Delasiauve (261), Traité de l'épilepsie, p. 85: "A la Salpêtrière . . . on les désigne vulgairement sous le nom d'état de mal." Trousseau (1032), Clinique médicale, p. 101: "Vous avez cependant entendu parler de faits dans lesquels des attaques ont duré deux, trois jours, et se sont terminées par la mort. C'est là ce qu'on a appelé, à la Salpêtrière et à Bicêtre, l'état de mal." According to Calmeil (197), De l'épilepsie, p. 13, this term goes back to the patients: "c'est ce que les malades appellent entre eux état de mal."

[23]Cf. Hunter (520), p. 165. In his detailed analysis of the history of status epilepticus, Hunter has shown that reports of this condition were very rare before epilepsy was studied in hospitals (p. 167) and remained rare until the introduction of potassium of bromide into the therapy of epilepsy (p. 168 ff.). See below, p. 298 f.

[24]Georget (406), Article Épilepsie, p. 210: "Mais, les cas de ce genre doivent être fort rares, car l'épilepsie est une affection fort commune, et sur des réunions nombreuses de malades, on n'en rencontre point qui offrent cet aura tel que le signalent les auteurs; on n'en trouve que quelques exemples, presque toujours les mêmes, dans les ouvrages." In addition he stated that one no longer heard of physicians curing epilepsy by surgical operations at the seat of the aura.

[25]Prichard (824), A Treatise on Diseases of the Nervous System, p.v.

commence in some extreme part, as in a foot or hand; a convulsive tremor, or sometimes a rigid contraction of the muscles, takes place, first at the extremity of the limb, and gradually ascends towards the head: when it reaches the head the paroxysm of coma and convulsion ensues."[26] To this description he added in a footnote: "This symptom is usually termed by medical authors the *aura epileptica*, and it is described by them as a sensation of a cold vapour affecting the part and rising upward. I have met with a great number of patients who have perceived the affection alluded to, but I never once heard it described in this way, though I have been very minute in my inquiries."[27] With the doubt of Galen's original observation and the connection of the term "aura" with symptoms of a quite different character, the way was now opened to an identification of "aura" with all possible warnings. Romberg (1795–1873), who mentioned "premonitory symptoms of a sensitive, motor, or psychical character,"[28] did not limit the use of the term to the sensitive group but, acquainted with Prichard's work, also talked of "motor aura."[29] Hasse stated that "the differentiation between a sensory, sensitive, and motor aura has been made."[30] In short, the old concept of "aura" was of scarcely more than historical interest.[31]

### b. Statistics

On December 31, 1813, Esquirol counted 389 epileptic women at the Salpêtrière and 162 epileptic men at the Bicêtre.[32] Of the latter, 119 were bachelors, 33 married, 7 widowers, and 1 divorced.[33] The assembling of such large numbers of epileptic patients in the hospital wards made the introduction of statistical methods possible and indeed stimulated them. One question which met with the interest of early statisticians concerned the influence of heredity. In 1825 Bouchet (1801–54) and Cazauvieilh (1801–49) approached it in a twofold manner. They tried to establish the proportion between healthy and ill forebears of epileptics. Among 110 epileptics they found 79[34] whose

---

[26]*Ibid.*, p. 88.

[27]The note continues: "It is generally represented as a convulsive tremor commencing in a limb. Sometimes there is even a perceptible convulsion of the large muscles of the limb," etc.

[28]Romberg (865), *A Manual of the Nervous Diseases of Man*, vol. 2, p. 197 (Sieveking's translation).

[29]*Ibid.*, p. 198.

[30]Hasse (461), *Die Krankheiten des Nervensystems*, p. 250: "Man hat eine sensorielle, sensible und motorische Aura unterschieden," etc.

[31]For the history of aura cf. Herpin (487), *Du pronostic et du traitement curatif de l'épilepsie*, pp. 389–420.

[32]Esquirol (329), *Des maladies mentales*, vol. 1, p. 292.

[33]Cf. *ibid.*, p. 301.

[34]The text gives 99, which seems a misprint.

relatives were free from nervous diseases, and 31 who had insane, epileptic, imbecile, or hysterical relatives. In another group of epileptics, they tried to fix the number of healthy and ill descendants. Here, however, they encountered great difficulties and these statistics extended over only 14 epileptic women.[35] Leuret (1797-1851), in 1843, arrived at quite different results. "In 106 epileptics I found but 7 with relatives affected by epilepsy: one had an epileptic father, brother, and sister; the second an epileptic father only; the third an epileptic mother and one sister; the fourth an epileptic mother and uncle; the fifth and sixth had epileptic mothers only; the seventh had one epileptic uncle."[36] In addition, Leuret made inquiries as to the number of relatives who had suffered from cerebral diseases other than epilepsy; the result was positive in only 8 cases.[37] Again, a few years later, in 1854, Moreau (1804-84) stated the very opposite. He found a great number of pathological incidents in the families of epileptics[38] and concluded that in practically all cases the origin of epilepsy could be traced to heredity.[39] But Moreau's statistics were based on the assumption that diseases could change their form when inherited. Hence, he not only took all nervous disorders into consideration[40] but believed that even phthisis might appear as epilepsy in the tainted offspring. With methods and results at such variance, it is hardly surprising that Delasiauve, in 1854, doubted whether the problem could be solved at all by statistical investigation.[41]

The age at which epilepsy manifested itself, the influence of menstruation, and similar data also interested the early statisticians. Concerning these matters it may, however, suffice to say that they were studied much more elaborately in the great monographs of the fifties and sixties of the nineteenth century. But there are a few inquiries on which we must dwell in more detail, because they reveal characteristic attitudes toward broader issues. There is first of all the attempt at finding the relative frequency of various determining causes of epilepsy. Bouchet and Cazauvieilh gave the following data:

---

[35] Bouchet et Cazauvieilh (140), *De l'épilepsie considérée dans ses rapports avec l'aliénation mentale*, pp. 39-41.

[36] Leuret (638), *Recherches sur l'épilepsie*, p. 34 f.

[37] *Ibid.*, p. 35.

[38] Moreau (708), *De l'étiologie de l'épilepsie*, p. 53: "Ainsi, pour 44 enfants épileptiques, nous trouvons 100 cas pathologiques répartis sur 83 parents;" *ibid.*, p. 54: "... pour 51 épileptiques (hommes adultes), 113 cas pathologiques répartis sur 115 parents;" *ibid.*, p. 55: "... 29 épileptiques (femmes) adultes, 71 états pathologiques divers répartis sur 57 parents."

[39] *Ibid.*, p. 20: "Il n'est aucun cas de cette maladies il en est du moins infiniment peu dont on ne puisse faire remonter l'origine à l'hérédité ainsi comprise."

[40] *Ibid.*, p. 21: "En résumé, les troubles nerveux, à quelque ordre qu'ils appartiennent, sous quelque forme symptomatique qu'ils nous apparaissent, depuis les plus simples jusqu'aux plus complexes, ne prédisposent pas moins à l'épilepsie que l'épilepsie elle-même."

[41] Delasiauve (261), *Traité de l'épilepsie*, p. 187.

| | | | |
|---|---|---|---|
| Fright | 21 | Dentition | 1 |
| Sorrow | 10 | Vexation | 1 |
| Masturbation | 3 | Blows on the head | 1 |
| Difficult menstruation | 3 | Artificial insolation | 1 |
| Consequence of childbed | 1 | Unknown causes | 26 |
| Critical age | 2 | | |
| | | TOTAL | 69[42] |

Beau's statistics, which were gathered at the Salpêtrière in 1833[43] and published in 1836, were similar although a little more detailed.[44] Cazauvieilh and Bouchet, as well as Beau, admitted only the causes which to them seemed probable. Leuret's figures are subjected to more critical considerations. Of his 106 epileptics he discounted 39 who could not even assign a probable cause to their disease. From the remaining 67 he obtained the following answers:

| | | | |
|---|---|---|---|
| Fear | 35 | Insolation | 1 |
| Masturbation | 12 | Sudden chill | 1 |
| Drunkenness | 6 | Injuries of the head | 1 |
| Wrath | 2 | Decreasing psoriasis | 1 |
| Misery | 2 | Difficult dentition | 1 |
| Fall | 2 | Heredity | 1 |
| Debauchery | 1 | | |
| | | TOTAL | 67[45] |

But then Leuret emphasized that the causes which appeared only once should not receive much consideration, particularly since they had not been followed promptly by an epileptic attack. He applied almost the same restriction to the causes which appeared in but two cases;[46] there remained only fear, masturbation, and drunkenness to be reckoned with.

The preceding statistics were used and enlarged by Moreau[47] in 1854, but by now scepticism as to their usefulness had advanced one more decisive step. Hasse (1855) classified them under "occasional causes," and, in reprinting Moreau's figures, he said: "It is, indeed, worth while to preserve this confused and thoughtless enumeration as given by the patients and their relatives. Who could not enrich this list with many 'causes' from his own experience!"[48] Obviously, the statis-

---

[42] Bouchet et Cazauvieilh (140), *De l'épilepsie*, p. 44. Here again a mistake must have been made somewhere, since the total of these figures is 70.

[43] Beau (91), *Recherches statistiques pour servir à l'histoire de l'épilepsie et de l'hystérie*, p. 328.

[44] *Ibid.*, p. 342.

[45] Leuret (638), *Recherches sur l'épilepsie*, p. 38. This figure is also wrong, since the total amounts to 66.

[46] Except wrath, which in both cases was followed almost immediately by the first epileptic attack.

[47] Moreau (708), *De l'étiologie de l'épilepsie*, pp. 108-10.

[48] Hasse (461), *Die Krankheiten des Nervensystems*, p. 266, footnote.

tical method alone could not yield any definite results about the etiology of epilepsy. Whether the factors furnished by the patients were
admitted as probable causes or not depended on the general views of
the statistician. For this very reason these statistics are of historical
interest because they reveal the frame of mind of both patients and
physicians.

As is to be expected, "fright" took first place. The etiological
relevancy of fright and "moral" causes in general was scarcely as much
as doubted. Doussin-Dubreuil (1762-1831), whose work *On Epilepsy
in General and Particularly that Determined by Moral Causes*, first
published in 1797, was republished as late as 1825, tried to explain the
influence of various emotional states. He believed that emotions forced
the heart to contract, thus impeding the excretion of substances
normally excreted through sweat or "insensible transpiration." These
substances would then affect the blood, other humors, and diverse
organs.[49] Doussin-Dubreuil did not belong to the hospital school of
the period; the members of the latter were not so easily given to inventing pathological theories. Maisonneuve even went as far as to say
that in many cases fear, wrath, and sadness were but the occasional
causes of an epilepsy, the essential and true cause of which consisted in
a plethoric condition, a defect of the humors, etc. But he added: "However, there is a great number of epilepsies which really have to be
attributed to violent passions of which they have been the consequence."[50] In the later part of the century, the frequency of causation
by fright was more generally doubted,[51] but then the doubt coincided
with the development of certain philosophical ideas concerning the
relation of body and mind which did not favor an emotional etiology of
disease.

One particular cause of epilepsy deserves notice: the alleged origin
from fright of the pregnant mother. Tissot had considered it impossible.
But although Tissot was still widely read in the early nineteenth
century, this factor appeared in Beau's statistics, Esquirol and Georget
definitely defended it,[52] and even Delasiauve and Trousseau (1801-67)

---

[49]Doussin-Dubreuil (297), *De l'épilepsie en général, et particulièrement de celle qui est
déterminée par des causes morales*, p. 144 f.

[50]Maisonneuve (661), *Recherches et observations sur l'épilepsie*, p. 141.

[51]Cf., e.g., Trousseau (1032), *Clinique médicale*, p. 100.

[52]Esquirol (329), *Des maladies mentales*, vol. 1, p. 291. Georget (406), Article *Épilepsie*, p.
208: "Un autre fait remarquable, et qui confirme la puissante influence de la frayeur, c'est que
la plupart des épilepsies de naissance coïncident avec un mouvement de terreur éprouvé par la
mère pendant la grossesse; reste à savoir s'il existe entre ces deux phénomènes des rapports de
causalité, ce qui nous paraît très-vraisemblable." With this should be compared the following
remark of a more recent investigator, Muskens (725), p. 234: "In my statistics on the etiology
of epilepsy, and in my observations of infantile convulsions, I have been impressed by the
number of cases where the mother's pregnancy was attended by emotional strain or disturbance."

admitted the possibility.[53] Compared to the eighteenth-century physicians, the French clinicians of the Salpêtrière and Bicêtre were less dogmatic and, consequently, more willing to submit to statistical evidence what had previously been decided by a priori reasoning. The general truth of this argument is best revealed by the attitude toward lunar influence upon epileptic attacks.

Tissot had rejected the possibility of lunar influence,[54] and Portal, who stands nearer to the eighteenth century than to the nineteenth, had expressed himself in a similar vein.[55] This sceptical attitude was no longer shared by all scientists and physicians. No less a physicist than Arago warned that such doubts were based on preconceived ideas rather than on true scientific arguments.[56] Romberg even said: "The planetary influence of the moon (especially of the new and full moon,) upon the course of epilepsy, was known to the ancients, and although here and there doubts have been raised against this view, the accurate observations of others have established its correctness."[57] He found such observations in the writings of Stahl and Mead, whereas he mentioned Esquirol as having said "that in the Parisian Hospitals no relation has been observed between the frequency of the fits and the phases of the moon."[58] The reference to Esquirol is correct,[59] although Esquirol himself did not supply statistics to prove his point. Yet his later colleagues did. Beau, intending to ascertain any possible influences of atmospheric variations upon epileptic attacks, had his patients under daily observation from October 7 to November 20, 1833. He then compared these observations with the meteorological data for the same period but was not able to establish any relation whatsoever.[60] Leuret justly criticized Beau for having made his investigations over much too short a period. He observed 70 patients daily for an entire year and noted the frequency of their attacks during the single months, during the seasons, and particularly at the various phases of the moon. He

---

[53]Delasiauve (261), *Traité de l'épilepsie*, p. 191; Trousseau (1032), *Clinique médicale*, p. 100.

[54]Cf. above, p. 229.

[55]Portal (819), *Observations sur la nature et le traitement de l'épilepsie*, p. 116: "Les opinions [i.e., concerning relation of epileptic attacks to phases of the moon] ont tellement varié à cet égard que l'on peut bien n'ajouter foi à aucune d'elles, et les regarder toutes comme de simples préjugés dont la médecine n'est malheureusement que trop pleine."

[56]Cf. Boudin (141), *Traité de géographie et de statistique médicales*, vol. 1, p. 8; cf. also *ibid.*, vol. 2, pp. 16–18. Daquin (255), *Philosophie de la folie*, who studied lunar influence on some of his patients, on p. 235 f. cited the case of a man, both epileptic and insane, where the moon exerted different influences on epilepsy and insanity. On Daquin cf. Nyffeler (744).

[57]Romberg (865), *A Manual of the Nervous Diseases of Man*, vol. 2, p. 205 (Sieveking's translation).

[58]*Ibid.*

[59]Cf. Esquirol (329), *Des maladies mentales*, vol. 1, p. 281.

[60]Beau (91), *Recherches statistiques* etc., p. 351 f.

counted the daily average of patients who had attacks during the waxing moon and compared it with the figures for the waning moon: no
difference could be found. He also tried to find out whether the phases
of the moon had any relation to the maximum and minimum figures of
attacks: again the result was negative. He concluded that the belief in
the action of the moon was without foundation in actual fact.[61] About
ten years later, Moreau of the Bicêtre submitted statistics which comprised 42,637 attacks of 108 male patients in the course of five years;
his results were equally negative.[62] Moreau's reasons for starting upon
this comprehensive statistical survey confirm our argument that the
hospital physicians of the nineteenth century were less dogmatic than
the practitioners of Enlightenment, though perhaps more accessible to
romantic influences of the period, which was so greatly interested in
somnambulism. Moreau blamed his contemporaries for denying what
their predecessors had affirmed without supporting their denial by
convincing reasons.[63] He himself had not doubted that the belief in the
influence of the moon upon epilepsy was a mere prejudice. But then he
realized that his point of view was not incontestable, particularly since
he had often had occasion to notice a coincidence between phases of
the moon and epileptic attacks. Hence, he decided that the matter
would still be worth serious examination.[64] As mentioned before, the
results confirmed his original disbelief, and his statistics were not without influence upon later authors, who quoted his findings.[65] From this
time on, the moon as a causative factor was scarcely ever mentioned in
textbooks.[66]

### c. Psychiatric Studies

The whole study of epilepsy was influenced by the special character
of the hospitals as lunatic asylums. Since many of the physicians were
psychiatrists, the psychic abnormalities of the epileptics met with
special interest. Esquirol and his pupils, Bouchet and Cazauvieilh,

---

[61] Leuret (638), *Recherches sur l'épilepsie*, pp. 43-48.

[62] Moreau (708), *De l'étiologie de l'épilepsie*, p. 94 f.: "Le tableau ci-contre contient le
nombre total des accès que 108 épileptiques ont éprouvés dans le cours de cinq années.

| | |
|---|---|
| Total des accès | 42,637 |
| Ont eu lieu pendant les phases lunaires | 16,324 |
| "   "   " dans l'intervalle | 26,313 |
| Différence en faveur des accès intermédiaires | 9,989." |

[63] *Ibid.*, p. 91: "Encore, pour être juste, devons-nous ajouter que ces auteurs se sont con-
tentés de nier ce que leurs devanciers avaient affirmé, sans apporter en faveur de leur opinion
aucune raison capable de porter la conviction dans les esprits."

[64] *Ibid.*, p. 90. Cf. above, on Arago, who expressed the same view about twenty years
before.

[65] Cf. Sieveking (926), *On Epilepsy and Epileptiform Seizures*, p. 40.

[66] Later statistical investigations of the subject have received relatively little attention,
although they have not always corroborated Moreau's results; cf. Hellpach (478), p. 283 ff.

stressed the close connection between epilepsy and insanity. Together with Calmeil, Esquirol studied the case histories of 385 women located in the ward for epileptics with a view to establishing the frequency of mental disturbances. But they realized that from this number 46 had to be deducted as suffering from hysteria.[67] The incidence of hysteria, particularly among women, and its possible influence upon the sex statistics of epilepsy were not overlooked. Joseph Frank (1771-1842), who had counted 35 men and 40 women among 75 epileptics, remarked that one would possibly find fewer women if one could distinguish those suffering from hysterical convulsions.[68] Esquirol found that no less than 4/5 of the remaining 339 epileptic women were mentally affected. In more detail his figures were as follows: 12 suffering from monomania, 30 from mania (some with tendency to suicide), 34 from fury, 145 demented, 8 idiots, 50 showing periodical loss of memory (*absences de mémoire*), exalted ideas, etc. The remaining 60 did not evince any definite deterioration of intelligence but were marked only by peculiarities of character.[69] Not only did Esquirol emphasize the psychiatric aspect of epilepsy, he also claimed that epileptic vertigo had a much stronger influence upon the brain than the grand mal.[70] This thesis, repeated by Foville (1799-1873),[71] was upheld by many later authorities.

If Esquirol studied the psychiatric aspect of epilepsy, Bouchet and Cazauvieilh drew attention to the incidence of epileptic attacks among the insane. In particular, they noted the occurrence of fits in advanced cases of dementia combined with general paralysis. Such fits had already been characterized as "epileptiform convulsions." Bouchet and Cazauvieilh, however, contended that these were really epileptic attacks belonging to what they considered "acute epilepsy."[72]

Among the various psychiatric complications mentioned by Esquirol, none was studied so carefully and assumed such far-reaching importance as the maniacal attacks from which epileptics were prone to suffer. This *furor epilepticus* had various names. Mead had stated that "the raving fits" of lunatics were usually associated with "epileptic symptoms," an observation which was corroborated by Tyson (1650-1708), the former physician at Bethlehem Hospital, who used to call this type of patient "epileptick mad."[73] Greding (1718-75) dis-

---

[67]Esquirol (329), *Des maladies mentales*, vol. 1, p. 284.

[68]Cf. Georget (406), Article *Épilepsie*, p. 207.

[69]Esquirol, *l.c.*, p. 284 f.

[70]*Ibid.*, p. 288.

[71]Foville (374), Article *Épilepsie*, p. 416

[72]Bouchet et Cazauvieilh (140), *De l'épilepsie* etc., p. 14 ff.

[73]Mead (676), *De imperio solis ac lunae*, p. 43: " . . . Edvardus Tyson, in nosocomio mente captorum Londini medicus, qui idcirco hoc modo aegrotantes *insanos epilepticos* appellare

tinguished a separate class of *Fallsüchtig Rasende*.[74] Later on we find
such designations as "epileptic mania," "epileptic delirium," and *fureur
épileptique*. The *furor epilepticus* was observed preceding the fits[75] as
well as following them, but it was also noticed that it might take place
independently of any classic fit. "This affection," said Prichard, "which
I shall distinguish by the term 'epileptic delirium,' generally appears
when the patient is expected to revive from the comatose state consequent on a severe fit; *but, in other instances, it appears without any
previous fit*.[76] The face is flushed, and the aspect of the patient is like
that of a man under intoxication; he attempts to start from bed and run
about, and on being withheld, vociferates and endeavours to overcome
resistance. Sometimes an appearance of maniacal hallucination displays
itself, but more generally the disorder resembles phrenitic delirium. It
commonly continues one, two, or three days, during which the patient
requires confinement in a straight waistcoat, and then gradually subsides, and the patient returns into his previous state."[77] Parallel with
the description of epileptic mania, other types of mental confusion also
found increasing attention. They were usually designated as epileptic
somnambulism or epileptic ecstasy. To quote Prichard again: "A more
unusual circumstance in the history of epilepsy is the appearance of a
species of somnambulism, or of a kind of ecstasis, during which the
patient is in an undisturbed reverie, and walks about, fancying himself
occupied in some of his customary amusements or avocations. This
takes place during the waking as well as the sleeping hours."[78] Prichard's observations are particularly important in this connection because
he anticipated the concept of what was later termed "psychic equivalents." He not only stressed the close connection of somnambulic and
ecstatic states with epilepsy but also remarked: "Where they do not
coexist with epilepsy, they often seem to stand in the place of it, and to
depend on those particular circumstances of the constitution which are
the fundamental causes of epilepsy."[79] Not much later it was clearly
stated that passing states of maniacal excitement, so-called *mania
transitoria*, might be considered substitutes for the more typical convulsive attacks.[80]

---

soleret." For English translation cf. Mead (678), *The Medical Works*, p. 180. It is of course
hardly possible to tell whether Tyson's patients were originally epileptics.

[74] Greding (423), *Sämmtliche medizinische Schriften*, vol. 2, p. 3.

[75] Cf. Portal (819), *Observations* etc., p. 55.

[76] Italics are mine.

[77] Prichard (824), *A Treatise on Diseases of the Nervous System*, p. 99 f.

[78] *Ibid.*, p. 100.

[79] *Ibid.*, p. 407.

[80] Meyer (691), *Ueber Mania transitoria*, p. 205: " ... Anfälle, in welchen die allgemeinen
Convulsionen zurückweichen, und die Tobsucht mehr und mehr als Haupterscheinung in den
Vordergrund tritt; zuweilen fehlen die Convulsionen gänzlich und *die Manie scheint gewisser-*

In a state of somnambulism the external activities appeared to correspond to dreams. Was it possible that the epileptic convulsions corresponded to subjective experiences usually forgotten afterward? The question was raised by an anonymous German author of 1825 who had had a vision of persons, enemies, who had put a chain around his breast and heart and against whom he defended himself with all his strength. Later he was told that he had collapsed on a chair "and then suffered an epileptic attack;" he had clenched his teeth, foamed at the mouth, and uttered loud cries. "Can it be," the article asked, "that epileptic movements are always accompanied by such fantasies? The fact that the victims do not recollect any such does not flatly contradict this suspicion; the differences in the sleeping state which follows the seizures can render remembrance of the attack easier or more difficult."[81]

Quite independently, the great physiologist Purkyně arrived at a similar conclusion. As a boy, he tells, he suffered from convulsions. In these attacks, "I had the impression that I was being turned around with the greatest velocity in the tremendous vortex of a sea of fire and had to fight against it with all my strength. To those around me this fight appeared as a convulsion."[82] Purkyně was concerned with the investigation of vertigo and believed that in most forms of epilepsy violent vertigo was an essential element of the disease. The movements of the body corresponded to this vertigo, and since the sensation of vertigo was the subjective side of a change in the condition of the brain, a study of the movements should indicate "the particular seat of the evil in the brain."[83] In contrast to the vague sense in which the term epileptic vertigo usually was employed, Purkyně was speaking of the

---

massen zu vikariiren" (italics mine). Interestingly enough, Meyer, *ibid.*, p. 207, also considered transitory states of heightened vivacity and rhetorical prowess as possible epileptic equivalents and cited Paul of Aegina in this connection. In the same year, 1855, Meyer (689), *Aus der Krampfkranken-Abtheilung der Charité*, p. 9, wrote: "Von gleich grossem Interesse für die Entwickelung der allgemeinen Krampfkrankheiten sowohl als der Geisteskrankheiten ist die häufige Verbindung des Wahnsinns mit allgemeinen Krämpfen. Nicht jener sekundäre stupide oder maniakalische Zustand, welchen man als eine Folge des vorangegangenen Anfalls aufgefasst hat, sondern die ebenso plötzlich und selbstständig, wie der Krampfanfall selbst, ausbrechende und abschneidende Tobsucht ist es, welche das irrenärztliche Interresse so sehr in Anspruch nehmen, da sie in ihrer Complikation gleichsam eine Brücke zwischen Krampf- und Geisteskrankheiten auf dem Gebiete der allgemeinen Neurosen bildet. Man kann nicht umhin diese maniakalische Anfälle den epileptischen gleichzustellen, und die Manie selbst für ein ebenso berechtigtes Element dieser Krankheiten zu halten, wie die Convulsionen. Nach West scheint diese gleichsam stellvertretende periodische Manie gerade bei Kindern häufig vorzukommen."

[81] Temkin and Temkin (729), pp. 567 and 568.

[82] Purkyně (831), *Beyträge zur näheren Kenntnis des Schwindels aus heautognostischen Daten*; p. 21. Cf. Vogel (1051), who has gathered this material and discussed its significance in detail. For Purkyně's life and work see Kruta (596a). Purkyně spoke of his boyhood attacks as "Fraisen" and "Eclampsia;" cf. above, pp. 29 and 100 and below, footnote 84.

[83] Purkyně (831), *Ueber die physiologische Bedeutung des Schwindels und die Beziehung desselben zu den neuesten Versuchen über die Hirnfunctionen*; p. 13.

true sensation of vertigo, when objects seemed to turn around the person. Some twenty years later, Purkyně returned to his boyhood experiences and concluded that "even epilepsy, which differs only gradually from eclampsia, may be accompanied by similar dreams of vertigo. To these the dreaming fantasy will supply motives in the shape of the most diverse images, according to the dreamer's individuality."[84]

The recognition of somnambulic and of maniacal states as epileptic manifestations had more than academic interest. The *furor epilepticus* was dangerous; patients in this condition might even commit murder.[85] The correct interpretation of such morbid states was therefore of great legal importance. Dangerous epileptics had to be certified, and they had also to be diagnosed in court, lest they be punished for their criminal acts. The neglect of this aspect in former times had two reasons. The epileptic had either been believed possessed, in which case he was cited before the spiritual rather than the civil powers; or the existence of epileptic attacks was overlooked and the case considered as one of "furor," "delirium," or "mania" without reference to epilepsy. An instructive example of this latter possibility is given in Foderé's comprehensive work on legal medicine, the first edition of which appeared at the end of the eighteenth century. What was here described as "periodic delirium" must have included many cases of epileptic mania, as can be seen from the following remark: "These paroxysms do not come on suddenly. Usually the patient feels their approach; they are preceded by a noise in the head and frightening dreams; then the patient feels something ascending from the lower parts of the body to the uppermost, almost as in the aura epileptica. He loses consciousness; he falls down; he is raised up again and is now raging."[86] A few years later epilepsy had come into its own. Delasiauve collected many examples of court procedures against epileptics, going as far back as 1808, when an epileptic murderer was acquitted and placed in a workhouse. One case under Delasiauve's own observation illustrates a diagnosis of epilepsy long after the crime. Confined to the Bicêtre for mental derangement, the patient had escaped and killed his wife. The counsel for the defense successfully pleaded insanity, and the patient was returned to the Bicêtre. He proved quite manageable except that twice, at intervals of approximately one year, he evinced a peculiar change lasting one or two days. His expression became ardent, his speech irritated, and he felt a violent urge to strike and destroy. Only

---

[84] Purkyně (831), *Wachen, Schlaf, Traum und verwandte Zustände*; p. 204 f. "Selbst die Epilepsie, die von der Eclampsie nur dem Grade nach sich unterscheidet, mag von ähnlichen Schwindelträumen begleitet sein, die die träumende Phantasie nach Verschiedenheit der Individuen durch die mannigfaltigsten Traumbilder motiviren wird."

[85] Cf. Portal (819), *Observations* etc., p. 11.

[86] Foderé (367), *Les lois éclairées par les sciences physiques*, vol. 1, p. 93.

later was it revealed that the patient had long been subject to nocturnal epileptic attacks.[87]

On one point, however, opinions differed. One school maintained that the existence of epilepsy as such was of importance for the decision of responsibility. This point of view found its most radical expression in the maxim that an epileptic could not be held responsible for criminal acts.[88] But others pointed out that this opinion would lead to absurd consequences, giving an epileptic a free hand to commit crimes. It was not epilepsy that interested the criminologist, but those attacks of mania which could occur in epilepsy as well as in other diseases.[89] This problem of epileptic insanity was to motivate the contributions of Morel and Falret of 1860.[90]

The majority of physicians were less occupied with legal problems than with collecting observations of the peculiar mental disturbances of epileptics. Bright, for instance, was able to diagnose a case of "Cerebral Congestion, with sudden temporary Delirium" as epileptic, although grand mal had never been observed. The patient had been subject to temporary feelings of heaviness and drowsiness all his life and had suffered from occasional fainting fits when about twelve or fourteen years old. A few weeks before his admission to Guy's Hospital "he was attacked with intense headache and a rigor, which continued all night." On the next day he was able to go back to work, but the headache repeated itself several times "till five days before his admission, when he became delirious, and wandered in the streets without hat or coat, walking in a state of complete unconsciousness from Clapham Common to Shoreditch, and was between four and five hours on the road." Then intelligence returned, but the patient again suffered from headaches until he was put under Bright's care on December 3, 1829.[91]

---

[87]Delasiauve (261), *Traité de l'épilepsie*, pp. 496, 161, and 486.

[88]Platner (800), *Opuscula academica*, p. 38 ff., insisted that an epileptic might not be guilty of a crime even if it seemed to show premeditation and intent to harm and even if at the time of the crime no suspicious signs of epilepsy or insanity had been noted (p. 39: "nulla epilepsiae ne dum insaniae suspicio apparuisset"). He motivated this opinion p. 39: "Nam . . . occulta esse solet insania epilepticorum, neque eo ipso tempore, quo maxima ejus vis in anima et efficientia est, aut sermonum, aut actionum inconcinnitate significatur . . . Caeterum qui amens est, nullo tempore non mentis expers est habendus: ergo etiamsi epilepticus, qua die et hora v. g. incendium fecerat, nullam morbi caduci accessionem habuisset, imo vero ex longo tempore vacuus omni molestia et recte valens fuisset, tamen medicis non magis sanus videbitur; apud quos tanta est epilepsiae suspicio, ut si quis vel semel aliquando ea tentatus fuit, ab eo nullam vel cerebri, vel animi commotionem et infirmitatem alienam putent." This extreme view was criticized by the editor, p. 39, footnote.

[89]Cf. Casper (206), *A Handbook of the Practice of Forensic Medicine*, vol. 4, pp. 100 and 188.

[90]See below.

[91]Bright (154), *Reports of Medical Cases*, vol. 2, part II, p. 522 f.

## 2. ANATOMICAL OPTIMISM AND PESSIMISM

Pinel listed epilepsy among the great class of "neuroses;" it belonged to the second order, as one of the "neuroses of the cerebral functions."[92] Such attempts at nosological classification, which followed in the wake of the works of Boissier de Sauvages and of Cullen, received a new impetus in the early nineteenth century, when it was believed possible to establish natural nosological systems. Pinel was one of the main representatives of this trend, and his pupil Maisonneuve tried to distinguish ten different species of epilepsy. Maisonneuve accepted the traditional division into idiopathic and sympathetic epilepsy, assigning five species to each of these two groups. Thus idiopathic epilepsy was congenital, spontaneous, plethoric, humoral, or caused by strong emotions; whereas the sympathetic form was produced by "irradiation" from external parts, the stomach, intestines, or uterus, to which "vaporous or hypochondric epilepsy" had to be added as a fifth species.[93] The whole elaborate system would be of little interest, if it did not at the same time contain some new elements. Speaking of sympathetic epilepsy originating from external parts, Maisonneuve described the sensitive aura, its spread to the brain with subsequent complete attack, and added: "The attacks of this species of sympathetic epilepsy are often incomplete in the beginning . . . but become complete with the years."[94] Thus, Maisonneuve definitely connected sensitive aura with partial epilepsy, which might become generalized in the course of time. The very term "partial epilepsy" was firmly established in the literature by Prichard, who devoted an entire chapter to the discussion "Of local convulsion, or partial epilepsy," including among others a case where partial epilepsy had involved the left arm without accompanying loss of consciousness.[95] Observations of partial convulsions, preceding or intermingled with general epileptic fits, are frequent in the literature of the day.[96] Bravais, in 1827, described *épilepsie hémiplégique*; Bright ob-

---

[92]Pinel (797), *Nosographie philosophique*, vol. 3, pp. 73 ff. and 597.

[93]Maisonneuve (661), *Recherches et observations sur l'épilepsie*, p. 50 f.

[94]*Ibid.*, p. 187 f.: "Sentiment de douleur, d'engourdissement ou de fourmillement, de chaleur ou de froid, se propageant du bras, de la jambe, ou d'un endroit quelconque de la surface du corps, ordinairement avec convulsions des parties, jusqu'au cerveau où il détermine l'accès complet d'épilepsie, à moins qu'on n'intercepte la communication entre la tête et l'endroit primitivement affecté. Les accès de cette espèce d'épilepsie sympathique sont souvent incomplets dans le commencement . . . mais ils se complètent avec l'âge."

[95]Prichard (824), *A Treatise on Diseases of the Nervous System*, p. 385 ff.

[96]Cf. Portal (819), *Observations*, p. 68 f., who reports the case of a tuberculous patient whose original symptoms were headaches, occasional vomiting, and emaciation. Convulsive movements first started in the face and fingers and later in the entire right arm; certain mental symptoms developed and finally some generalized attacks occurred.

served the occurrence of impaired sight in cases of partial epilepsy[97] and recognized impaired vision as a forerunner of cerebral disease.[98] We shall have to come back to these observations in more detail.

Accepting the division of epilepsy into idiopathic and sympathetic, Maisonneuve was only being consistent when he tried to refute Le Pois and others who had denied the possible origin of epilepsy from outside the brain.[99] It is true, the theory of sympathetic epilepsy found a new adversary in Georget, a resolute critic of tradition. Georget maintained that he had never observed a case of sympathetic epilepsy, i.e., where the disease had its cause somewhere else than the brain. Together with his older predecessors he believed that the various sensations felt in more distant parts of the body might just as well have been formed in the brain itself.[100] Yet, on the whole, the situation remained much as it had been in the eighteenth century. Doubted by a few, the existence of sympathetic epilepsy was accepted by the majority. What changed, however, were the theoretical explanations concerning the disease, and in order to understand the more important of these changes it will be best to start out with a résumé of the older doctrine as it had crystallized in the work on epilepsy by Portal (1742-1832).

Portal's book was published in 1827, i.e., nearly at the end of the period under discussion. Moreover, Portal was acquainted with the more recent publications of the French physicians, Bouchet and Cazauvieilh, and others. Yet at the time when his book appeared, Portal was eighty-five years old. Much of his experimental research had been done in 1771, one year after the appearance of Tissot's monograph on epilepsy, and it is therefore not astonishing to see Portal formulate old ideas. He even thought that under normal conditions the cerebral membranes were scarcely sensitive, a statement in support of which he cited experiments performed by himself.[101]

Portal collected a great many clinical data and post-mortem reports, for he was a great believer in the anatomical method and quick to find a satisfactory explanation of the case if he could discover some definite anatomical change. He had to admit that sometimes dissection revealed no lesion either in the brain or anywhere else in the body. This, however, he deemed understandable, if one considered the soft nature of the substance of the brain and the imperfect state of our knowledge of its structure.[102] Epilepsy always had its seat in the brain, particularly in

[97]Bright (154), *Reports of Medical Cases*, vol. 2, part II, p. 516.

[98]Cf. *ibid.*, p. 536.

[99]Maisonneuve (661), *Recherches*, p. 40 f. Cf. also Doussin-Dubreuil (297), *De l'épilepsie*, p. 38 ff.

[100]Georget (406), Article *Épilepsie*, p. 214 f.

[101]Portal (819), *Observations sur la nature et le traitement de l'épilepsie*, pp. 47-48.

[102]*Ibid.*, p. 108 f.

its medullary part, and from here it propagated itself via the nerves to various parts of the body. This was true of idiopathic as well as of sympathetic epilepsy. In the latter the nerves were molested by some pathological condition; the morbid impression was transmitted to the brain, where it produced the symptoms of the many kinds of sympathetic epilepsies.[103] So much for the general theory of epilepsy. How Portal imagined the details of the process can be understood from his analysis of those cases—very frequent in his opinion—where bloody obstructions are found in the arteries, veins, and sinuses of the brain, its ventricles, etc. In all these cases he thinks circulation in the brain has been impeded and "this organ has been irritated and more or less compressed." Compression and irritation are progressively transmitted to the medullary substance, whence follow convulsions, disturbance of mental functions, sleep, and loss of memory.[104]

This vague yet coherent theory of epilepsy was a late modification of Haller's ideas. In 1827 it could no longer exert any considerable influence. Yet there was no other theory which could find general approval. Brown's system, which had also developed from Haller's work on irritability, had been in vogue at the end of the eighteenth century and, particularly in Germany, in the early nineteenth century as well. Brown (1735-88), who grouped diseases into sthenic and asthenic, according to whether there was too much or too little irritability and stimulation, considered epilepsy an asthenia.[105] Such a classification might please physicians of the romantic era in German medicine, for they looked for fundamental principles on which to base a speculative system of medicine.[106] But pathologists interested in more detailed physiological and clinical analysis had to go elsewhere. There were various attempts made in various directions, but little was achieved in the way of uniform results. In contrast to Portal's optimism, others were clearly sceptical of the results of the anatomical method. Esquirol described a number of autopsies, but his conclusion was negative: "Let us admit frankly that up to now pathological anatomy has shed little light on the immediate seat of epilepsy."[107] But at least he had hopes

---

[103] *Ibid.*, p. 119: "L'épilepsie a toujours son *siége* dans le cerveau où elle y est *idiopathique*; tout semble prouver qu'il réside particulièrement dans la substance médullaire de cet organe, duquel, moyennant les nerfs, elle se propage dans toutes les parties du corps qui jouissent d'une sensibilité plus ou moins exquise; d'où, par suite des affections morbides très-diverses qui peuvent les molester, leur impression contre nature se transmet au cerveau et y produit les symptômes des nombreuses espèces d'épilepsies qu'on a appelées *sympathiques*. Ce n'est qu'ainsi qu'on peut les admettre." (Italics in the text.)

[104] *Ibid.*, p. 2.

[105] Brown (169), *The Elements of Medicine*, vol. 2, p. 259.

[106] Cf., e.g., Röschlaub (860), *Untersuchungen über Pathogenie*, 3. Theil, p. 514 f.

[107] Esquirol (329), *Des maladies mentales*, vol. 1, p. 313.

for the future,[108] whereas Georget's doubts were of a more fundamental nature. He too emphasized that autopsies had led to no satisfactory results concerning the immediate cause of the disease. "This
cause clearly consists in a particular disposition of the brain, since
epilepsy is characterized by disturbances in the functions of this organ;
but up till now the researches of pathological anatomy have not been
able to discover this disposition of the cerebral structure."[109] Georget
found that encephalitis characterized by epileptiform attacks had been
taken for epilepsy and the pathological changes of the former had been
related to epilepsy, or else the two diseases had not been distinguished
at all. This was the "double error" which Georget criticized in
Morgagni's chapter on epilepsy and to some extent in Greding's observations. To the alleged findings of other authors he objected on the
grounds that in the majority of cases brains of epileptics, if not affected
by inflammation, showed no noticeable alterations at all, and that the
same findings that could be obtained in a few epileptics could also be
observed in persons free from epilepsy. For the rest, changes in the
brains of epileptics were to be expected as a result of the attacks, which
led to irritation and acute and chronic inflammation.[110]

Anatomical pessimism was counterbalanced, on the other hand, by
very concrete statements concerning the seat of epilepsy. In all the
bodies of epileptics that he had dissected, Joseph Wenzel (1768-1808)
had found the pituitary gland and the surrounding area in an abnormal
condition. Hence, he concluded that disease of the pituitary gland was
the general cause of epilepsy. This broad statement was soon contradicted,[111] but, although rejected by the majority, Wenzel's claims
occupied pathologists for a considerable time, and Sieveking in 1858
still thought it worth while to include a detailed account of them in his
monograph on epilepsy.[112] How inconclusive, however, all the accumulated anatomical material regarding the seat of epilepsy was could be
learned in 1826 from Burdach's (1776-1847) work *Of the Structure
and Life of the Brain*. The third volume of this publication contained
vast statistical material on the relation of all kinds of pathological
changes in the brain to various forms of nervous disturbances. In these
statistics epilepsy appears together with general convulsions. Burdach's
tables extend over 1,911 anatomical abnormalities observed in the brain

---

[108] He added, *ibid.*: "Cependant il ne faut pas se décourager, la nature ne sera pas toujours
rebelle aux efforts de ses investigateurs."

[109] Georget (406), Article *Épilepsie*, p. 217.

[110] *Ibid.*, p. 217 f.

[111] Cf. Burdach (186), *Vom Baue und Leben des Gehirns*, vol. 3, p. 468; Romberg (865), *A
Manual of the Nervous Diseases of Man*, p. 207.

[112] Sieveking (926), *On Epilepsy and Epileptiform Seizures*, pp. 139-49.

(i.e., from the medulla oblongata on).[113] The number of cases of epilepsy investigated anatomically was 476.[114] Thus the proportion of lesions in general convulsions and epilepsy to the total number of cerebral lesions was 476 : 1,911, i.e., 1 : 4.01. More important are the figures for general convulsions compared to the general incidence of lesions in the main divisions of the brain. Here it appears that the highest figure refers to the pallium (plus membranes): general convulsions were present in 1 : 4.63 of all lesions of this part. However, the differences between the figures for the various parts were very small.[115] More detailed anatomical analysis showed that in absolute figures the lateral ventricles were most frequently affected in general convulsions and epilepsy, with 86 of the total of 476. And of these 86 pathological changes, not less than 63 consisted of a serous effusion. The cerebral hemispheres proper represented the next highest number, 66, and here again serous effusion stood at the top with 22. The figures are not very surprising. Burdach's statistics were mainly compiled from literature where cases of hydrocephalus, head injuries, and other organic diseases had long found particular attention. Besides, these maximum figures did not point to a definite seat; the cerebellum, for instance, was also found affected in 42 cases.[116]

Sceptical because of general considerations and cautioned by many unsuccessful attempts, most investigators of this, as well as of the following, period abandoned the quest for "the seat" of epilepsy altogether. Sometimes resignation was more pretended than real, as for example in the case of Bouchet and Cazauvieilh.[117] These authors had not made epilepsy as such the subject of their research; rather, they wanted to establish the relationship between this disease and insanity. We have mentioned some of their clinical suggestions, and their pathological findings and hypotheses were not less significant. Among 18 autopsies performed on epileptics they found hardening of the brain in 11 cases, softening in 4, and ordinary consistency in 3 (where, however, the patients had died during the attack, and where at least congestion of the brain had been present[118]).[119] Partly on the authority of Lallemand (1790–1853),[120] partly on the basis of their own reasoning,

[113] Burdach (186), *Vom Baue und Leben des Gehirns*, vol. 3, table 1, p. 297.

[114] *Ibid.*, table 20, p. 312.

[115] *Ibid.*, table 35, p. 320.

[116] *Ibid.*, p. 278 and table 20, p. 312.

[117] Bouchet et Cazauvieilh (140), *De l'épilepsie*, etc., p. 5: "En rapprochant ces diverses autopsies, notre intention n'est pas précisément de chercher le siége de l'épilepsie ou de l'aliénation," etc.

[118] *Ibid.*, p. 9.

[119] *Ibid.*, pp. 6–7.

[120] *Ibid.*, p. 9.

the authors concluded "that the congestion, hardening, and softening of the brain constitute the same alteration, but in different degrees or at different stages."[121] What process, then, went on in the brain of the epileptic? In an epileptic attack the blood was carried to the brain, as was proved by the exterior aspect of an epileptic as well as by autopsies of patients who had died during the attack, and the "congestion" led to chronic inflammation.[122] Autopsies of insane patients showed similar changes, particularly in the superficial parts of the brain. The alterations in both epilepsy and insanity could therefore be interpreted as representing inflammations. From this the general conclusion to be drawn concerning the seat of mental alienation and epilepsy was as follows: "Since we have seen the former [i.e., insanity] correspond to alterations of the gray substance and the latter [i.e., epilepsy] to alterations of the white substance or of dependent parts, we should place the former, after the example of MM. Delaye and Foville, in the superficial gray substance and the latter in the white substance."[123]

The interpretation of epilepsy as an inflammatory process, an idea stimulated by Lallemand's work, was of passing interest. The assignment of epilepsy to the white substance of the brain was more or less in harmony with the views of Portal and earlier authorities. To relate epilepsy to congestion of blood in the brain was nothing original either; Prichard, too, considered congestion of cerebral blood vessels its immediate cause.[124] More important was Bouchet and Cazauvieilh's attempt to establish a mutual anatomical relationship between insanity and epilepsy. By assigning insanity to the gray substance they confessedly followed Delaye and Foville's ideas, according to which the cerebral cortex was the seat of intellectual functions.[125] By placing epilepsy immediately underneath, they tried to explain the interrelation between epilepsy and insanity. Yet this explanation necessitated a pathological *tour de force*, such as the interpretation of epileptiform fits of paralytics as "acute epilepsy."[126] Foville pointed out that Bouchet and Cazauvieilh had gone too far.[127] Only where epilepsy was complicated by mental symptoms or where dementia was complicated by general paralysis and epileptic attacks, could it be assumed that

---

[121] *Ibid.*, p. 10.

[122] *Ibid.*, p. 7.

[123] *Ibid.*, p. 13: "Et si, d'après ce nombre de faits, nous osions préciser le siége de l'aliénation mentale et le siége de l'épilepsie, comme nous avons vu la première correspondre à des altérations de la substance grise et la seconde à des altérations de la substance blanche ou à des parties dépendantes; nous placerions la première, à l'exemple de MM. Delaye et Foville, dans la substance grise superficielle, et la seconde dans la substance blanche."

[124] Prichard (824), *A Treatise on Diseases of the Nervous System*, p. 101.

[125] Cf. Soury (939), p. 526.

[126] Cf. above, IX-1c.

[127] Foville (374), Article *Épilepsie*, p. 418 f.

processes going on in reverse directions accounted for the alterations of the white and gray substances of the brain.[128]

In order to appreciate the significance of the work of Bouchet and Cazauvieilh, Foville, and others, it has to be remembered that by this time the question of the localization of higher nervous functions had again become an object of physiological dispute. Even in the eighteenth century the author of the article on epilepsy in the *Encyclopédie* had been puzzled at "the disposition of the brain in which the paths serving distribution of the nervous fluid to the sense organs are completely closed or considerably obstructed, whereas those serving the distribution of the same fluid to the organs of motion remain open and receive it abundantly, very quickly and without order."[129] But as long as consciousness, intellectual functions, and the initiation of movements were rather indiscriminately placed in the entire brain, and particularly as long as no special functions were assigned to the cerebral cortex, it was not necessary to account anatomically for the psychic and motor aspects of epilepsy. Now, however, Haller's doctrine was disintegrating. Gall and Spurzheim had given strong support to the idea of functional localization, particularly on the surface of the brain.[130] "From strict anatomy" Charles Bell (1774-1842) had drawn the conclusion "that the cineritious and superficial parts of the brain are the seat of the intellectual functions."[131] If it were true that higher nervous functions were localized, then the problem of epilepsy became very complicated. Foville clearly recognized the difficulties implied for the pathology of epilepsy. "In other words," he asked, "why is it that in consequence of a suddenly developed derangement the portion of nervous centers which presides over intelligence and sensibility is annihilated in its action, whereas the portion which presides over the voluntary movements is so much excited as to produce horrible convulsions?"[132] Foville thought that the state of science at his time did not yet allow an answer.[133] But the question was well put by him, and during the next period most theories of epilepsy tried to explain how different parts of the brain could be affected so as to produce the contrasting symptoms of the attack of grand mal.

---

[128]*Ibid.*, p. 423 f.

[129]*Encyclopédie* (321), vol. 12, p. 692. The article which is signed "d" (Diderot?) is remarkable for its considerable dependence on Boerhaave.

[130]Cf. Soury (939), p. 497 ff., and Young (1114), ch. 1.

[131]Charles Bell (97), *Idea of a New Anatomy of the Brain*, p. 33.

[132]Foville (374), Article *Épilepsie*, p. 417: "En d'autres termes, pourquoi, par suite d'un dérangement subitement développé, la portion des centres nerveux qui préside à l'intelligence et à la sensibilité est-elle anéantie dans son action, tandis que celle qui préside aux mouvements volontaires se trouve assez violemment excitée pour produire d'horribles convulsions?"

[133]*Ibid.*

# X
# Second Period: 1833-1861

## 1. THE REFLEX THEORY

It is doubtful whether Marshall Hall (1790–1857) should be named as the discoverer of reflex action, since this discovery had been anticipated by Descartes, Willis, Whytt, Prochaska and others.[134] It is, however, certain that only after Hall's communication did reflex action become a widely accepted hypothesis for the explanation of epilepsy. Using the term *centric* for such phenomena as took their origin from the central nervous system, Hall distinguished as *eccentric* those where the exciting causes were "distant from the nervous centres"[135] and where reflex action came into play. He believed this distinction to be important for the pathology of diseases like chorea, epilepsy, and asthma, some cases being of centric others of eccentric origin. Regarding epilepsy, the matter seemed rather simple to him. "Epilepsy," he said, "is plainly of two kinds: the first has a centric origin in the medulla itself; the second is an affection of the reflex function, the exciting cause being eccentric, and acting chiefly upon the nerves of the stomach or intestines, which consequently form the first part of the reflex arc."[136]

It is easy to see that Hall's eccentric epilepsy was nothing but the sympathetic form of epilepsy, now given a new and apparently solid physiological basis. For some time, the term "sympathetic" still remained

---

[134] For the over-all history of the notion of reflex action see Fearing (347); for a critical discussion of the origins of the concept, especially regarding the claims for Descartes, see Canguilhem (199).

[135] Hall (450), *On the Reflex Function of the Medulla Oblongata and Medulla Spinalis*, p. 637.

[136] *Ibid.*, p. 654 f.

in use; later on it was replaced by the term "reflex" epilepsy. Since reflex action was considered a property of the medulla oblongata and the medulla spinalis, it is also easy to see why Hall associated eccentric epilepsy with these anatomical structures. Moreover, as early as the seventeenth century, Charles Drélincourt (1633-94), the teacher of Boerhaave, had provoked epileptiform convulsions in a dog by driving a needle into the fourth ventricle of the brain.[137] Older observations of this kind had been confirmed and generalized by Flourens (1794-1867), whose findings were widely accepted by the physiologists of Hall's generation.

In a memoir published in 1823, Flourens laid down some basic rules concerning irritability and sensibility of the central nervous system. The latter was not a homogeneous system; different functions could be assigned to different parts. In particular, the cerebral hemispheres and the cerebellum were not irritable; irritability pertained to the spinal cord, its continuation (the medulla oblongata), and its end (the corpora quadrigemina).[138] These parts alone had the property of immediately exciting muscular contractions,[139] and of these parts, Flourens emphasized the medulla oblongata.[140] The cerebral hemispheres, on the other hand, were the exclusive seat of volition and sensation,[141] just as co-ordination of movement was placed in the cerebellum. However much physiologists of the succeeding forty years corrected these statements in details, the majority agreed that movements could not be elicited by stimulation of the cerebral hemispheres, that this response could only be obtained from the basal ganglia and particularly the medulla oblongata. The pallium thus remained reserved for the higher nervous functions of consciousness.

Hall, therefore, seemed justified in assigning epilepsy to the medulla, in as far as epilepsy is a convulsive disease. But the epileptic attack does not manifest itself by convulsions alone. It implies loss of consciousness and of voluntary movements. Within the theory of Flourens, this meant involvement of the cerebral lobes, and Foville's question, how different parts of the brain could be affected so as to account for the different symptoms of the epileptic fit, was more pertinent than ever.

Hall himself hit upon an explanation which in principle became a pattern, though untenable in detail. He believed that centric epilepsy

---

[137]Drelincurtius (299), *Experimenta anatomica*, canicid. 3; p. 8: "Acu in cerebelli ventriculum compulsa inter primam vertebram et os occipitis, canis, *ceu epilepticus*, ter quaterque concussus est universe, sed mox expiravit."

[138] Flourens (365), *Recherches physiques sur les propriétés et les fonctions du système nerveux dans les animaux vertébrés*, p. 346. On Flourens and his experiments cf. Young (1114) ch. 2.

[139]*Ibid.*, p. 347.

[140]*Ibid.*, p. 369.

[141]*Ibid.*, p. 354.

was caused by some disease within the cranium or the spine, acting directly or indirectly upon the "true spinal marrow,"[142] i.e., the spinal cord and those parts of the brain that responded to stimulation. Eccentric epilepsy, on the other hand, led to a secondary affection of the whole brain with venous congestion "and the consequent effusion of serum."[143] Of course, he had to account for the cause of this congestion and he suspected its source in "a forcible closure of the *larynx* and *expiratory efforts*"[144] at the beginning of the convulsive attack. It was soon pointed out that Hall's *trachelismus* and *laryngismus* could not explain those cases where the attack began with loss of consciousness.[145] Criticism of Hall occupied many minds in the middle of the last century and tended to obscure the fact that most workers had to follow in a direction similar to his. The essential feature of this pattern was that one part of the brain caused the convulsions, whereas the loss of consciousness was attributable to another part. Changes in the blood supply, it was supposed, formed the connecting link, and the change in color of the patient from paleness to extreme lividity made this assumption probable. Clinical and experimental observations seemed to give it a scientific justification.

It had been known for a long time that extreme loss of blood could lead to epileptic attacks. In 1836 Astley Cooper (1768–1841) made known an experiment which proved the possibility of provoking epileptiform attacks by temporary anemia, even without actual loss of blood. He tied the carotid arteries of a rabbit and then, with the thumbs, compressed the vertebral arteries. "Respiration almost directly stopped: convulsive struggles succeeded; the animal lost its consciousness, and appeared dead. The pressure was removed; and it recovered, with a convulsive inspiration. It laid upon its side, making violent convulsive efforts; breathed laboriously; and its heart beat rapidly. In two hours it had recovered; but its respiration was laborious."[146] The experiment seemed to prove the connection between loss of consciousness, convulsions, and changed blood supply of the brain.

These concepts formed the basis for some contributions to the pathology of epilepsy which were to become authoritative in the fifties of the last century. According to Henle (1809–85), the epileptic convulsions were provoked by an increased turgor at the base of the brain.

---

[142] Hall (449), *On the Diseases and Derangements of the Nervous System*, pp. 319–20.

[143] *Ibid.*, p. 325.

[144] *Ibid.*, p. 323.

[145] It is, however, interesting to see that at the beginning of the present century, Hughlings Jackson explained certain "lowest level fits" (laryngeal crises in tabes dorsalis) very much in the manner of Hall. Cf. Jackson (552), *Neurological Fragments*, p. 185.

[146] Sir Astley Cooper (236), *Some Experiments and Observations on Tying the Carotid and Vertebral Arteries*, p. 465.

The loss of consciousness, on the other hand, depended either on increase or decrease of the blood flowing in the hemispheres. In "plethoric" epilepsy, both the convex surface as well as the base of the brain were congested with blood. In "anemic" epilepsy, on the other hand, the collapse of the hemispheres was the primary phenomenon, leading to a subsequent turgor at the base.[147] The epileptic attack was therefore largely dependent upon the condition of the blood vessels and might result from a cramp of their muscles.[148]

Henle's views were criticized by Brown-Séquard[149] (1817-94), who experimented on the spinal cord of animals, particularly of guinea pigs. If a transverse section of a lateral half of the spinal cord was made, the animals showed convulsions, strongly reminiscent of epileptic attacks. Brown-Séquard did not claim that these convulsions were "truly epileptic,"[150] but they had at least to be considered as epileptiform, and from these artificial attacks he therefore drew cautious conclusions concerning epilepsy in man. The attacks in the animals could be provoked by various irritations, e.g., by pinching the skin of the face or neck in certain areas. This seemed to be a case of reflex action, and Brown-Séquard inferred "that it is in the cutaneous ramifications of certain nerves of the face and neck that resides the faculty of producing convulsions in the animals upon which I have injured the spinal cord."[151] Brown-Séquard's experiments led to a renewed assertion of the existence of sympathetic epilepsy. The beneficial results from ligatures or local surgical treatment of the parts whence an aura started seemed to confirm the theory which his experiments had suggested. He collected a great many such cases from literature[152] and thought that success of the treatment was due to the blocking of the fatal reflex arc. Even where no aura was felt, some kind of local irritation might still be the cause of epilepsy, and he advised inquiring for such zones in every case.[153]

---

[147]Henle (481), *Handbuch der rationellen Pathologie*, 2. Band, 2. Abtheilung, p. 46: "Die Verbindung der Bewusstlosigkeit mit epileptischen Krämpfen kann also nur dadurch zu Stande kommen, dass entweder Decke und Basis des Gehirns gleichzeitig, nur jene im vorwiegenden Maasse, von Blut überfüllt werden oder dass Collapsus der Hemisphären von Turgor der Basis begleitet wird. Man darf den epileptischen Krampf der ersten Art einen plethorischen, den der zweiten einen anämischen nennen . . . "

[148]*Ibid.*, pp. 48-49.

[149]Brown-Séquard (170), *Experimental and Clinical Researches Applied to Physiology and Pathology, Boston Medical and Surgical Journal*, vol. 56, p. 220.

[150]*Ibid.*, vol. 55, p. 342.

[151]*Ibid.*, p. 340.

[152]Cf. *ibid.*, pp. 421-27 and 457-61.

[153]*Ibid.*, vol. 56, p. 114: ". . . it becomes evident that it is of the greatest importance to try to find out, in epileptics who have no aura epileptica, if there is not a part of the skin or of a muscle from which arises an unfelt irritation causing the fits."

Brown-Séquard drew attention to reported changes in the spinal cord in man,[154] but in spite of his experiments with animals he combated the belief in the existence of "spinal epilepsy." Against various authors like Copland, he contended that their description of spinal epilepsy represented a confusion of various diseases.[155] He readily admitted the possibility of epilepsy from alterations of the cord,[156] and he emphasized that epilepsy might arise from any part of the nervous system.[157] The main point, for Brown-Séquard, was that epilepsy in all its forms was a reflex phenomenon: "The so-called *centric* and *eccentric* causes of excitation of epileptic fits, both act on, or through the sensitive side of the cerebro-spinal centres, and consequently both act on the reflex faculty of these centres, so that they both ought to be called reflex excitations."[158] In most cases of epileptics, he believed, certain parts of the cerebro-spinal axis had an increased reflex excitability, so that any slight irritation could lead to the beginning of an attack.[159]

Brown-Séquard developed his theory further, incorporating into it his own researches and those of Claude Bernard on the vaso-motor functions. Pallor of the face and loss of consciousness were among the first phenomena of an epileptic fit. They had, therefore, to be accounted for, as well as the convulsions. Brown-Séquard proposed the following hypothesis. As soon as the spinal cord and the base of the brain are excited, the sympathetic nerve fibers leading to the head are irritated. Some of them make the blood vessels of the face contract and the patient becomes pale. Others, innervating the blood vessels of the brain, cause the blood to be expelled, particularly from its small arteries, and "the brain proper loses at once its functions, just as it does in a complete syncope."[160] The decrease of blood is compensated by its accumulation at the base of the brain and in the spinal cord. Since respiration is already impeded, this blood contains little oxygen, but much carbon dioxide. By its qualitative change and the pressure which it exerts, the base of the brain and the spinal cord are stimulated and convulsions are provoked.[161]

Many of the features of Brown-Séquard's theory can be found again in the work of Schroeder van der Kolk (1797–1862), who was well acquainted with the former's experiments.[162] To some extent

[154]Cf. *ibid.*, vol. 55, p. 377.

[155]*Ibid.*, vol. 56, p. 55 f.

[156]*Ibid.*

[157]*Ibid.*, vol. 55, p. 377.

[158]*Ibid.*, vol. 56, pp. 435–36.

[159]*Ibid.*, p. 436 f.

[160]*Ibid.*, pp. 475–76.

[161]*Ibid.*, p. 476 ff.

[162]Schroeder van der Kolk (902), *On the Minute Structure*, etc., p. 218 ff.

Schroeder van der Kolk simplified and concentrated Brown-Séquard's deductions, but he also introduced new elements, carrying the reflex theory of epilepsy to a certain conclusion. Guided by his anatomical researches and impressed by the fact that the medulla oblongata is the center of many reflex actions, Schroeder van der Kolk regarded "an exalted sensibility and excitability of the medulla oblongata"[163] as the first cause of epilepsy. From here convulsions arose as reflex movements. The loss of consciousness was a result of the influence of the medulla oblongata upon the vaso-motor nerves of the brain and of the subsequent disturbance of circulation in this organ.[164] If the disease lasted for a long time, organic vascular changes took place in the medulla oblongata, leading to hardening, fatty degeneration, and softening, and the patient thus became incurable. Together with the medulla, the brain became similarly affected and mental changes occurred.[165] Apart from allocating the seat of epilepsy to the medulla oblongata, Schroeder van der Kolk assumed an underlying regularity in the production of attacks which he compared to the discharges of an electric battery.

> The special seat and starting-point of these convulsive movements is situated in the ganglionic cells of the medulla oblongata, which, as reflex ganglia, possess the peculiar property, that when once brought into an excited condition, they may more or less suddenly discharge themselves and communicate their influence to different nervous filaments. After their discharge, a certain time is again required to bring them to their former degree of excitability, and to render them capable of fresh discharges, just as we see to be the case with electric batteries, or in the phenomena of an electrical fish.[166] Hence, a slight attack of epilepsy, whereby these cells are not completely discharged, is usually followed more quickly by a second attack, while a longer free interval generally succeeds to a severe fit.[167]

As we have said before, changes in the blood supply of the brain were considered an important factor in the reflex theory of epilepsy. Shortly before the appearance of Schroeder van der Kolk's treatise,

---

[163]*Ibid.*, p. 250 (Moore's translation).

[164]*Ibid.*, p. 230.

[165]*Ibid.*, p. 250.

[166]This was not a mere simile. Speaking of the functional change of the medulla oblongata he added (p. 237): "whereby this part more rapidly answers every stimulus in abnormal reflex movements, or transfers its accumulated nervous or electrical force to the nerves. . . ." Considering the contemporary advances in the electrophysiology of muscles and nerves it is not astonishing to find such views expressed by Schroeder van der Kolk, Todd (cf. below) and others. Radcliffe (835), *Lectures on Epilepsy*, etc., p. 115 f., even went so far as to believe that by loss of blood or the change caused in blood by suffocation, a reversal was effected "in the electrical relations of the exterior and interior of the nerve-fibres" of the medulla oblongata and hence general convulsions brought about.

[167]Schroeder van der Kolk, *l.c.*, p. 283 (Moore's translation).

Kussmaul (1822–1902) and Tenner had further elucidated the role of the blood supply in researches that were mainly directed to epileptic convulsions following profuse hemorrhage. Much of their work consisted in disproving some of Hall's deductions, while others of their findings had a positive bearing upon the contemporary concept of epilepsy. One of their results was that general convulsions consequent upon hemorrhage must have their origin within the cranium, while the spinal cord could practically be disregarded.[168] Experiments performed after removal of certain parts of the brain convinced them that these convulsions proceeded not "from the non-excitable, but from the excitable parts of the brain," i.e., "from the motor centres situated behind the thalami optici."[169] The brain proper situated before these parts might react to anemia by loss of consciousness, etc., and this alone might account for the incomplete attack.[170] But a complete attack presupposed an alteration of the entire brain.[171] On the other hand, these authors rejected the idea of epilepsy resulting from a congestion of the brain.[172] Altogether their findings supported the view "that epileptic convulsions can be brought about by contraction of the blood-vessels induced by the vaso-motor nerves."[173]

Kussmaul and Tenner believed that the convulsions observed in animals had been the consequence of a "sudden interruption in the nutrition of the brain."[174] Yet though some forms of epilepsy in man might be referred to the same process, it could not be considered the real cause of epilepsy. "The sudden arrest of nutrition acts, as it appears to us, only indirectly by producing certain molecular alterations of the brain-substance, which are in necessary connexion with it; but these alterations may likewise be brought about by chemical and nutritive agencies of another description";[175] poisons, for example.[176] Here Kussmaul and Tenner met with the work of other investigators, like Harley, who had studied convulsions resulting from poisons.[177]

If we disregard the greater and lesser differences of all these theories and focus upon the concepts dominating the pathology of epilepsy

---

[168] Kussmaul and Tenner (602), *On the Nature and Origin of Epileptiform Convulsions*, etc., p. 57.

[169] *Ibid.*, p. 69 (Bronner's translation).

[170] *Ibid.*, p. 107.

[171] *Ibid.*, p. 84.

[172] *Ibid.*, p. 91 ff.

[173] *Ibid.*, p. 101 (Bronner's translation); cf. also p. 108.

[174] *Ibid.*, p. 89 (Bronner's translation).

[175] *Ibid.* (Bronner's translation).

[176] *Ibid.*, p. 90.

[177] Cf. *ibid.*

around 1860, we find: reflex action, cerebral angiospasm, and changes
in the molecular state of the brain through malnutrition or poisoning.
In all these theories, several parts of the central nervous system were
believed to be affected, either simultaneously or in succession; in none
of them was the cause of epilepsy attributed to definite structural
changes of a definite organ. Even Schroeder van der Kolk, who at least
assigned the seat of epilepsy to the ganglionic centers of the medulla
oblongata, ascribed epilepsy to increased irritability of these centers,
not to morphological alterations. This is confirmed by the deliberate
statements of the contemporary authors, who are almost unanimous in
rejecting the possibility of a strictly anatomical explanation. Of course,
it was realized that organic changes in the brain could lead to epilepsy.
But in these cases, it was said, the organic lesions had to be considered remote causes producing the disposition to the disease, rather
than directly responsible agents. Furthest in this respect went Kussmaul
and Tenner, who rejected the very idea of an anatomically localized
seat of the disease. To uphold such a view, they argued, would mean to
presuppose the existence of an anatomical center of life, a revival of
Cartesian views, altogether incompatible with the results of modern
physiology. The pathology of epilepsy had once more become a problem of physiological rather than anatomical research.

## 2. NOSOLOGICAL DOUBTS

During the early part of the nineteenth century the most valuable
contributions to the medical history of epilepsy were made by physicians associated with hospitals and lunatic asylums. During the second
third of the century, a reaction set in, for it was realized that observations made in hospitals did not necessarily give a true picture of the
disease. Marshall Hall was one of the early critics. Epilepsy from
diseases within the cranium or spinal canal he admitted often to be
incurable. These were the cases frequently met in institutions, and
hence observers of the disease who gathered their material at such
places inclined to the belief that epilepsy could not be cured.[178] When
Herpin in 1852 published a work which included observations of private patients, he arrived at a much more optimistic view than had
prevailed among the former generation.[179] Herpin's book created quite
a sensation, and it was partly under its influence that after the middle

---

[178]Hall (449), *On the Diseases and Derangements of the Nervous System*, p. 320.

[179]Herpin (487), *Du prognostic et du traitement curatif de l'épilepsie*, p. 510: "Que la
médecine peut intervenir utilement chez les trois quarts des malades; qu'elle peut en guérir plus
de la moitié, et procurer une amélioration plus ou moins durable dans un cinquième des cas;
enfin que le nombre des épilepsies rebelles aux traitements dirigés avec persévérance est d'un
quart seulement."

of the century some physicians were inclined to emphasize the limitations of hospital statistics.[180]

Such criticism did not, however, put an end to the statistical investigation of epilepsy. On the contrary, this method now found an almost unprecedented use in the great monographs of Moreau, Delasiauve, Sieveking, Reynolds, and others. The source material available had increased. For one thing, surveys of military conscripts were available in greater number. Rayer in 1822 published figures for the French Département de l'Oise, which in 1820 counted 372,476 inhabitants.[181] During the four-year period of 1816-19 a total of 7,507 men had been called to the colors, of whom 1,496 had been rejected for various reasons, including 28 on account of epilepsy.[182] Boudin's study, in 1857, included a table showing the number of epileptics exempt from military service in France each year between 1831 and 1853. The figures ranged from 269 in 1831 to 135 in 1853, a decrease which Boudin ascribed to greater justice in the recruiting system.[183] Sieveking computed the occurrence of epilepsy among English soldiers as approximately "4 out of every 3000 soldiers."[184] Similar statistics from other countries also became available at this time.[185] The statistical material was further increased by reports of the Registrars,[186] and thus it became possible to approximate the incidence and mortality of epilepsy among the population. Such calculations were of importance in various respects. The more reports were obtained, the more probable it appeared that neither climatic nor national peculiarities had any decisive influence upon the occurrence of epilepsy.[187] Thus, the comparative statistics gathered from all over the world supplemented and corrected the many limited statistics concerning the influence of climate, seasons, winds, etc., which had been computed during the middle of the century.[188]

[180]Cf. Hasse (461), *Die Krankheiten des Nervensystems*, p. 256; Sieveking (926), *On Epilepsy and Epileptiform Seizures*, p. 63 f.

[181]Rayer (838), *Histoire de l'épidémie de suette-milaire*, p. 25, footnote 2.

[182]*Ibid.*, pp. 50-53.

[183]Boudin (141), *Traité de géographie et de statistique médicales*, vol. 2, p. 449.

[184]Sieveking, *l.c.*, p. 79.

[185]Cf. Hirsch (494), *Handbuch der historisch-geographischen Pathologie*, dritte Abt., p. 372 ff.

[186]Cf. Sieveking, *l.c.*, p. 77 ff.

[187]Cf. Hirsch, *l.c.*, pp. 374-75.

[188]These statistics usually referred to the influence of climatic factors upon the frequency and severity of the attacks. Delasiauve (261), *Traité de l'épilepsie*, p. 117, for instance, stated that contrary to expectation, north and west winds were correlated with exacerbations of the disease, whereas south and east winds coincided with a diminution of its intensity. Hasse (461), *Die Krankheiten d. Nervensystems*, p. 259, on the other hand, pointed to the fact that all these influences had found different evaluations and that even the statistical investigations had led to contradicting results. At any rate, no lasting results were obtained, and in the following decades observers tended to neglect those aspects altogether. The inadequacy of a statistical approach is

Yet a disturbing thought began to occupy the minds of the investigators. Statistics are of value only if the subject under investigation is clearly defined. But was that the case with epilepsy? What should be considered as epilepsy and investigated statistically? Here the answers began to differ radically. For, in the meantime, the nosological concept of epilepsy had disintegrated, and it had become necessary again to define its meaning.

The clinical descriptions of grand mal epilepsy given in the middle of the last century come near those of modern textbooks. A tonic and a subsequent clonic stage were usually distinguished,[189] a distinction to which but few authors objected.[190] The headaches of epileptics were studied and even a special name *cephalalgia epileptica* proposed.[191] Salaam convulsions were described.[192] Reflexes were examined as far as they were known at the time.[193] Some observers claimed to have found albumen and sugar in the urine after the fit, an observation that was denied by others.[194] The blood was analyzed for carbonate of ammonia in a case of "renal epilepsy"—with negative result.[195] Here we find the modest beginnings of laboratory research, which, in the course of time, was to submit almost every substance of the body to careful examination.

But the impression of steady progress in the study of epilepsy is destroyed as soon as nosological questions are touched upon. We have already mentioned the doubts which had arisen earlier concerning sympathetic epilepsy, and it is worth noticing that such doubts came chiefly from clinicians. Hasse (1810-1902), for example, was very sceptical about the accuracy of alleged cases of epilepsy from the periphery of the body. He thought it peculiar that such observations were chiefly to be found in the older literature and were scarcely ever made in modern times.[196] The existence of sympathetic or eccentric

---

admitted by Petersen (787), p. 150, who strongly emphasizes the influence of meteorological factors.

[189]Cf. Herpin (487), *Du pronostic et du traitement curatif de l'épilepsie*, p. 378 f.; Trousseau (1032), *Clinique médicale*, p. 93; Reynolds (842), *Epilepsy*, p. 103 f.

[190]E.g., Hasse (461), *Die Krankheiten des Nervensystems*, p. 252.

[191]Cf. Sieveking (926), *On Epilepsy and Epileptiform Seizures*, p. 47 f.

[192]W. J. West, a practitioner of Tunbridge, England, reported on his own infant child. West (1087), *On a Peculiar Form of Infantile Convulsions*, p. 725: " . . . I took the child to London, and had a consultation with Sir Charles Clarke and Dr. Locock, both of whom recognised the complaint; the former, in all his extensive practice, had only seen four cases, and, from the peculiar bowing of the head, called it the 'salaam convulsions;' . . . ." Lennox (632), vol. 1, p. 145, cites a case described by Tissot and credits Newman with having introduced the term *epilepsia nutans* in 1849. For other synonyms see Janz (561), p. 3.

[193]Cf. Romberg (865), *A Manual of the Nervous Diseases of Man*, p. 199; Hasse, *l.c.*, p. 254.

[194]Cf. Hasse, *l.c.*; Reynolds, *l.c.*, p. 114.

[195]Cf. Todd (1026), *Clinical Lecture on a Case of Renal Epilepsy*, p. 130.

[196]Hasse, *l.c.*, p. 269.

epilepsy was, on the other hand, asserted again and again by the representatives of the reflex theory of epilepsy, especially Hall, Brown-
Séquard, and Schroeder van der Kolk. This is understandable, since
such cases lent themselves more than any others to this interpretation.
Even Pflüger in his work on the sensible functions of the spinal marrow
illustrated his theory of reflex conduction by a case reported by the
surgeon, Dieffenbach, where a glass splinter in the hand had led to
epileptic seizures, only to be cured by the removal of the splinter.[197]

Yet whatever doubts were raised regarding the existence of sympathetic epilepsy, they were of a subordinate nature compared with
another difficulty. It will be remembered that long before, the term
"symptomatic epilepsy" had been introduced to designate those cases
where epileptic attacks appeared among the symptoms of other
diseases. Thus, there seemed to be three kinds of epilepsy: (1) idiopathic, originating from the brain itself; (2) sympathetic, having
its seat somewhere else in the body; and (3) symptomatic, occurring in
dentition, smallpox, and other complaints. In Esquirol's outline, both
idiopathic and sympathetic epilepsy were subdivided into several
species. Idiopathic epilepsy, for instance, might be produced by an
external force causing fracture of the skull, or by a disease of the skull,
meninges, or brain, or by the influence of "moral causes," like fright.
Sympathetic epilepsy, on the other hand, would include among its
species all the old categories of *epilepsia plethorica, polyposa, humoralis, metastatica, scorbutica, syphilitica, uterina* and others.[198]

This classification was without logic. Why should syphilitic epilepsy
be classified as sympathetic and epilepsy during smallpox as symptomatic? Or, again, if an organic lesion, a tumor perhaps, developed in the
brain, consequent epileptic attacks would, according to definition, be
considered idiopathic epilepsy. But the tumor might be a syphilitic
gumma; would it then provoke sympathetic epilepsy? Besides, if it was
granted that epilepsy was a disease of the nervous system, then fits
subsequent to a fractured skull were just as little idiopathic as those
arising from a disease somewhere else in the body.

There were two ways out of these difficulties. Either the whole
traditional classification had to be abandoned altogether, or its meaning
had to be changed. Both ways were taken and led to two contradicting
concepts of epilepsy.

Sieveking (1816–1904) was one of the most radical representatives
of the first view. He cited "the impossibility of rigidly carrying out the
distinction between essential and nonessential, idiopathic or symptomatic epilepsy" as an argument for "discarding such an arrange-

---

[197]Pflüger (790), *Die sensorischen Funktionen des Rückenmarks der Wirbelthiere*, p. 89 f.
[198]Esquirol (329), *Des maladies mentales*, vol. 1, p. 314 f.

ment."[199] He did not even admit any basic difference between epilepsy and eclampsia and convulsions of children; to him they all appeared variations of the same disease.[200] This view was partly based on the uncertain pathology of the disease, partly on the similar form of attacks in all such cases. But even so, Sieveking had to draw the line somewhere. In reporting some of the cases which Prichard had described as "partial epilepsy" and where consciousness was not lost, Sieveking found an "opportunity of expressing a doubt of the propriety of classing any convulsive affection with epilepsy, in which there is not at the same time decided evidence of a coexistent affection of the mental powers."[201]

By far the majority of physicians tried to modify the meaning of the older terms. It would be confusing to discuss all the varieties of schemes proposed. Most agreed on one point, viz., a redefinition of idiopathic epilepsy. If this term was to be clear at all, all cases where epilepsy was connected with any other disease or any definite lesion inside or outside the brain had to be excluded. Thus, Delasiauve (1804–93), for example, arrived at the following classification: "1. *Essential* or *idiopathic epilepsy*, manifesting itself merely in functional deviations, without lesion, corresponding to simple nervous afflictions and, in a word, constituting a veritable neurosis. 2. *Symptomatic epilepsy*, belonging to a more or less appreciable cerebral lesion, the convulsive spasm being here the symptom and not the disease. 3. Finally a third epilepsy, called *sympathetic*, produced by the irradiation of abnormal impressions which can have their seat in all parts of the body except the brain or its appendages."[202] In this scheme, symptomatic and sympathetic epilepsy were considered on a par with idiopathic epilepsy, all three forms constituting "epilepsy." On the other hand, the name epilepsy could be reserved for idiopathic epilepsy considered as a disease entity *per se*, as was done by Russell Reynolds (1828–96).

Reynold's book on epilepsy deals with idiopathic epilepsy alone. In as far as he uses the terms symptomatic and sympathetic, he does so only in deference to convention and in order to separate true epilepsy from these other convulsive disorders. "In this volume I propose treating only of epilepsy proper, viz., of that form of idiopathic convulsions to which I believe alone the name of epilepsy ought to be applied."[203] Epilepsy and "idiopathic," "essential," or "simple" epilepsy are synonyms to him. As early as 1855, he had stated that if all cases

---

[199]Sieveking (926), *On Epilepsy and Epileptiform Seizures,* pp. 162–63.

[200]*Ibid.,* pp. 32, 120 and 174 ff.

[201]*Ibid.,* p. 25.

[202]Delasiauve (261), *Traité de l'épilepsie,* p. 37.

[203]Reynolds (842), *Epilepsy,* p. 27.

usually called epilepsy could be distributed amongst the various other diseases, then the term epilepsy should be dropped altogether. If, however, we were "compelled to recognise the existence of many, or even of a few, cases distinct from any more general condition of systemic or local disease, then we must employ the term epilepsy in a restricted sense, implying only those cases which, in the present state of medical science, are irreducible."[204] This was a definition *per exclusionem*, i.e., it depended upon the diagnostic exclusion of definite causes like tumors, blood diseases, and "eccentric irritations."[205] It was only logical that Reynolds rejected such concepts as renal epilepsy, uterine epilepsy, "epilepsy from tumour of the brain" and complained that we "find these confounded together with the simple or idiopathic affection."[206]

In support of his stand, Reynolds could, of course, point out how frequently epileptic symptoms alone were observed and no organic lesions of any kind found at the post-mortem examination. In addition, he tried to show that the pathology of the disease also justified his view. On the whole, he agreed with Schroeder van der Kolk that the medulla oblongata was the organ whence convulsions as well as loss of consciousness took their origin, the latter through an induced contraction of the cerebral blood vessels.[207] The question then arose as to what kind of morbid change took place in the medulla oblongata. The answer was that the disturbance was "functional,"[208] i.e., "an undue readiness of disturbance in the centre of reflection."[209] This in turn was the result of a change in the nutritive processes going on in this organ.[210] Reynolds did not see any reason why such changes should not occur primarily and thus constitute an idiopathic disease, "*a morbus per se*."[211] Where tumors or other diseases existed, they did not produce convulsions directly. They could only act as remote causes of some change in the nervous centers, a change which, in turn, represented the proximate cause.[212] Why then should it not be possible for these changes to develop primarily, on the basis of heredity or other factors which produced just this disease, epilepsy?

With Reynolds the concept of idiopathic epilepsy reached the climax of its metamorphosis. Of course, the anatomical and physiological

---

[204] *Ibid.*, pp. 32-33.
[205] *Ibid.*, p. 33.
[206] *Ibid.*
[207] *Ibid.*, p. 244.
[208] *Ibid.*, p. 245.
[209] *Ibid.*, p. 249.
[210] *Ibid.*, p. 260. Reynolds did not, however, exclude the spinal cord entirely.
[211] *Ibid.*, p. 29.
[212] *Ibid.*, p. 23.

interpretations have changed in the course of time, but the arguments offered for the existence of idiopathic epilepsy, i.e., epilepsy as a genuine disease, different from other diseases with epileptiform manifestations, have essentially remained the same. The stages in the history of this term represent an interesting example of the metamorphosis of a concept. For Galen, idiopathic epilepsy was the type which developed as a primary disease of the brain. For Tissot and many others, including Esquirol, gross lesions in the brain or its surroundings seemed demonstrable examples of idiopathic epilepsy. Now these cases were excluded rigorously, and idiopathic epilepsy became a *morbus per se* with unknown etiology.

If we compare the diametrically opposed views of Sieveking and Reynolds, we can easily understand that statistics, based on such different concepts, were bound to lead to different results. Yet in spite of statistical and theoretical divergences, there was one point where both arrived at somewhat similar consequences. Owing to the undeveloped state of diagnostic technique, Reynolds had to rely on clinical observations in order to exclude cases which were not idiopathic. He registered various features which in his opinion distinguished epileptic from other convulsions.[213] For instance, in "genuine epilepsy" he had never observed the convulsions actually limited to one side, whereas in convulsions connected with uremia and organic disease of the brain "it is common to observe the spasms actually limited to one lateral half of the body, or even to one limb."[214] He did not believe, moreover, that "simple epilepsy" was followed by paralysis.[215] Above all, he thought that convulsive paroxysms where consciousness was retained should not be considered epileptic at all.[216] Thus, both Sieveking and Reynolds were led to exclude certain epileptiform attacks, particularly where the convulsions were localized and consciousness preserved. This explains why Hughlings Jackson called these attacks, which we now usually connect with his name, "epileptiform."

## 3. THERAPY

The history of the treatment of epilepsy between 1800 and 1860 mirrors the history of its pathology. There existed an interesting interaction between the empirical attitude, tending to give various remedies a fair trial, and the possibility of observing results in a great number of hospital patients. Even as late as 1861, Reynolds, impressed by the

---

[213] For the distinguishing marks of "convulsions symptomatic of cerebral disease" cf. *ibid.*, pp. 301–2.

[214] *Ibid.*, p. 108.

[215] *Ibid.*, pp. 166 and 227.

[216] *Ibid.*, p. 81.

older enthusiastic reports, recommended a new trial of mistletoe.[217] Other physicians reviewed the entire list of traditional remedies, adding more or less interesting historical remarks.[218] Still others attempted a more systematic study of the comparative effects of different drugs. Each spring and autumn at the Salpêtrière, Esquirol submitted thirty epileptic patients to treatment with some new remedy. In this way he studied the effectiveness of bloodletting, cathartics, baths, cauterization, and all kinds of antispasmodic and even secret medicaments. He prepared his patients carefully for this experiment, certain cure being promised to them. The result was the same in all cases. Each new remedy suspended the attacks for a certain time, ranging from a fortnight in some individuals to a maximum of three months in others. The inference to be drawn seemed inevitable. It was not so much the remedy as the confidence in it which caused the passing remission.[219]

The effect of such a "moral treatment" had, of course, been known long before. But observations like those of Esquirol, where the drug appeared as the least important therapeutic measure, shook the confidence of many of the earlier nineteenth-century physicians. Repeatedly, profound scepticism was expressed in the efficacy of any remedies whatsoever.[220] This was more than the eighteenth century distrust of specifics recommended as sure cures of the disease. The new scepticism extended to all pharmacological and surgical treatment and, instead, emphasized the relative benefit of supervising the hygiene of the patients.[221]

Therapeutic scepticism and prognostic pessimism were likely to go hand in hand. Herpin denounced such pessimism as unfounded. Epilepsy was a curable disease and there existed potent drugs for its treatment, above all, *selinum palustre* and zinc oxide.[222] But neither the general optimism of Herpin nor his faith in zinc oxide[223] made any lasting impression. Delasiauve subjected Herpin's data to scathing criticism, doubting the correct diagnosis in some cases and the soundness of the cure in others.[224] Still, Herpin exerted a certain stimulating

[217]Reynolds (842), *Epilepsy*, p. 321.

[218]Cf. particularly Delasiauve (261), *Traité de l'épilepsie.*

[219]Esquirol (329), *Des maladies mentales*, vol. 1, p. 318 f.

[220]Cf. Delasiauve (261), *Traité de l'épilepsie*, p. 444; Meyer (689), *Aus der Krampfkranken-Abtheilung der Charité*, p. 18 f.; Westphal (1091), *Tracheotomie bei Epilepsie*, p. 17. *Spicelegia epileptica* (943), p. 441, claimed that any new treatment would often postpone attacks.

[221]Cf. Esquirol, l.c., p. 329; it must, however, be added that, long before Esquirol, Heberden (468), *Commentaries on the History and Cure of Diseases*, p. 164, had expressed trust in the healing power of nature rather than in remedies.

[222]Herpin (487), *Du pronostic et du traitement curatif de l'épilepsie*, p. 613.

[223]Herpin's praise of the *salinum palustre* received little attention.

[224]Delasiauve (261), *Traité de l'épilepsie*, p. 283 ff.

effect, and zinc remained among the drugs used for epilepsy and found its defenders.[225]

Much more contested as remedies were preparations of silver, especially silver nitrate given internally. In some cases, severe poisoning resulted. A woman who had been treated elsewhere with nitrate of silver for eighteen months died at the Salpêtrière. The dissection showed that the mucous membrane of the stomach had been partly destroyed; at some points the peritoneum alone remained intact, while at others, the stomach was completely perforated.[226] Argyrism was a common result of this type of treatment. Todd complained of the fact that so many patients showed in the discoloration of their faces the indelible marks of the ineffective treatment they had undergone.[227]

There was a great number of other remedies of which the pros and cons were discussed: turpentine,[228] indigo, belladonna,[229] inhalations of chloroform,[230] and many more; indeed, most monographs on epilepsy of this period devoted considerable space to a critical catalogue of various drugs. Empiricism was the resort of those who confessed ignorance of the nature of epilepsy. "Since we know nothing of the nature of the disease," said Georget, "we cannot establish precise indications; it is empiricism alone that will be able to guide the physician."[231] Those, however, who believed that they knew more about epilepsy sometimes drew practical conclusions from their pathological hypotheses.

There was, first of all, the domain of sympathetic epilepsy, which traditionally had given frequent indications for surgical intervention. Early in the century, Joseph Frank reported one case which was often quoted in later literature.[232] A man of twenty-three had been injured at the scrotum. The inflammation and other troubles having been cured, nightly pollutions set in for which cold baths were prescribed. During one of these baths, the patient suffered vehement convulsions which repeated themselves every day. When the patient was admitted to the hospital, it was observed that the testicles "were drawn up" after each attack, the left epididymis being very tender. Castration was advised and performed, and eleven years after the operation the man was still free from epileptic attacks. The testicles upon inspection showed no

---

[225] Cf. Sieveking (926), *On Epilepsy and Epileptiform Seizures*, p. 217.

[226] Cf. Georget (406), Article *Épilepsie*, p. 222.

[227] Todd (1026), *Clinical Lecture on a Case of Renal Epilepsy*, p. 155.

[228] Cf. Foville (374), Article *Épilepsie*, p. 427.

[229] Cf. Trousseau (1032), *Clinique médicale*, p. 145.

[230] Cf. Reynolds (842), *Epilepsy*, p. 322.

[231] Georget (406), Article *Épilepsie*, p. 225.

[232] Cf., e.g., Romberg (865), *A Manual of the Nervous Diseases of Man*, p. 221.

pathological change. This was an extreme case of surgical treatment of sympathetic epilepsy, given full credit by Brown-Séquard[233] in his almost exhaustive account of surgical successes ranging from simple ligatures to sections of nerves and amputation. The theory held by this author, viz., that many cases of epilepsy originated from the skin,[234] led him to recommend cauterization with a red-hot iron, even where injury of the head had preceded the outbreak of the disease and trephining seemed indicated. A case communicated to him by Van Buren of New York seemed to support this view. A woman had received a blow upon her head and had developed epileptic fits several months afterward. When admitted to the New York Hospital, she was suffering from headaches, the pain always commencing in a small spot over the middle of the right parietal bone, which was also sensitive to pressure. The bone was laid free at this place and its surface being found elevated and roughened, the morbid portion was removed by trephining. On the eighth day after the operation, fits occurred again, and at the same time erysipelas developed. The fits returned on two following days and then ceased; the erysipelas was cured. Brown-Séquard reasoned that removal of the bone could not have caused the cure of epilepsy, since attacks had occurred afterward. Therefore, he believed, the effect must have been produced either by the erysipelas or, much more likely, by changes in the skin, due to the operation.[235]

Brown-Séquard's account of this case shows that physicians were still prone to talk of the cure of epilepsy when the attacks had disappeared for a few months,[236] although it was well known that remissions for an even longer time could frequently be observed.

This case is an illustration in the nineteenth century of trephining for traumatic epilepsy and diseased bone of the skull. The indication usually rested on the suspicion of mechanical irritation or compression of the brain or on a local injury that could be seen or felt.[237] In Anglo-Saxon countries the operation was performed with relative frequency,[238] and here again the surgeons of the United States were foremost. Benjamin W. Dudley (1783–1870), who popularized the operation among American surgeons, had five cases—all of them cured or

---

[233] Brown-Séquard (170), *Experimental and Clinical Researches*, etc., (*Boston Med. and Surg. Journal*), vol. 55, p. 426.

[234] Cf. above, p. 281.

[235] Brown-Séquard, *l.c.*, pp. 458–60.

[236] The patient had been operated upon, May 10, 1856, and had been last seen in November of the same year.

[237] Cf. Echeverria (309), *De la trépanation dans l'épilepsie par traumatismes du crâne*, and Cutter (250).

[238] Cf. the statistics as given by Echeverria, *l.c.*, p. 655 ff.

improved—to his credit.[239] This was pointed out in a survey article on the surgical treatment of epilepsy published in 1852 by Stephen Smith. While expressing doubts about the effect of such measures as setons, issues, cauterization, moxas, scarification, amputation of the extremity (if the seat of an aura), division of nerves, and ligation of arteries[240] (including the carotid),[241] Smith thought differently about trephining where a proper indication existed.[242] He tabulated a total of twenty-seven cases where the operation had been performed in the United States, and he summed up the result as follows: "Unrelieved, none. Relieved, but not cured, 3. Immediate relief after operation, and no further note of result, 2. Relieved for one month or under when last seen, 3; between one and six months, 3; between six months and one year, 6; between one and five years, 3; set down *cured*, but lapse of time from date of operation to time last seen not given, 7."[243] But even here Smith was not convinced that all cases recorded as successful really were so. He noticed with regret "the unjustifiable haste of surgeons in reporting their cases, before sufficient time has elapsed after the operation to give a rational opinion as to its success."[244]

Similar observations were made by John Shaw Billings in his review of 1861, which comprised seventy-two cases, though not all from the United States.[245] Sixteen cases ended fatally; cure was reported in forty-two, while four were said to have remained unchanged and ten were improved.[246] Apart from this, Billings made the remarkable statement that, according to information received, Dr. McDowell of St. Louis had performed the operation "over one hundred times in epileptic cases, but with what result, I am unable to state."[247]

---

[239] Smith (931), *The Surgical Treatment of Epilepsy*, p. 232; cf. Cutter (250), p. 190. Dr. Gert H. Brieger kindly drew my attention to Smith's article.

[240] Smith (931), p. 234.

[241] *Ibid.*, p. 229.

[242] *Ibid.*, p. 233.

[243] *Ibid.*, p. 242.

[244] *Ibid.*, p. 234 f., Van Buren (1044), *Trephining in Epilepsy*, in 1860, thought trephining a simple and harmless operation, its bad reputation being caused by the often hopeless nature of the injuries for which it was performed. Interestingly enough, in the case which gave rise to the particular communication, "no abnormal local condition had been recognized" during the operation, and it must be inferred that such a condition had been diagnosed pre-operatively, or that the patient, a boy with attacks every week, had been operated upon without any specific indication—a not very likely eventuality. Subsequently, the boy had no attacks for three weeks, but especially in view of the unrevealing operation, Van Buren warned that the time was too short to claim a cure. The notice was written in the third person, and was signed by C. Echeverría (311), *On Epilepsy*, p. 353, endorsing Van Buren's opinion expressed himself "in favor of trephining the skull for the relief of epilepsy due to local injury to the head."

[245] Billings (112), *The Surgical Treatment of Epilepsy*; see also French and Darling (378).

[246] Billings, p. 337.

[247] *Ibid.*

French surgeons were averse to the operation, and it created quite a sensation when Broca in 1866 dared to trephine a case of traumatic epilepsy.[248] Incidentally, Broca was assisted by Lucas Championnière (1843-1914)[249] who was soon to become the French protagonist of Listerism and modern brain surgery.

A hundred and thirty years ago bleeding was practiced as an old and traditional therapeutic measure. In as far as it was based on rational grounds at all, the theory of congestion of the brain seemed to lend it some support. This theory also justified ligatures of arteries and compression of the carotids. Then Marshall Hall introduced the notion of "laryngismus." Since he believed that closure of the larynx was responsible for the severe cerebral congestion, it was but logical to assume that tracheotomy would prevent the consequences of "laryngismus" and would cure epilepsy.[250] Some cases were reported where this operation seemed to have had good results.[251] Brown-Séquard was among those who, in principle at least, upheld the soundness of Hall's proposals, but believed that the same result could be obtained by cauterization of the larynx with nitrate of silver, a view which he tried to prove experimentally in animals.[252] Others, however, pointed out that tracheotomy was a dangerous procedure without effect upon epilepsy.[253] Kussmaul and Tenner's work suggested not only that spasm of the glottis was a rare cause of epileptic convulsions,[254] but that "all theories are false which assert the epileptic attack to be derived from a sudden determination of blood, whether active, passive, or mixed."[255] One of their practical conclusions was that "the debilitating method of treating epilepsy, especially by *abstracting* blood, should almost always be rejected,"[256] a conclusion which harmonized with the general disfavor into which bleeding was gradually falling.[257]

In the opinion of most contemporary physicians, skin eruptions and, particularly, acute febrile diseases had a beneficial influence upon epilepsy. During acute diseases, epileptic attacks were seen to have stopped—although the lasting effect upon the course of epilepsy was

---

[248] Cf. Broca (162), *Trépanation du crâne*, etc., p. 508 ff.

[249] Cf. Lucas-Championnière (650), *Trépanation du crâne*, etc., p. 230.

[250] Hall (449), *On the Diseases and Derangement of the Nervous System*, p. 279.

[251] Cf. Westphal (1091), *Tracheotomie bei Epilepsie*, p. 7 ff.

[252] Brown-Séquard (171), *Experimental Researches*, pp. 80-84.

[253] Cf., e.g., Westphal, *l.c.*; *Spicelegia epileptica* (943), p. 442, reported on one of Marshall Hall's tracheotomized cases where the operation had proved futile.

[254] Kussmaul and Tenner (602), *On the Nature and Origin of Epileptiform Convulsions*, etc., p. 94.

[255] *Ibid.*, p. 108.

[256] *Ibid.*, p. 106.

[257] On this point cf. Bryan (178) for the United States.

doubtful.[258] On the other hand, it was claimed by some, though refuted by others, that epileptics were less susceptible to infectious
diseases.[259] Such views went back to the times of the Hippocratic
physicians, and the thesis that quartan fever would cure epilepsy was
repeated almost dogmatically by some authors.[260] The wish to produce
an intermittent fever artificially had been voiced in the days of Antiquity. Arnald of Villanova had believed it possible, and around 1840 a
Belgian physician, Selade, invented a new method of inducing "intermittent fever" in some patients. Having two chronic epileptics under his
care toward the end of winter, he exposed them half-clad to intense
cold for an hour daily. After exposure, the patients were immediately
put into a warm bed, whereupon perspiration set in. This procedure was
followed for a fortnight and both cases were "cured," one showing no
repetition of the disease for four years, the other having a relapse after
two years but being cured again by the same method.[261] This original
therapeutic approach was hailed as encouraging—but rejected on account of the obvious risks involved.[262]

Thus, therapeutic endeavors both empirical and rational in the
middle of the last century seem to be best summarized by the following
contemporary statement: "Perhaps no disease has been treated with
more perfect empiricism on the one hand, or more rigid rationalism on
the other, than has epilepsy. Unfortunately, both methods have often
and completely failed; the former, as it must do in a certain proportion
of the cases; the latter in a still larger number, because the theories
upon which it has rested have often been abundantly wrong."[263] The
same author, Reynolds, prefaced his chapter on the prognosis of epilepsy by the opposing views of two authorities:

> "J'en ai guéri un très grand nombre."—Tissot.
> "Elle conduit presque infailliblement à l'incurabilité par de lentes
> dégradations."—Delasiauve.[264]

By contrasting the optimism of the eighteenth century physician
Tissot with the pessimism of his own contemporary, Delasiauve,
Reynolds wanted to indicate that "the prognosis of epilepsy in the
present day is, it would seem, less favourable than was that of the last
century."[265] At about the same time, Watson (1792-1882) told his

---

[258] Cf. Hasse (461), *Die Krankheiten des Nervensystems*, p. 259 f.

[259] Cf. Reynolds (842), *Epilepsy*, p. 229 f.

[260] Cf., e.g., Delasiauve (261), *Traité de l'épilepsie*, p. 139.

[261] Cf. Delasiauve, *ibid.*, p. 418 f.

[262] Cf. Delasiauve, *ibid.*; Hasse, *l.c.*, p. 285.

[263] Reynolds, *l.c.*, p. 318.

[264] *Ibid.*, p. 312.

[265] *Ibid.*

medical readers that they might, perhaps, encourage their patients by referring to the epileptics Caesar, Mohammed, and Napoleon. But they themselves should have no illusions and should not attach any importance to these historical examples.[266] Yet even if we disregard Herpin's exaggerated optimism, it would not be true to say that the attitude of all physicians in the middle of the century was one of defeatism. Men like Todd and Sieveking admonished their colleagues not to lose confidence and to consider it their duty to try their utmost in this disease.[267] And then a new drug appeared which, even if it did not cure epilepsy, at least offered greater relief than any drug before.

Bromide of potassium owed its introduction into the therapy of epilepsy to a rather doubtful theoretical concept. On May 11, 1857, Sieveking read a paper on epilepsy before the Royal Medical and Chirurgical Society of London,[268] and in the ensuing discussion Sir Charles Locock (1799–1875) made the following comments. He had come across the report of a German physician showing that bromide of potassium produced temporary impotency in men.[269] This gave him the idea of trying the remedy in hysteria in young women. Satisfied with his results, he then prescribed the drug in cases of "hysterical epilepsy" where the epileptic attacks "only occurred during the catamenial period, except under otherwise strong exciting causes." Out of about fourteen such cases he cured epilepsy in all but one.[270] From this report it would appear that Locock had not thought of using the bromide as a general remedy for epilepsy[271] but had concentrated upon the troubles in the sexual sphere and cases of what Prichard had called "uterine epilepsy."[272] It was still in this sense that Reynolds, four years later, interpreted Locock's suggestion without himself having any positive results to report.[273] Even as late as 1866, Althaus (1831–1900) credited tincture of henbane rather than bromide of potassium with the best results in suppressing epileptic attacks.[274]

---

[266]Watson (1067), *Lectures on the Principles and Practice of Physic*, p. 346.

[267]Cf. Todd (1026), *Clinical Lecture on a Case of Renal Epilepsy*, p. 156; Sieveking (926), *On Epilepsy and Epileptiform Seizures*, p. 203 ff.

[268]Sieveking (925), *Analysis of Fifty-two Cases of Epilepsy*, p. 527.

[269]I infer from Hunter (520), p. 169, that the reference is F. Butzke, *De efficacia bromi interni experimentis illustrata* (Berlin, 1829) which, however, I have not found suggestive.

[270]Sieveking, *l.c.*, p. 528.

[271]Sieveking (926), *On Epilepsy and Epileptiform Seizures*, p. 221 f., gives a similar report of Locock's comments without making it quite clear whether he himself limited the use of drugs to "hysterical" epilepsy only.

[272]Prichard (824), *A Treatise on Diseases of the Nervous System*, p. 141 ff.

[273]Reynolds (842), *Epilepsy*, p. 332 f.

[274]Althaus (27), *On Epilepsy, Hysteria, and Ataxy*, p. 29 f.

The new drug owed its popularity to Wilks (1824-1911), as he himself indicated.[275] The remarkable success of iodide of potassium in epilepsy due to syphilis, combined with the fact that it was often difficult to be certain of this cause, had induced him to begin treatment with this preparation. By way of experiment he changed to the bromide of potassium. "About this period [c. early 1859] also, the bromide was recommended by Sir C. Locock as a remedy having some influence over the ovary in females, and therefore curative of those epileptiform affections which might be due to an irritation of this organ." Wilks doubted the theory but thought that in case of positive results, the remedy ought to be "equally good for all cases, whether men or women."[276]

By the mid-seventies, the drug had become so popular that 2.5 tons of bromide were used every year at the National Hospital Queen Square.[277] Bromism must have been rampant and was taken into the bargain. Hammond in New York treated a boy of fourteen with 120 grains of bromide of potassium as his daily allowance. He demonstrated the patient, who had shown marked mental improvement and was free of attacks, with the words: "As you see he is broken down in appearance, has large abscesses in his neck, and is altogether in a bad condition. But this is better than to have epilepsy."[278]

Any sanguine expectations of now possessing a remedy that would cure epilepsy were not fulfilled,[279] and the gradual withdrawal of the drug was advised to avoid severe recurrences. The introduction of bromide of potassium coincided with an increased interest in status epilepticus, which, though described and named much earlier, had not received anything like the attention given to it in the seventies. If its former rare citation can be taken as an indication of its rare occurrence, more than a fortuitous coincidence between this condition and the introduction of effective anti-convulsant therapy suggests itself.[280]

---

[275]Cf. Wilks (1105), *Observations on the Pathology of Some of the Diseases of the Nervous System*, p. 231, footnote.

[276]Wilks (1103), *Bromide and Iodide of Potassium in Epilepsy*, p. 635.

[277]Holmes (509), p. 21.

[278]Hammond (453), *Clinical Lectures on Diseases of the Nervous System*, p. 217.

[279]A short note on *Bromide of Potassium in Epilepsy* (165), published in early February 1864 and reporting the use of bromide of potassium at the Hospital for Paralysis and Epilepsy stated: "There can be no question as to its very great value in diminishing the number of fits . . . but it is very doubtful whether it effects a cure."

[280]This is the conclusion to which Hunter (520) has been led on the basis of a thorough analysis of the historical literature, for which his article should be consulted. As examples I mention Browne (174), p. 32, and Obersteiner (746).

# PART SIX

# SIX

# THE NINETEENTH CENTURY: THE AGE OF HUGHLINGS JACKSON

# XI
# Jackson's Forerunners

## 1. THE SITUATION AROUND 1860

Seen in retrospect, the history of epilepsy between 1800 and 1860 reflects some of the major medical trends characterizing those years. The enthusiasm for gross pathological anatomy and its co-ordination with clinical observation, the appreciation of statistical data, the growing scepticism regarding treatment by drugs, the progress of neurophysiology in general, all can be recognized in the approaches to epilepsy. Without the discovery of the law of Bell and Magendie as an anatomical basis for reflex function, and without the elucidation of nervous vasoregulation, the theories of the mid-century could hardly have been formed. As is to be expected, the following twenty-five years or so, to which the remaining chapters are devoted, show a similar relationship between medicine and epilepsy. But while general trends form the background against which the particular history of epilepsy developed, they do not explain all that was thought and done. Individual physicians and scientists act within their time, which offers them possibilities and imposes limitations. If outstanding, they also leave their stamp on their time; they contribute in ways which are not self-evident, and their significance is not exhausted by particular discoveries and inventions often duplicated by others. In the history of epilepsy, John Hughlings Jackson played such a role, and 1861 is the year in which his activity began.

Hughlings Jackson's work was connected largely with the National Hospital for the Relief and Cure of the Paralysed and Epileptic from 1862 till 1906. Here he could study a considerable number of epileptics, many of them ambulatory, and enjoyed the contact with eminent neurologists: Brown-Séquard, Radcliffe,

Reynolds, Sieveking among the older generation, and Ferrier and
Gowers among the younger. Gowers was his assistant and, later on, his
junior colleague.[1] In the same year in which Jackson joined the National Hospital, Jean-Martin Charcot was appointed physician at the
Salpêtrière in Paris.[2] Charcot combined clinical observation with intensive gross and microscopic anatomical investigations, and in the
following years he was able to present his classic descriptions of a
number of important neurological diseases. In 1865 the medical faculty
of Vienna entrusted to Theodor Meynert (1833–92) the teaching of
"the structure and function of the brain and of the spinal cord with
reference to their diseases."[3]

These few data show that during the sixties neurology was beginning
to establish itself. In this development Jackson played a leading part.
To bring out his significance, the work of those whose ideas and observations came closest to his will have to be discussed, and this will be
done most conveniently under the headings of Jacksonian epilepsy
named after him, and of dreamy state, a designation associated with
him. Under various names, both conditions had been described long
before, yet the fact that he did not discover either of them by no means
diminishes his specific merits. When Gowers stated that "a new era in
the study of epilepsy" may be said to have commenced with Jackson's
investigations, he was referring to the onset of attacks and to initial
subjective sensations.[4] But in adding that Jackson's main merit lay in
the mode of his investigation he passed a judgment that can be extended to Jackson's entire work on epilepsy.

Hughlings Jackson did not dominate neurological thought during the
early decades of its modern phase, nor did his work simply supersede
that of his predecessors. But the influence of his ideas has proved more
enduring than that of others and also more far-reaching, even to our
own time.

It may be helpful first to sketch the state of neurological knowledge
around 1860, a sketch which can be very brief if negatives are used.
Gall's theory of cerebral localization of functions was widely dis-
credited. In agreement with Flourens, the cerebral cortex was associated with volition and intelligence—though not necessarily with consciousness. Regarding the functions of the subcortical ganglia and the
paths whereby the latter are connected, ignorance and uncertainty
prevailed, although theories were not lacking and will have to be
touched upon later. The cellular composition of ganglia was known and

---

[1] Holmes (509), p. 47.
[2] Guillain (441), p. 15.
[3] Lesky (634), p. 374.
[4] Gowers (420), *Epilepsy and Other Chronic Convulsive Diseases*, p. 40.

the connection of nerve cells and nerve fibers well established. However, the neuron theory was still to come; its elaboration fell into the eighties.

There was talk about nerve-force or nerve-power,[5] which was a conveniently neutral expression for the unknown nature of nervous action. Nerve current and muscle current, i.e., the resting potentials of nerves and muscles, had been explored, and what is now called action potential was known as "negative variation." After the work of Bernstein, in 1868, had led to a better understanding of its nature, the idea of recording the negative variation of the brain soon presented itself; indeed, in 1875, Caton registered "the electric currents in the brain" in rabbits.[6] For the history of epilepsy within the period under consideration, this anticipation of the electroencephalogram was of no consequence.[7] Most of the work that will be discussed was of a clinical nature.

## 2. JACKSONIAN EPILEPSY

### a. Bravais and Bright

In *A Study of Convulsions* (1870) Hughlings Jackson proposed to deal with "those [convulsions] in which the fit begins by deliberate spasm on one side of the body, and in which parts of the body are affected, one after another."[8] This is the clinical definition of what has come to be called "Jacksonian epilepsy." Obviously, the chain of those who noted convulsions of this kind goes at least as far back as Aretaeus. Herpin, in 1852, collected a large number of pertinent observations from the literature,[9] and in a book completed in 1865 gave many examples from his own practice.[10]

When coining the expression "Jacksonian epilepsy," Charcot claimed priority for Bravais, who, in 1827, had published a thesis under the title of *Investigations on the Symptoms and the Treatment of Hemiplegic Epilepsy.*[11] Jackson himself accepted Bravais' priority for the descrip-

---

[5] See below, p. 312.

[6] Caton (210), *The Electric Currents of the Brain.*

[7] Cf. Brazier (149) for the subsequent history of the electroencephalogram.

[8] Jackson (556), *Selected Writings*, vol. 1, p. 8.

[9] Herpin (487), *Du pronostic et du traitement curatif de l'épilepsie*, p. 382 ff., where he included all such cases under the heading of aura.

[10] See below, p. 324.

[11] Charcot (215), *Leçons du mardi à la Salpêtrière*, p. 15: "Il arrive quelquefois, à la suite des attaques d'épilepsie partielle, qu'il se produit des attaques de paralysie.

"Ce phénomène de l'épilepsie partielle a été pour la première fois décrit et distingué de l'épilepsie ordinaire par un nommé Bravais qui était interne dans cet hôpital. Cela date de 1827 ou 1828.

"Mais dans ces derniers temps, un savant anglais, Mr. Jackson de Londres, est revenu sur se sujet et il a traité la question d'une façon si particulière qu'il m'est arrivé quelquefois

tion of unilateral seizures.[12] Therefore, the work of Bravais merits more detailed consideration, as does that of Bright, which belongs to the same period.

Bravais did not aim at increasing the number of previous observations, but at establishing a new type of disease.[13] In the majority of cases of "hemiplegic epilepsy," he maintained, one side of the body only was attacked by convulsions[14] which were often followed by more or less severe paralysis of the side affected.[15] Having thus defined his subject, Bravais tried to distinguish it from general epilepsy and, on the other hand, describe its main varieties. The stress which he put upon the nosological point of view led him to an overemphasis of the distinction between general and hemiplegic epilepsy, for he neglected the transitions from one form to the other. All the more valuable were his observations of the varieties of "hemiplegic" epilepsy, of which he distinguished five: (1) Where the attacks began in the head; (2) in the arm; (3) in the foot; (4) where the "aura" started from an abdominal or thoracic organ; (5) where it depended upon a local disease of the nerves.[16] Of these five varieties he studied more particularly the three first mentioned, paying special attention to the course the attack followed. The attack might begin with localized spasms or an aura; these two symptoms Bravais treated as virtually equivalent. A few of his remarks on hemiplegic epilepsy from the arm may best serve to illustrate his approach.

> In the majority of cases the patients know that their hands, their forearms, their arms are affected in the first place, either by spasms or by a particular aura. . . . Many amongst them are subject to incomplete attacks in which the arm alone is affected; they complain to their physician of experiencing jerking, numbness, nervous twitching in the diseased limb, either during the day or at nightfall.[17]

---

d'appeler cette affection l'épilepsie Jacksonienne et le nom lui en est resté. C'était Justice. Je ne m'en repens pas. J'ai fait un peu de tort à Bravais, mais enfin l'étude de Mr. Jackson est si importante que véritablement il méritait bien d'attacher son nom à cette découverte. Si on pouvait fusionner Bravais et Jackson, le français et l'anglais et dire l'épilepsie Bravais-Jacksonienne, ce serait plus juste; il est vrai que ce serait un peu long!" For an English translation see Guillain (440), p. 124. See also Charcot et Pitres (217), *Contribution à l'étude des localisations dans l'écorce des hémisphères du cerveau*, p. 4.

[12]Jackson (556), *Selected Writings*, vol. 1, pp. 148, footnote 1; 414 and 424.

[13]Bravais (148), *Recherches sur les symptômes et le traitement de l'épilepsie hémiplégique*, p. 6.

[14]*Ibid.*, p. 7: "Nulle part, d'ailleurs, je n'ai lu cette assertion, fondée sur l'expérience, *que l'épilepsie débutant par un seul membre est en général limitée à la moitié du corps.*" Cf. also *ibid.*, p. 23.

[15]*Ibid.*, p. 12: "Un autre indice de cette maladie, c'est la paralysie du côté affecté dans l'intervalle des accès; . . . Le temps de cette faiblesse musculaire est variable; elle peut durer quelques instants, quelques heures, des journées entières, ou enfin se convertir en une véritable paralysie."

[16]*Ibid.*, p. 16.

[17]*Ibid.*, p. 24.

If the attacks return at regular periods or if by a happy chance the physician is a witness, these are the symptoms one observes: At first, convulsions of the arm and forearm, then of the muscles of the lower limb, of the face, of the neck and finally of the wall of the chest and of the abdomen. . . .

Do the convulsions begin with the muscles of the shoulder and of the arm, or with those of the hand and the flexors of the fingers? The attack is too prompt and observation too difficult for me to have been able to solve this question. . . . Which is the order in which the muscles of the lower limb, of the head and the neck, of the wall of the great cavities of the trunk contract? It seemed to me that the flexor, extensor, and rotator muscles of the head convulse before the muscles which move the mouth sidewards, the patient inclining the head towards the shoulders before the mouth is split to the ear on the same side.[18]

Even if Bravais' observations did not always agree with those of Jackson forty years later, the clinical data which interested them and which they observed were largely the same. In so far Bravais anticipated Jackson. But he did not venture upon an explanation of what he had observed. Richard Bright (1789–1858), on the other hand, combined the clinical approach with the anatomical and reached conclusions which made him one of the closest forerunners of Jackson.

Many of the cases of epilepsy which Bright observed in Guy's Hospital showed definite changes in the cortex of the cerebral hemispheres. Two of these cases deserve more than passing reference.

George Osborne had been suffering from headaches for more than ten years. "In August last . . . he fell down in an epileptic fit, which has since returned at irregular intervals, and has occasionally been accompanied by paralysis, of greater or less duration, of the right side." At the time of his admission (November 7, 1827) he was affected by peculiar attacks of tremor. "This tremor generally begins in the foot, running up the leg to the thigh, and occasionally extending to the body and head, when he is deprived of the power of speech, but is aware of what is passing at the time. The vision is occasionally defective, and he closes the lid of the left eye involuntarily and unconsciously. . . . His right leg is so far paralyzed that he evidently drags it after him in

---

[18]*Ibid.*, p. 25: "Si les attaques reviennent à des périodes régulières, ou si, par une cause fortuite, le médecin en est témoin, voici les symptômes qu'on observe. D'abord, convulsions du bras et de l'avant-bras, ensuite des muscles du membre inférieur, du visage, du cou, et enfin des parois de la poitrine et du ventre.

"Les convulsions débutent-elles par les muscles de l'épaule et du bras, ou ceux de la main et les fléchisseurs des doigts? L'accès est trop prompt, et l'observation trop difficile pour qu'il m'ait été possible de résoudre cette question . . . .

"Quel est maintenant l'ordre dans lequel se contractent les muscles du membre inférieur, de la tête et du cou, des parois des grandes cavités du tronc? Il m'a semblé que les muscles fléchisseurs, extenseurs et rotateurs de la tête se convulsent avant les diducteurs de la commissure des lèvres; le malade inclinant la tête contre l'épaule avant d'avoir la bouche fendue jusqu'à l'oreille du même côté."

attempting to walk."[19] The later history of the patient until the time of his death (October 19, 1828 at St. George's Hospital) tells of repeated partial as well as complete attacks, the latter often preceded by "a peculiar cramp-like sensation"[20] ascending from the leg. At one time "he experienced temporary loss of sight, and brief accessions of double vision."[21] The post-mortem report contains the following passage of importance: "From between the under surface of the dura mater and its investing arachnoid membrane, there grew up a tumour of the consistence of softish cheese, and of the size of a small almond; in the course of its development it had pushed forward the two laminae of the arachnoid, the pia mater, and the cortical substance of the brain, without, however, producing any ulceration or softening of these parts, and had thus indented itself into the upper part of the posterior lobe of the left hemisphere of the brain."[22] Bright's closing remark is: "In this case the most decided aura was experienced in connection with organic disease within the skull."[23]

In the other patient, Rigby Chamberlain, the history stated "that nearly two years ago he fell from a cart upon his head, and was brought to this Hospital in a state of insensibility, and had since been subject to occasional fits of an epileptic character. He had experienced a fit three days before his admission, when, as on former occasions, the left side of his body became weak and almost powerless, with greatly impaired sensation; he lost his sight for several hours, and bit his tongue."[24] Some fits occurring in the Hospital were described as follows: "They generally begin by an agitation of the left leg, accompanied by a peculiar sensation which passes up the thigh and body till it reaches the head, when he loses his recollection, is convulsed for about an hour, then sleeps for half an hour, and awakes quite unconscious of what has happened to him."[25] The patient, who had first been admitted to the Hospital on April 28, 1830, applied again on July 2, "stating that he has had a return of his complaint, which was brought on by seeing another man in a fit."[26] At this time Bright closed the case with the remark: "In this case we have another exemplification of the frequently observed fact, that in cases where the disease is in all probability entirely dependent on mischief going on within the cranium, the first indications of the attack are felt in some distant part of the body."[27]

---

[19]Bright (154), *Reports of Medical Cases*, vol. 2, part 2, p. 538.
[20]*Ibid.*
[21]*Ibid.*, pp. 540-41.
[22]*Ibid.*, pp. 541-42.
[23]*Ibid.*, p. 542.
[24]*Ibid.*, pp. 544-45.
[25]*Ibid.*, p. 545.
[26]*Ibid.*
[27]*Ibid.*

But the case had an aftermath. On February 18, 1831, the patient was brought to the Hospital "in a most violent paroxysm, of which he had frequent returns."[28] On April 5 "he complained of frequent returns of a peculiar sensation in the left leg, with considerable and almost constant pain."[29] On the 18th it is stated that "He has had no return of fits, and the pain in the left leg is much less; but he complains that the foot of that side is in a constant state of perspiration. He often talks of a kind of 'twittering' sensation in the leg, rising half way up the body."[30] A few days later the patient died from a "severe cynanche tonsillaris." The dissection revealed a very thick and heavy skull. "The dura mater looked healthy externally; but when it was cut and turned back, it was found to be thickened and ossified in small portions at the posterior part of the falx, where it was inserted into the tentorium; and there it adhered so firmly to both the posterior lobes of the cerebrum, but chiefly to the left, that considerable portions, including the whole thickness of the cineritious substance, tore away with the membrane: this disease extended over a surface of two or three inches altogether, and some depression of the convolutions extended on the left side still further. The arachnoid was slightly opake, and so firm, that, together with the pia mater, it was easily drawn off in one sheet."[31] At the end of his epicrisis Bright could say: "I have already said . . . that epilepsy generally depends upon irritation on the surface of the brain, and that it is often connected with unusual thickness of the skull."[32]

We have related these two cases in such detail because they show the range of Bright's observations and conclusions. Looking at the contemporary neurological literature, Bright found an authoritative support in Foville's views on the functional preponderance of the gray matter of the brain.

> It is an idea entertained by Dr. Foville, that the cineritious is the more active part of the brain generally, with regard to all its functions; and that the medullary part is more particularly employed in the conveyance of the motions and sensations, or whatever else may be acted upon or produced in the cineritious part. And, supposing for a moment this to be the case, we might expect that lesion of the cineritious substance would produce disordered action in that part; and that such action might be transferred to the distant parts of the body, producing disordered and involuntary motions: whereas, if the great injury were done in the substance of the brain, the means of communication with the active part being cut off, paralysis might result, more or less mingled with convul-

---

[28] *Ibid.*, p. 643.
[29] *Ibid.*
[30] *Ibid.*
[31] *Ibid.*, pp. 643–44.
[32] *Ibid.*, p. 644.

sion, in proportion as the cineritious substance is more or less involved.[33]

We are now prepared to understand the diagnostic acumen which Bright revealed a few years later (1835) in a case of "Fatal Epilepsy, from Suppuration between the Dura Mater and Arachnoid, in consequence of Blood having been effused in that situation."[34] The patient was in a "fair state of health" (although suspected of a past history of syphilis) "when, suddenly, his right arm was affected with a kind of cramp; and this feeling seemed to rise toward his face: he then fell insensible, and came to himself in about three-quarters of an hour."[35] During the following few days he suffered from similar attacks, and on the evening of the day preceding his admission he had seven fits. "Since that time the right arm had been weak, and affected with a tingling sensation, but not paralyzed. The leg of that side was free. The right cheek felt numb; and the tongue, when protruded, inclined a little to the right side. He had very severe headache."[36] The day following his admission, the patient had a long fit with frothing at the mouth and convulsion of the whole right side, but he "appeared to be sensible during the whole of the paroxysm. His power of articulation was destroyed for several hours after the fit, but it returned: when it left him, he appeared feverish and irritable."[37] Bright now gave it as his opinion "that these fits were owing to some *local disorganization affecting the membranes and cineritious portion of the brain on the left side, and probably influencing the deep-seated parts about the posterior portion of the corpus striatum.*"[38]

The short subsequent history of this case, which ended with the death of the patient, and a post-mortem finding indicated in the title of the communication need not interest us here. What interests us is the reason on which Bright based his early diagnosis. This was so clearly stated that it had best be given in his own words. "My reason, then, for supposing that the epileptic attacks, in this case, depended rather on a local affection than on a more general state of cerebral circulation or excitement, was, *the degree of consciousness which was observed to be retained during the fits:* for although we meet with great variety in this respect, yet, in two cases which have occurred to me, the fact of the patient generally remaining conscious has been a remarkable feature;

---

[33] *Ibid.*, p. 514 f.

[34] Bright (153), *Cases Illustrative of the Effects Produced when the Arteries and Brain are Diseased*, p. 36.

[35] *Ibid.*

[36] *Ibid.*, p. 36 f.

[37] *Ibid.*, p. 37.

[38] *Ibid.* (italics in text).

while, in each, the injury on which the fits depended was of a local, rather than a constitutional or a general character."[39] Even more interesting is the second argument which Bright adduces. "With regard to the other parts of the diagnosis—the temporary paralysis of one side, and the permanent weakness, favoured the view of decided organic lesion. *The epileptic character seemed to point to the membranes and surface of the brain, as the parts most affected*; for of this connection I have pretty well satisfied myself, by an extensive induction of facts: and the circumstance of the right hand having suffered more than the leg, and the speech having been affected, directed my views to the posterior, rather than the anterior portion of the left hemisphere."[40]

Summarizing briefly, it can be said that Bright studied cases of "Jacksonian epilepsy," observed their connection with impaired sight, paresthesia and weakness of the convulsed parts, noticed the presence of consciousness, and associated these symptoms with local lesions affecting the surface of the brain (membranes and cortex) on the side opposite to the one convulsed. Moreover, Bright did not separate these cases from "epilepsy," even if he tried to point out their clinical and anatomical peculiarities.

### b. Todd, Carpenter, and Wilks

Bravais' thesis was little read, and even Bright's observations did not receive the attention they deserved among the physicians of the following generation. Those who studied similar cases gave them a new interpretation which was to explain much of Jackson's early work. For this we may cite Robert Todd (1809-60), physician to King's College Hospital, with whose writings Jackson was acquainted and whom he repeatedly quoted in his early papers.

Todd used the term "epileptiform"—it had been used before[41]—for the following kind of fits: "One arm, or both arm and leg on one side, become seized with convulsive movements, quite of the clonic or epileptic kind. These come in paroxysms; the paroxysm lasts a variable time, and then subsides; leaving more or less general exhaustion and disposition to sleep; but consciousness is not impaired. Yet there can be no doubt that such fits may pass into the true epileptic fit; for it is not rare to see a very complete epileptic fit commence with some local derangement of sensation or motion, or both." He had observed these symptoms in cases "of meningeal disease, especially . . . when the pia

---

[39] *Ibid.*, p. 39 (italics in text).

[40] *Ibid.*, p. 39 f. (italics in text).

[41] Cf. above, p. 266. The English edition of Tanquerel des Planches' work on lead poisoning (992), p. 293 f., discusses "convulsions or epileptiform movements" as a variety of the convulsive form of encephalopathy. They were distinguished from "lead epilepsy" proper, of which Tanquerel had observed thirty-six cases (*ibid.*, p. 289).

mater has been previously affected."[42] No doubt, Todd was well acquainted with "Jacksonian" attacks and knew of their connection with morbid changes of the surface of the brain, particularly on the side opposite to that convulsed.[43] We might now expect Todd to harmonize his pathological knowledge with his physiological views and to ascribe to the cerebral cortex a direct influence upon motor functions. Indeed, he stated that he had noticed "slight convulsive twitching of the muscles of the face" upon electric irritation of the hemispheric lobes, and he believed "that a disturbed state of the hemispheric lobes . . . may, *in some degree* at least, contribute to the development of the convulsions."[44] In contrast to many of his contemporaries, he even attributed a primary role to the cerebral hemispheres in the development of the epileptic paroxysm. But this role referred to the psychic rather than to the convulsive component of the fit.

Todd was much interested in epileptiform convulsions appearing in the course of uremia or as a consequence of poisoning. This gave him the clue to his "humoral theory of epilepsy."[45] "I hold that the peculiar features of an epileptic seizure are due to the gradual accumulation of a morbid material in the blood, until it reaches such an amount that it operates upon the brain in, as it were, an explosive manner; in other words, the influence of this morbid matter, when in sufficient quantity, excites a highly polarised state of the brain, or of certain parts of it, and these discharge their nervous power upon certain other parts of the cerebro-spinal centre in such a way as to give rise to the phenomena of the fit."[46] On the basis of this theory, he explained the variety of attacks. If the poisonous or morbid material affected the hemispheres alone, the epileptic vertigo resulted. "If it affect primarily the region of the quadrigeminal bodies, or if the affection of the hemispheres extend to that region, then you will have the epileptic fit fully developed."[47]

Todd's humoral theory contains some features worth noticing. The idea of morbid material accumulating in the blood and affecting the brain in an explosive manner is reminiscent of Willis' views.[48] The notion of a discharge, derived from the analogy with the Leyden jar, connects his theory with that of Schroeder van der Kolk.[49] The most

---

[42]Todd (1027), *Clinical Lectures on Paralysis*, etc., p. 395.

[43]Cf. *ibid.*, p. 124.

[44]Todd (1028), *The Lumleian Lectures for 1849*, p. 28 (italics in the text). Jefferson (563), p. 118 ff. has discussed Todd's experiments in detail.

[45]Todd (1026), *Clinical Lecture on a Case of Renal Epilepsy*, etc., p. 129.

[46]*Ibid.*

[47]*Ibid.*

[48]Cf. above, VII-1.

[49]Cf. above, X-1.

notable feature distinguishing him from the adherents of the reflex theory is the insistence upon the cerebral hemispheres as the primary seat of the paroxysms. Otherwise, he agrees with most pathologists of his day in assigning one seat (the hemispheres) for the disturbances of consciousness, and another (the quadrigeminal bodies) for the convulsions.[50]

However, these hypotheses did not suffice for an explanation of "epileptic hemiplegia," that is, epileptic attacks combined with weakening or paralysis of the affected side. Todd used the term "epileptic hemiplegia" for cases which bore a marked similitude to those of Prichard and of Bravais and are now called Todd's paralysis.[51] He assumed that the epileptic attack left the brain in an exhausted condition "apt to continue as one of weakened nutrition."[52] If these after-effects were confined to the convolutions of the brain, "mental power, memory, perception suffer,"[53] that is to say those faculties which were ascribed to the cortex. But if deeper parts were involved, viz., "the deeper parts of the white matter of the hemisphere, and the corpora striata and optic thalami, then we have hemiplegic paralysis."[54]

With Köllicker, Todd, Bowman, and Carpenter, the corpus striatum was cast in a role hereto assigned to the cerebral cortex. The older theory[55] was summarized very clearly by Carpenter in the following words: "It has usually been considered that the Cerebrum acts directly upon the muscles, in virtue of a direct continuity of nerve-fibres from the grey matter of its convolutions, *through* the Corpora Striata, the motor tract of the Medulla Oblongata, the anterior portion of the Spinal Cord, and the anterior roots of the nerves; and that in the performance of any voluntary movement, the Will determines the

---

[50]Todd (1028), *The Lumleian Lectures for 1849*, p. 28 f.: "The part of the encephalon primarily disturbed, is the hemispheric lobes: if the disturbance do not go beyond a certain point, the phenomena are limited to loss of consciousness and impaired intellectual action, with more or less of sopor. But if the disturbance be considerable, then the tubercula quadrigemina and mesocephale become involved, and *epileptic convulsions* are produced" (italics in text).

[51]Cf. Todd (1027), *Clinical Lectures on Paralysis*, etc., p. 248 f. Cf. Prichard (824), *A Treatise on Diseases of the Nervous System*, p. 60: ". . . others, who recover from a severe fit, or from frequently repeated fits of epilepsy, are often found to labour under hemiplegia, or other modifications of palsy."; Cf. Hunter (520), p. 165. For Bravais cf. above, footnote 15.

[52]*Ibid.*, p. 300.

[53]*Ibid.*

[54]*Ibid.*

[55]Bell (97), *Idea of a New Anatomy of the Brain*, p. 29: "From the medullary matter of the hemispheres, again, there pass down, converging to the crura, Striae, which is the medullary matter taking upon it the character of a nerve; for from the Crura Cerebri, or its prolongation in the anterior Fasciculi of the spinal marrow, go off the nerves of motion." Cf. also Bell (98), *The Nervous System of the Human Body*, p. 215. As Carpenter (203), *Principles of Human Physiology*, p. 490, formulated it, the older theory was in harmony with the doctrine of Gall and Spurzheim who believed that fibers originating in the pyramids and reinforced by fibers from the pons and the crura cerebri reached the cerebral convolutions; cf. Temkin (1003), p. 285 f.

motor force to the muscles or set of muscles, by whose instrumentality it may be produced."[56] This view was challenged in the forties.

It was now claimed that the fibers from the hemisphere ended in the corpus striatum and that from the corpus striatum a different set of fibers started out to the parts further below, while the very existence of transient fibers was greatly doubted.[57] Anatomically, the corpora striata were now considered the origin of the motor tract. True, it was commonly admitted that stimulation of these bodies did not provoke motor reactions, but their motor function seemed probable on account of the pathological anatomy of paralysis.[58] Their influence upon the motility of the organism was deemed so important that Todd made them the chief center of volition, while the cerebral cortex was reserved for "intellectual action."[59] William B. Carpenter (1813–85), who largely shared Todd's opinions and who was one of the most popular physiological authors around the middle of the last century, incorporated these views in what became known as Dr. Carpenter's theory of the function of the sensori-motor ganglia. As formulated by Broadbent in 1866, this theory contended "that the thalamus is the organ of conscious sensibility, to which all impressions made on peripheral sensory nerve-fibres must be transmitted in order to be recognized as sensations, and the corpus striatum the organ or instrument of voluntary motion,—the downward starting point of volitional motor impulses, or it might be said of all cerebral motor impulses. These two ganglia are again associated . . . in sensori-motor action, impressions reaching the thalamus being passed on to the corpus striatum, and giving rise to automatic movements differing from those which have their centre in the cord, only in being accompanied by sensation."[60] The relationship of the thalamus to the corpus striatum on each side appeared analogous to that of the posterior and anterior horns of the gray matter of the spinal cord. At a time when really very little was known about the physiology of the brain, such an analogy with the

[56] Carpenter (203), *Principles of Human Physiology*, p. 508.

[57] Cf. Todd and Bowman (1030), *The Physiological Anatomy and Physiology of Man*, pp. 215 f. and 308. Cf. also Kölliker (589), *Manual of Human Histology*, vol. 1, p. 435 ff., and Carpenter (203), *Principles of Human Physiology*, pp. 490 and 508.

[58] Todd (1029), *Physiology of the Nervous System*, p. 722 M: "The invariable occurrence of paralysis as the result of lesion, even of slight amount, in the corpora striata, must be regarded as a fact of strong import in reference to the motor functions of these bodies."

[59] *Ibid.*, p. 723 E: "That the cerebral convolutions, with the fibres which connect them to the corpora striata and optic thalami, constitute the centre of *intellectual action.* That the centre of *volition* consists primarily of the corpora striata . . ." (italics in the text).

[60] Broadbent (158), *An Attempt to Remove the Difficulties Attending the Application of Dr. Carpenter's Theory of the Function of the Sensori-motor Ganglia to the Common Form of Hemiplegia*, p. 468. Cf. Carpenter (203), *Principles of Human Physiology*, pp. 490 and 508. On the development of the knowledge about the basal ganglia see Schiller (895). Walshe (1061) has analyzed the role Carpenter assigned to the sensory ganglia in relation to consciousness.

anatomical substratum of spinal reflex action must have been enticing.[61]

From theories like these there was but a short step to associating epileptic convulsions with the corpora striata. John Simon (1816-1904), for instance, in 1850, assigned the loss of consciousness to the "convoluted surface of the cerebrum" and believed that the general clonic convulsions implied "the excitement of some aggregative centre of motion," i.e., the cerebellum or the corpus striatum.[62] And in 1866 Samuel Wilks extended Bright's and Todd's ideas[63] to a point which was an almost complete break with the accepted theory of irritation of the medulla oblongata and the pons Varolii. Commenting upon a case of epileptic convulsions, where a tumor had been found in the pons, he said: "I have no hesitation in saying that for one such case fifty might be found in which the morbid changes producing these symptoms occupy the surface."[64] Morbid changes in the cortex of the brain, according to Wilks, accounted for practically all cases of epilepsy whether partial or general. "It appears to me that, from clinical and post-mortem observations, as well as from all analogy, we cannot but conclude that the *fons et origo mali* is in the cineritious substance of the brain. I believe that in this region a commotion occurs which would, perhaps, be analogous to a palpitation affecting the heart, and that this irritates the ganglia below, which form the summit of the motor tracts."[65]

At that time Hughlings Jackson had already entered upon his investigations of epilepsy. His work was referred to by Wilks,[66] and a few years later Jackson was to combine the various trends in a new synthesis. We have dwelt upon the work of his British predecessors, because the starting point of his research would otherwise not be understandable. Yet in giving due weight to the contributions of Jackson's forerunners we must keep in mind that they formed but a minority. "Dr. Carpenter's theory" was not generally accepted.[67] How great the uncertainties regarding the anatomy and physiology of the central

---

[61]Cf. Carpenter, *ibid.*, p. 490. Young (1114), pp. 111 f. and 212-21 has discussed the development of these thoughts in detail with results which do not quite agree with mine.

[62]Simon (929), *General Pathology*, p. 152.

[63]Cf. Wilks (1105), *Observations on the Pathology of Some of the Diseases of the Nervous System*, pp. 228 and 230 where he refers to Bright and Todd.

[64]*Ibid.*, p. 227.

[65]*Ibid.*, p. 229 (italics in text).

[66]*Ibid.*, p. 154, footnote.

[67]Dalton (251), *A Treatise on Human Physiology*, p. 368, speaking of the anterior pyramids as continuation of the anterior columns of the cord, in 1867 wrote: "They pass onward, underneath the transverse fibres of the pons Varolii, run upward to the corpora striata, pass through these bodies, and radiate upward and outward from their external surface, to terminate in the gray matter of the hemispheres." For Wilks see below, p. 333.

nervous system were[68] is indicated by the fact that the course of the so-called pyramidal motor tract was ascertained only after Flechsig's studies of 1876. These uncertainties have to be taken into account when authors do not always seem to be consistent even with themselves. Moreover, the majority paid little attention to partial convulsions caused by gross anatomical lesions in the brain. In 1868 Nothnagel (1841-1905) postulated the existence of a *Krampfcentrum* in the substance of the pons.[69] In 1872 he reformulated the theory of the dual nature of the epileptic attack. Excitement of the vaso-motor center and of the motor centers were co-ordinated factors. The former caused anemia in the brain,[70] and thereby coma, while the latter accounted for the convulsions.[71] The subsequent course of the attack was explained by venous hyperemia inside the skull.[72]

### 3. THE DREAMY STATE (PSYCHOMOTOR EPILEPSY, TEMPORAL LOBE EPILEPSY)

#### a. Morel, Griesinger, Falret

What Jackson came to call "dreamy states" and the "uncinate group of fits" comes close to the "psychomotor" epilepsy and "temporal lobe" epilepsy of today.[73] He thus established categories, the great significance of which was recognized only long after his death. But, as was the case with Jacksonian epilepsy, here too descriptions of cases assignable with more or less certainty to these categories go back to Antiquity. There is even a suggestive passage in the book *On the Sacred Disease*, where the author says: "And I know that many persons in their sleep groan and cry out, while others seem to be choked and still others get up and flee outside and are deranged until they wake up afterwards

---

[68]Cf. Greenblatt (425), p. 364.

[69]Nothnagel (740), *Die Entstehung allgemeiner Convulsionen vom Pons und von der Medulla oblongata aus*, p. 9.

[70]Sometimes also as *Epilepsia vasomotoria* in the periphery of the body as described by Voisin; cf. Nothnagel (742), *Ueber den epileptischen Anfall*, p. 317.

[71]Nothnagel, *ibid.*

[72]*Ibid.*, p. 320.

[73]Symonds (986), p. 634 ff. Details are discussed below. For the history of temporal lobe epilepsy see Bailey (75) and Hassler (462), p. 231 f. Griesinger (see below, footnote 115) had already spoken of psychomotor symptoms ("psycho-motorische Symptome"); in 1902 Ira Van Gieson presented a communication on "A Case of Psycho-motor Epilepsy" before the annual meeting of the American Neurological Association [(30), p. 345, where the title only is given]; and five years later Turner (1035), pp. 130 and 138, spoke of "psychomotor fits." Cf. Bailey (75), p. 10. When Gibbs, Gibbs, and Lennox (410), p. 380, in 1937 began to use this term, they did so on the basis of electroencephalogram studies. As these authors (409), p. 300, explained it: "... we have observed a third type of electrical activity, distinct from those of petit mal and grand mal, which occurs in seizures ordinarily classed as psychic variants, or equivalents. In these attacks the patient, though he may perform apparently conscious acts, is not subject to command; he may exhibit involuntary tonic movements; he may display psychomotor disturbances of a surly, unpleasant sort, and on recovery he has complete amnesia for the events which occurred in the attack." Later on, Lennox (632), vol. 1, pp. 227-321, used the term to include automatisms as well as hallucinations and "psychic seizures."

healthy and sensible as before, only pale and weak, and this not once but often."[74] Conceivably, this referred to "nightmarish psychomotor seizures."[75] But if so, the Hippocratic author apparently did not associate such paroxysms with the sacred disease, for he expressly cited them among the wondrous doings "which yet nobody thinks to be sacred."[76]

Hallucinations and automatisms of all kinds, states of rage, and acts of violence were noticed often enough in the literature from Aretaeus to the nineteenth century. There is obvious continuity from Esquirol, Prichard, Bright, Delasiauve, Brierre de Boismont to Morel, Falret, Griesinger, and Herpin, whose work is to be discussed next. Yet there is also a hiatus; for the influential voices after 1860 were those of Morel, Falret, and Herpin, rather than those of earlier writers.

Both Benedict Augustin Morel (1809-79) and Jules Falret (1824-1902) were psychiatrists and directors of asylums. Their epileptic patients were in advanced stages of the disease or showed features which made their social sequestration desirable. The epileptic who had committed acts of violence was a subject of theoretical and practical concern for them.[77] Morel, in particular, studied the life and the character of his patients. As his friend Lasègue[78] put it: "One must do justice to him and admit that he was the first, or one of the first, to discern the epileptic within epilepsy; and instead of limiting himself to the description of the attacks, he has recounted the biography of the patient."[79]

Morel found irritability and anger to be salient features of the epileptic character.[80] Any trifle could provide "epileptic anger," which might last one to two hours and repeat itself again and again during the day.[81] But there also existed epileptic fury, which appeared in two forms: either in continuity with an epileptic attack, i.e., preceding or following it,[82] or, without such continuity, bursting forth "like lightning and being condensed in terrible deeds."[83] This was said in 1853.[84]

---

[74]Hippocrates (491), ed. Littré, vol. 6, p. 354, 4-10, 12; Grensemann (429), p. 60, 13-19.

[75]Lennox (632), vol. 1, p. 253 f., where he cites a case showing some similarities.

[76]Hippocrates (491), ed. Littré, vol. 6, p. 354, 1 and Grensemann (429), p. 60, 10-11. However, a little later in the book, similar symptoms are mentioned which the magicians ascribe to Hecate and the Heroes, presumably as manifestations of the sacred disease; cf. above, I-3.

[77]See above, p. 270.

[78]Cf. Ackerknecht (8), p. 5.

[79]Lasègue (613), Morel—sa vie médicale et ses oeuvres, p. 595.

[80]Morel (711), Etudes cliniques, t. 2, p. 322: "L'irritabilité et la colère sont les traits saillants du tempérament de ces malades."

[81]Ibid., p. 321.

[82]Preictal and postictal in modern parlance.

[83]Morel, ibid., p. 321.

[84]Morel (713), Traité des maladies mentales (of 1860) repeats much of what was said in 1853 verbatim.

In 1860 Morel published an article in which he described "larval" or "masked" epilepsy (*épilepsie larvée*). Ordinarily, epilepsy manifested itself in convulsive attacks, falls, and vertigoes. But the disease could also exist in a masked form which was diagnosed by the main symptoms of epileptic insanity. Morel gave a long list of these symptoms, which was largely taken from his picture of the epileptic character.[85] Masked epilepsy could exist by itself without any attacks of ordinary epilepsy, though it was by no means less dangerous. On the contrary, patients who months or years later, in addition, acquired ordinary seizures generally became less violent.

Falret's article appeared around the same time as that of Morel, which it even quoted in the last installment[86] and to which it was rather close.[87] The mental disorders (Falret spoke of *troubles intellectuels*) of epileptics were assigned to three categories: There existed passing trouble before, during, or after a convulsive attack, to which it stood in the relation of a mere epiphenomenon. Second, there existed disorders ordinarily met in epileptics during the intervals between the attacks, i.e., the epileptic character. The third category comprised the more or less prolonged delirium to which the name epileptic insanity (*folie épileptique*) was appropriate.[88]

The first category included various premonitory symptoms and, in particular, "more immediate mental prodromes, a kind of intellectual aura,[89] which precede the convulsive attack by a few minutes only and which, in some manner, constitute its first symptom." For instance, there were epileptics "in whom the same idea, the same reminiscence, or the same hallucination arises spontaneously at the moment of the invasion of every attack and infallibly precedes its appearance."[90] He added that very often "this reminiscence, this idea or this image are the reproduction of the idea or the sensation which has provoked the first attack in this patient."[91]

In the vast majority of cases, Falret thought, intellectual disturbances could be observed during the attack; indeed, absolute loss of con-

---

[85]Morel (710), *D'une forme de délire*, etc. p. 840. On the epileptic character see more below. In 1872–73 the Société médico-psychologique (934) devoted several sessions to masked epilepsy.

[86]Falret (343), *De l'état mental des épileptiques*; vol. 18, p. 442. The article appeared in three installments in December 1860 and April and October 1861. The reprint in Falret's (344), *Etudes cliniques sur les maladies mentales et nerveuses* of 1890 shows some changes.

[87]Morel (710), *D'une forme de délire*, p. 840, mentions a visit to a patient together with Falret who, in turn, (343), vol. 17, p. 482, mentions Morel.

[88]Cf. Falret (343), *De l'état mental des épileptiques*, vol. 16, pp. 663, 668, and 671; see below, footnote 97.

[89]Falret, *ibid.*, vol. 16, p. 664: ". . . il est d'autres prodromes intellectuels plus immédiats, sorte d'aura intellectuelle . . . ."

[90]The examples cited include a number of purely sensory phenomena.

[91]*Ibid.*, p. 664 f.

sciousness was an essential characteristic of the disease. Nevertheless, there existed certain incomplete or aborted attacks where this rule did not hold good.

> During these aborted attacks the patients, who have no rapport with the external world, utter certain incomprehensible sounds or articulate a few incoherent words which seem to indicate a painful anxiety or deep fright. In these incomplete attacks, which hold the middle between the simple epileptic vertigo and the great convulsive attacks, the patients also have only partial convulsive movements, such as involuntary contractions of certain muscles of the face or of the limbs, automatic movements (*mouvements automatiques*) of swallowing, chewing action, etc. Hence these attacks are incomplete from the point of view of abnormality of movement, as well as of loss of consciousness. After the attacks have ceased, some of these patients have retained a more or less vague memory of the ideas that preoccupied them while the attacks lasted. They have declared that at the time they were under the influence of a painful dream, in a state of profound mental suffering, and dominated by a vague feeling of violent pangs of conscience or of an insurmountable misfortune, the reason of which they were unable to penetrate.[92]

The statement is a conglomerate of various sources. Falret named John Cheyne[93] and the anonymous German author whose report, under the title of *Phantasies during an Epileptic Attack*, had appeared in 1825.[94] He also cited Griesinger's textbook of psychiatry that had been published in its first edition in 1845.[95]

Griesinger, probably Falret's main source, also had referred to Cheyne and to the anonymous German author and, in addition, to Jean Pierre Falret (1794–1870), the father of Jules, who in his courses had discussed at length a variety of epilepsy with "suspension of comprehension and convulsive phenomena consisting in successively repeated motions of swallowing with alternative elevation and lowering of the lower jaw."[96]

---

[92] *Ibid.*, p. 665 f.

[93] *Ibid.*, p. 666. Cf. Cheyne (219) article, *Epilepsy*, p. 77. Cheyne died in 1836, and his article belongs to the early part of the nineteenth century.

[94] Cf. above, p. 268 and Temkin and Temkin (729).

[95] Cf. Griesinger (432), *Die Pathologie und Therapie der psychischen Krankheiten*, p. 287 f.

[96] Billod (113), *Recherches et considérations relatives à la symptomatologie de l'épilepsie*, p. 407: "M. Falret, mon maître . . . a, dans son cours de clinique et de pathologie générale des maladies mentales et des affections nerveuses, fixé l'attention . . . sur une variété d'épilepsie que je n'ai vue mentionnée nulle part . . . . Le signe pathognomique de cette variété est la concomitance des deux symptômes suivants: suspension de l'intelligence et phénomènes convulsifs consistant *en mouvements successivement répétés de déglutition* avec élévation et abaissement alternatifs de la mâchoire inférieure" (italics in the text). This seems to be a description of what Penfield and Kristiansen (784), p. 26, have called "unconscious masticatory seizures." Trousseau (1032), *Clinique médicale*, p. 106 f. "Il en est chez lesquels tout consiste en une sorte de mâchonnement, suivi d'un bruit guttural analogue à celui que produit la déglutition quand elle se fait à vide."

Falret's main interest was in the third category of mental disorders, epileptic insanity,[97] which he divided into *petit mal intellectuel* and *grand mal intellectuel*, as counterparts to the petit mal and grand mal of the convulsive attacks. *Petit mal intellectuel* usually was associated with vertigoes and the grand mal type with the convulsive grand mal. The delirious types could precede or, more often, follow the convulsive attacks; less frequently they appeared in the intervals between the latter, in persons who were recognized as epileptic.[98] Finally, "the epileptic delirium, with the psychic characteristics proper to it, ... occurs in patients who are not considered as presently affected by epilepsy. In this case either vertigoes or nightly attacks which have passed unnoticed are really demonstrated; or, on the contrary, these somatic symptoms do not exist at the time when the patients are observed but have taken place before or will show up later in the course of their life. Under these circumstances, the epileptic delirium *substitutes* somehow for the epileptic convulsions and is, so to speak, but another manifestation of the same disease in a different form."[99] Falret viewed convulsions on the one hand and delirium on the other as the two manifestations of the same morbid entity,[100] and by maintaining that the psychic form could be present when the convulsive form was absent, he followed Morel's doctrine of larval or masked epilepsy.[101]

Falret claimed that *petit mal intellectuel* was not easily confounded with the grand mal. "The calm of the movements, the partial lucidity of the ideas, in short the semblance of reason which are observed in epileptics suffering from *petit mal intellectuel* contrast in the highest degree with the maniac agitation, the extreme disorder of their actions, and the incessant loquacity of those affected by the grand mal." But he immediately pointed out how much the two had in common and that there were numerous intermediary states, "which tend to show that, in reality, only a simple difference of degree exists between these two varieties of epileptic insanity."[102]

Falret's preoccupation with the psychiatric aspects of epilepsy influenced his physiological views of the disease, expressed in a critique of the reflex theories of the preceding period. Mental symptoms were

---

[97]Falret (343), *De l'état mental des épileptiques*; vol. 16, p. 671: "Accès de délire plus prolongés, méritant spécialement le nom de folie épileptique."

[98]Falret (343), vol. 16, p. 679, and vol. 17, p. 490.

[99]*Ibid.*, vol. 16, p. 679: "Dans ces circonstances, le délire épileptique *se substitue* en quelque sorte aux convulsions épileptiques, et n'est, pour ainsi dire, qu'une autre manifestation de la même maladie, sous une forme différente" (italics mine). This whole passage is lacking in Falret (344).

[100]Falret (343), vol. 17, p. 485.

[101]*Ibid.*, vol. 18, p. 442, cites Morel's article.

[102]*Ibid.*, vol. 16, pp. 677 and 678.

more important than epileptiform convulsions, which he thought rare, and the loss of consciousness was the main element of the epileptic attack. He, therefore, rejected all theories which placed the seat of epilepsy in the medulla oblongata and, instead, reinstituted the brain, admitting that the double course of the attack—sensory loss and motor hyperactivity—was as yet incomprehensible.[103]

Of considerable interest is Falret's emphasis on the automatism prevailing in many epileptic phenomena. He talked not only of the automatic movements of deglutition. The epileptic who, in a state of post-ictal delirium, attempted or committed suicide, homicide, arson, had not the slightest responsibility for "violent acts committed by him in the midst of this completely automatic, though short, delirium."[104] In the *petit mal intellectuel* the patient left his home and his work; he was absent-minded, his thought was dulled, he had fits of despair and of unprovoked anger, various impulses followed one another at brief intervals, he had a desire of destroying himself and the things that came under his hands; he was extraordinarily forgetful, had complete lapses of memory, headaches, giddiness (*étourdissement*); he noticed luminous sparks, visions, frightening objects. "It is in the midst of this state of mental anxiety, of instinctive or automatic impulses and of extreme confusion of ideas,[105] that the epileptics, pushed as they say by an invincible force that dominates their will," commit all kinds of destructive acts. "They strike mechanically (*machinalement*), without motivation, without interest, without knowing what they do or, at least, with a very vague consciousness of their actions."[106] In judging the mental condition of an epileptic the forensic physician must take into account, among other things, the characteristics of the acts performed during such seizures, "characteristics which can be summed up by saying that these acts are violent, automatic, instantaneous and not motivated."[107]

In rare exceptions these acts were not free of motives, calculation, and premeditation. "Sometimes, indeed, an attack of *petit mal intellectuel* suddenly arouses in the heart of an epileptic a feeling of jealousy, of vengeance, or of anger towards a definite person and then pushes him immediately into action, while in his normal state he had succeeded in suppressing this feeling."[108]

---

[103]Falret (344), *Théories physiologiques de l'épilepsie*, pp. 305-37. The article had originally been published in 1862. Albers (17) in Germany echoed Falret's views.

[104]Falret (343), vol. 16, p. 667: ". . . des actes violents commis par lui au milieu de ce délire tout à fait automatique, quoique de courte durée."

[105]*Ibid.*, vol. 18, p. 434 f.: "C'est au milieu de cet état d'anxiété morale, d'impulsions instinctives ou automatiques, et de confusion extrême des idées . . . ."

[106]*Ibid.*, p. 435.

[107]*Ibid.*, p. 440: "caractères que l'on peut résumer en disant que ces actes sont violents, automatiques, instantanés et non motivés."

[108]*Ibid.*, p. 436.

Automatism, especially since the essay by Baillarger (1809-90) of 1845, was not a novel idea in French psychiatry, and it harmonized with the notions of "unconscious cerebration" developed by Carpenter in England.[109] Casuistic material on automatic actions of epileptics was accumulating in many parts of the world, for instance, in Germany, in the dissertation of Griesinger's pupil Höring, published in 1859.[110] We read of a young man who in the preceding two to three years had experienced relatively few attacks of grand mal but a great many mild attacks of which he remembered nothing. He

> suddenly falls into a state of deep dreaming and stretches his hands in front of him. These together with his head (which is turned to the right) and the upper part of his trunk begin to tremble. Often all is over in a minute, or within a few minutes. At other times he runs away during the attack and talks gibberish, or he searches, as in a dream, in all his pockets, as if he were missing something, and he himself says that something has fallen down, or he makes scrubbing and rubbing motions on his trousers, or hides his hands in his sleeves and talks of the possibility of breaking off his fingers and so on; sometimes he answers if addressed during this dream state,[111] but usually wrongly. Whatever form this slight attack may take, at its end he usually closes his eyes, seems to sleep for a few minutes, and then has no idea of what happened.[112]

Another patient, for about an hour following the attack "remains somewhat mentally disturbed: he undresses, inappropriately starts praying, and so on; some time later he becomes sleepy."[113]

In the introduction Höring pointed out that in medical practice the concept of epilepsy as "occasional convulsions with loss of consciousness" proved too narrow. There existed many "cases of incompletely developed epilepsy,"[114] when consciousness was not altogether lost, and some hardly showed any convulsions.

Comparisons with a dreamlike state suggested themselves. Griesinger himself, in 1868, even used the term "psycho-motor symptoms" in what he called "epileptoid conditions." In certain patients "psycho-motor symptoms are added; mild twitchings in the hands, the bulbi,

---

[109]Baillarger (74), *Théorie de l'automatisme*, cf. also Baruk (83a), pp. 94 and 117. On the notion of "unconscious cerebration" cf. Carpenter (203), *Principles of Human Physiology*, p. 589.

[110]Höring (501), *Über Epilepsie*. The title page has "Unter dem Praesidium von Dr. W. Griesinger," and in the preface Höring expressed his thanks to his teacher, Professor Dr. Griesinger, who had advised him in the present work. Griesinger, in turn, cited this dissertation in the second edition of his textbook (404), p. 404, footnote.

[111]"in diesem Traumzustande."

[112]Höring (501), *Über Epilepsie*, p. 19.

[113]*Ibid.*, p. 21.

[114]"Fälle unvollständig entwickelter Epilepsie."

around the mouth, rigidity in the neck, tension in the abdominal muscles; as one patient expressed it, his 'body' acted independently: only with difficulty could it be moved by his will, and so on."[115] Movements of the lips or of swallowing, even if slight, and words mumbled every time without being remembered afterward hardly allowed any doubt of the epileptoid nature of the vertigo. In the great majority of his male epileptoid patients, Griesinger observed "sexual weakness" and "in rare cases long-lasting decidedly morbid sexual excitement."[116]

Obviously, terms reappear in the history of epilepsy without necessary historical connection. To some extent, the phenomena themselves seem to suggest names; at other times, names imply theories. In the seventeenth century Sennert had spoken of "little" and "incomplete" epilepsies;[117] major and minor seizures have proved convenient names to the present times;[118] a patient of Herpin talked of momentary "absences."[119] To these few examples of what seem to be spontaneously recurrent names must be added those which imply a theory. Sennert referred to the little epilepsies as "incomplete" ones, others also did so, and Herpin devoted an entire book to incomplete attacks of epilepsy. This name not only conveys the impression of something less massive than a grand mal, it also includes the notion of something not fully developed, something aborted, something that has stopped or has been made to stop before it could reach perfection. In his work of 1852, Herpin had arranged his cases in a series descending from intensive grand mal to a mere cramp of a few fingers of one hand.[120] The purpose of this arrangement was to elucidate the area between the two extremes: complete convulsive seizure and vertigo.[121]

Herpin's work of 1852 suggested that imperfect fits comprised both motor and psychic phenomena. His book of 1867, which appeared posthumously (he had died in 1865), dealt with partial seizures, petit

---

[115] Griesinger (433), *Ueber einige epileptoide Zustände*, p. 329: "Bei einer Minderzahl von Kranken kommen eigentlich motorische, bei mehreren aber psycho-motorische Symptome hinzu; leichte Zuckungen in den Händen, den Bulbis, um den Mund, Starrheit im Nacken, Spannung in den Bauchmuskeln; ein Kranker drückt sich aus: sein 'Körper' sei selbständig thätig, er könne nur noch schwierig durch den Willen bewegt werden u. dergl."

[116] *Ibid.*, pp. 324 and 329: "Bei der sehr grossen Mehrzahl der männlichen Kranken besteht *sexuelle Schwäche* [spaced in the text], in seltenen Fällen eine lange dauernde, ganz krankhafte sexuelle Aufregung." Cf. Peters (786). Dr. Dietrich Blumer has drawn my attention to this aspect of temporal lobe epilepsy.

[117] Sennert (913), *Institutionum medicinae*, lib. II, pars 3, sect. 1, c. 9; vol. 1, p. 374: ". . . affectus quidam reperiuntur, qui et ipsi epilepsiae accensendi sunt, velut parvae quaedam et imperfectae epilepsiae, aut certe via ad epilepsiam. . . ."

[118] Penfield and Kristiansen (784), p. 16.

[119] Herpin (487), *Du prognostic et du traitement curatif de l'épilepsie*, p. 65.

[120] *Ibid.*, p. 441 ff; cf. also p. 70.

[121] *Ibid.*, p. 449.

mal, and what would now be called psychomotor attacks. From a clinical point of view, Herpin was Jackson's closest forerunner; at the same time his opinions, just because they went in a different direction from those of Jackson, help to set off the latter's originality.

### b. Herpin

Théodore Herpin (1799-1865) was a pupil of Laennec and a great admirer of Louis, to whom his book of 1867 was dedicated.[122] It was based on his observation of 300 patients from his own private practice and defended the following thesis. In at least half of the cases, the disease did not begin with major attacks but with milder forms, such as localized cramps, visceral spasms, or vertigoes. In most of these patients, one to five years passed before the appearance of major attacks. During this interval, treatment was most promising; the medical world ought to learn how to recognize the epileptic nature of the early phenomena. The symptoms that preceded the onset of major seizures, the initial symptoms with which major attacks began, and all the minor attacks appearing in the intervals between complete attacks were the main object of Herpin's study. Varied as the initial phenomena and the minor attacks might be, they showed a remarkable constancy in each individual patient. Fundamentally, they were the same thing: the as yet incomplete or aborted epileptic attack.

The traditional classification of epilepsy into idiopathic and sympathetic was no longer valid for Herpin. It had rested on physiological differences; Galen had distinguished the forms of epilepsy according to whether the seizures had their origin in a disease of the brain or in the involvement of an otherwise healthy brain by sympathy or irritation from ascending substances. Herpin claimed to go back to the ancient division into epilepsy from (a) an external part; (b) from the uterus, mouth, stomach, etc.; or (c) from the head or brain. Actually, however, he stripped the old scheme of its essence, leaving only the topographical differences regarding the onset of the attacks and thus adapting it to his own mode of thinking. An epileptic attack consisted of convulsions of voluntary muscles, of spasms of the visceral muscles, and of suspension of the senses and of consciousness. Accordingly, peripheral onsets, visceral onsets, and cerebral onsets formed the three chapters of the book.

There was consistency in this approach which did not admit a distinction between "real" epilepsy and other forms. The book is very modern in concentrating on the modes of onset of seizures. Although

---

[122] For biography cf. Müllener (717), pp. 69-72. Herpin's (487), *Du prognostic et du traitement curatif de l'épilepsie* of 1852 has been mentioned above, p. 285. Cf. Janz (561), p. XIII f., for Herpin's work on epilepsy.

Herpin's own interest was greatest in epileptic vertigo,[123] and although his book is famous for the delineation of what would now be called psychomotor attacks, it must not be overlooked that it also dealt with "Jacksonian epilepsy" and other forms. A few examples will illustrate Herpin's catholicity.

A consumptive ten-year-old girl "is seized by short and frequent episodes (accès) of cramp in the left arm without other nervous symptoms." Herpin tells the girl's attending physician that these are "incomplete episodes (accès) of epilepsy, and that some day she will have complete attacks if one does not succeed in curing these first occurrences (accidents). Indeed," he adds, "little by little, and in spite of the incredulity of my colleague, the tonic convulsion spreads over the whole left side of the body and is accompanied by jerky movements. Later, the convulsions become generalized, sometimes without loss of consciousness; and, finally, complete attacks appear, but very rarely." Herpin then describes in detail the kind of attack without loss of consciousness from which the girl now suffers.[124]

Regarding a visceral onset, there is, for instance, the case of a lady whose attacks have the following prelude: "First a sort of blow in the epigastrium followed by tension, constriction of the stomach; she is frightened and calls out; her heart beats forcefully and fast; she then flees to her room to escape notice; her thoughts begin to be confused; her words are incoherent; she sits down. The pupils are already dilated and fixed, she loses her sight, then her hearing, and consciousness disappears with the onset of tonic convulsions. The head turns to the right, the mouth is pulled in the same direction, and the eyes are turned upwards. The patient utters a cry and falls."[125]

Of the 300 epileptics who furnished the data for Herpin's book, 183 (61 per cent) showed attacks or incomplete episodes (accès) beginning with disturbance or suspension of the senses, mental troubles, and loss of consciousness. In 49 of these 183, the initial symptoms had their seat in the sense organs. Fifty-four had attacks or vertigo beginning with mental trouble or some "cerebral malaise." In another 54, "loss of the feeling of existence" was so complete at the very beginning that the patients did not remember any initial symptom. In the remaining 26 cases the incident began with a shock.[126]

This last category, to which Herpin devoted a special section, has as its prelude "a jolt (secousse) which shakes the whole body, as an elec-

---

[123]Herpin (486), *Des accès incomplets de'épilepsie*, p. 160, admitted having gone into such details that a résumé was needed, which he proceeded to give forthwith. See Appendix I for an English translation (by C. Lilian Temkin) of this résumé.

[124]*Ibid.*, p. 47 f.

[125]*Ibid.*, p. 91.

[126]*Ibid.*, p. 105 f.

tric shock would; this comparison is repeated by all patients who know from experience what an electric discharge is like."[127] The jolt can also be partial and limited to one or two arms, or to a single finger.[128] Often a psychic disturbance, even loss of consciousness, accompanies these jolts.

Of the many varieties of seizures with "cerebral onset" which Herpin described and which included all kinds of sensations and hallucinations, those with intellectual disturbances and with immediate loss of consciousness deserve notice.[129] One patient declared: "The trouble is purely intellectual; I am neither dazed nor giddy; I can still read words, but I no longer grasp their meaning. This is a most distressing condition; it seems to me that one part of my intellect witnesses the disorders of the other." To this Herpin added: "It would be impossible to define the partial delirium more clearly."[130]

In cases beginning with complete loss of consciousness, the mind does not necessarily abdicate completely, and co-ordinated movements may well be present.[131] One patient upon entering a church had an attack. Without being aware of it, he went through passages, climbed stairs, crossed a courtyard, went along one street and was turning into another when he began to regain awareness and found himself about 300 feet from the place where he must have lost consciousness.[132]

Herpin was not in charge of an asylum. He knew that epileptics could commit violent acts, but this did not preoccupy him as it did Morel and Falret. He was interested in epilepsy, not in psychiatry at large; his aim was therapy, his method clinical observation and numerical analysis. Pathological anatomy interested him, but where it might have given him a decisive lead, he shrank back.

Herpin rejected the belief that lesions in the peripheral parts where a sensation seemed to be located or where convulsions began could cause epilepsy.[133] One case from the literature[134] and one case with periph-

---

[127] *Ibid.*, p. 163.

[128] *Ibid.*, p. 168. The relationship of Herpin's observations to myoclonus epilepsy is discussed by Janz (561), p. 135 f.

[129] For more details see below, Appendix I.

[130] Herpin, *op. cit.*, p. 111.

[131] *Ibid.*, p. 121.

[132] *Ibid.*, p. 199 f.

[133] *Ibid.*, p. 30 f. In other words, he denied the existence of what was then called sympathetic or reflex epilepsy.

[134] A soldier had received a sabre wound on the head, followed many years later by convulsions. At first these affected the right little finger only; gradually they involved elbow, shoulder, and head; then there were complete epileptic attacks. A post-mortem dissection revealed on the left parietal bone the trace of the sabre wound to which a protuberating and seemingly carious piece of bone corresponded on the inside of the skull. In the same spot a large sanguine tumor existed subdurally. The tumor, embedded in the brain, reached almost as far as the base of the skull and strongly compressed the left ventricle. Herpin, *op. cit.*, p. 31 f. quoted this story from Odier's *Manuel de médecine pratique* (3ᵉ éd.; Geneva, 1821), p. 189.

eral onset from his own practice showed organic causes located in the brain. Several of his patients had more or less pronounced hemiplegic weakness of the part where the convulsions began; others also suggested cerebral lesions. "Thus," he wrote, "the facts tend to demonstrate that in the case of so-called sympathetic external epilepsy, the affection will often show itself to be bound to an organic lesion of the brain. Moreover, the localization of the first symptoms being always the same and their appearance isolated seem a priori to indicate a local cause which, as soon as it is not found in the organs that are the seat of these symptoms, must reside in a definite and unilateral point of the nervous centers. Epilepsies with peripheral onsets ought, therefore, more than the others, to have anatomical lesions of these centers for their cause." After having gone thus far, Herpin stops. "But it is necessary to guard against generalizing this origin too much. . . ."[135] There follow arguments against such generalization; he points to twelve cures in his own practice, of which two go back more than fourteen years, and other patients are on the road to health; since the attacks ceased a rather long time ago, the existence of organic lesions of the brain is not to be presumed in these cases.[136]

Hughlings Jackson, who had become acquainted with Herpin's book of 1852 at a relatively early date in his career, did not come across Herpin's work of 1867 until near the time when his own contribution to epilepsy was all but completed.[137] Then he advised the younger neurologists to study Herpin's writings carefully, and himself quoted copiously from Herpin's observations, for he wished to convince the readers of his earlier reports that they were not mere collections of scientific curiosities. "I wish to show by the quotations from Herpin that statements essentially the same as those I make were made by a great authority long ago."[138]

Jackson's generous admission that many of his own statements had been anticipated by Herpin was founded in fact as far as clinical observation was concerned. So much the preceding pages will have borne out. But here the similarity ended. Herpin remained a clinician studying the course of epilepsy and the opportunities for treatment. His observations as such, anatomical, physiological, and pathological, were valid, regardless of any hypotheses. This cannot be said of Jackson, whose clinical observations directed him to anatomy, physiology, and pathology, and then back to the bedside. The fact that he reasoned rather than dissected or experimented does not alter the essential scope of his work.

---

[135] Herpin, *op. cit.*, p. 36.

[136] *Ibid.*

[137] Jackson (556), *Selected Writings*, vol. 1, p. 469. The article is of 1899.

[138] *Ibid.*, p. 471.

# XII

# John Hughlings Jackson

In 1859 John Hughlings Jackson (1835-1911) came to London at a crucial point in his career.[139] He intended to give up medicine and to devote himself to a literary life; however, Jonathan Hutchinson persuaded him to revise this decision and succeeded in keeping him for medicine.[140] What Jackson's intellectual leanings at that time were, we do not know. Perhaps he stood under the influence of Laycock, with whom he had come into contact at the York Medical School,[141] and who, as early as 1840, had extended the theory of reflex action to the brain.[142] Perhaps he was acquainted with the ideas of Alexander Bain (1818-1903), one of the ablest protagonists of association psychology, and with those of George Henry Lewes (1817-78), one of the outstanding English positivists, for later Jackson was to quote these and other names in support of his own ideas.[143] Possibly he had already read Herbert Spencer (1820-1903), whose

---

[139] Jackson's life and career till 1864 have been re-examined by Greenblatt (424 and 425) who has traced the influences, both personal and scientific, to which Jackson was exposed.

[140] Hutchinson in Jackson (552), *Neurological Fragments*, p. 28, and Greenblatt (425), p. 354 f. Hutchinson said that Jackson intended "to engage in a literary life." It is unclear whether this should be understood in the light of Hutchinson's subsequent remark about the possibly greater gain to the world if Jackson "had been left to devote his mind to *philosophy*" (italics mine).

[141] I have in mind metaphysical interests, such as documented by Laycock (616), *An Essay on Hysteria*, ch. 5, p. 149 ff. For the possible date of Jackson's personal contact with Laycock see Greenblatt (425), pp. 348 f. and 352 f.

[142] See Amacher (28) for Laycock's ideas on reflex action and Greenblatt (425), *passim*, for Laycock's influence on Jackson.

[143] Jackson (556), *Selected Writings*, vol. 1, p. 167; cf. Greenblatt (425), p. 373. On Bain's influence cf. Young (1114), ch. 3.

*Principles of Psychology* had appeared in 1855, a book that became a veritable gospel for Jackson.[144] There is nothing to contradict the assumption, made probable by Jackson's later work, that from the beginning he inclined toward agnosticism regarding the relation of body and mind. Jackson never turned philosopher in the strict sense of the word, although he reverted to philosophy through the medium of neurology.

But in 1859 Jackson's dedication to medicine seemed complete. He became associated with various London hospitals, gave lectures on physiology,[145] and started his literary career in 1861 as a medical reporter rather than as a speculative thinker.

In that part of Jackson's work which bears directly on epilepsy,[146] we can distinguish three periods: the years from 1861 to 1863, during which he found his focus of interest; the period from 1864 until the appearance of his *Study on Convulsions* in 1870, during which he evolved step by step his own point of view; and the period after the *Study of Convulsions*, a period of revision, elaboration, and broadening of judgment.

Jackson's first publication on epilepsy concerned *Cases of Epilepsy Associated with Syphilis*. It contained reports from various hospitals and from medical literature, including, for instance, one of the cases which Todd had described and analyzed in his *Clinical Lectures on Paralysis*.[147] This first publication of Jackson's was indicative of his entire later work, for it related to unilateral epilepsy. "In most of the following cases," Jackson wrote, "the convulsions were limited to one side, and in one of them the epileptic fit was not complete, there being no loss of consciousness,"[148] and some of them, as we may add, showed lesions on the surface of the brain. In this year and the next (1861 and 1862), there followed more reports dealing with methods of treatment and, in 1863, cases which were under the direct care of Jackson.[149] Here again, most exhibited unilateral convulsions or localized spasms before the onset of the fully developed attack, and some showed defects of sight. "As a clinical fact, this [i.e., temporary defect of sight] is common in cases of epilepsy in which the convulsions are

---

[144]Cf. Langworthy (612), p. 575. Greenblatt (425), p. 373, however, has not been able to find a reference to Spencer before 1864, when Jackson quoted from an article published by Spencer in 1857 (and republished in 1858).

[145]Cf. Taylor in Jackson (552), *Neurological Fragments*, p. 3.

[146]For an analysis from a modern neurological point of view cf. Walshe (1062).

[147]Cf. Jackson (539), *Cases of Epilepsy Associated with Syphilis*, p. 649, and Todd (1027), *Clinical Lectures on Paralysis*, etc., pp. 381 ff. and 398 ff.

[148]Jackson, *ibid.*, p. 648.

[149]Cf. bibliography in Greenblatt (425), pp. 374-76.

unilateral."[150] The forms of aura and the progress of the convulsions were carefully described in Jackson's characteristic manner, which considered the minutest detail worth noticing. By 1863 Jackson had come to a definite conclusion regarding the morbid anatomy of unilateral convulsions. "In very many cases of epilepsy, and especially in syphilitic epilepsy, the convulsions are limited to one side of the body; and, as autopsies of patients who have died after syphilitic epilepsy appear to show, the cause is obvious organic disease on the side of the brain, opposite to the side of the body convulsed, frequently on the surface of the hemisphere."[151] Convulsions associated with syphilitic disease of the brain had been noticed as far back as the Renaissance. In the early sixties, epileptiform seizures in sufferers from general paralysis were studied carefully by Westphal[152] —but the syphilitic nature of this disease had not yet been demonstrated. Through his association with such leading British syphilologists as Hutchinson and Wilks, Jackson contributed to the pathology of this disease just as he contributed to the knowledge of epilepsy.[153] By 1863 he had joined the ranks of Bravais, Bright, Todd, and the others who had been studying partial convulsions. He had reached the same conclusions regarding the clinical and anatomical phenomena of these cases of epilepsy. He had developed his method of clinical analysis but had not yet made any decisive step beyond the knowledge of his forerunners. Such theoretical views as occurred reflected the opinions of Todd and Brown-Séquard;[154] he even seemed to accept the medulla oblongata as the primary seat of epilepsy.[155]

It is true that in 1863 he published (for private circulation) a pamphlet entitled *Suggestions for Studying Diseases of the Nervous System on Professor Owen's Vertebral Theory*, where he also discussed "epilepsies." In elaboration of Richard Owen's (1804–92) view of the segmental nature of the skull, he assumed that the vertebrae of the skull corresponded to a segmentation of bones, nerves, blood vessels, and muscles. Epilepsy could differ according to the vertebra affected. For instance, part of the medulla oblongata and the vagus nerve were the neural element of the occipital vertebra controlling the heart. There

---

[150]Jackson (558), *Unilateral Epileptiform Seizures, Attended by Temporary Defect of Sight*, p. 588.

[151]Jackson (544), *Convulsive Spasms of the Right Hand and Arm Preceding Epileptic Seizures*, p. 110.

[152]Westphal (1090), *Einige Beobachtungen über die epileptiformen und apoplektiformen Anfälle der paralytischen Geisteskranken.*

[153]Cf. Greenblatt (425), p. 360.

[154]Brown-Séquard with whom Jackson was associated at the National Hospital for the Paralysed and Epileptic, Queen Square, had persuaded Jackson to devote himself to neurology. Cf. Taylor and Hutchinson in Jackson (552), *Neurological Fragments*, pp. 3 and 29.

[155]Cf., e.g., Jackson (544), *Convulsive Spasms of the Right Hand*, etc. p. 110.

existed an interplay between ganglionic masses and the blood vessels which they regulated and from which, in turn, they received their nourishment. Therefore, a stoppage of the heart would affect the nutrition of the medulla oblongata and lead to epilepsy—in this case petit mal.[156] This was epilepsy of the occipital vertebra; other vertebrae had other epilepsies. "The full epileptic process" was "epilepsy of all the vertebrae." Any epilepsy was loss of function of the respective nervous part, "probably as Dr. Brown-Séquard points out, the contraction of the blood-vessels diminishing the quantity of the blood."[157]

Fantastic as the whole theory may sound now, it was not entirely out of line with Jackson's clinical experience and with opinions then current. He set great value on the examination of the eyes and was one of the first English physicians to recommend the use of the ophthalmoscope in neurological disorders. In a case of transient blindness in which subsequent headache was the only other symptom and in which the eyes showed no abnormality, his diagnosis "epilepsy of the retinae" probably depended on "contraction of the blood-vessels of the retinae."[158] This was another epilepsy depending on regional blood supply. Jackson then asked whether "in cases in which loss of sight is followed by the epileptic paroxysm, may we not say that the contraction of the blood-vessels has begun in an outpost of the cerebral circulation (the retina being supplied by branches of the same vessels as the brain, these vessels being supplied by the same vaso-motor nerves), and that, on extension to the other branches of the carotid, the 'brain's blindness,' loss of consciousness supervenes?"[159] This may be an illustration of the following remark that occurs in the Suggestions, and for which Jackson apparently did not depend on anybody else.[160] "In epilepsy, the sensitive fibres going to a diseased part of the brain, act not according to their proper correlation, producing a simple reflex action, but, as it were, the stimulus runs on to another part of greater or more central vitality, and induces diseased action."[161]

We now come to the important year, 1864, in which Jackson published his first major article on aphasia, and in which he also took a step forward in his concept of the pathology of epilepsy. These two sides of

---

[156] This puzzling explanation of petit mal by cardiac arrest may be an analogy with the syncope of the Adams-Stokes syndrome.

[157] The quotations are from Greenblatt's (425), p. 368 f., excerpt from Jackson's *Suggestions*, which was not available to me. A very extensive historical analysis of the *Suggestions* is given by Greenblatt (424), pp. 41–72, to which I am indebted for my understanding of this rare publication.

[158] Jackson (554), *Observations on Defects of Sight in Brain Disease*, p. 923.

[159] *Ibid.*

[160] Greenblatt (424), p. 67 ff., who has pointed out the significance of the following remark has not been able to find it in other writers of that time.

[161] Greenblatt (425), p. 369.

his activity were intimately connected. Three years before, Paul Broca had studied the case of an epileptic[162] suffering from motor aphasia and had localized the seat of the speech defect in the left third frontal convolution of the brain.[163] We may disregard in our context how far Jackson agreed or disagreed with Broca. It may suffice to say that at the very outset of his article he emphasized that "the convolution of articulate language of Broca is but one of many convolutions supplied by the left middle cerebral artery."[164] This artery also supplies the corpus striatum, and morbid changes in this artery seemed to explain a number of cases where unilateral convulsions were combined with defects of speech. In the first case, the patient suffered from "epileptic hemiplegia," loss of speech, and a valvular disease of the heart. Jackson conjectured that cases of this kind might be caused by emboli plugging the middle cerebral artery. The diminished blood supply would bring about the convulsions, for Jackson accepted Radcliffe's view "that convulsions depend on enfeebled power of the nervous centres, or diminution of blood supply, rather than on increased irritability or on congestion."[165] In the second case, unilateral seizures were combined with passing defects of speech. For the latter, Jackson coined the expression "epileptic aphemia." In this case no valvular disease could be diagnosed, so Jackson suggested that a spasm had been induced in the middle cerebral artery. Such spasm by reflex action might also, in his opinion, explain the cases of epileptic hemiplegia as observed by Todd, where, upon autopsy, the surface of the brain was found to be diseased.[166] To these cases Jackson linked a third type where unilateral convulsions and defects of speech were combined with an aura of disagreeable smell at the onset of the attack.[167] "When . . . we further consider that the left middle cerebral artery supplies (1) the roots of the olfactory bulb; (2) the corpus striatum; and (3) the hemispheres, we can readily understand how the three strangely associated symptoms should occur together in plugging of that vessel; and I submit that temporary spasm of the vessels in that arterial region would account for the three temporary symptoms in epileptiform seizures." Jackson realized that these views differed from the usual explanations. Regarding his assumption of spasm, he could defend himself by pointing out that "the theory of contraction of the blood-vessels in epilepsy is the established theory of

---

[162]Broca (160), *Remarques sur le siège de la faculté du langage articulé*, p. 343: "Il était sujet, depuis sa jeunesse, à des attaques d'épilepsie."

[163]*Ibid.*, p. 353.

[164]Jackson (550), *Loss of Speech*, p. 28.

[165]Jackson (551), *Loss of Speech, with Hemiplegia on the Left Side*, p. 167.

[166]Jackson (546), *Epileptic Aphemia*, etc., p. 167.

[167]Jackson (559), *Unilateral Epileptiform Seizures Beginning by a Disagreeable Smell*, p. 168.

the day. My view is only different in limiting it in certain cases to certain arterial regions of the brain."[168] Regarding the current opinion that epilepsy pointed to a diseased medulla oblongata, he did not exclude this possibility, "but" he added, "post-mortem examination shows that in unilateral convulsions the middle cerebral artery itself, or some part of the brain in its range, is diseased too."[169]

Jackson's conviction that the corpus striatum was the part affected in convulsions hardened in the following years. In 1866 Wilks, with whom Jackson was acquainted, hinted at the possibility that fibers of the motor tract might run downward directly from the cerebral cortex, and that damage to the hemispheres might cause epileptic fits without necessary intervention of the corpus striatum.[170] Yet as late as 1868, Jackson "believed the corpus striatum to be the part discharged in *convulsions* beginning unilaterally."[171] He did not doubt that the convolutions contained "processes representing movements,"[172] nor did he definitely deny involvement of the cortex. But his attention was focused upon the parallelism between unilateral epilepsy and hemiplegia.[173] In hemiplegia certain muscles were paralyzed and in unilateral epilepsy convulsed. Here was a good opportunity for comparison. If nerve tissue was destroyed, the muscles would be paralyzed, and if the nerve tissue were damaged so as to become unstable, the muscles would act in a disorderly fashion.[174] Later, Jackson found two convenient terms for designating the fundamental difference. Paralysis in ordinary hemiplegia was due to "destroying lesions"; convulsions, on the other hand, to "discharging lesions."[175] Where a discharging lesion existed, the gray matter would discharge from time to time explosively. After the discharge the gray matter would be exhausted, and this exhaustion would account for the paralysis in cases of epileptic hemiplegia.

Jackson's clinical analysis of unilateral epilepsy had taught him that a certain order prevailed in the onset and spread of the convulsions. Most frequently they started in the arm, and in that case the thumb and forefinger were affected first. "The order of frequency in the parts first affected is according to the order of 'intelligence,' so to speak."[176] How could this order be accounted for? Here Spencer had offered a possi-

---

[168] *Ibid.*

[169] Jackson (551), *Loss of Speech with Hemiplegia on the Left Side*, p. 167.

[170] Wilks (1105), *Observations on the Pathology of Some of the Diseases of the Nervous System*, pp. 168 and 169. Cf. above, p. 315.

[171] Jackson (556), *Selected Writings*, vol. 1, p. 38 (italics in text).

[172] *Ibid.*

[173] Cf., e.g., Jackson (553), *Note on Lateral Deviation of the Eyes*, etc., p. 311.

[174] Jackson (556), *Selected Writings*, vol. 2, p. 217.

[175] *Ibid.*, vol. 1, pp. 94 and 95.

[176] *Ibid.*, vol. 2, p. 216.

bility of understanding which Jackson accepted and elaborated. "As every student of the nervous system knows," Spencer wrote, "the combination of any set of impressions, or motions, or both, implies a ganglion in which the various nerve-fibres concerned are put in connection. To combine the actions of any set of ganglia, implies some ganglion in connection with them all. And so on in ever-ascending stages of complication: the nervous masses concerned, becoming larger in proportion to the complexity of the co-ordinations they have to effect." A few lines further on, Spencer added that "no physiologist . . . can long resist the conviction that different parts of the cerebrum subserve different kinds of mental action. Localization of function is the law of all organization whatever: separateness of duty is universally accompanied with separateness of structure: and it would be marvellous were an exception to exist in the cerebral hemispheres."[177] Jackson now assumed that all the parts of the body were represented "in *every* part of the corpus striatum and optic thalamus," but that the muscles involved in elaborate movements were "those most largely represented *throughout* these centres." Apart from this "localisation of superiority," as he called it, there also existed a "localisation of specialty . . . certain parts of the motor centre specially superintending certain movements."[178] On this latter principle it might be understood why spasms sometimes began in the foot or other parts than thumb and index-finger.

It was but one step now to the *Study of Convulsions*, in which Jackson outlined his views on unilateral convulsions in a more systematic way than before. At some time between 1868 and 1870, it occurred to him that instability of the gray matter of the cerebral convolutions might account for the convulsions. If we remember that long before Jackson had thought of disturbances in the region of the middle cerebral artery supplying some convolutions as well as the corpus striatum, the shift of emphasis is not so very startling.[179] Nor did he disregard the corpus striatum in favor of the cortex. For many years to come, the corpus striatum was still considered by him as a starting point of fits. Yet in 1870 he wrote: "Palsy depends on destruction of *fibres*, and convulsion on instability of *grey matter*. As the convolutions

---

[177]Spencer (941), *The Principles of Psychology*, pp. 606–7. Cf. also Jackson (555), *Remarks on the Disorderly Movements of Chorea and Convulsion*, etc.

[178]Jackson (556), *Selected Writings*, vol. 2, p. 216 (italics in text).

[179]Nevertheless, on the supposition that Jackson wrote the *Study on Convulsions* before the appearance of Fritsch and Hitzig's experiments, I am not able to account for the almost sudden shift of emphasis from the corpus striatum to the cortex. A possible hint is given in the following passage from his (547) *Epileptic or Epileptiform Seizures Occurring with Discharge from the Ear*, p. 591: "In convulsions beginning unilaterally, we may compare and contrast the hemispasm with hemiplegia: in other words, we may compare the effects of discharge of, *or through*, the corpus striatum with the effects of destruction of the corpus striatum" (italics mine).

are rich in grey matter I suppose them to be to blame, in *severe* convulsions at all events; but as the corpus striatum also contains much grey
matter I cannot deny that it may be sometimes the part to blame in
slighter convulsions. Indeed, if the discharge does begin in convolutions,
no doubt the grey matter of lower motor centres, even if these centres
be healthy, will be discharged secondarily by the violent impulse received from the primary discharge. Now both these parts—the corpus
striatum and many convolutions—are supplied by one artery, the
middle cerebral or Sylvian, and this artery circumscribes the region I
speak of."[180]

It would be repetitious to analyze the *Study of Convulsions* in detail;
it will suffice to give a brief summary of those parts which deal with the
"cause" of unilateral convulsions. Jackson distinguishes four "causes"
which are highly characteristic for his point of view.[181] There is first of
all "the seat of the internal lesion" to be considered, i.e., the existence
of a localized lesion in the cortex (or corpus striatum) which causes the
localized spasms. The muscular group affected points to the localization
of the morbidly changed nerve tissue, while the "condition" of the
muscles reveals the "functional nature" of the change. By the latter,
Jackson means whether the nerve tissue is destroyed or whether it is
unstable, a difference marked by either palsy or choreatic or convulsive
movements of the muscles. The functional nature of the change in
nerve tissue is the second cause. He separates it carefully from the third
cause, the "pathological process" which has brought about the functional change, and which can be an embolus, a tumor, syphilitic disease,
or any other coarse disease. The fourth and last cause is the "circumstances which determine the paroxysm," the provocative or exciting
cause in the conventional terminology of pathologists. Jackson's explanation of the mechanism by which exciting causes produce convulsions is so important that it had best be given in his own words.

> We may say of all nerve tissue, healthy and diseased, that it
> acquires by nutrition a condition of unstable equilibrium, but dis-
> charge in health is a consequence of excitations which are *special*.
> The discharge of a *highly unstable* patch in disease may, I believe,
> be brought about by very general excitations. That is, I presume,
> the belief of those who attribute fits to excitement, flatulence,
> etc. . . . All these general causes, I presume, act by altering the
> circulation in the head, during which alteration the equilibrium of
> the unstable patch is upset. I suppose this must be the explanation
> of the effect which dyspepsia, fright, etc., have in "causing" con-
> vulsion limited to one side. They can only alter the bodily condi-
> tion generally. They cannot, at least, pick out one side of the

---

[180] Jackson (556), *Selected Writings*, vol. 1, p. 9 (italics in text).
[181] *Ibid.*, p. 23 ff.

brain. They must affect both its sides equally, and yet the equilibrium of the side diseased only will be upset, because on that side only is there nerve tissue which is in a condition to explode on slight and general provocation. I believe such general conditions are only exciting causes of the paroxysm—that they only determine the beginning of the discharge, which when begun leads to further and further discharges in the vascular region in which the unstable nerve tissue lies.[182]

Thus, we have followed Jackson's work on unilateral epilepsy from its beginnings, in 1861, to 1870. This phase of his work left a lasting impression. In 1870 Fritsch and Hitzig published their investigations *On the Electric Excitability of the Cerebrum*. They discovered the motor area of the hemispheres in dogs; they demonstrated that localized groups of muscles could be irritated by the application of weak electric currents upon a very small region of the hemisphere and that application of stronger currents or prolonged application would lead to convulsions as an after-effect. These convulsions might begin locally and develop into "well characterized epileptic attacks."[183] Here indeed was experimental proof for Jackson's clinical observations and pathological inferences. Then Ferrier's (1843–1928) experimental work followed and anatomical investigations of the conductive fibers, all of which gave a sound basis for Jackson's contention that localized convulsions indicated localized injuries of the convolutions, and that the convulsions might spread if the discharge involved more and more nervous tissue. Ferrier insisted that as a result of his and Jackson's work the dualistic pathology of epilepsy should be abandoned.[184] But recognition of "Jacksonian epilepsy" did not necessarily mean acceptance of Jackson's views on epilepsy in general.

Unilateral convulsions dependent on coarse disease had been considered atypical cases of epilepsy. Whether the existence of idiopathic epilepsy was admitted or not, it was the seizure with generalized convulsions and loss of consciousness, or at least a minor seizure with

---

[182] *Ibid.*, p. 35 (italics in text).

[183] Fritsch and Hitzig (381), *Ueber die elektrische Erregbarkeit des Grosshirns*, p. 18.

[184] Ferrier (353), *Experimental Researches in Cerebral Physiology and Pathology*, p. 90: "And now that the motor signification of the grey matter of the hemispheres is clearly demonstrated, it is not necessary to assume that the medulla oblongata is the primary seat of the motor disturbances, while the psychical symptoms are only subordinate to changes induced in the circulation of the brain by a primary affection of the medulla itself." Statements like these were attacked by the followers of the more traditional doctrine. With reference to Hitzig's experiments, Nothnagel (741), *Epilepsy and Eclampsia*, p. 207, wrote that they "must of course be entirely disregarded in the inquiry as to the causation of epilepsy, although these experiments were repeated by Ferrier and others, and even made use of in theories of epilepsy" (Emerson's translation). As late as 1881, Bubnoff and Heidenhain (180), *Ueber Erregungs-und Hemmungsvorgänge innerhalb der motorischen Hirncentren*, still thought it necessary to prove the direct electric excitability of the cortex. In their excursus on epilepsy, pp. 170–74, they counted with the possibility that the cortex, in turn, might stimulate something like a *Krampfzentrum* in the region of the pons and the medulla oblongata (p. 173).

dimmed consciousness, which the pathologists before Jackson tried to explain in the first place. Jackson chose the very opposite approach. Unilateral convulsions were the simplest form of epileptic attacks, and it was from them that the study of epilepsy had to proceed. This meant a radical break with the usual concept of epilepsy. The new departure was already indicated in terms like "epileptic aphemia," which Jackson began to use in 1864.[185] Two years later he began to attack the nosological concept of epilepsy vigorously.

> Indeed, Dr. Jackson suggests that the word "epilepsy" should be degraded, and be used to imply the condition of nerve tissue in sudden and temporary loss of its function, whether that be loss of sight, loss of consciousness, or "running down of tension" in those parts which govern muscles. For it is not unlikely that the condition of nerve tissue is the same or similar (although this is not taken for granted) when a patient loses sight for, as he says, half a minute, or has temporary loss of consciousness, or becomes unable to talk for a short time, or has spasm of the hand, or of the side of the face, or of the leg, or of all three on one side. Probably, too, in cases in which a man all at once passes into a violent rage from no apparent cause, or into a state somewhat like somnambulism, in which he may walk a mile or two, or walk into a canal, or in which he takes off his boots in church, or undresses himself in the streets, there is epilepsy—using the word in the new sense—of some parts of the hemisphere.[186]

All such nosological entities as "genuine epilepsy" and "chorea" were, therefore, impediments rather than a guide for correct understanding. They misled the student into comparisons with more or less artificial entities, whereas he should in every case try to find out what functional changes in the nervous system might account for the symptoms of the patient. For such considerations as these the *Study on Convulsions* dealt with unilateral convulsions only and yet claimed to be a methodical study of the subject in general.[187] And considerations like these, as well as the insight won into the nature of convulsions, led Jackson a little later (1873) to the following broad definition of epilepsy: *"Epilepsy is the name for occasional, sudden, excessive, rapid and local discharges of grey matter."*[188] According to this definition there was no one disease epilepsy, but many epilepsies, an expression Jackson frequently used. Even "a sneeze is a sort of healthy epilepsy" as Jackson said,[189] and migraine certainly also belonged in this group. In a modi-

---

[185] Cf. above, p. 332.

[186] Jackson (541), *Clinical Remarks on Cases of Temporary Loss of Speech*, etc., p. 442. Cf. also Jackson (556), *Selected Writings*, vol. 1, p. 4 f.

[187] Jackson (556), *Selected Writings*, vol. 1, p. 8.

[188] *Ibid.*, p. 100.

[189] *Ibid.*, p. 96.

fied form, Jackson had returned to an idea already found in his *Suggestions* of 1864.[190]

Jackson's task now was to explain different forms of epilepsies anatomically and physiologically. In 1866 already, he suggested that in "cases of sudden and temporary loss of consciousness in which convulsive movements were slight, or perhaps absent, the disorder of function was chiefly in the range of the anterior cerebral artery."[191] After 1870 he wrote more frequently and more extensively on other than unilateral epilepsies. Cases where consciousness was lost at the outset of the attack he saw as "beginning in the *very highest* nervous centres of the cerebral hemisphere."[192] In other words, genuine epilepsy was not essentially different from unilateral epilepsy. In the latter the discharge started in a cerebral area which represented muscular movements; and if in an attack beginning unilaterally, consciousness was lost, a higher area representing the most varied muscular movements as well as mental operations had become involved. In genuine epilepsy, with sudden loss of consciousness and general convulsions, it was the other way round. In a somewhat similar way he also explained "temporary mental disorders after epileptic paroxysms,"[193] from states of slight confusion to attacks of homicidal mania. All actions performed in such conditions were automatic, and their explanation rested on the principle of "dissolution" which Jackson had taken over from Spencer.[194] On the principle of evolution, voluntary actions were the most varied, and the last to develop. If the reverse process of dissolution set in, the highest coordinating centers would be affected first and the automatic actions alone would go on. This was the case in mental disorders after paroxysms. Voluntary control was lost and mere automatisms, i.e., unconscious actions, remained. The slighter the paroxysm removing control the more complex the automatism afterward. From a medical point of view it did not matter whether the automatic acts were harmless or violent. These theories on mental disorders were significant because they illustrated the principle of abnormal movements and actions resulting from inhibition of higher controlling centers, and because in Jackson's opinion they paved a way for the understanding of insanity.

We have done no more than indicate some of the milestones on Jackson's new road of investigation in the years between 1870 and 1875. That it was a new road he was fully aware. "I have not simply

---

[190]Cf. above, p. 330 f.

[191]Jackson (542), *Clinical Remarks on the Occasional Occurrence of Subjective Sensations of Smell*, etc., p. 660.

[192]Jackson (556), *Selected Writings*, vol. 1, p. 121 footnote.

[193]*Ibid.*, pp. 119-34. Cf. especially pp. 122-24.

[194]According to Broadbent (159), p. 309, Jackson began to mention evolution from 1868 on. As Jackson himself stated, he had taken over the term of "dissolution" from Spencer's *First Principles*. Cf. Jackson (556), *Selected Writings*, II, p. 5.

repeated accepted doctrines with slight variations and new illustrations. Working on a novel method, I run continual risk of making novel blunders. But in thinking for one's self there are certain kinds of blunders which almost must be made. And it is always easy to avoid appearing to go far wrong if one does not go far from the beaten track."[195] This new road was the study of epilepsies as departures from health,[196] as disease considered as an experiment of nature parallel to the artificial experiment of the physiologist.[197] It was the purely scientific—though highly speculative—approach, and the continuous redefinitions, corrections, and broadening of aspect which appear in his writings are a consequence of his travelling along new paths.

The purely physiological in contrast to the nosological study of epilepsy prevailed in Jackson's work until about the middle of the seventies. At this time Jackson began to feel that his definition, though sound from a scientific point of view, did not satisfy practical demands. Influenced by an article by Moxon,[198] he now believed in the necessity for two kinds of classification, a scientific and an empirical. He illustrated the difference by alluding to the botanist and gardener. The former classifies plants scientifically, the latter from a utilitarian point of view. Medicine as a science needs a classification that advances knowledge; medicine as an art must have a clinical, practical, even if arbitrary, classification. Speaking anatomically and physiologically, epileptic vertigo, petit mal, and grand mal are but differences in strength of a discharge "beginning in and spreading from the same parts of the brain."[199] Yet speaking empirically, they are the three classes of "epilepsy proper."[200] From this the "epileptiform or epileptoid" group—"(1) Convulsions beginning unilaterally. (2) Unilateral Dysaesthesia (migraine). (3) Epileptiform Amaurosis, etc."—has to be differentiated.[201]

Thus the old distinction between epilepsy proper and epileptiform seizures was readmitted by Jackson. It did not contradict his scientific definition, yet there was no connecting link between the two. About ten years later he had to make another concession to older beliefs: he had to acknowledge "that *some* convulsions . . . depend on lesions of the pons or medulla oblongata."[202] Convulsions of this kind, for instance laryngismus stridulus in children, were neither epileptic nor epileptiform. To include them in any general classification necessitated

[195]Jackson (556), *Selected Writings*, vol. 1, p. 78.

[196]*Ibid.*, p. 4 ff.

[197]*Ibid.*, p. 77 ff.

[198]Cf. *ibid.*, p. 190.

[199]*Ibid.*, p. 193.

[200]*Ibid.*, p. 199.

[201]*Ibid.*, p. 200.

[202]*Ibid.*, p. 348 (italics in text).

the adoption of a more comprehensive term, and Jackson chose the very old-fashioned term "fits," On the other hand, it also required the adoption of a very broad view of "the hierarchy of centres of the nervous system."[203] This he found in the concept of "evolutionary levels" elaborated from Spencer's ideas, which had played an ever increasing role in Jackson's thought since the late sixties.[204] The Lumleian Lectures *On Convulsive Seizures* present his theory of epilepsy in an advanced form. Before considering them we must, however, remember that by 1890, the year when they were read, the work of Charcot, Horsley, Macewen, Sherrington and many other neurologists and surgeons had supplied Jackson with a host of new data which he could use to give anatomical precision to his doctrines.

The central nervous system consists, for Jackson, of three levels, each of them sensorimotor and each representing "impressions and movements of all parts of the body."[205] The lowest level consists of the spinal cord, the medulla oblongata, and the pons, roughly speaking, the " 'spinal system' of Marshall Hall."[206] It represents the simplest movements. The "motor province" of the middle level "is composed of centres of the Rolandic region (so-called 'motor region' of the cerebral cortex), and, possibly, of the ganglia of the corpus striatum also. It represents complex movements of all parts of the body from eyes to perineum (re-represents)."[207] The highest level (i.e., its "motor province") is formed by the centers of the prefrontal lobes, the "organ of mind." They are the "acme of evolution," and this level "re-re-represents" all movements, which here become most complex.[208]

Discharges may start from any of the three levels; hence there are three kinds of fits: lowest level fits, middle, and highest level fits. This evolutionary classification (if we may use this expression) can be translated into the language of the clinician. Lowest level fits are "pontobulbar fits,"[209] which comprise "respiratory fits" (e.g., the experimental convulsions of Kussmaul and Tenner), "*fits produced by convulsant poisons*" (e.g., by camphor or absinthe), and "*a condition for fits consequent on certain injuries of the cord or sciatic nerve* in guinea-pigs" (such as produced by Brown-Séquard).[210] Discharges starting in the lowest level need not be limited to it. Through the intermediation of ascending fibers, centers of higher levels can also be discharged. Connec-

---

[203] *Ibid.*, p. 413.

[204] Cf. above, footnote 194.

[205] Jackson (556), *Selected Writings*, vol. 1, p. 413.

[206] *Ibid.*

[207] *Ibid.*, p. 414.

[208] *Ibid.*

[209] *Ibid.*, p. 415.

[210] *Ibid.*, p. 416 f.

tions between cells of the same level, and between different levels, allow any discharge, wherever it may start, to spread and involve neighboring as well as more distant parts of the cerebral nervous system. This is particularly important in considering middle and highest level fits, where the original discharging lesion may be confined to a few cells.[211]

Middle level fits are *epileptiform* seizures, and highest level fits are *epileptic* seizures. Epileptiform fits are those which we now usually designate as Jacksonian epilepsy.[212] For obvious reasons, Jackson did not employ this term, nor did he permit the designation of cortical epilepsy. "I do not use the term 'cortical epilepsy,' because both epilep*tic* and epilep*tiform* seizures are, to my thinking, cortical fits"[213]—though starting from (hypothetically) different parts of the cortex. Using the term epileptic as distinct from epileptiform, Jackson, on his own admission, reverted to the common nomenclature. "I formerly used the term 'epilepsy' generically for all excessive discharges of the cortex and their consequences ... I now use the term 'epilepsy' for that neurosis which is often called 'genuine' or 'ordinary' epilepsy, and for that only."[214] But the practical concession to clinical diagnosis did not mean any scientific concessions. On the contrary, the essay *On Convulsive Seizures* and some other articles, e.g., *On Post-epileptic States*, written not long before, show that in Jackson's opinion epileptiform and epileptic seizures could be explained on closely parallel lines. What was true of epileptiform attacks was also true of epileptic attacks, the difference in symptoms being mainly due to differences in the seat of the discharging lesion.

Epileptiform fits start from a definite place. Adopting a term of Seguin's, Jackson calls the place of onset "the signal symptom."[215] The fits may vary in range and may involve the whole body, but it is always the signal symptom which localizes the original discharging lesion and which, therefore, is of utmost importance to the brain surgeon.[216] Sometimes crude sensations are felt in the place of onset before the start of convulsions.[217] To understand this phenomenon it is necessary to keep in mind that (according to Jackson) all levels are sensorimotor.

---

[211] *Ibid.*, p. 417 f.

[212] Strictly speaking the term "epileptiform" was a misnomer for this type of fits. Epileptiform attacks are those which look like ordinary epileptic attacks, though not caused by epilepsy. Whatever we may think of the nosological concept underlying such a definition, the term epileptiform should not be used (as in Jackson) for attacks which are somehow different from ordinary fits. Their designation as "Jacksonian attacks" offered a convenient way out of these difficulties.

[213] *L.c.*, p. 415.

[214] *Ibid.*, p. 416, footnote 1.

[215] *Ibid.*, p. 424.

[216] *Ibid.*, p. 428.

[217] *Ibid.*, p. 425.

There are provinces which are predominantly motor, like the motor region of the middle level and the prefrontal lobes of the highest level, while others are predominantly sensory. But no part is exclusively motor or sensory; hence sensations may precede the appearance of epileptiform as well as epileptic attacks (various forms of aura in the broad sense). If, on the other hand, the discharge takes place in a predominantly sensory province, as is the case in migraine, sensations will predominate.

The cells of the discharging lesion are diseased. Their disease is brought about by "morbid nutrition,"[218] which in turn can be the effect of various pathological processes. Their morbid condition causes the cells to discharge excessively and too readily. These cells have become a "mad part," and while the discharge spreads, other "sane cells" are made to "act madly." "The more excessive the discharge the severer the fit."[219] In principle this explains the varieties of both epileptiform and epileptic fits. If there is excessive and swift discharge in the middle level, resistance of neighboring stable cells will be easily overcome, and the convulsions will quickly extend over a wide range of the body.[220] If the discharge starting from the highest level is relatively slight, a slight loss of consciousness will result, and the attack will have the form of the petit mal. If, on the other hand, the attack is excessive, a severe epileptic fit with loss of consciousness and violent convulsions will take place.[221]

The symptoms mentioned so far are the direct consequence of the overactivity of diseased cells. After these cells have discharged, they lose their function temporarily and form a "negative lesion."[222] Therefore, paralysis, "sensory or motor, or both,"[223] is present after every seizure, whether epileptiform or epileptic. In epileptiform fits, the paralysis is limited in range, while in epileptic fits it extends over the whole body. "Indeed, I submit that the whole condition of bodily impotence after a severe epileptic fit is paralysis, and that, speaking generally, there is really more paralysis than is found after severe epileptiform seizures."[224]

Paralysis and coma are not the only result of the negative state of the diseased cells. The latter in addition lose control over lower centers. The cells of these lower centers are perfectly healthy, they do not

[218] *Ibid.*, p. 429.
[219] *Ibid.*, pp. 432 and 433.
[220] *Ibid.*, p. 433 f.
[221] *Ibid.*, p. 432.
[222] *Ibid.*, p. 429.
[223] *Ibid.*, p. 421.
[224] *Ibid.*, p. 445.

discharge excessively. Yet, being no longer under control, they become overactive. Hence we have a combination of negative and positive symptoms. In epileptiform fits paralysis may exist, while at the same time the tendon reflexes are increased.[225] In epileptic fits all the degrees of post-epileptic states may be explained on the basis of this principle, and the explanation of post-epileptic states, moreover, forms a pattern for the explanation of insanities in general.

For the understanding of post-epileptic states the assumption of three levels does not suffice. They all proceed from lesions of the highest centers and all involve disturbances of consciousness. But the degree to which consciousness is impaired varies, and in order to explain this variance, Jackson imagines the highest centers to be made up of four layers which, as he frankly admits, do not correspond to any structural division of the cortex.[226] But the principle of evolution on which the division into three levels was assumed also holds good with regard to the layers of the highest centers. Therefore, morbid processes can also be explained as the reverse process, viz., dissolution of higher layers while the evolutionary lower layers remain functioning.

If the first layer, subsequent to discharge, is incapacitated, the dissolution has reached its first depth. Consciousness is now impaired but not lost, since the second layer remains active. The patient suffers from a "confusion of thought," a condition which includes the "dreamy state."[227] If dissolution reaches the second depth, the patient loses consciousness. Yet his actions are not completely stopped, since the third and fourth layer have not been affected. Such a patient might present the picture of epileptic mania. If dissolution reaches the third layer, the patient is in a coma and his "vital operations" alone persist.[228] It is easy to see how Jackson could adapt this schema to insanities in general. There is one point above all which he stresses again and again: In post-epileptic states as well as insanities, the actions of the patient, that is the positive symptoms, are correlated to those layers which have remained intact.[229] It is just the part which is healthy—though out of control—that accounts for the insane behavior. Compared to a normal person in whom all the layers act smoothly, the

---

[225] *Ibid.*, p. 444.

[226] *Ibid.*, p. 380.

[227] For details see below.

[228] Jackson, *l.c.*, p. 380.

[229] The underlying principle, as Jackson (556), *Selected Writings*, vol. 1, p. 123 footnote 1, stressed, had been developed by Monro, Laycock, Anstie, and Thompson Dickson. *Ibid.*, p. 184, he cited Anstie's (37), *Stimulants and Narcotics*, p. 80, assertion that apparent stimulating action of certain drugs actually consisted in the removal of controlling influences. Anstie, *ibid.*, pp. 78–81, had in mind alcohol, opium, and hashish, whose immediate effect was paralyzing rather than stimulating.

mental patient is certainly "insane." But the insanity is simply the result of dissolution of higher, and overactivity of lower, layers. "The insane man is a different person from his sane self,"[230] that is, he acts as might be expected from a person living on a lower evolutionary plane.

Jackson's theory, which accounted for all kinds of convulsive "fits" as well as for insanity, was strictly neurological. The unity of this theory rested heavily on speculation. Of this fact Jackson was fully aware. He knew that his distinction of evolutionary levels and layers was schematic and not supported by anatomical data. The whole concept of evolution so fundamental for his views was, after all, a theory rather than a fact. But in details, Jackson owed much to an assembly of information from various sources, as is shown by the development of his concept of "dreamy state" and its relationship to an uncinate group of fits. In a reminiscing vein Jackson, in 1888, confessed that he had formerly underrated the dreamy state. He quoted from a publication of 1875 in which he had described a patient's harmless automatism in the latter's own words: "[my sister-in-law found me] standing by the table mixing *cocoa* in a dirty gallipot, half-filled with bread and milk intended for the cat, and stirring the mixture with a mustard-spoon, which I must have gone to the cupboard to obtain."[231] Jackson had failed to mention that "at the onset of his fits the patient had 'a sort of dreamy state coming on suddenly.' "[232] The analogy with "dreams" had certainly been in Jackson's mind (and that of others before him), for in the same article of 1875 he said of such "mental automatism" that the patients' acts were external signs of "epileptic dreams."[233] He argued against the assumption of a masked epilepsy and contended that these automatisms were preceded by epileptic fits possibly too slight to be discovered. "The highest or controlling centres" having been put out of use, lower nervous centers became overactive.[234]

It seems that Jackson accepted the term "dreamy state" from his patients, perhaps the one just mentioned. In a short report of 1876 a number of expressions, obviously used by patients, for the "so-called intellectual aura" are mentioned from Jackson's case-books: " 'Old

---

[230] Jackson (556), *Selected Writings*, vol. 1, p. 383.

[231] The patient's original story [Jackson (556), *Selected Writings*, vol. 1, p. 126] continued: "This caused them to send for my friends, to whom I talked, showing no surprise that they were there, and entirely unconscious of what I had been doing until told this morning."

[232] Jackson (556), *Selected Writings*, vol. 1, p. 390.

[233] *Ibid.*, vol. 1, p. 122.

[234] *Ibid.*, p. 122: "There is what is called the *masked* epilepsy, described by Falret" (italics in the text). The neurologist Jackson was interested in the explanation of automatisms rather than in the social significance of the acts (crimes) which fascinated Morel, Falret, and Maudsley.

scenes revert.' 'I fell in some strange place' (a boy expressed it—'in a strange country'). *'A dreamy state.'* 'A panorama of something familiar and yet strange.' 'If I were walking along and had a fit, I should think 'Oh, I saw that before!' "[235] Jackson objected to calling such experiences intellectual aura, because they were not comparable to ordinary warnings, like crude sensations of smell, which resulted from the epileptic discharge of the highest center. Rather, he thought, they were owing to overactivity of next lower centers, as yet untouched by the discharge. Careful investigation might reveal various symptoms preceding "these vague 'reminiscenses' or 'reveries.' "[236]

Jackson's terminology and way of thinking were reflected in an article of 1886 by Dr. James Anderson with the descriptive title: *On Sensory Epilepsy. A case of basal Cerebral Tumour, affecting the Left Temporo-Sphenoidal Lobe, and giving rise to a Paroxysmal Taste-sensation and Dreamy State.* The patient had "a rough bitter sensation" in his mouth which preceded the feeling of something passing along the arm, shoulder and back of the brain," frequently accompanied by shivering. In the early stages of his illness, he always saw a childhood scene: a neighbor scolding him while he was there with other children to play. After this scene had ceased to appear, the patient still heard voices engaged in conversation.[237] Dr. Anderson believed that "the first part of the cortex involved by the tumour" was "the tip of the gyrus uncinatus," where Ferrier had located the centers of taste and smell.[238] Jackson, who for several weeks had had the patient under his care at the London Hospital,[239] stated that this was the only time that a necropsy had shown a local morbid change in a case of dreamy state.[240] Later, more necropsy results became available with involvement of the uncinate gyrus and of a wider area of the temporal lobe, with olfactory sensations or tasting movements, with or without mental automatisms,[241] so that around 1898 Jackson began to speak of the "uncinate group of epileptic fits."[242] Admittedly, this was a very inexact anatomical designation, "for some cells of different parts of a region of which this gyrus is part" were included. Primarily, this group comprised crude sensations of smell or of taste, or movements like chewing and

---

[235] *Ibid.*, p. 274 (italics mine). *Ibid.*, p. 386, Jackson repeats that the "adjective 'dreamy' " is sometimes used by the patients.

[236] *Ibid.*, pp. 274 f., cf. also p. 386.

[237] See Anderson (32), *On Sensory Epilepsy*, p. 385 f.

[238] *Ibid.*, p. 394.

[239] *Ibid.*, p. 388.

[240] Jackson (556), *Selected Writings*, vol. 1, p. 386 f.

[241] *Ibid.*, pp. 408–11, 458–63.

[242] *Ibid.*, pp. 462 and 467.

smacking of the lips. As to the dreamy state, it existed "in the paroxysms of many, *not of all*, cases of the uncinate group of epileptic
fits."[243]

Such details throw some light on the way in which Jackson's work
proceeded. They must not becloud the fact that Jackson's neurological
account of epilepsy and insanity rested on philosophical views which
had their limitations, as becomes clear when his contribution is viewed
within the context of neurology and psychiatry around 1880.

---

[243] *Ibid.*, p. 467 (italics mine). See also Jackson (552), *Neurological Fragments*, pp. 174-79,
and Feindel and Penfield (348) pp. 605-6. Janz (561), p. 167 ff., has discussed the development of Jackson's views regarding dreamy states and the uncinate group of fits in considerable
detail.

# XIII
# The End of the Falling Sickness?

## 1. IDIOPATHIC EPILEPSY

The recognition of Jacksonian epilepsy as a type of seizure associated with gross organic disease of the brain separated it from the majority of cases of epilepsy, which did not reveal gross organic disease. For some time past, sclerosis in the region of the temporal lobe had been suspected in genuine epilepsy. In 1825, Bouchet and Cazauvieilh had collected a number of cases with changes in the Cornu Ammonis.[244] The discussion was revived by Meynert (1833-92) in 1867,[245] and in 1880 the whole literature on the role of the Horn of Ammon was reviewed by Sommer, who believed that its lesions were associated with sensory symptoms.[246] But leading authorities of the early eighties were not willing to accept Meynert's results.[247] However much pathologists might continue looking for

---

[244]Bouchet et Cazauvieilh (140), *De l'épilepsie considérée dans ses rapports avec l'aliénation mentale*, p. 515 ff. and synopsis on pp. 540-42. Induration of the horn of Ammon was noted in four cases, softening in one.

[245]Meynert (695), *Der Bau der Gross-Hirnrinde*, p. 59: "Ein Rindengebeit (die Hakenwindung) besteht einzig aus den Pyramiden. An eine eminente motorische Störung (Epilepsie und epileptiforme Krämpfe) knüpft sich constante Erkrankung dieses Rindengebietes." In 1876 Meynert (696), *Skizzen*, p. 14, insisted that indurations in the neighborhood of the posterior horn of the lateral ventricle exerted a morbid influence upon the vascular innervation and irritability of the brain. This was related to his view of epilepsy as hyperesthesia of a vascular center.

[246]Sommer (936), *Erkrankung des Ammonshorns als aetiologisches Moment der Epilepsie.*

[247]Gowers (420), *Epilepsy and Other Chronic Convulsive Diseases*, p. 199 f. Strümpell (966), *Lehrbuch der speciellen Pathologie und Therapie der inneren Krankheiten*, vol. 2, 1., p. 415. Eulenburg (333), *Lehrbuch der Nervenkrankheiten*, p. 634. For some of the subsequent discussion see Turner (1035), pp. 173-78, Bratz (147), Corsellis (241), Falconer et al. (340).

anatomical changes,[248] idiopathic epilepsy could not be traced to gross organic disease of the brain, and Jacksonian epilepsy, therefore, remained a type per se.

Physiological methods also failed to explain the etiology of idiopathic epilepsy. Some information was gathered by means of experiments with convulsant drugs such as absinth. For instance, through a window made in the skull of dogs Magnan observed the circulatory status of the brain and found vaso-dilatation rather than constriction at the stage corresponding to loss of consciousness and tonic convulsions in man.[249] Experiments of this kind broadened the knowledge obtained from various toxic forms of epilepsy, such as uremia (internally) and lead poisoning (externally), which had been well studied for many decades[250] and which, possibly, had even been observed in Antiquity.[251] So much was clear: epilepsy unaccompanied by visible changes in the brain had many causes which, as their very number indicated, had to be considered exciting causes only. Heredity, however, formed a predisposing cause, as was generally admitted in scientific as well as in popular literature.[252]

The statistics of the time suggested inheritance in about 30 per cent.[253] This high figure, with which few other diseases could compete, seemingly offered supporting evidence for the existence of a distinct disease, the result of some as yet unknown condition of the brain and evidenced by disordered function.

The heredity of idiopathic epilepsy raised some interesting problems. What was inheritable and how? As to the first part of the question, the prevailing opinion did not insist on the transmission of epilepsy as a specific disease. As earlier in the century, all kinds of disorders appearing in the family, including even consumption, were considered.[254] The second question, viz., how the neuropathic taint was passed on, was even more difficult to answer and usually did not receive any clear answer at all.

---

[248]Echeverria (311), On Epilepsy, represents a valiant effort.

[249]Magnan (659), Leçons cliniques sur l'épilepsie, p. 15.

[250]Cf. Tanquerel des Planches (992), Lead Diseases.

[251]Paulus of Aegina (778), ed. Heiberg III, 43, 5; vol. 1, p. 239, transl. by Adams (779), vol. 1, p. 534, describes a form of epidemic colic which in many cases terminated in "epilepsy." I owe this reference to the courtesy of Dr. Lloyd Stevenson.

[252]Cf. Kipling's (583a), The Post that Fitted, above, Part Three, footnote 152.

[253]Gowers (420), Epilepsy, p. 8; his own figures indicated nearly 36 per cent.

[254]See above, IX-1b. Cf. Echeverria (311), On Epilepsy, p. 191 ff. On p. 175 he writes: "Lucas, Moreau de Tours, Baillarger, Morel, Herpin, Guislain, Griesinger, Briquet, Trousseau, and several more, have adduced facts establishing such successive transformation of every kind of neurosis into epilepsy, insanity, hysteria, locomotor ataxy, paralysis, etc., from parent to offspring." Gowers, l.c., pp. 7-12, while excluding apoplexy and hemiplegia, still seriously discusses the relationship to phthisis.

Hughlings Jackson injected a much needed critical note. Nervous disease, by definition, should be disease of the nervous tissue, which meant of the ganglionic cells. But in many allegedly nervous diseases, e.g., in hemiplegia or in softening of the brain, the pathological changes began in non-nervous tissues, and the nerve cells were affected secondarily.[255] "The hypothesis in possession," Jackson wrote, "is that epilepsy is owing to changes beginning in the nervous elements of nervous organs."[256] He countered this by a different hypothesis: "the cells suffer secondarily, as a consequence of arterial disease; . . . there is thrombosis or embolism of small arteries in most cases of epilepsy proper."[257] On this hypothesis, epilepsy was not inherited *qua* nervous disease.

Implicitly, Jackson's hypothesis constituted a denial that genuine epilepsy was an idiopathic disease in the Galenic sense, viz., a primary disease of its anatomical substratum. In Galen's time the brain was the substratum, and idiopathic epilepsy was a disease of the brain in contrast to sympathetic epilepsy, where the brain was affected secondarily. By the late nineteenth century, the nerve cells of the brain had become the anatomical substratum; consequently, epilepsy should be considered idiopathic when these cells were primarily diseased. If they were affected by disease of surrounding tissues or of their blood vessels, the resulting epilepsy would have been named sympathetic by Galen; Jackson's contemporaries called it symptomatic, for the term sympathetic epilepsy had been preempted in the meantime. Sympathetic epilepsy had become synonymous with reflex epilepsy.[258]

But this consequence of Jacksonian doctrine was not drawn by his contemporaries. Idiopathic epilepsy was a functional disease of the nervous system, characterized by fits of convulsions and disturbance of consciousness. Authors differed in making convulsions or disturbed consciousness the leading characteristic.[259] Whether the disease was designated as idiopathic, genuine, or essential epilepsy was relatively unimportant. From a nosological point of view, idiopathic epilepsy and epileptiform convulsions retained the position they held before Hughlings Jackson's work had made its impact. Jackson himself had ad-

---

[255] Jackson (556), *Selected Writings*, vol. 1, pp. 175, 230, and 294.

[256] *Ibid.*, p. 294.

[257] *Ibid.*, p. 294 f. Jackson took pains to stress that this was an unproved hypothesis, and that Brown-Séquard's experimentally produced hereditary epilepsy in guinea pigs was an argument for the hereditary character of the disease epilepsy; cf. *ibid.*, p. 231.

[258] Voisin (1053), *Epilepsy*, p. 606: "Lorsqu' une cause excitante quelconque produit l'épilepsie en agissant sur l'axe cérébro-spinal, par l'intermédiaire d'un nerf sensitif ou du grand sympathique, l'épilepsie est dite réflexe ou sympathique."

[259] Gowers (420), *Epilepsy*, p. 1, speaks of epilepsy as a chronic convulsive disease, whereas Strümpell (966), *Lehrbuch*, p. 404, makes disturbances of consciousness the leading symptom.

mitted the practical necessity of an empirical classification of epilepsy, although scientifically speaking he allowed epilepsies only.

"It is generally admitted," Handfield Jones wrote in 1870, "that the essential change in Epilepsy is purely functional, that if we could examine the normal organs of a sufferer at an early stage of his malady, we should be unable by any scrutiny in our power, to detect any lesion whatever."[260] Ten years later, more was known about convulsions and less about epilepsy as a morbus per se. Nor were Jackson's clinically founded speculations equally palatable for all. Neurologists and psychiatrists, while commonly accepting Jacksonian epilepsy, individually used as much or as little of Jackson's theories as fitted their own opinions. Jacksonian epilepsy could be discussed among diseases of the motor cortex of the brain, and epilepsy among neuroses without known anatomical foundation, and then analogies might be drawn from the former to the latter. On the other hand, Magnan accepted Jackson's explanation of epileptic insanity. "The discharge," he wrote, "according to Jackson's theory, for a certain time paralyzes the action of one or of several of the superior nervous centres, and the suppression of the directing action then allows the development of greater automatic action."[261]

Gowers' *Epilepsy and Other Chronic Convulsive Diseases*, which first appeared in 1881, was the most important contemporary book written in English on the cause, symptoms, and treatment of epilepsy. That Jackson's experience and views were given considerable attention is to be expected in view of the close proximity of the two men. The following paragraph from Gowers' chapter on "Pathology" offers insight into the concordance between them.

> The conclusion, then, is that all the phenomena of the fits of idiopathic epilepsy may be explained by the discharge of grey matter; that the hypothesis of vascular spasm is as unneeded as it is unproved; that there are no facts to warrant us in seeking the seat of the disease elsewhere than in the grey matter in which the discharge commences; that this is in most cases within the cerebral hemispheres, probably often in the cerebral cortex, although possibly in some instances lower down, even in the medulla oblongata; that epilepsy is thus a disease of grey matter, and has not any uniform seat. It is a disease of tissue, not of structure.[262]

Nevertheless, Gowers' approach to epilepsy was different from Jackson's. Gowers tried to cover the subject as a whole rather than limit

---

[260]Jones (568), *Studies on Functional Nervous Disorders*, p. 304.

[261]Magnan (659), *Leçons cliniques sur l'épilepsie*, p. 25. Explaining automatism and referring it to "the perceiving cerebral centres," he says (p. 3) of the latter: "Ceux-ci sont rendus indépendants par l'*ictus* épileptique, *lésion dé-chargente* des Anglais, qui frappe, qui annihile pour un temps les centres les plus élevés des hémisphères" (italics in the text).

[262]Gowers (420), *Epilepsy*, p. 211.

himself to the areas of personal contribution; he based his discussion on a relatively large number of cases (1,450) which had been under his care, mainly at the National Hospital for the Paralyzed and Epileptic, and throughout the book he analyzed this material statistically.

As the title indicates, the book was not limited to epilepsy. Epileptic attacks, Gowers said, were but one class of "the chronic convulsions which are recognized as of 'functional' origin." Hysterical attacks formed the other class.[263] Right away, Gowers tried to differentiate the features of the two classes. In epilepsy the convulsions were of a random character, and the attitudes of the limbs did not resemble those during voluntary movements. In contrast, in severe hysterical attacks, the convulsive movements had "a quasi-purposive aspect, they are *co-ordinated* in character, although excessive in degree."[264] Gowers preferred the terms "hysteroid" and "co-ordinated convulsion" to avoid the connotation of "hysterical" and the confusing name of "hystero-epilepsy," which Charcot had used.[265] Unfortunately, as Gowers admitted, it was not always possible neatly to separate severe hysteroid convulsions from epileptic ones. Well-co-ordinated movements also appeared in sequence to epileptic fits, and there were "rare cases in which the attacks are actually of a nature intermediate between the two."[266]

Even since the electroencephalogram has facilitated the separation of epileptic attacks from others, the difficulty in which Gowers and his contemporaries found themselves can be appreciated. The difficulty was, above all, of a practical nature. The theoretical dichotomy between epilepsy and hysteria met with obstacles in medical practice. But on what presumptions did the dichotomy itself rest? This question leads back to the falling sickness and involves the philosopher Hughlings Jackson.

## 2. EPILEPSY AND HYSTERIA

Among his contemporaries, Hughlings Jackson certainly was one of the strictest adherents of the doctrine of psychophysical parallelism. From Laycock he had accepted the principle that even the highest nervous arrangements in man functioned according to the law of reflex action. "What are physiologically reflex actions are anatomically sensori-motor arrangements. The same is true of the centres which are the substrata of mental states in man."[267] Hence came his emphasis on the sensorimotor

---

[263] *Ibid.*, p. 1.

[264] *Ibid.*, p. 2 (italics in the text).

[265] *Ibid.*, p. 2 f.

[266] *Ibid.*, p. 3, cf. also pp. 176 ff., 217 f., and 227 ff. On p. 229, the diagnostic characters of epileptic and hysteroid fits are presented in tabular form.

[267] Jackson (556), *Selected Writings*, vol. 1, p. 239.

character of all nervous centers. But with Spencer he contended that the anatomy and physiology of the substratum of the mind in no way explained consciousness and mental processes: we know of the existence of a parallelism between physiology and psychology, but nothing of any connection between these two realms. He believed it a grave error on the part of materialists to assume that mind can be a *product* of the body.[268] "There is no physiology of the mind any more than there is psychology of the nervous system."[269]

Jackson took great pains to stress his rejection of materialistic metaphysics. But having made clear the fundamental difference between physiology and psychology, he categorically made physiology alone the physician's province. "A medical man's aim should be to deal with what are called diseases of the mind (really diseases of the highest cerebral centres) as materialistically as possible. But to be thoroughly materialistic as to the nervous system we must not be materialistic at all as to mind."[270] In other words, the physician ought to approach mental diseases as a neurologist, and not as a psychologist. Nevertheless, Jackson did not deny the importance of psychological observations. Disturbances of consciousness and abnormalities in behavior indicated that something was wrong with the patient, and allowed inferences as to the seat and nature of the nervous disease. In this respect, psychological knowledge was desirable and necessary, but—and this is the decisive point—merely in order to recognize symptoms, not in order to *understand* the patient's behavior. "On the basis of mere concomitance, mental symptoms (synonymously abnormal states of consciousness) are, strictly speaking, only signs to physicians of what is not going on or of what is going on wrongly in part of a patient's material organization."[271]

These philosophical views of Jackson were in accordance with his explanation of epilepsy, including post-epileptic states. They, furthermore, agreed with his ideas concerning emotional and psychic factors as possible causes of epilepsy. Jackson admitted that fear could lead to an epileptic fit, but it was not the psychological fact of fear, nor its psychological content, which might bring about an attack. It was the general change in the body concomitant with a strong emotion that led to a discharge of the unstable nerve cells.[272] The epileptic patient had a discharging lesion, that is, part of his brain was organically diseased. To assume that fear or any other psychological condition could directly

---

[268] *Ibid.*, p. 367.
[269] *Ibid.*, p. 417.
[270] *Ibid.*, p. 367.
[271] *Ibid.*, p. 417.
[272] Cf. above, p. 335 f.

cause organic changes of nerve tissue would run counter to all of Jackson's basic principles.

Jackson's position with regard to the psychical causes of epilepsy, though more clearly defined and consistent than that of the great majority of physicians, represented a common attitude. The many "moral" causes, compiled by earlier statisticians, were demoted to the rank of accidental and provoking causes. The belief that epilepsy was an organic disease prevailed, regardless of whether the seat of the disturbance was looked for in the cortex or the medulla oblongata and pons. In many respects this attitude resembled that of the iatromechanists and iatróchemists of two hundred years before. The great systematists of the seventeenth century had assumed that the epileptic attack was a necessary consequence of pathological changes in the central nervous system, and that the attack was bare of biological purpose or psychological meaning.[273] In this belief the medical men of the later nineteenth century concurred, though in detail their ideas were more biological compared with the crude mechanical and chemical concepts of their predecessors. Though Jackson, for instance, maintained that convulsions had their cause in the brain, he denied that these convulsions were a mere aggregate of muscular contractions. The brain represented *movements*, some more automatic, others less. The whole idea of evolution and dissolution depended on this assumption. Therefore, the epileptic fit was a combination of *movements*, such as the patient was wont to make in his life.[274] A study of these movements was necessary in every case in order to ascertain the seat of the nervous lesion, although no psychological meaning could be attributed to them.

We have now reached the limitations of Jackson's doctrine. It demanded of the neurologist that he be a student of human behavior without compelling him to understand the psychological meaning of the acts. The neurologist might well be satisfied with this restriction and leave the rest to the psychiatrist, were it not for hysteria. Psychoses did not necessarily concern the neurologist—but hysteria did. In the nineteenth century, hysteria was eminently a neurological problem, and some of the main students of hysteria were not psychiatrists: Benjamin Brodie was a surgeon, and Charcot and, later, Freud were neurologists. The surgeon had to know whether anything was anatomically wrong that he could set right, or whether the complaint was nervous and outside his competence. The neurologist dealt with palsies and spasms, with anesthesias and paresthesias; he had to know whether the complaint could or could not be explained by a recognizable lesion of the nervous system. It is difficult to obtain a clear picture of Jack-

---

[273] Cf. above, VII-1.

[274] Jackson (556), *Selected Writings*, vol. 1, p. 431 f.

son's ideas on hysteria. He warned that hysteria might be wrongly diagnosed, where a careful search would reveal the post-epileptic nature of the peculiar behavior.[275] This chance remark would mean that he did not consider hysterical fits as automatisms on a par with epileptic dreamy states, Gowers' assertion to the contrary.[276] But Jackson also quoted Handfield Jones to the effect that grand mal represented epilepsy as the type which shaded off "on one side by the *petit-mal* into mere vertigo, on another, into hysteria and choreic convulsion, on a third, into delirium, catalepsy, and somnambulism, on a fourth, into neuralgia."[277]

Whatever Jackson's view of hysteria may have been, it is hard to understand how his theory could go beyond a mere demarcation line setting off hysterical convulsions as not epileptic. This state of affairs was not very satisfactory, and a different approach supplementing a purely neurological philosophy recommended itself.

During the first half of the nineteenth century, it was as yet a matter for discussion whether hysteria was not merely a variety of epilepsy.[278] It was even maintained anew that hysteria originated from the uterus.[279] In short, the old debate regarding the relationship between epilepsy and hysteria was still continued much in the spirit of the preceding period. Toward the middle of the century the debate centered chiefly around the problem of what older authors had called *epilepsia uterina* and the French authors called *hystéro-épilepsie*. On the whole there was agreement that a hysterical person might also suffer from epilepsy and that the attacks might sometimes be hysterical, sometimes epileptic. These were the *accès distincts*, where a differential diagnosis was possible. In addition, some authorities claimed the existence of *accès complexes*, where epileptic and hysterical symptoms were combined so as to make a distinction between the two diseases

---

[275] Jackson (556), *Selected Writings*, vol. 2, p. 10: "Unless we have studied many kinds of actions after epileptic seizures of different degrees of severity, and especially actions after the slightest, we shall overlook the epileptic nature of some of our patients' cases altogether; for example, we may mistake epilepsy for hysteria."

[276] Gowers (420), *Epilepsy*, p. 217: "The fact that these [i.e., hysteroid] seizures may succeed attacks of epileptic *petit mal* has been regarded by Hughlings Jackson as evidence that the hysteroid convulsion (like the automatic action, p. 118) is always due to the release of lower centres from the control of the higher by the temporary discharge of the latter." Unfortunately, Gowers does not cite any exact reference to Jackson. On p. 118, Gowers sets forth his theory of post-epileptic hysteria. These attacks depend on two factors: a cerebral discharge making lower centers act in an insubordinate manner, and a previous morbid state of the brain "such as leads to the manifestations of hysteria, apart from epilepsy."

[277] Jackson (556), *Selected Writings*, vol. 1, p. 203. The quotation is from Jones (568), *Studies on Functional Nervous Disorders*, p. 285.

[278] Calmeil (197), *De l'épilepsie*, etc. p. 8: ". . . puisqu'on dispute chaque jour pour savoir si le mal hystérique n'est pas une nuance de l'épilepsie."

[279] Cf. Cesbron (214), p. 60 ff.

impossible.[280] Gowers was inclined to accept the existence of a combined form, whereas Charcot insisted on a complete separation of
hysteria and epilepsy.[281]

In order to understand the position taken by Charcot, some clinical
and etiological data gathered by physicians of the preceding generation
have to be considered. We single out Todd and Briquet, the former
because his work was studied by Jackson and the latter because Charcot
accepted many of his fundamental concepts. Presented with a case "of
a highly-developed hysterical paroxysm or fit"[282] which resembled
epilepsy more than any other convulsive disease, Todd drew attention
to the following facts. The movements "were combined and regular,
and directed to an end and by a purpose."[283] Consciousness was not
completely lost, "the apparent insensibility" depended "upon an
intense concentration of the attention on one particular object."[284]
And from the past history of the case he cited that the patient "was a
highly-excitable, hysterical person, who has been subjected to moral,
and perhaps physical influences also, well calculated to keep up that
state."[285] The essential criterion of Todd's diagnosis of hysteria as
against epilepsy was the presence of psychological factors in the etiology, as well as the symptomatology, of the case.

Briquet (1796–1881) offers a more elaborate theory of hysteria. The
disease, he contends, may occur in men, but is predominantly a disease
of women. To fulfill her noble mission in life, woman has been endowed with great sensitiveness and is easily moved emotionally. This
makes her readily disposed to hysteria. Any painful and disagreeable
impressions affect the emotional centers of the brain. This portion of
the brain will react, and the outward manifestations of this reaction will
correspond to the painful emotions which caused the disorder.[286] "To
sum up, an attack of hysteria is nothing but the reaction of that part of
the brain which receives emotional impressions. The reaction is expressed outwardly by an exaggeration or perversion of those acts
through which these impressions are habitually manifested externally."[287] In other words, the symptoms of hysteria are in some way

---

[280] Cf. Landouzy (610), *Traité complet de l'hystérie*, p. 144 f. But even Landouzy believed
that few cases of "accès complexes" would remain if the symptoms of epilepsy and hysteria
could be analyzed better.

[281] Cf. Charcot (216), *Leçons sur les maladies du système nerveux*, I, p. 369 f.

[282] Todd (1027), *Clinical Lectures on Paralysis*, etc. p. 470.

[283] *Ibid.*, p. 467.

[284] *Ibid.*, p. 469.

[285] *Ibid.*, p. 470.

[286] Briquet (155), *Traité clinique et thérapeutique de l'hystérie*, pp. 100 f. and 116.

[287] *Ibid.*, p. 398.

related to its causes, among which emotional factors hold a pre-eminent place. This is also one characteristic which distinguishes hysterical from epileptic convulsions. In hysteria "the convulsions correspond to the expression of the passions, sensations or ordinary acts of life."[288] In epilepsy, on the other hand, "the convulsion is a kind of tetanus without resemblance to the movements which take place under physiological conditions."[289]

We must, however, beware of imputing a purely psychological explanation of hysteria to Briquet, or of minimizing the role which he assigned to the brain. True, his ideas about the seat of emotions are very vague, and it is hard to understand why only disagreeable passions and emotions should affect the brain and produce hysterical symptoms. Nevertheless, the fact remains that in his belief the hysterical attack is directly a result of the affection of the brain.[290] So it might be argued that psychology had no more place in his theory of hysteria than in Jackson's later theory of epilepsy. But this would mean overlooking two main points. In Jackson's theory of epilepsy, anatomical and physiological speculations form the cornerstone of the whole system. If they are removed, the whole system collapses. This is not the case with Briquet's or Charcot's assumptions regarding the seat of hysteria. The refutation of these assumptions does not invalidate the rest of the theory, particularly the fundamental role of passions and emotions. Moreover, these "moral" causes do not act indirectly via the concomitant general change in the body. The reaction of the patient depends on the psychological content of the emotions. The physician who has to treat a hysterical patient must analyze the circumstances of her life and remove conditions which cause mental pain, sadness, and unhappiness.[291]

Generally speaking, the etiological explanation of epilepsy and hysteria followed opposite directions. An anatomical substratum for both diseases was assumed to exist in the central nervous system. In epilepsy the trend was to look for organic causes which might affect the brain, whereas in hysteria an ever increasing emphasis was laid on emotional factors.

In the days of Briquet and Charcot, historical interests were strong among French physicians, particularly psychiatrists. In 1845 Calmeil published his fundamental work *On Madness*, tracing the various cultural manifestations of psychic disturbances from the fifteenth to the

---

[288] *Ibid.*, p. 390.

[289] *Ibid.* The contrast indicated by Briquet is well illustrated by a comparison between Figs. 5 and 6.

[290] *Ibid.*, pp. 398 and 600 ff.

[291] *Ibid.*, p. 633.

eighteenth century. What the past had attributed to possession and divine ecstasy he interpreted in the light of the psychiatric knowledge of his days. Many outbreaks of psychic epidemics he diagnosed as hysterical,[292] but Calmeil's concept of hysteria was still limited, and he used it side by side with such terms as *démonopathie* and *théomanie.*[293] With Briquet the concept of hysteria widened and comprised most instances where convulsive movements had been recorded.[294] Trying to account for the epidemic spread of hysterical attacks, Briquet had recourse to the impression made upon the imagination of a hysterical person. "It is very probable that in several of these epidemics particular circumstances determined the form of the symptoms of the hysterical persons seized first. Then, through the involuntary influence upon the mind and the tendency to imitation, the hysterical persons who came afterwards had symptoms similar to those who had them first, and these in turn influenced the others."[295] This explanation was strikingly similar to the one given in the eighteenth century for the spread of "simulated epilepsy." Here too, the epidemics of what had been considered epilepsy had been attributed to the power of imagination.[296] The explanation was the same but the diagnosis of the disease had changed, for these convulsions were now considered hysterical. In relating Boerhaave's experience at the orphanage of Haarlem, for instance, Briquet denied the epileptic nature of the disorder and explained it as hysterical.[297] To distinguish sharply between epilepsy and hysteria in the past, as well as in the present, became a point of view adopted by an ever increasing number of medical men. No one contributed more to this tendency than Charcot and the school inspired by him.

A perusal of Charcot's lectures on hysteria, delivered in the early seventies, makes it clear that he was, in many respects, dependent on Briquet.[298] How far the latter's influence extended and what Charcot's general ideas on hysteria were need not interest us here. We shall confine ourselves to Charcot's work on *hystéro-épilepsie* and to that of his pupil, Richer, who devoted a comprehensive monograph to it. Charcot takes up the older distinction between *hystéro-épilepsie à crises distinctes* and *à crises combinées.* He admits the existence of the former but denies the existence of fits in which the two neuroses are combined.

---

[292] Calmeil (196), *De la folie*, II, p. 155.

[293] *Ibid.*, I, 86.

[294] Briquet (155), *Traité clinique et thérapeutique de l'hystérie*, p. 338 ff.

[295] *Ibid.*, p. 376.

[296] Cf. above, VIII-1a.

[297] Briquet, *l.c.*, p. 388.

[298] Cf., e.g., Charcot (216), *Leçons sur les maladies du système nerveux*, I, p. 372.

The alleged *crises combinées* or *attaques-accès*, as they were called in the jargon of the Salpêtrière, are of a purely hysterical nature.[299] They are attacks of *hysteria maior* or *grande hystérie*, which constitute an extreme form of ordinary hysteria.[300]

The great hysterical attack is preceded by an aura followed by the epileptic phase (cf. Fig. 6). In this phase, tonic convulsions predominate and the patient may really resemble a true epileptic. But in the next phase, *la phase clonique*, the hysterical character of the whole seizure is evident. "Then the hysteria is supreme: one sees the great movements of an intentional character supervene, and contortions which sometimes express the most varied passions, fright, hatred, etc. At the same time the *delirium of the attack* breaks out."[301] The attacks end with sobbing, crying, laughing, etc.

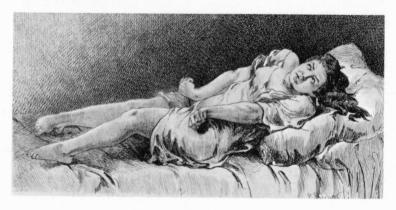

Fig. 6

Grande hystérie, "epileptoid period." (Richer, *Études cliniques sur l'hystéro-épilepsie ou grande hystérie*, Paris 1881, plate II.)

The study of his hysterical patients confirms for Charcot an observation of Valentiner's: certain cases of hysteria present in rudimentary form the features fully developed in the convulsive epidemics.[302] One patient illustrates the dancing mania, another is "possessed" or can be compared to the "jerkers" at a Methodist camp-meeting. Following in the footsteps of Charcot, Richer compares the clinical picture of the *grande hystérie* with the accounts given of the convulsionists and certain cases of ecstasy. The comparison shows him that the symptoms are essentially the same and that the etiology is similar. Strong emotions

---

[299]*Ibid.*, pp. 369-72.
[300]Richer (846), *Études cliniques sur l'hystéro-épilepsie ou grande hystérie*, p. xi.
[301]Charcot, *l.c.*, p. 374 (italics in text).
[302]Cf. *ibid.*, p. 342.

are not only an important factor in the genesis of hysteria but may even determine the character of the main symptoms, and the religious excitement of the past accounts for the necessary emotional element. Besides, he takes the "nervous contagion" of hysterical symptoms for an established fact.[303]

Richer's historical studies have a definite clinical purpose. They aim at proving that the *"grande hystérie* is a perfectly well-characterized morbid entity"[304] whose fundamental features were the same in the past as they are in the present.[305] It must neither be attributed to supernatural powers, nor must it be mistaken for epilepsy, with which it has nothing in common.

Charcot and Richer re-interpreted the phenomena of possession in terms of a natural disease, *grande hystérie*. Hysteria now was the counterpart to epilepsy that possession had been in centuries past. Possession was a magico-theological concept, whereas hysteria was a natural one. However, both had in common the establishment of a category of abnormal, yet understandable, behavior with somatic symptoms. Possession was a disease of the soul manifesting itself through the body, and with Freud the doctrine of hysteria developed to the point where it was ready to take over this role. Around 1880 this point had not yet been reached, but the tendency was there. Convulsive disorders in schools, convents, and women's wards,[306] diagnosed as mass hysteria, had once been viewed as possession. The falling down no longer united epilepsy and psychogenic convulsive disorders. But the detachment with which Jackson and other neurologists viewed epilepsy as a problem in neurophysiology and neuropathology did not mean the elimination of all psychology from the study of epilepsy.

### 3. CRIME, RELIGION, AND THE EPILEPTIC CHARACTER

In spite of the role he had assigned to automatisms in epilepsy, Falret had admitted that in exceptional cases the *petit mal intellectuel* might free the patient from normal inhibitions and might lead to acts of jealousy or anger against certain individuals.[307] Ten years later, a case

---

[303] Richer, *l.c.*, p. 615 f.

[304] *Ibid.*, p. 615.

[305] *Ibid.*, p. 615 and p. xvi.

[306] Cheyne (219), *Epilepsy*, p. 83, with the addition by Robley Dunglison. Laycock (616), *An Essay on Hysteria*, p. 47, describes an epidemic of "imitation hysteria" (with and without convulsions) in a woman's surgical ward.

[307] See above, p. 321. In his analysis of van Gogh's disease, Gastaut (401) has shown that the diagnosis of *épilepsie non convulsivante* was made by Dr. Félix Rey, a fellow student of Dr. Aussoleil, who graduated with a thesis on *épilepsie larvée* (p. 200). According to Gastaut, Dr. Rey's diagnosis reflected the ideas of Morel and Falret (p. 201), van Gogh having actually suffered from attacks of *petit mal intellectuel* (p. 212 ff.) as well as *grand mal intellectuel* (p. 214). Van Gogh's maniacal states were induced by terrifying hallucinations (p. 214) and the automatisms were more or less motivated (p. 215). Some of the features attributed to "epileptic character" by authors of the nineteenth century are discernible in Gastaut's description

was tried in Rochester, New York, which looked like an illustration of this exception.[308]

David Montgomery was an industrious, abstemious, religious young cartman who, since childhood, had suffered from epileptic attacks and was called "crazy" and "daft Davy." At the age of eighteen he married a prostitute, and although they had a baby, his wife apparently refused to live with him permanently. On a Saturday night after a week of repeated seizures he still was in an excited state and laboring under delusions. Yet at nine o'clock, all three of them went home peacefully. On Sunday morning Montgomery hit his wife in her sleep with an ax and tried to commit suicide afterward. For hours he remained in an obvious state of excitement but gave an otherwise uncontradicted account of the events. He and his wife had intercourse during the night, which he had spent sleeplessly. Allegedly he had tried to make her promise to live with him, but she refused. Questioned about his motive for the murder (his wife died of the injury), he said, "because she had run with other men" and "I loved her so well I could not live without her, and all I want is, that they will let me go to the grave with her, and come back and hang me." Regarding the details of his deed he stated: "I stood with the ax about five minutes looking at her, and seemed impelled to strike her, and though I did not want to, I had to strike the blow." To an interrogating police detective he remarked: "My temper got the upper hand of me."[309] These statements were made in course of the morning, up to about four hours after the murder. In the early afternoon Montgomery fell asleep, and when roused he neither knew that he was in jail, nor remembered the events.[310]

In his testimony Dr. William A. Hammond expressed the opinion that "deliberation takes away the idea of an insane act."[311] If Montgomery had deliberated, he was not to be judged insane. Moreover, Dr. Hammond declared that he had never "known a case of an epileptic fit or seizure when, during the continuation of it, the party will be spoken to and will answer and then relapse into the same condition, and being spoken to again will answer and relapse again."[312]

---

of van Gogh's behavior. Interestingly enough, van Gogh noted religious episodes even after he had become a convinced agnostic, a fact which puzzled and perturbed him. Cf. Gastaut (401), p. 223, and Riese (849a), p. 205, note 5.

[308]The following account is based on Echeverria (308), *Criminal Responsibility of Epileptics, as Illustrated by the Case of David Montgomery.* Fink (359), pp. 41–46, has reviewed the attitudes of American authors on the criminal responsibility of epileptics. (I am indebted to Dr. Gert Brieger for this reference.)

[309]Echeverria, *l.c.*, pp. 349–50.

[310]*Ibid.*, p. 350.

[311]*Ibid.*, p. 369.

[312]*Ibid.*, p. 370. Dr. Hammond, as Echeverria, *ibid.*, p. 371, indicates, previously had published an account of the trial in the *Journal of Psychological Medicine* for January 1872, which, however, I have not seen.

In Dr. Echeverria's opinion, however, Montgomery had not only suffered repeated epileptic attacks before the night of Saturday but must have suffered another seizure upon getting up on Sunday morning.[313] The whole episode had ended only with his falling asleep in jail. From the literature, Echeverria cited cases where epileptics had asked to be forcefully prevented from criminal acts to which they were driven by an irresistible impulse.[314] For an explanation, Echeverria appealed to reflex action, which, even in a healthy state, usually was not under our control. In epilepsy, "the reflex faculty of the nervous system is carried to the highest morbid pitch," which accounted for "the extremely violent and uncontrollable reactions peculiar to the disease."[315] Epileptics were unconscious of their acts; "unconscious cerebration" exhibited itself in a high degree.[316]

It is remarkable that in the early seventies the question of consciousness was still put in the form of an alternative: conscious or unconscious. Maudsley suspected that "the metaphysical notion of consciousness as a definite invariable entity which must either be or not be" was still exerting its influence.[317] Perhaps it was the forensic question of the criminal responsibility of the epileptic that kept the alternative alive. Jackson got away from the alternative and allowed various degrees of impairment of consciousness.[318] But his explanation of the insanity of epileptics focused upon mental disorders after epileptic paroxysms; on his own admission he was not an alienist.[319]

A different theory, based on the notion of "psychic equivalents," came to rival Jackson's explanation. As early as 1862, Hoffmann said that "the epileptic attacks can be lacking altogether, and yet by means of its peculiar symptoms the insanity may reveal itself as an equivalent of epilepsy, especially of the convulsions and of the coma."[320] Al-

---

[313]Echeverria, *op. cit.*, p. 421: "... it may be fairly assumed that Montgomery might have had an epileptic seizure on getting up, before or after he was cutting the kindling for the fire."

[314]*Ibid.*, p. 409. Echeverria, who was physician in chief of The New York Hospitals for Epileptics and Paralytics and had received his M.D. degree from Paris, was very well acquainted with the French literature on epilepsy in all its aspects.

[315]*Ibid.*, p. 415 f.

[316]Echeverria (312), *On Epileptic Insanity*, p. 47 f. and *passim*, categorically defends the unconscious nature of acts conditioned by epilepsy, yet insisting [Echeverria (308), *Criminal Responsibility of Epileptics*, p. 418] "that design, a premeditation, is not any more incompatible with epileptic insanity than with any other form of insanity." For the contemporary notion of unconscious cerebration see Carpenter (203), *Principles of Human Physiology*, p. 589.

[317]Maudsley (674), *Responsibility in Mental Disease*, p. 239.

[318]Jackson's ideas of consciousness have been discussed frequently; I mention here only Cobb (229) and Riese (849 and 850).

[319]Jackson (556), *Selected Writings*, vol. 1, p. 120.

[320]Hoffmann (502), *Ueber die Eintheilung der Geisteskrankheiten in Siegburg*, p. 372: "Die epileptischen Anfälle können endlich ganz fehlen und dennoch kann die Geisteskrankheit durch ihre eigenthümlichen Symptome verrathen, dass sie ein Aequivalent der Epilepsie, insbesondere

though Hoffmann listed the diagnostic symptoms for these equivalents, he hardly introduced any new species of attacks. But in 1875, P. Samt elaborated the theory of "psychic equivalents" so as to assure it lasting attention. He praised Falret for having established epileptic insanity as a specific psychiatric entity,[321] though he did not accept Falret's classification. Instead, Samt divided epileptic insanity into two main forms: post-epileptic insanity and psychic equivalents. The latter, which were not bound to any ordinary epileptic manifestations, could be simple, recidivous, or protracted. The diagnosis had to rest solely on symptomatology, development, and cause. Stupor, extreme violence, severe anxious delirium, and multiform defects of memory were the main pathognomonic symptoms.[322]

The very first of Samt's case histories, presenting a simple psychic equivalent, had some analogous features to the case of Montgomery as far as memory was concerned.[323] The patient was a medical student who had never suffered from epileptic attacks of any kind, though there was insanity in the family. After an incubation period of two days (malaise, insomnia, trembling hands) the patient suffered a paroxysm during which he made several homicidal attempts upon his friends. Afterward, when brought to a room, offered a cigar, and engaged in conversation he knew that he had attacked his room fellows, expressed satisfaction over not having killed anybody, and readily agreed to be taken to a hospital. On the way he had suicidal tendencies, admitted an urge to kill—he would do it if he had a weapon at hand, "I would have no choice, I would have to do it"[324]—but he also was anxious and thought himself persecuted. This anxiety continued throughout the night, and he saw himself surrounded by a mass of people who beat him. Irritation and anxiety lasted for about another twenty-four hours. At this time, however, he no longer knew what he had done during the

---

der Convulsionen und des Coma, sei. Man muss die intermittirenden Geisteskrankheiten darauf ansehen, namentlich diejenigen, wo die Anfälle kurz sind und schnell einander folgen. Man beachte dann die Aura, den partiellen Tetanus, die bleierne Schwere der Körpertheile, die anscheinend im Parenchym der Nervencentra auftretenden Schmerzen, das bisweilen, besonders beim Einschlafen, den Kranken befallende Todesgefühl, den plötzlichen Ausbruch der psychischen Symptome, mitten im Satz der Rede, in einem angefangenen Gestus, die Stupidität, begleitet von Wuth oder incohärentem Delirium, beide ganz oder grossentheils unerinnerlich, die schnelle Rückkehr zur Besinnung, die Hoffnungsfülle und Sorglosigkeit bald nach dem Anfall u. dgl." It is hard to judge whether Hoffmann used the term "equivalent" in elaborating the views of Meyer (cf. above, Part Five, footnote 80), or whether he was stimulated by Falret, as Samt admittedly was.

[321]Samt (885), *Epileptische Irreseinsformen*; vol. 5, p. 394: "Wie bekannt, hat zuerst Jules Falret in seiner ausgezeichneten Abhandlung: de l'état mental des épileptiques die specifische Natur des epileptischen Irreseins dehauptet."

[322]*Ibid.*, vol. 6, p. 196 f. On p. 214 Samt subdivided epilepsy into twelve categories.

[323]Although in Samt's classification Montgomery's case would have belonged to post-epileptic insanity.

[324]Samt, *op. cit.*, vol. 5, p. 400: "Ich könnte nicht anders, ich müsste es thun."

paroxysm, though he remembered his feelings of anxiety and having wrestled with one of his friends. He also remembered having been in the room where he smoked a cigar, but what he had actually told about the preceding events while in the room was now completely blotted out. From the fact that in the room the patient related his deeds, Samt inferred that he was conscious during his homicidal attacks, "since there is no reason for assuming that unconscious acts could be remembered afterwards."[325] Samt also raised the question whether the subsequent "partial defect of memory"[326] was genuine or simulated. Many other similar cases confirmed his belief in the reality of partial defects. During a paroxysm, Samt explained, the "intensity of consciousness" was low, and what was still remembered shortly afterward could be forgotten with rising intensity.[327]

Samt's detailed clinical descriptions of more than forty cases of epileptic insanity revealed a remarkable concomitance of violence and religious ecstasy. Together with others, Samt attributed the violence to anxiety and to frightful hallucinations. But a considerable number of Samt's patients also thought they were in heaven; they addressed the physicians and attendants as divine beings and usually ascribed to themselves some heavenly status. Samt spoke of the "god-nomenclature" which such patients used for their surroundings.[328] He received much information from them during the period when their subjective experiences were still fresh in their memory.

Others published reports of a similar kind. These stories show a striking resemblance to medieval and Renaissance tales of prophesying epileptics.[329] To give an example, a patient was diagnosed as suffering from genuine epileptic attacks, followed by a state of mental twilight and confusion. Several times a year, usually before or after an accumulation of seizures, rarely without them, he fell into an irritated and excited state, condemned his godless environment, mistook others for devils, thrashed out, and wished to be crucified for the true faith. At the height of his ecstasy he saw God face to face and declared himself Christ, God's true warrior, prophet, and martyr. The author added that "consciousness is considerably dimmed during this delirious time, but still amenable to impressions from the external world. Accordingly

---

[325] *Ibid.*, p. 406; cf. also, p. 419.

[326] *Ibid.*, "partieller Erinnerungsdefekt."

[327] *Ibid.*, vol. 6, p. 142 f. On this basis Samt also explained the case of a patient who remembered the figments of his deliriums, but had forgotten talking about them to the physician, whom he did not recognize.

[328] *Ibid.*, p. 154: "... die Gott-Nomenclatur der Umgebung bei sonst fast vollständig negativer sprachlicher Reaction scheint mir specifisch." Incidentally, on this page Samt also used the expression "psycho-motorische Reaction."

[329] See above, V-2.

there does not exist any defect of memory afterwards. The patient remembers his divine visions and does not correct them."[330]

To these views of the late nineteenth century on aggressive acts and religious ecstasies during epileptic states, must now be added the descriptions and evaluations of the epileptic character. With the increasing psychiatric interest, the behavior of epileptics between attacks, as well as their emotional and intellectual fate in course of the disease, came under closer scrutiny. Authors who were not psychiatrists dwelled less on these changes. For instance, Gowers' description of the mental state of epileptics was rather brief: "In its slighter form there is merely defective memory, especially for recent acquisitions. In more severe degree there is greater imperfection of intellectual power, weakened capacity for attention, and often defective moral control. Mischievous restlessness and irritability in childhood may develop into vicious and even criminal tendencies in adult life. Every grade of intellectual defect may be met with, down to actual imbecility."[331] This sober summary contrasted with Maudsley's dramatization of the mental anguish of epileptics suffering from attacks of maniacal insanity. "It is one of the saddest experiences of asylum life to witness the pitiful fate of those patients who have not sunk below the consciousness of their condition. Gentle, amiable, and industrious through their long intervals of lucidity, they hope against hope that each recurring paroxysm will be the last; they eagerly try all remedies, in the hope of curing the disease; they see others leave the asylum restored to health, and confidently anticipate that their turn will also come; but confidence wanes as the attacks recur, the mind is slowly weakened by the storms of fury through which it passes, and they sink finally into the apathy of dementia—a state of mere oblivion, in which they cease to hope or care more."[332]

In accounting for the development of the epileptic character, authors of the mid-century, especially French authors, were willing to allow considerable influence to social conditions. "Usually, the epileptic is avoided; on all faces he reads his sentence to isolation. Everywhere he goes, menacing and insurmountable obstacles arise to his obtaining a position, to his establishing himself, to his relationships, and to his very livelihood; he has to say good-by to his dreams of success, for the masters even refuse him work in their shops; good-by to his dreams of marriage and fatherhood, good-by to the joys of the domestic hearth. This is death to the spirit." Billod, the author of those lines, thought that many changes in the epileptic's character could be attributed to these conditions, if, in addition, the acquired impressionability of the

[330]Krafft-Ebing (594), *Lehrbuch der Psychiatrie*, vol. 2, p. 192.

[331]Gowers (420), *Epilepsy*, p. 121.

[332]Maudsley (674), *Responsibility in Mental Disease*, p. 228 f.

brain was taken into account. In a footnote he remarked that where favorable economic and social conditions obliterated many of the obstacles, the modifications of the epileptic's character were also less noticeable.[333] Howden, a British author, suggested a psychological explanation of the epileptics' religious inclinations. In their hopeless condition they sought the consolations religion offered.[334]

According to Morel, suffering had a share in the pathogenesis of epileptic mental disturbance. For its unfortunate victims, epilepsy was nothing imaginary that could be more or less assuaged by friendly council and by the help of science. "It is an incessant suffering whose fateful periodicity accumulates an ever greater amount of irritability in their nervous system. The latter phenomenon expresses itself not only in the form of perversion in their ideas and feelings, it also manifests itself by the most serious lesions in the physiological realm."[335] Irritability was at the base of the epileptic character, and suffering produced and magnified the latter. The epileptic furor, on the other hand, was not inherent in the disease; it was an accident which the progressive improvement of our asylums could modify, just as the furor of sufferers from mania had been modified.[336] Complete separation of epileptics and maniacs, added walks in the gardens reserved for the former, and application to work had already brought about considerable improvements.[337]

Morel's name is prominently connected with the idea of degeneracy, which, around the middle of the nineteenth century, increasingly engaged the minds of pathologists, psychiatrists, anthropologists, and sociologists.[338] In the form which Morel gave to it, the theory, with and without modifications, remained influential into the twentieth century, though anatomically, physiologically, and nosologically it was ill-

---

[333] Billod (113), *Recherches et considerations relatives à la symptomatologie de l'épilepsie*, p. 419: "On fuit généralement l'épileptique; il lit sur tous les visages sa condemnation à l'isolement. Partout, sur ses pas, s'élèvent menaçants et insurmontables des obstacles à son placement, à son établissement, à ses relations, à sa *subsistance*; adieu pour lui les rêves de fortune, car les maîtres d'atelier lui refusent même du travail; adieu les rêves d'époux et de père, adieu les jouissances du foyer domestique. Il est frappé de mort morale" (italics in the text). *Ibid.*, footnote: "Est-il besoin de dire qu'il faut éliminer ici certains épileptiques, dont la position de fortune et d'entourage est exceptionnelle, en ce qu'elle aplanit bon nombre des obstacles que j'ai énumérés? Dans ce cas, d'ailleurs, on peut remarquer que la modification du caractère est moins sensible."

[334] Howden (517), *The Religious Sentiment in Epileptics*, p. 483.

[335] Morel (713), *Traité des maladies mentales*, p. 702: "... c'est une douleur incessante, réelle, dont la périodicité fatale accumule dans leur système nerveux une dose de plus en plus grande irritabilité. Ce dernier phénomène ne se traduit pas seulement sous la forme de perversion dans les idées et dans les sentiments, mais se manifeste par les lésions les plus graves dans l'ordre physiologique."

[336] Morel (711), *Etudes cliniques*, p. 330.

[337] *Ibid.*, p. 321 f.

[338] In this connection see Genil-Perrin (405), Ackerknecht (8), p. 55 ff., Wettley (1092), Leibbrand-Wettley (623), p. 524 ff., Burgener (188).

defined. Alcoholism and other chronic poisoning, and physical and moral squalor caused a deterioration which tainted the descendents, leading to mental disease, idiocy, and extinction of the line. Epilepsy fitted well into this picture. It had a strong hereditary tendency; and it could be caused by absinth, alcohol, and lead poisoning, all prominent among the degenerating causes. It could also appear first within the descendents of degenerates. "The rule of progressive degeneracy . . . proves true very often, so that with a relatively mild neuropathic morbid condition in the first generation, possibly epilepsy will arise in the second and severe mental disease in the third."[339] Many criminals were said to be epileptic, and criminals were readily considered a separate type of man. "All persons who have made criminals their study, recognize a distinct criminal class of beings, who herd together in our large cities in a thieves' quarter, giving themselves up to intemperance, rioting in debauchery, without regard to marriage ties or the bars of consanguinity, and propagating a criminal population of degenerate beings."[340] Alcoholic and epileptic degeneration affected these beings in large proportion.[341]

With the advancing nineteenth century the tendency to approach social problems in biological terms gained momentum. In Cesare Lombroso's (1836-1909) version of the theory of degeneracy this showed itself not only in making the born criminal a special type of man but in finding almost any kind of similarity between him and the epileptic. They shared physiognomic signs, degenerative stigmata, and, above all, psychological traits.[342] Epilepsy united the criminal and morally insane in one natural family.[343]

Lombroso broadened the biological, social, and cultural role of the epileptic by accepting Moreau de Tours' transformation of the ancient doctrine of the great melancholic. Now cerebral irritability was the common organic cause of great original intellectual and psychic power on the one hand and of nervous disorders on the other.[344] This theory

---

[339]Eulenburg (333), *Lehrbuch der Nervenkrankheiten*, p. 636.

[340]Maudsley (674), *Responsibility in Mental Disease*, p. 29.

[341]Letourneau in his preface to Lombroso (644), *L'homme criminel*, p. IV: "Les dégénérescences alcoholiques ou épileptiques les frappent dans une large proportion." In an article, *The Hereditary Nature of Crime*, J. B. Thomson (1019), p. 492, offered the following statistical information for the prison of which he was the surgeon: "Out of a population of 5,432 no less than 673 were placed on my registers as requiring care and treatment on account of their mental condition. The forms of mental disorder were—

    Weak-mindedness or Imbecility in    580
    Ditto and Suicidal                    36
    Epileptic                          57."
The incidence of epileptics among the criminals was barely over one percent.

[342]Lombroso (644), *L'homme criminel*, ch. 14; p. 583, where he entered in great detail upon what he called "the natural history of the epileptic."

[343]*Ibid.*, p. 583: ". . . l'épilepsie, qui réunit et fond les fous moraux et les criminels—nés dans une même famille naturelle."

[344]Moreau (709), *La psychologie morbide*, pp. V and 38 f.

allowed Lombroso to account for the epileptic not only as a criminal but also as a genius. All genius was epileptic as well as cognate to the criminal. One may argue whether Lombroso glorified or vilified the epileptic. However, if his thesis is stripped of its untenable assumptions, it reveals the endeavor to reduce behavior which deviates from the norm in two, socially opposite, directions to a uniform physiological explanation.

Research had shown that epilepsy was a localized irritation of the cerebral cortex on a degenerative basis, yet the cortex was also the substratum of the mind and its functions. Hence, one could conclude that the creativity of genius was "a form of degenerative psychosis belonging to the family of epileptic affections."[345] Indeed, genius and epilepsy had many features in common: hereditary affliction, inclination to criminality, frequency of suicide, religiosity, vagabondage, and many more.[346] Very often the notorious absentmindedness of great men was but an epileptic "absence."[347] Genius showed ruthlessness and a loss of moral sense, which Lombroso illustrated in the case of Napoleon, who, to him, was an epileptic.[348]

Most important perhaps was the alleged analogy between the epileptic attack and the moment of inspiration which genius experienced. Lombroso analyzed creative inspiration by citing descriptions from the literature.[349] Buffon was credited with the statement that after long consideration of a subject, "it gradually unfolds and develops itself; you feel a slight electric shock strike your head and at the same time seize you at the heart; that is the moment of genius."[350] Foremost in showing how inspiration and epileptic attack intermingled were the confessions of Mohammed and of Dostoievski. The famous passages from Dostoievski's *Demons* and *The Idiot* were cited at length, and Lombroso said that one might call the kind of fit they described "psychic epilepsy."[351]

Epilepsy, Lombroso thought, was not just an accident in the genius, "but a true *morbus totius substantiae*," a disease of his whole sub-

---

[345] Lombroso (646), *The Man of Genius*, p. 336.

[346] *Ibid.*, p. 336 f.

[347] *Ibid.*, p. 337. Lombroso here names Tonnini as his authority.

[348] *Ibid.*, pp. 38 and 342–47. Lombroso relied on the psychological portrait of Napoleon by Taine and concluded (p. 347): "This is the completest view of Napoleon ever given by any historian. To any one acquainted with the psychological constitution of the epileptic, it becomes clear that Taine has here given us the subtlest and precisest pathological diagnosis of a case of psychic epilepsy, with its gigantic megalomaniacal illusions, its impulses, and complete absence of moral sense." Actually, Taine (989), *L'origine de la France contemporaine*, vol. 1, pp. 62–75, characterized Napoleon as "the great survivor of the 15th century" (p. 64), as a man of strong passions which sometimes expressed themselves organically.

[349] Lombroso (646), *The Man of Genius*, p. 22 ff., also p. 339.

[350] *Ibid.*, p. 339, footnote. No source is given for this; moreover, it is not put in quotation marks.

[351] *Ibid.*, p. 341.

stance.[352] Such a statement was too sweeping to be supported by the relatively small number of names of great men who had suffered from manifest epileptic convulsions. The difficulty was solved by pointing out the broadened clinical concept of epilepsy. Today, "many cases of headache (hemicrania) or simple loss of memory, are now recognized as forms of epilepsy . . . ." Lombroso then reminded his readers of "the numerous men of genius of the first order who have been seized by motor epilepsy, or by that kind of morbid irritability which is well known to supply its place. Among these we find such names as Napoleon, Molière, Julius Caesar, Petrarch, Peter the Great, Mahomet, Handel, Swift, Richelieu, Charles V, Flaubert, Dostoieffsky and St. Paul."[353] The frequency of epilepsy among the very great suggested its wide diffusion among all men of genius, and it helped Lombroso to form the notion of "the epileptoid nature of genius."[354]

Some of the names on Lombroso's lists were known from the days of the Renaissance. For the others, the direct evidence for epilepsy he offered often was distressingly slight. For instance, he simply referred to Flaubert as a known epileptic without mentioning or describing the attacks from which the novelist suffered.[355] There was a striking discrepancy between biographical carelessness and far-reaching theoretical superstructure. Obviously, these theories were not the result of induction. The idea of the epileptic nature of genius was a product of Aristotelian tradition, of neurophysiological theory, of the belief that civilization could be explained biologically, and of the conviction that much of the civilization of the time was sickly and degenerate.

The alleged ties which the theory of degeneracy in general and Lombroso's theory in particular established between epilepsy and criminality were by no means generally accepted as binding all epileptics. The violent aggressiveness of those prone to it during seizures could contrast markedly with meek and gentle behavior during intervals, except that many epileptics were inclined to excessive irritability. Yet, although criminality was not considered an overt feature of the epileptic character, epileptics were not absolved of all blemishes. "They" were accused of egoism, brutality, and duplicity. "They" were said to incline to religiosity and a show of piety which contrasted unpleasantly with their attitude toward their environment. Here, too,

---

[352] *Ibid.*, p. 348.

[353] *Ibid.*, p. 337 f.

[354] *Ibid.*, p. 336, see the heading of the chapter. It should be noted that a link between genius and epilepsy was not accepted unanimously. Crichton Browne (174), *Notes on Epilepsy and Its Pathological Consequence*, p. 20, rejected it categorically and thought the disease a handicap to the epileptic genius.

[355] *Ibid.*, p. 39. Flaubert's contemporaries, Du Camp and Goncourt, spoke of epilepsy, whereas Dr. René Dumesnil explained the attacks as hystero-neurasthenia; see Shanks (922), p. 162 f., and Tarver (993), p. 32.

the religiosity of their character was not to be confused with religious hallucinations during seizures.

Morel drew attention to the religious propensity of epileptics and its association with shameful behavior,[356] and hardly any subsequent author dealing with the epileptic character failed to mention it. One of the most pointed formulae was found by Samt, who spoke of the "poor epileptics who have the prayer book in their pocket, the dear Lord on their lips, and an excess of meanness inside."[357] It is not quite clear whether Samt's reference to the "poor epileptics" was meant seriously or ironically. But even if it carried sympathy, the rest of the formula did not. He and most other authors couched their descriptions in words of moral rejection and revulsion. The "bigotry and suffering mien stand in strange contrast to the irritability, quarrelsomeness, brutality and moral defectiveness . . . ."[358]

Such words came mostly from those who were in charge of epileptics confined to mental institutions. To what degree the sentiments they reveal and the conditions of institutionalized life in the later nineteenth century, when bromides were still the most powerful remedy and the seton was still used and recommended, helped to stamp what was described as the epileptic character can hardly be ascertained.[359] The epileptic was generally considered a sick person who was not responsible for the deterioration of his state. The unfriendly words were emotional reactions rather than deliberate moral judgments of the human beings. This suggests itself by comparison with the frequently open condemnation of hysterical persons, chiefly women. Samt's article

---

[356]Morel (713), *Traité des maladies mentales*, p. 701.

[357]Samt (885), *Epileptische Irreseinsformen*, vol. 6, p. 147: ". . . genug, die armen Epileptischen, wie sie wohl in jeder Anstalt zu treffen sind, welche das Gebetbuch in der Tasche, den lieben Gott auf der Zunge, aber den Ausbund von Canaillerie im ganzen Leibe tragen." Read in the context of the entire paragraph, the passage sounds sarcastic rather than sympathetic.

[358]Krafft-Ebing (594), *Lehrbuch der Psychiatrie*, vol. 2, p. 182. The criticism and even hostility in depicting the epileptic character on the part of some authors was noted by Victor von Weizsäcker (1073), p. 359: ". . . einige Autoren schildern den Charakter des Epileptikers mit unverkennbarer Kritik, ja sogar mit dem Unterton feindseliger Abneigung." Cf. Janz in Tellenbach (996), p. 17.

[359]Williams (1106), p. 40, has gone so far as to say: ". . . the epileptic temperament in my view is the sort of temperament which we all would have if we were treated as the majority of epileptics used to be treated. It was described in the bad old Victorian days when people with epilepsy were incarcerated in mental hospitals for which they were totally unfitted, and from which they could not escape. It was a state of mind of a prisoner of a war without end." The asylum directors of the period apparently thought differently. At least Morel (711), *Etudes cliniques*, vol. 2, p. 314, footnote, maintained that "the epileptic insane would have a greater chance of recovery, if they were placed earlier in an environment where they would find *the calm and the rest* which are so necessary for the irritability of their nervous system" (italics mine). It has also been pointed out that asylums must have housed a relatively large number of cases of psychomotor epilepsy [cf. Janz (561), p. 274], which touches on the question how far this type is especially prone to changes of character. Cf. Glaser (413) and Peters (785). For the seton see Echeverria (311), *On Epilepsy*, p. 326, and Hammond (453), *Clinical Lectures on Diseases of the Nervous System*, p. 218.

dealt with men only, because he believed that in the vast majority of women epilepsy was hystero-epilepsy, requiring separate considera-tion.[360] If he spoke harshly of male epileptics, he expressed himself still more harshly with regard to women: "In this connection I call to mind some hystero-epileptic females whom, amongst ourselves, I am wont to designate as hystero-epileptic canailles, females of whose baseness every institution will have had sufficient experience."[361] The recognition of hysteria (together with neurasthenia and similar conditions) as a real disease, in contrast to the earlier disbelief and suspicion that viewed the victim as an imaginary patient, was praised as an advance of recent neuropathology by Erb in 1884.[362] But four years later no less a physi-cian than Clifford Allbutt (1836–1925) still could write: "Take a hysterical person, man or woman, in its common and, so far, proper sense; take it to mean a person of feeble purpose, of limited reason, of foolish impulse, of wanton humours, of irregular or depraved appetites, of indefinite and inconsistent complaints, seeing things as they are not, often fat and lazy, always selfish; or to take it in less degree, one capricious, listless, wilful, attractive perhaps, yet having always the chief notes of hysteria—selfishness and feebleness of purpose; and if such persons . . . have or have had anaesthesia, unreal epilepsy, unreal syncope, unreal palsy, unreal cramps, then set down such a person as hysterical, but forget not, nevertheless, to cure mind and body."[363] Allbutt's "unreal" epilepsy presupposed the contrast to "real" epilepsy, a natural disease. Here again, in the moral sphere, epilepsy and hysteria stood in a relationship somewhat similar to that which had once ob-tained between epilepsy on the one hand and witchcraft and possession on the other. The purposeful element in attacks of *grande-hystérie* pointed to a wilful, and therefore condemnable, behavior, just as the commerce with devils and demons had been condemned at an earlier time.[364]

## 4. THE WORLD OF THE EPILEPTIC

The increasing attention which the later part of the nineteenth century paid to the religious behavior of the epileptic showed a remarkable parallel to earlier preoccupations with prophesying epileptics. The

---

[360] Samt (885), *Epileptische Irreseinsformen*, vol. 5, p. 420.

[361] *Ibid.*, vol. 6, p. 147, footnote: "Ich erinnere hierbei an manche hystero-epileptische Frauenzimmer, welche ich für den Hausgebrauch gewöhnlich als hystero-epileptische Canaillen zu bezeichnen pflege, Frauenzimmer, deren Nichtswürdigkeit jede Anstalt zur Genüge erfahren haben wird."

[362] Erb (325), *Ueber die neuere Eutwicklung der Nervenpathologie*, p. 19.

[363] Allbutt (24), *On Visceral Neuroses*, p. 21. Cf. also Veith (1046), p. 195, on the aversion to hysterical patients.

[364] Fischer-Homberger (362), has pointed out the common bond of misogyny which made the hysterical woman of modern times a secularized witch.

metaphysical approach had, of course, changed radically. The question then had been whether in their attacks epileptics were prone to have a true revelation of things not reached by ordinary experience. The question now concerned the subjective truth of what the epileptic claimed to see and to hear and the possible social significance of his beliefs. The interest in such matters was not restricted to psychiatrists, to whose reports we previously referred; it also was reflected in the work of historians and of literary men. The changing evaluation of Mohammed's revelations from the early forties of the century is a mirror of changing thoughts about the epileptic and his world.

Western tradition, it will be remembered, had shaped the story of Mohammed as an epileptic and hence an impostor. Gibbon had dismissed the story as a calumny. Now, when Carlyle lectured on heroes and hero worship, he chose Mohammed to illustrate the hero as prophet.[365] Epilepsy was not even mentioned; to Carlyle a hero could not be an impostor.

Psychiatrists also moved away from this diagnosis. Epilepsy was denied by Dr. Beau, who saw in Mohammed a monomaniac. This in turn was contested in a report to the French Academy of Medicine by a number of outstanding psychiatrists: Jules Falret, Ferrus, and Renauldin. They saw Mohammed as a firm believer in his apostolate, a great lawgiver, and a great statesman. They rejected the diagnosis of epilepsy; but whereas Dr. Beau had wished to replace it by ecstatic states of an insane person, they thought the ecstasies simulated. "If [Mohammed] deceived the people by alleged visions, by pretended revelations to which he attributed a celestial origin, and which caused his enemies to give him the insulting title of impostor, it certainly happened with pure and sincere intentions, as the Koran proves; it was done to reform his nation and to take it out of the state of brutishness and of ignorance in which it stagnated."[366]

The time of the dogmatic rejection of Mohammed as a fraud had obviously passed and was succeeded by a historical interest in his person and a study of the Islamic tradition. In 1843 the German orientalist, Gustav Weil, published a book on *Mohammed the Prophet*, in which he too accorded sincerity to Mohammed. According to Weil, Mohammed's reasoning made him conceive of himself as the apostle of a pure faith. Then his vivid phantasy did the rest, making him see an angel with divine revelation. "Such self-deception is all the more understandable in Mohammed, since as an epileptic he formerly deemed himself possessed by evil spirits according to the prejudices of his time. Now he could easily ascribe to the supernatural companionship with

---

[365] Carlyle (202), *On Heroes, Hero-Worship, and the Heroic in History*, lecture 2.
[366] Falret et al. (345), *Mémoire sur Mahomet*, p. 798.

angels the loss of consciousness which probably recurred most frequently after great mental efforts concerning some important question, and he could consider as a heavenly revelation what stood clearly before his soul after his awakening."[367] Weil offered the traditional biographical material in evidence of Mohammed's epilepsy, and his remarks reached the Anglo-Saxon world through a note in Washington Irving's *Life of Mahomet*.[368]

Some twenty years later, another German biographer, Sprenger, reinterpreted the biographical material. Epilepsy, he thought, was unlikely, because Mohammed's attacks were not marked by amnesia. In Sprenger's opinion, Mohammed suffered from hysteria, an illness whose victims tended to mimic the symptoms of other diseases. Since malaria was rife in Mohammed's environment, his attacks usually resembled a fever. "His face turned pale, he trembled and he shivered, and finally large drops of sweat on his face announced the arrival of the crisis."[369]

The examples adduced so far corroborate the impression that the medical evaluations of Mohammed rested heavily on the interpreter's religious and philosophical orientation, as well as on the nosological fashions of the day, and not just on the material on hand. Mohammed became a hysterical person when the diagnosis of hysteria became more fashionable. Weil had not declared Mohammed's visions and inspirations epileptic hallucinations, but this step was made soon when the subjective experiences of epileptics and especially their religious sentiments attracted the increasing attention of psychiatrists.[370] Cases were cited which showed parallels with what tradition had ascribed to Mohammed. The following extracts are from a letter which an epileptic patient wrote to his wife.

> I then thought that I was caught up by the hair of my head, and brought through the air to a beautiful country, which was surrounded by beautiful green grass parks, and those parks were full of young lambs, . . . I then asked the person supposed to be in my company, where was God. His reply was in Heaven. I then said this was Heaven. He then said that this was only a kitchen to Heaven, and none can enter into Heaven but those that are pure and perfect. He, the visionary man,[371] said that this was the place that saints were made perfect in. He then told me the number that had entered since our Saviour went there . . . .[372]

---

[367]Weil (1071), *Mohammed der Prophet*, pp. 42–45.

[368]*Ibid.*, footnote; Irving (534), *Life of Mahomet*, p. 38, note.

[369]Sprenger (947), *Das Leben und die Lehre des Mohammed*, vol. 1, p. 208.

[370]Cf. Moreau (709), *La psychologie morbide*, p. 552 ff., and above, XIII-3, where the situation is discussed in more detail.

[371]It is not clear whether "the visionary man" is part of the letter or an explanation by its editor, Dr. Howden.

[372]Howden (517), *The Religious Sentiments in Epileptics*, p. 489.

Patients of this kind were convinced of the reality of what they had heard and seen. They believed that their soul had temporarily absented itself from the body and had visited the land of the spirits.[373] Their experiences, it was said, did not differ from those of many religious enthusiasts who had founded new sects—Mohammed among them.[374]

The story of the epileptic Mohammed was thus reasserted, but whereas it had once served the purpose of discrediting Mohammed as a prophet, it now served to establish his good faith, with the understanding, however, that he had taken hallucinations for reality. A reassertion also came on grounds of personal insight from Feodor Mikhailovich Dostoievski (1821-81), whose epileptic attacks began with an ecstatic aura which has become famous in psychiatric literature.

The following account is by Sophie Kovalevskaya, who, as a child, had known Dostoievski. In her presence, in 1865, he talked about his disease and its alleged beginning at the time of his exile in Siberia, when he was unexpectedly visited by an old friend.[375]

> That was just on the night before Easter Sunday. But in the joy of meeting, they forgot what night it was and sat through it at home, talking and noticing neither time nor fatigue, drunk with their own words. They talked about what was to both of them dearer than anything else—about literature, art, and philosophy; finally

---

[373] *Ibid.*, pp. 487-88.

[374] *Ibid.*, p. 495: "There is strong evidence that Mahomed was an epileptic, and that, though a man of undoubted power and strong religious feeling, he founded his pretensions as a medium of revelation on visions which appeared to him during epileptic trances." Howden bolstered this opinion by citing Gustav Weil from Washington Irving's *Life of Mahomet*. Maudsley (674), *Responsibility in Mental Disease*, p. 243, who utilized Howden's article, also mentioned Mohammed. Most modern orientalists have abandoned the belief in the epileptic nature of Mohammed's inspirations. All biographical data apart, it is indeed hard to imagine that the Koran, a body of religious, legal, and social instruction should largely be the product of a succession of hallucinatory epileptic attacks. If, however, it were claimed that Mohammed was epileptic, but that his original visions only were associated with the disease, the value of the biographical tradition as a source of information for the diagnosis would altogether be weakened. The case of Mohammed is instructive because it illustrates the danger of diagnosing epilepsy in history with disregard of the historical setting, merely on the basis of behavioral similarities. Only recently has the alleged bond between shamanism and epilepsy been dissolved. Various so-called primitive peoples seem to be better able to distinguish between epilepsy and ecstatic states than they had been credited with. Thus Butt (1069), p. 39, contrasting an older account with her own observations writes: "During my research I encountered two, possibly three, Akawaio who were subject to fits. None of them were shamans and Akawaio do not consider that epileptics have any part to play in shaman activity." The attitude toward epileptics among "primitives" seems to vary with the tribe; cf. Koty (592), pp. 61, 100, 114, 115, and 123. The whole material on shamanism and its relation to disease has been appraised by Eliade (319), p. 23 ff.; see also Ackerknecht (7), and Rosen (872), pp. 55-58. Findeisen (358), p. 165, considers any association between shamanism and epilepsy as belonging to the realm of mythology. Nevertheless it remains possible that sporadically sufferers from temporal lobe epilepsy played the role of shamans or prophets.

[375] The following account is from Kovalevskaya (593), p. 90 ff.; cf. Alajouanine (16), p. 212. For this whole section on Dostoievski cf. Tellenbach (996) for papers and reports presented at a seminar on *Epileptikergestalten Dostojewskijs*; cf. also Minkowski and Fusswerk (704). These two publications contain many interesting points, though I am not able to share the philosophical orientations of all the authors.

they touched on religion. The friend was an atheist, Dostoievski a believer; both were passionately convinced, each in his way. "God exists, he exists," Dostoievski finally cried, beside himself with excitement. At the same moment the bells of the neighboring church rang for Easter matins. The air was vibrant and full of sound. "And I felt," Feodor Mikhailovich [Dostoievski] narrated, "that heaven had come down to earth and had absorbed me. I really perceived God and was imbued with Him. Yes, God exists,—I cried,—and I do not remember any more."

Having reached this point of his narrative, Dostoievski identified his own experience with Mohammed's visit to Heaven, which tradition connected with the flight from Mecca to Jerusalem. According to legend, all this had happened in one moment.[376] Dostoievski had a French translation of the Koran in his library; his wish to possess this book went back to the days of his exile.[377] He probably read Sura XVII, 1, and he was obviously acquainted with the legendary embellishments.

"All you, healthy people," he [Dostoievski] continued, "do not even suspect what happiness is, that happiness which we epileptics experience during the second before the attack. In his Koran Mohammed assures us that he saw paradise and was inside. All clever fools are convinced that he is simply a liar and a fraud. Oh no! He is not lying! He really was in paradise during an attack of epilepsy, from which he suffered as I do. I do not know whether this bliss lasts seconds, hours, or months, yet take my word, I would not exchange it for all the joys which life can give."

The story of Mohammed is also mentioned in *The Idiot* and the *Demons*, the novels in which Dostoievski makes two of his heroes, Prince Myshkin (in *The Idiot*) and Kirillov (in the *Demons*), suffer from the same kind of aura.[378]

Dostoievski's interest in Mohammed is understandable on purely human grounds. How far this identification with the great founder of a great religion enhanced Dostoievski's sense of his own mission, and whether it could possibly have influenced the character of his aura is a question for biographers of the novelist and political thinker. The fact remains that his own affliction, far from making him suppress all men-

---

[376] For the Western tradition of this story see Cerulli (213), p. 333. Gibbon (408), *Decline and Fall*, ch. 50; vol. 2, p. 665, speaks of "the tenth part of a night."

[377] Dostoievski (296), *Idiot*, p. 729, footnote to p. 257. According to Carr (204), p. 64, the Koran was among the books Dostoievski asked his brother to send him in 1859.

[378] See Appendix II. In both novels Dostoievski compares the subjective time of Mohammed's visit to paradise with the objective time which, as Dostoievski said, was less than it took for Mohammed's upset water jug to empty itself. I have not been able to trace the direct source for the story of the water jug. Possibly it refers to the jug of water belonging to a caravan which, according to Ibn Ishāq (525), *The Life of Muhammed*, p. 184, Mohammed emptied on his nightly journey; cf. Muir (721), vol. 2, p. 221. Dostoievski's association of his own ecstatic experience with that of Mohammed has long been noticed; cf. Clark (223), pp. 47 and 49, and Voegele and Dietze (1050), p. 135.

tion of epilepsy, allowed Dostoievski to draw on his experience for his novelistic use of epileptic figures, at least in the case of Prince Myshkin and Kirillov. A third major epileptic character, Smerdyakov, is introduced in *The Brothers Karamasov*. Whereas Myshkin and Kirillov are saintly types, Smerdyakov is the murderer of old Karamasov, his master and, probably, also his father. He is the son of an idiot girl and the grandson of an alcoholic. Dostoievski portrays him in a manner calculated to arouse disgust in the reader and likely to evoke the picture of a degenerate.

The genesis and nature of Dostoievski's own epilepsy is still a matter for debate. Sophie Kovalevskaya remarked that according to a different version, "Dostoievski acquired the falling sickness in consequence of a birching he had to undergo as a punishment during his penal servitude." She could not decide which the true version was, since doctors had told her "that it is typical of almost all persons who suffer from this disease to forget how it began and constantly to let their imagination run away with them in this respect."[379] Indeed, Trousseau remarked that little store was to be set by the epileptics' own accounts of what caused their disease. "The patients repeat what they have heard their relatives say."[380] At any rate, even before his deportation to Siberia, Dostoievski was already under medical treatment by his physician-friend Dr. Yanovski, and the nature of his disease seems to have been diagnosed by 1848.[381] How much further back in time his attacks went is not quite clear. Freud has given them a psychogenic explanation, connecting them with the assassination of Dostoievski's father by the latter's peasant serfs.[382] Around the time of the undoubted manifestations of his illness, Dostoievski used to borrow medical books from Dr. Yanovski, "particularly those which dealt with diseases of the brain and of the nervous system, with mental diseases, and with the development of the skull according to the old system of Gall, which was then in vogue.[383]

The pathography of Dostoievski and his work are of concern here only in as far as they form elements in the history of epilepsy. Apart from the aura of his grand mal attacks, Dostoievski's character and behavior showed some peculiarities that agreed with the picture of an epileptic as traced at his time. After his attacks, he suffered from " 'extraordinary anguish' " and from an "unbearable mystical ter-

---

[379] Kovalevskaya (593), p. 90.

[380] Trousseau (1032), *Clinique médicale*, p. 100.

[381] Cf. Yarmolinski (1112), ch. 5, pp. 55-62, Mochulsky (706), p. 6. To his superior in Siberian exile and friend, Baron Vrangel, Dostoievski (294), p. 299, declared that he had the first seizures in Petersburg and that the disease had become worse in prison. Cf. *ibid.*, p. 265, the reminiscences of D. V. Grigorovich, describing a seizure Dostoievski suffered when attending a funeral.

[382] See Freud (379), also reprinted in Wellek (1074), pp. 98-111.

[383] Yanovski as quoted by Grossman (435), p. 94.

ror."[384] He was highly irritable, suspicious, given to vehement outbursts (Sophie Kovalevskaya has described a jealous scene he made at a social gathering[385]), and, of course, he was a deeply religious person. The very depth of his religious feeling distinguished it from the shallow display usually attributed to epileptics. His fervent religiosity combined with his ecstatic visions harmonized with the contemporary interpretation of epileptic prophets. Indeed, there was a prophetic tone in much of what he said and wrote.[386]

Nevertheless, however great a part epileptics were assigned in his novels, the purpose of these novels was not the portrayal of epileptics. The disease of Prince Myshkin, Kirillov, and Smerdyakov was used in as far as it helped the aim of the story, and Dostoievski utilized it rather freely. There are small touches which have their counterpart in the medical literature of the time. For instance, of Prince Myshkin it is said: "His eyes were large, blue, and steady; there was something quiet but heavy in their look, something full of that strange expression from which a few people at first glance guess the presence of the falling sickness."[387] A particular look of epileptics had been noted by the ancient physiognomists, and in 1843 Billod had written that their "look has a characteristic expression which, no doubt, it owes to a dilatation often unequal, of the pupil, which is somewhat more than physiological and has become habitual."[388] Maudsley spoke of "the heavy, lost look so often seen in confirmed epileptics."[389] Shortly after having introduced Prince Myshkin as an epileptic, Dostoievski makes him tell that he [Myshkin] had been sent abroad "because of some peculiar nervous illness, in the nature of the falling sickness or St. Vitus dance, a kind of tremblings and convulsions."[390] At the time, epilepsy and chorea were seen in close proximity and mentioning them together was by no means strange.[391]

---

[384]Mochulsky (706), p. 385. For the feeling of anguish see above, p. 319.

[385]See Dostoievski (294), p. 327 ff.

[386]Dostoievski's prophetic attitude was noted by de Vogüé (1052), *The Russian Novel*, *passim*.

[387]Dostoievski (296), *Idiot*, p. 6.

[388]Billod (113), *Recherches et considérations relatives à la symptomatologie de l'épilepsie*, p. 420.

[389]Maudsley (674), *Responsibility in Mental Disease*, p. 168.

[390]*Idiot*, l.c., p. 7: "... po kakoi-to strannoi nervnoi bolezni, vrodi paduchei ili vittovoi plyaski, kakikh-to drozhenii i sudrog."

[391]Maudsley (674), *Responsibility in Mental Disease*, p. 41: "Chorea, again, which has been described fancifully as 'an insanity of the muscles,' is a nervous disease which exhibits sometimes a close relation of descent to insanity or epilepsy ...." P. 42: "In like manner insanity might truly be described as a chorea or convulsive disease of the mind, the derangement being in nerve centres whose functions are not motor but mental, and whose derangements therefore display themselves in convulsions not of the muscles but of mind." See also Gowers (420), *Epilepsy*, pp. 183-88. Alajouanine (16), *passim*, has analyzed the variety of seizures to which Dostoievski was subject and which, knowingly or not, he depicted in the characters of his novels.

The ecstatic aura gave to Myshkin metaphysical depth and to Kirillov a more than intellectual relationship to the besetting idea of God. Without his psychic attacks, Kirillov would hardly have been placed among the epileptics (he denied being one), and even with all the well-known traits of the disease Myshkin remains a peculiar epileptic. He is sufficiently restored to health to become an actor, however innocent, in an extremely complicated plot of intrigue, passion, and crime. "By a happy chance," as a critic put it, the disease "has destroyed that part of the intellect which is the seat of all our defects: irony, arrogance, selfishness, avarice; while the noble qualities are largely developed."[392] Then, abruptly, he falls into a complete, incurable state of mere vegetative existence. He and the other epileptics remain the creation of Dostoievski, whose stature as a novelist is not diminished by directing Prince Myshkin's epilepsy in accordance with the aim of *The Idiot*, the picture of "a human being of positive beauty."[393]

The Western discoverers of Dostoievski in the eighteen-eighties did not escape the impression which few of his readers are likely to be spared, that of entering a morbid world.[394] The literary interpretation of Dostoievski's novels, following their discovery and translation, belongs to a period largely outside the limits of this book. There is, however, a question which is pertinent here in view of a structural parallel between the life of an epileptic with its seizures and the course of a Dostoievskian novel with its unbearable tensions discharging themselves in violent scenes.[395] Dostoievski was epileptic; his novels were the creation of his mind, temper, and imagination; hence their world is the product of that unique epileptic, Dostoievski, in whom disease, personal experiences, and creativity were inseparably interwoven.[395a] This is not quite the same as considering the world of Dostoievski an epileptic world. And just because Dostoievski's influence exerted itself so strongly upon future generations, it is all the more important for a

---

[392]De Vogüé (1052), *The Russian Novel*, p. 188.

[393]Dostoievski (293), *Pis'ma*, p. 71: "Glavnaya mysl' romana izobrazit' polozhitel'no prekrasnovo cheloveka" (from a letter to S. A. Ivanova). Stollreiter-Butzon (962) believes to recognize in Prince Myshkin the features of an epileptic personality as analyzed by Bräutigam (145), and contrasts this with the claims for positive beauty of a Christ-like figure. But even if Dostoievski really envisaged a parallel between Prince Myshkin and Christ, he hardly went as far as identifying the two. Regarding Prince Myshkin's aggressiveness as attested by his account of an execution, I believe this to be an example of his peculiar role as a spectator who insists on seeing things as they are [cf. Rosenberg (873), pp. 159 and 173]. An evaluation of Dostoievski's characters must, I think, also take into account differences in the standards of behavior prevailing in Russian society of about 1860 and Western European society a hundred years ago.

[394]De Vogüé (1052), *The Russian Novel*, p. 198: "... we call him ... the Shakespeare of the madhouse." De Vogüé's book was instrumental in spreading understanding for Dostoievski's significance. Cf. Wellek (1074), pp. 2 and 10.

[395]Zweig (1120), pp. 178–80; cf. literature cited above in footnote 375, also Janz (561), p. 419 f., Vogel (1051a), Alajouanine (16), p. 214.

[395a]Cf. Alajouanine (16), pp. 215–18.

history of epilepsy not to lose sight of other views on life, literature, and epilepsy, existent at his time.

In an essay on the brothers Goncourt, who, together with Flaubert and the young Zola, belonged to the rising school of French naturalism, Paul Bourget remarked that for the Goncourts life "was almost reduced to a series of epileptic attacks between two nothings." Bourget said this in view of the philosophy of absolute fatalism which made of life a sad and dangerous adventure, a useless effort condemned in advance.[396] Lombroso picked up Bourget's remark about the Goncourts but added: "And the Goncourts always wrote autobiography."[397] Lombroso imputed epilepsy to the brothers Goncourt; he quoted from a letter to Zola, in which Edmond Goncourt wrote that "our whole work . . . rests on nervous disease . . . we have extracted these pictures of the sickness [of Charles Demailly] out of ourselves . . . ." Lombroso also cited a passage from the brothers' *Journal* attributing their work [*Soeur Philomène*] to "a superior will . . . which guided the pen," so that the novel surprised them like something which was in them, but of which they were unconscious.[398] The creations of the Goncourts were considered by Lombroso as pathognomonic for the epileptic brothers, just as Dostoievski's work has been seen as an expression of his disease.

Lombroso's version of the degenerate epileptic influenced Zola's portrayal of Jacques Lantier in *The Human Beast* (1890). In Jacques, sexual desire is mixed with an irresistible impulse to cut the woman's throat. Eventually, his mistress becomes a victim of his supposed atavism, of the pathological reawakening of the cave man.

Zola did not expressly call Jacques Lantier an epileptic, but to contemporary physicians this diagnosis seemed clear. Lombroso himself is said to have praised Zola for describing in Jacques "a criminal epileptoid vertigo."[399] The Paris physiologist, Dr. Héricourt, while criticizing the notion of atavism and altogether blaming Zola for being carried away by Lombroso's theories,[400] wrote of Jacques Lantier: ". . . he is an epileptic, only his epilepsy is psychical, and his attacks, instead of

---

[396] Bourget (143), *Edmond et Jules de Goncourt*, p. 170: "Aperçue sous cet angle de fatalisme absolu, la vie humaine n'est plus qu'une aventure triste et dangereuse, un effort inutile et condamné par avance. Pour les frères de Goncourt, en particulier, elle se réduit presque à une série d'attaques d'épilepsie entre deux néants." In the edition used, the essay is dated 1885, but it has an appendix (p. 193) dated 1882. Babbitt (72), *Literature and the American College*, p. 176: "Life itself has recently been defined by one of the lights of the French deliquescent school as 'an epileptic fit between two nothings.' "

[397] Lombroso (646), *The Man of Genius*, p. 343.

[398] Lombroso (645), *L'homme de génie*, pp. 461 and 468, footnote 2. It should be noted that in reality *Charles Demailly* does not depict an epileptic.

[399] Zola (1119), *La bête humaine*, editorial notes by Henri Mitterand who, on p. 1752, states that, according to Lombroso, "Zola avait fort bien décrit, en Jacques Lantier, un 'vertige criminel épileptoïde' . . . ." On p. 1026 Zola said that Jacques' good looks were marred by too strong a jaw, a stigma which Lombroso had listed among those of the born criminal; cf. *ibid.*, p. 1763, the editorial note to this passage.

[400] Héricourt (484), *La 'bête humaine' de M. Zola*, p. 714.

being convulsive, take the form of an impulse which is always the same. At first he is able to resist it, but eventually, activated by favorable circumstances, it ends by completely beclouding the sick man's reason, by taking hold of his whole being in a generalized cerebral convulsion, and by satisfying itself . . . . The impulses, as we know, are in the first place hereditary defects, and Mr. Zola takes care to tell us this."[401]

One scene in particular depicts Jacques as suffering from epileptic vertigo as this was understood. Jacques follows a young woman into a railway car and decides on the very spot where he will plunge the knife. But then an acquaintance enters and engages him in an irrelevant conversation. "And from this moment on, everything became confused."[402] Afterward, Jacques was not sure whether he had followed the woman; he remembered throwing his knife into the Seine; he also must have eaten somewhere. When he came to himself, he was lying fully dressed across his bed. He awakened bewildered from a heavy sleep as if after a dead faint.

Zola's portrait of Jacques Lantier is not limited to externals. The reader is acquainted with Jacques' feelings when he desperately resists the compulsive urge, yet is attracted by images of murder and blood. Zola tries to show the inner life of this epileptic, but apart from what belongs to the province of his "disease" (as Jacques thinks of it) Jacques' world is that of the naturalist author. As far back as 1873, Maudsley, musing about "the mental characteristics of the epileptic neurosis," noted the "singularly vivid imagination, which is apt sometimes to occupy itself with painful or repulsive subjects. Probably," he continued, "the invention of the modern sensational novel, with its murders, bigamies, and other crimes, was an achievement of the epileptic imagination."[403] "The epileptic imagination" was probably taken in a generic sense and was credited to all authors with starkly realistic tendencies. It is very unlikely that Maudsley was thinking of Dostoievski, who, in 1873, was as yet practically unknown in England.[404] Yet the description obviously fitted him. The conclusion to be drawn is that to some contemporaries at least the epileptic Dostoievski was a member of a much wider group of authors whose novels reflected their alleged epileptic traits.

The preoccupation with epilepsy as a frame of mind had still another witness in Friedrich Nietzsche (1844-1900). Nietzsche speculated

---

[401] *Ibid.*, p. 713; cf. also Mitterand's note in Zola (1119), p. 1751.

[402] Zola (1119), *La bête humaine*, p. 1212: "Et, à partir de ce moment, tout se brouilla, il ne put jamais, plus tard, rétablir les faits exactemente." However, this scene is the only one where a confused state and amnesia are clearly mentioned.

[403] Maudsley (674), *Responsibility in Mental Disease*, p. 243.

[404] According to Muchnic (716), p. 7, interest in Dostoievski was aroused in England after his death (1881) only. Mr. I. Irvine has kindly brought Muchnic's book to my attention.

about "people with intellectual convulsions,"[405] who were impatient
with themselves, whose own work gave them brief burning satisfaction
followed by desolation and bitterness. They thirsted for absorption in
something outside themselves, in God, in images of passionate life, or in
deeds. And so, Nietzsche asked, with Pascal, might not the urge to act
be, after all, a flight from one's self? The proposition could indeed be
proven: one should consider, of course "with a psychiatrist's knowledge
and experience, that four of the men most thirsty for action of all time
were epileptics (Alexander, Caesar, Mohammed and Napoleon), just as
Byron, too, was subject to this disease."[406]

In speaking of people with intellectual convulsions (or cramps),
Nietzsche was not very original, for epileptic metaphors were not rare
at the time. Jackson himself mentioned the expression "convulsions of
ideas," which was used for insanity in general and for seizures of epileptic insanity in particular.[407] In the same work of 1880-81 in which
Nietzsche's remark occurred, he also referred to St. Paul as the founder
of Christianity, taking it for granted that the apostle was an epileptic.
As Nietzsche saw him, Paul, the zealot of the Jewish Law, actually
wished to free himself from it, and he succeeded by recognizing in Jesus
the annihilation of the Law. This idea appeared to him "together with a
vision, as it was bound to happen in an epileptic: to him, the furious
fanatic of the Law who internally was deadly tired of it, Christ
appeared in a lonely street, the lustre of God on his face, and Paul
heard the words: 'why do you persecute *me*?' "[408] From St. Paul,
Nietzsche turns to Christianity as such, for which all morality is
grounded in the religious rebirth of the sinner, "that ecstatic minute ... when man experiences the 'breakthrough of grace' and the
moral miracle." Nietzsche inquires after the physiological meaning "of
such a sudden, irrational, and irresistible turn, such a change of lowest

---

[405]Nietzsche (734), *Morgenröthe*, par. 549; p. 341: "Jene Menschen der intellectuellen
Krämpfe, welche gegen sich selber ungeduldig und verfinstert sind . . . ."

[406]*Ibid.*: ". . . man erwäge doch, mit dem Wissen und den Erfahrungen eines Irrenarztes, wie
billig,—dass Vier von den Thatendurstigsten aller Zeiten Epileptiker gewesen sind (nämlich
Alexander, Cäsar, Muhammed und Napoleon): so wie auch Byron diesem Leiden unterworfen
war." Nietzsche was no more critical in attributing epilepsy than was Lombroso. Maudsley
(674), *Responsibility in Mental Disease*, p. 243, had also stressed "the immense energy, such as
was exemplified in Mahomet, Napoleon, etc." as a mental characteristic in epilepsy.

[407]Jackson (556), *Selected Writings*, vol. 1, p. 122: "It has been said that the patient who is
subject to attacks in which there is convulsion of muscles may at another time have an attack in
which there is 'convulsion of ideas,' and corresponding excess of external action (mania)."
Jackson may be referring to Maudsley, who used this expression, e.g. (674), p. 156:
". . . homicidal impulse as a convulsive idea springing from a morbid condition of nerve element . . . ."

[408]Nietzsche (734), *Morgenröthe*, par. 68; p. 63 (italics in the text). St. Paul was not
generally accepted as having been an epileptic. Renan (839), *Les apôtres*, p. 171, conceded that
the famous "thorn in the flesh" of Saul (II Corinthians 12: 7) probably referred to some illness,
but on pp. 175-85, where he related the circumstances of St. Paul's conversion, Renan did not
mention or suggest epilepsy. Cf. above Part Four, footnote 89.

misery and most profoundly pleasurable feeling." He leaves the answer to the psychiatrist after asking suggestively, "was it, perhaps, a masked epilepsy?"[409]

At that time, Nietzsche had not yet discovered Dostoievski. The discovery came in 1887,[410] the time of his latest writings. In the *Antichrist*, Nietzsche attacked the gospel which presented "a world as if out of a Russian novel in which the scum of society, nervous disease, and 'childlike' idiocy seem to have a rendez-vous."[411] In reading of childlike idiocy it is hard not to think of Prince Myshkin. "What a pity," Nietzsche said a few lines later, "that no Dostoievski lived in the vicinity of this most interesting decadent, I mean somebody sufficiently perceptive of the touching attraction of such a mixture of the sublime, morbid, and childlike."[412] The decadent who presented this touching attraction was Jesus himself. A Christ-like feature in Prince Myshkin had been seen before Nietzsche,[413] but to Nietzsche it was left to degrade Christ by seeing in him a Prince Myshkin.[414] For Nietzsche epilepsy served as an instrument of destruction of both the faith and the faithful. The man of faith appeared to him no longer capable of honestly facing the question of true or untrue. Hence, he was the opposite of the strong, liberated mind. He who was convinced became a fanatic, a Savonarola, Luther, Rousseau, Robespierre, Saint-Simon—all their minds were sick, they were "epileptics of the idea."[415]

What a contrast in perspective between Nietzsche's epileptics of the idea and Jackson's sufferers from discharging lesions and dreamy states! The contrast does not lie in scientific explanations but in the evaluation of the disease. Zola, Nietzsche, and Dostoievski, each in his own way dealt with epilepsy within the world of social intercourse and human values, in contrast to Jackson, for whom this world was not much more than an index of biological processes. Jackson's great achievement was the aligning of the epilepsies with modern physiology of the human nervous system, based on discharges of ganglionic cells and the co-ordination of human behavior with an evolutionary anatomy of the brain and spinal cord. He did this with great scientific imagination, but apart from such sympathies as he might have had for his patients as a physician, he was indifferent to whether their behavior was ridiculous,

---

[409]Nietzsche, *l.c.*, par. 87, p. 80.

[410]Kaufmann (575), p. 280, footnote 9.

[411]Nietzsche, *Der Antichrist*, par. 31, in Podach (814), p. 112.

[412]*Ibid.*

[413]De Vogüé (1052), *The Russian Novel*, p. 188.

[414]Kaufmann (575), p. 298: "It seems plain that Nietzsche conceived of Jesus in the image of Dostoyevsky's conception of *The Idiot*."

[415]*Der Antichrist*, par. 54; Podach (814), p. 143: ". . . die grossen Attitüden dieser kranken Geister, dieser Epileptiker des Begriffs . . ."; cf. Kaufmann (575), p. 311. In this connection, cf. Maudsley's and Jackson's speaking of "convulsion of ideas," cf. above, footnote 407.

pathetic, or criminal. Zola could and, for all we know, did, enthusiastically agree with Jacksonian science, yet the significance of the particular epileptic he drew lies in the latter's place in a human society conceived in terms of inexorable natural law. It is easy to imagine Hughlings Jackson criticizing the portrait of Jean Lantier *qua* epileptic; but his work does not readily reveal whether a debate on naturalism would have interested him. The experiment of imagining Prince Myshkin as Jackson's patient and comparing Jackson's notes on this case with Dostoievski's *Idiot* seems ludicrous, not because of a clash of contradictions but because of utter incongruity.

If we do not look upon man at the end of the nineteenth century as isolated in national and professional departments, Jackson, Gowers, Samt, Falret, Lombroso, Dostoievski, Zola, Nietzsche, and others, all represent facets of the knowledge of and about epilepsy. In as far as the history of the Falling Sickness is the history of epilepsy between the competing claims of body and soul, of physical forces and mental powers, of individual rights and social restraints, these facets depicted the stage of that history near the close of the last century.

# Epilogue

Today, more perhaps than ever before, we feel the need for finding a synthesis of the somatic and psychological, the individual and social factors which coexist in all disease. This need also stimulates our historical work: it urges us to find unity in the history of disease and to bring together the threads which the past itself may have left loose and independent of one another. The history of a disease, therefore, is more than a record of its coming and going, of its clinical manifestations, of the impressions it made upon man, of the knowledge man acquired of it, of the theories he formed about it, and the means he employed against it. The history of a disease is also a moulding of all those elements into a unit implied when we talk about the disease, experience it, study it, and thus add to its history, so that eventually a new historical synthesis becomes necessary. The ideal history of a disease is a blend of its natural history, as far as it has revealed itself in the past, and its human history, if this term may be used to designate what man knew, thought, and did about it.

Have we then really traced the history of a disease? The very existence of a disease "epilepsy" is doubted; indeed, we are taught that there are only "epilepsies." Yet we would not be speaking of epilepsies were it not for something that is expressed by the plural form. The history of epilepsy is the development of this something, differently defined at different times. But, the argument continues, we have not described any coming and going of epilepsy, or any impressive changes in its clinical manifestations, except perhaps epileptic attacks appearing with the introduction of syphilis into

Europe (if really it was introduced). Moreover, by limiting ourselves to Western civilization, we have foregone the right to speak of *the* history of epilepsy, which knows no national or cultural boundaries. We have merely dealt with the human history of epilepsy in the West. The limitation to the West must be admitted. Without it, we might possibly have found greater variations in the past appearance of the disease, though this is not likely. The fact that so many types of epileptic attacks were described in Antiquity already suggests the existence of brain mechanisms which have been relatively stable, historically speaking, though released by different physical and psychic stimuli with varying historical roles. In short, the natural history of epilepsy as it revealed itself in the past is not very different from what it is today. It merges into the human history.

Altogether, the isolation of the past natural history of a disease from its human history is an abstraction. To some extent it is necessitated by methodology; there will hardly be investigators in full command of both the scientific and the historical methods. Moreover, there is the legitimate practice of many medical scientists to start with their subject as given by tradition and then to devote themselves to the approaches offered by modern science. Nevertheless, the isolation of natural history from human history remains an abstraction. Diseases do not exist without their victims, who, as human beings, live in historically changing societies and experience their illnesses differently. And when the modern medical scientist undertakes the study of a disease, he starts with concepts which are neither of his invention nor offered by Nature. Whether he knows it or not, they bear the imprint of his predecessors, they are historically shaped. The Hippocratic physician who wished to discuss the disease "epilepsy" had to refer to the so-called sacred disease, and to reject the magic connotations. Thanks to his Greek ancestors, the modern physician takes epilepsy as the name for a natural process. Thanks also to events which we set out in detail, he no longer has to deal with epilepsy as the medley of conditions going under the name of the falling sickness. Even as late as 1872, Morel reported of the nursing Sisters of a French asylum that, while recognizing the social behavior of a patient as epileptic, they added: "but she does not fall."[416] The fall to them was still the guiding symptom. It gradually ceased to be so when the grand mal attack no longer dominated the picture of epilepsy to the degree it had in earlier times.

In terminating our history of epilepsy at this point, we have—quite apart from all other shortcomings—failed to fulfill the demands of an ideal history of the disease. But a continuation would have required an

---

[416] Société médico-psychologique (934), *De l'épilepsie larvée*, t. 9, p. 157: "Les religieuses me disent: 'elle est méchante comme une épileptique, mais elle ne tombe pas.' "

integration of cultural, intellectual, social, and scientific matters which did not promise to be successful under the short perspective of the twentieth century. Apart from such general considerations, there were also reasons against a continuation along merely scientific lines after Hughlings Jackson.

Jackson's principles of the study of epilepsy were publicly vindicated by the achievements of William Macewen (1848-1924) and Victor Horsley (1857-1916). On August 13, 1886, Horsley addressed the Section on Surgery of the British Medical Association on "Advances in the Surgery of the Central Nervous System," and the reporter of *The Lancet* referred to this address as "what may truly be called *the* surgical paper of the meeting."[417] Three patients were demonstrated after successful operation. "Epileptiform fits" had been the main clinical symptoms, caused by injury in two cases and a tumor in the third. Horsley dwelt on the experimental work on monkeys that had made exact diagnosis possible. Both Charcot and Hughlings Jackson were present, and each congratulated Horsley on his "brilliant" and "admirable" success.[417]

Two years later, William Macewen, before the meeting of the same society in Glasgow, reported on his work in brain surgery, the successful beginnings of which had antedated that of Horsley, though his earlier publications seem to have aroused relatively little attention.[418] Macewen probably was the first surgeon to localize the cerebral focus by inference from the motor or sensory signs. The first case was that of "a convulsion," accompanied by loss of consciousness, beginning on the right side, gradually involving the whole body, and followed by right-sided hemiplegia and aphasia of two hours' duration. Macewen diagnosed an abscess "in the immediate vicinity of Broca's lobe" and proposed to open it. Unfortunately, permission was refused and the patient died. But permission was granted to perform the operation posthumously, the abscess was duly found as diagnosed, which gave "poignancy to the regret that the operation had not been permitted during life."[419]

In subsequent years a number of cases with focal epilepsy were operated upon successfully. In cases so complicated as to make an exact pre-operative anatomical diagnosis impossible, Macewen advised: "To lay bare a certain known convolution on a cerebral surface and observe the results of its stimulation."[420] But here he seems to have been antici-

---

[417]*Surgery* (980), pp. 346-47. The paper was published in full under the title *Brain-Surgery* (512). Cf. Jefferson (563), pp. 150-69, article on *Sir Victor Horsley, 1857-1916.*

[418]Cf. Jefferson (563), pp. 132-49: *Sir William Macewen's Contribution to Neurosurgery and Its Sequels.*

[419]Macewen (656), *An Address on the Surgery of the Brain and Spinal Cord*, p. 303.

[420]*Ibid.*, p. 305.

pated by Horsley.[421] However that may be, defining the focus by artificial stimulation during the operation has become an integral part of cerebral surgery in epilepsies amenable to this treatment.

Apart from exact anatomical diagnosis before and during the operation, the surgical treatment of epilepsies had to rely on the acceptance of Lister's antiseptic principles published in 1867. This acceptance came more or less slowly in various countries; in the Anglo-Saxon world it came only in the late seventies. Then again progress had to await the professionalization of neurosurgery. What appears as a triumph of preceding work in our context, appears as a mere beginning in the perspective of subsequent developments. This, of course, also holds generally true. With the beginning of modern neurology a reasonably comprehensive clinical basis for the study of epilepsy had been established. The rediscovery of the Mendelian laws at the turn of the century began to substitute exact genetic studies for loose speculations on heredity and degeneracy. In 1912 phenobarbital (luminal) was introduced into the treatment and was followed by sodium diphenylhydantoin (dilantin) in 1938 and later by other potent drugs. Beginning in the thirties, the study of the electroencephalogram has become an essential diagnostic tool, which in course of time has led to a sharper differentiation of epilepsy from other diseases and to changes in the classification of the epilepsies. Concomitantly, a more perceptive psychological analysis of epileptics has been cultivated than was known in the asylums of the nineteenth century. All this, together with improved care and a social outlook which has discarded much superstitious dread, has created a climate in which many epileptics can live hopeful, happy, and productive lives.

Yet a recital of milestones in the fight against epilepsy does not yet constitute history. In the scientific history of epilepsy, as in the scientific history of diseases in general, the laboratories have come to play an increasingly large part. The experimental history of epilepsy reaches back at least to the sixteenth century; it gathered momentum with Flourens' experiments of 1823 and entered its modern stage in 1870 with Fritsch and Hitzig's experiments on dogs, followed by those of Ferrier on monkeys. How close the ties between physiological experiment and the surgical treatment of epilepsy had become evinces from the fact that Horsley, the surgeon, co-operated with Schäfer, the physiologist, and Beevor, the neurologist, in experiments on monkeys extending Ferrier's research.[422] The direct irritability with faradic cur-

---

[421] Cf. below, footnote 424, cf. also Walker (1058), p. 294.

[422] Cf. Horsley and Schäfer (514), *A Record of Experiments upon the Functions of the Cerebral Cortex*; Beevor and Horsley (94), *A Minute Analysis*, etc. p. 163: ". . . the sequence in the movement of the joints is fundamentally similar to that which had been arrived at from

rent of the human cerebral cortex had been demonstrated by Bartho-
low in 1874 under tragic circumstances. The feeble-minded patient,
who suffered from a fatal illness, died a few days after the conclusion
of the experiments.[423] Twelve years later, Horsley used weak faradic
stimulation to ascertain the area to be excised.[424] What has served as a
practical guide for more effective treatment has contributed scientifically to the knowledge of the function of the human brain.

Research on the cerebral mechanisms of epileptic attacks and neurophysiological research are so intimately interwoven that the history of
the former must either presuppose the knowledge of the latter or concomitantly deal with it. A similar relationship exists with regard to
electrophysiology, biochemistry, and pharmacology: the history of
epilepsy cannot be followed separately from the history of these
branches of science. The understanding of the electroencephalogram is
associated with the knowledge of the electrophysiology of ganglionic
cells and synapses. Here too, the beginnings reach back to a period
already discussed, to the interpretation of the "negative variation" as an
accompaniment of nervous activity and to the early tracing of electric
currents in dogs' brains. The electroencephalogram can relate deviations
from the normal picture to foci in certain regions of the brain. For
instance, in many cases of psychomotor epilepsy it pointed to the
region of the temporal lobe. But it does not explain what it is that is
going on in the cells and their surroundings that makes them behave
abnormally. Jackson and his predecessors agreed that nutritional
changes must be involved. When they spoke of epilepsy as a functional
disease, they implied that no structural changes could be observed. But
the dimensions of structure have changed; the ultrastructure of cells has
now to be taken into account. Biochemistry having become allied with
genetics, the study of cellular metabolism in epilepsy includes disorders
of enzyme action of a genetic as well as an acquired nature. Where
Jackson's contemporaries could no more than guess at the metabolic
processes in nervous tissues, answers now are expected in qualitatively
precise and quantitatively exact terms. There have to be added those
investigations that concern the psychological interpretation of epileptics with the tools of experimental and dynamic psychology. All this
has then to be correlated with the clinical studies.

Though incomparably more is known than was the case in 1890, a
level has not yet been reached where the scientific explanation of

---

clinical observation by Dr. Hughlings Jackson in cases of epilepsy, in which he had recorded the
'march' of the movements of the joints."

[423] Cf. Walker (1057), p. 110.

[424] Horsley (513), *Remarks on Ten Consecutive Cases*, etc., p. 864, referring to case no. 5:
"October 19th, 1886. Trephining over 'facial centre,' and removal of cortex composing that
centre as determined by faradism at the time."

epilepsy presents a harmonious picture in which all true results fall into place and from which all false results are eliminated.[425] Writing the scientific history of epilepsy to the present must necessarily include a multitude of contributions whose bearing is as yet uncertain. Even the part we covered is not quite free from such uncertainties, although the distance from our own days permitted us to use as an unavowed frame of reference what is now by and large undisputed.

Many data toward a history of epilepsy since 1890 have been contributed by various authors,[426] and the day may soon come for a new historical synthesis of epilepsy. The Falling Sickness may then no longer be an appropriate title, and epilepsy may have ceased to appear as a paradigm of the suffering of both body and soul in disease.

---

[425] Walker's (1059) survey of problems to be investigated implicitly gives a summary of problems not solved yet.

[426] To the works of Lennox (632), Janz (561), and Szondi (988) with their many historical references have to be added historical works on neurology, psychiatry, and neurosurgery by Haymaker (466), Kolle (590), and Walker (1058), and articles dealing with the history of epilepsy by Purpura (832) and Wenger (1082).

**APPENDICES**

# Appendix I

Th. Herpin (486), *Des accès incomplets d'épilepsie*, pp. 160-61. (translated by C. Lilian Temkin).

The frequency of the vertigoes as an epileptic phenomenon, their numerous varieties, the interest their study affords for the physiology of the nervous system, and even for psychology, have involved us in details which we do not regret, but which may have caused the reader to lose sight of the ensemble of phenomena that constitute these incomplete attacks. We shall, therefore, retrace in broad outline the picture of the progressive steps in these episodes, or, in other words, give a résumé of what we have said about them.

*Résumé*—The vertigoes, beginning with a perturbation of a sense or with its suppression, with a psychic disturbance or with physical sensations in the head, end rapidly in complete suspension of consciousness, if they did not begin with such suspension. Once consciousness is lost, the episode may not develop further; at the mildest level the patient, giving no sign of comprehension, remains standing or continues to walk, pupils dilated, the face pale. At the medium or severe levels, he is very momentarily deprived of his senses. The vertigo is most often complicated by a pharyngeal spasm and by buccal noises or movements; minor facial convulsions, most often exclusively tonic, may also occur. Then each level may be marked by the greater or smaller degree of contracture, with or without partial jerks. When the trunk is involved, the cry, the fall, and the signs of a less pronounced asphyxia than in full attacks join the usual symptoms of vertigo. In short, vertigo may differ from the complete attack only in the non-generalization of the clonic convulsions, the contracture being extended to all the muscles. There is seldom any emission of saliva, and it is almost never frothy. Involuntary urination is still rarer and occurs only at the most advanced levels. Biting [of the tongue] is one of the most exceptional symptoms. Neither ecchymotic marks nor bruises are found afterward. The duration of the vertigo, properly speaking, is usually a minute at most, though it may be as much as two minutes. In the mild forms, patients immediately resume their activities; at a more advanced level, the return of understanding is preceded by a brief stupor. Still further up the scale of intensity, the return is marked by a slightly soporous state, the revival of the senses, then a short period of incoherence, sometimes with violence and malice. After the most complete vertigoes, particularly if they occur frequently and if the disease is of long standing, the period of return may be as long as a quarter of an hour, an hour, even two hours. It then takes on the appearance of somnambulism: without their being conscious of it, the patients silently perform the actions of ordinary life, though not quite correctly. They may unknowingly not only act, but speak, their speech being not too unreasonable and betraying only occasionally a slight mental disarray. They may conduct themselves in such a way that a person, if not forewarned, would not suspect that moments later they would know nothing of all that has happened.

# Appendix II

In Dostoievski's *The Possessed* (*Besy*), the ecstatic aura[1] is described in detail in a conversation between Kirillov and Shatov.

> "There are seconds, occurring five or six at a time, and you suddenly feel you have fully attained the presence of eternal harmony. This is nothing worldly; I do not mean that it is something heavenly, but something which a man, in a worldly sense, cannot bear. One must either change physically or die. It is a clear and indisputable sensation—as if you suddenly became aware of all nature and suddenly said: yes, this is true. When God created the world he said at the end of every day of creation: 'yes, this is true, this is good.' This . . . this is not a tender emotion but simply joy. You forgive nothing because there is nothing to forgive. It is not that you love, oh— this is higher than love. What is most awful is that it is so terribly clear and such a joy. If it lasts more than five seconds, the soul will not endure it and must vanish. In these five seconds I live a lifetime, and for them I shall give away my whole life because it is worth it. To endure ten seconds one must change physically. I believe man should stop having children. To what purpose are children, to what purpose is evolution, once the goal is reached? In the Gospel it says: that they will not give birth on resurrection, that they will be like God's angels. A hint. Does your wife bear children?"
>
> "Kirillov, does that happen often?"
>
> "Sometimes every three days, sometimes once a week."
>
> "You do not have the falling sickness?"
>
> "No."

---

[1] For this term cf. Alajouanin (16), p. 216.

"Then it will come. Take care, Kirillov. I heard that the falling sickness begins just so. An epileptic described to me in detail this warning sensation before the attack, exactly like you. He too set five seconds and said that it is impossible to endure more. Remember Mohammed's pitcher, which had not time to empty itself while he flew on his horse all over his paradise. The pitcher—that is your five seconds; it reminds one too much of your harmony, and Mohammed was an epileptic. Take care, Kirillov, the falling sickness!"[2]

Prince Myshkin, the hero of *The Idiot*, pondered the fact

that in his epileptic condition there was one phase before the attack itself (provided the attack came during waking hours) when suddenly in the midst of sadness, mental darkness, oppression, his brain momentarily was as if set on fire, and all his vital forces strained themselves at once, in an unusual outburst. His consciousness and feeling of being alive became almost tenfold during these moments, which repeated themselves like lightning. His mind, his heart were illuminated with an unusual light; all excitement, all doubts, all troubles were at once as if at peace, solved in some higher calm full of clear harmonious joy and hope, full of intelligence and final reason. Yet these moments, these flashes were nothing but the presentiment of that final second (never more than a second) with which the attack itself started. This second was, of course, unbearable.

Later, when reflecting on these experiences, Myshkin is aware of their being morbid, "and if so, it is by no means a higher existence, rather, on the contrary, it must be reckoned as the very lowest." And yet: " 'What about its being a disease?' he decided in the end, 'what has the fact of this being an abnormal tension to do with it, if the result itself, if the minute of sensation as remembered and considered in the healthy state proves in the highest degree harmonious, beautiful, gives an unheard of and hitherto unthought of feeling of completeness, measure, conciliation, and rapturous and gracious fusion with the very highest synthesis of life?' " Myshkin fully realizes the subjective nature of his experiences, yet he has no doubt that this is "beauty and grace (*molitva*)" and really "the highest synthesis of life." He cannot admit any doubts because "during that moment he did not dream any visions as from hashish, opium, or wine, which lower reason and pervert the soul, which are abnormal and unreal." In other words, Myshkin defends the reality of his "unusual intensification of self-consciousness" by pointing out the absence of hallucinations. In so far, Myshkin's aura is not of the visionary type. Yet he himself expresses a relationship to

[2]Dostoievski (296), *Besy*, Part iii, ch. 5, 5; t. vii, p. 614 f.

potential vision during "that final second." "Probably," he says, "this is the same second, not long enough for the upset water jug of the epileptic Mohammed to empty itself, while he, in that same second, had time to view the entire abode of Allah."[3]

[3]Dostoievski (296), *Idiot*; Part ii, ch. 5; t. vi, pp. 255-57.

BIBLIOGRAPHY

# BIBLIOGRAPHICAL ABBREVIATIONS

The raised Arabic figure at the end of a book title indicates the edition if stated on the title page.

| | |
|---|---|
| Abh. | Abhandlungen |
| *Bull. Hist. Med.* | *Bulletin of the History of Medicine* |
| C.M.G. | Corpus Medicorum Graecorum |
| *JAMA* | *The Journal of the American Medical Association* |
| Loeb | The Loeb Classical Library |
| *Pauly-Wissowa* | *Paulys Real-Encyclopädie der classischen Altertumswissenschaft*, Neue Bearbeitung herausgegeben von Georg Wissowa, Stuttgart, 1894 ff. |
| S.B. | Sitzungsberichte |
| *Sudhoffs Arch.* | *Archiv für Geschichte der Medizin*, and its successor |
| U.P. | University Press |
| *Virchows Arch.* | *Archiv für pathologische Anatomie und Physiologie und für klinische Medicin*, and its successor |

1 Abercrombie, John. *Pathological and Practical Researches on Diseases of the Brain and the Spinal Cord.*[2] Edinburgh, 1829.

2 Abt, Adam. *Die Apologie des Apuleius von Madaura und die antike Zauberei.* Giessen: Töpelmann, 1908. [Religionsgeschichtliche Versuche und Vorarbeiten, IV, 2.]

3 Abulqasim. *De chirurgia*, ed. Johannes Channing, vol. 1. Oxford, 1778.

4 _____. *Liber theoricae nec non practicae Alsaharavii, qui vulgo Acararius dicitur.* Augsburg, 1519.

5 Ackerknecht, Erwin H. "Death in the history of medicine." *Bull. Hist. Med.* 42 (1968): 19–23.

6 _____. *Medicine at the Paris Hospital, 1794–1848.* Baltimore: The Johns Hopkins Press, 1967.

7 _____. "Psychopathology, primitive medicine and primitive culture." *Bull. Hist. Med.* 14 (1943): 30–67.

8 _____. *A Short History of Psychiatry.*[2] transl. from the German by Sula Wolff. New York–London: Hafner, 1968.

9 Adie, W. J. "Pyknolepsy: a form of epilepsy occurring in children, with a good prognosis." *Brain* 47 (1924): 96–101.

10 Aelianus, Claudius. *De natura animalium libri XVII*, rec. Rudolph Hercher. Leipzig, 1864.

11 Aetius Amidenus. *Libri medicinales V–VIII*, ed. Alexander Olivieri. Berlin: Academia Litterarum, 1950. [C.M.G., VIII, 2.]

12 Agilon, Walter. *Gualteri Agilonis summa medicinalis*, ed. Paul Diepgen. Leipzig: Barth, 1911.

13 Agricola, Georgius. *De re metallica libri XII* [also included: De animantibus subterraneis, lib. I. De ortu et causis subterraneorum, lib. V. De natura eorum quae effluunt ex terra, lib. IV. De natura fossilium, lib. X. De veteribus et novis metallis, lib. II. Bermannus sive de re metallica, dialogus, lib. I.]. Basel, 1657.

14 Agrippa ab Nettesheim, Henricus Cornelius. *De occulta philosophia libri tres.* n.p., 1533.

15 Ahrens, Karl. *Muhammed als Religionsstifter.* Leipzig, 1935. [Abh. für die Kunde des Morgenlandes, XIX, 4.]

16 Alajouanine, T. "Dostoiewski's epilepsy." *Brain* 86 (1963): 209–18.

17 Albers. "Synoptische Darstellung der neuen Schriften über Epilepsie. Unter Benutzung von J. Falret Theories physiologiques." *Allgemeine Zeitschrift für Psychiatrie und psychisch-gerichtliche Medicin* 19 (1862): 545–86.

18 Alberti, Michael. *Systema jurisprudentiae medicae*, vol. I. Halle, 1736. Vol. IV. Leipzig: Goerlitz, 1760.

19 Albertus Magnus. *De animalibus libri XXVI*, herausgegeben von Hermann Stadler, 2 vols. Münster i. W.: Aschendorff, 1916–20. [Beiträge zur Geschichte der Philosophie des Mittelalters, XV–XVI.]

20 Aldrovandi, Ulysses. *Monstrorum historia* . . . Bartholomaeus Ambrosinus . . . volumen composuit, Marcus Antonius Bernia in lucem edidit propriis sumptibus. Bologna, 1642.

21 Alexander of Tralles. *Alexander von Tralles*, Original-Text und Übersetzung von Th. Puschmann, I. Band. Vienna, 1878.

22 Alī Ibn Abbās. *Liber totius medicine . . . quem sapientissimus Haly filius abbas . . . edidit, regique inscripsit, unde et regalis dispositionis nomen assumpsit.* Lyons, 1523.

23 'Alī b. Rabban-al-Ṭabarī. *Firdausu 'l-Hikmat or Paradise of Wisdom*, ed. M. Z. Siddiqi. Berlin, 1928.

24  Allbutt, T. Clifford. *On Visceral Neuroses.* London, 1884.
25  Alsarius a Cruce Genuense, Vicentius. *De morbis capitis frequentioribus.* Rome: Gulielmus Facciottus, 1617.
26  Alström, Carl Henry. *A Study of Epilepsy in Its Clinical, Social and Genetic Aspects.* Copenhagen: Munksgaard, 1950. [Acta Psychiatrica et Neurologica, Suppl. 63.]
27  Althaus, Julius. *On Epilepsy, Hysteria, and Ataxy.* London, 1866.
28  Amacher, M. Peter. "Thomas Laycock, I. M. Sechenov, and the reflex arc concept." *Bull. Hist. Med.* 38 (1964): 168-83.
29  Amatus Lusitanus. *Curationum medicinalium centuriae quatuor.* Basel, 1556.
30  American Neurological Association. *Semi-Centennial Anniversary Volume 1875-1924.* American Neurological Association, 1924.
31  *The Ancren Riwle; a Treatise on the Rules and Duties of Monastic Life,* ed. and transl. by J. Morton. London, 1853.
32  Anderson, James. "On sensory epilepsy. A case of basal cerebral tumour, affecting the left temporo-sphenoidal lobe, and giving rise to a paroxysmal taste-sensation and dreamy state." *Brain* 9 (1887): 385-95.
33  Andrae, Tor. *Mohammed: the Man and His Faith,* transl. by Theophil Menzel. London: Allen and Unwin, 1956.
34  _____. *Die Person Muhammeds in Lehre und Glauben seiner Gemeinde.* Stockholm, 1917.
35  "Anonymi carmen de herbis," ed. F. S. Lehrs, in: *Poetae bucolici et didactici.* Paris, 1862.
36  Anonymus Christianus. *Hermippus, de astrologia dialogus,* ed. G. Kroll et P. Viereck. Leipzig, 1895.
37  Anstie, Francis E. *Stimulants and Narcotics.* London, 1864.
38  Antonini, G. *I precursori di C. Lombroso.* Turin: Bocca, 1900.
39  Antonius Musa. *Antonii Musae de herba vetonica liber. Pseudoapulei herbarius. Anonymi de taxone liber. Sexti Placiti liber medicinae ex animalibus,* etc., eds. Ernestus Howald et Henricus E. Sigerist. Leipzig—Berlin: Teubner, 1927. [Corpus Medicorum Latinorum, IV.]
40  Apollodorus. *The Library,* with an English transl. by Sir James G. Frazer, 2 vols. Loeb, 1921.
41  Apollonius. "Historiae mirabiles," in: *Rerum naturalium scriptores Graeci minores,* vol. I, ed. O. Keller. Leipzig, 1877.
42  Appianus. *Roman History,* with an English transl. by H. White, vol. III. Loeb, 1913.
43  Apuleius. *Apulei apologia,* with introduction and commentary by H. E. Butler and A. S. Owen. Oxford: Clarendon Press, 1914.
44  _____. *The Metamorphoses, or Golden Ass of Apuleius of Madaura,* transl. by H. E. Butler, vol. II. Oxford: Clarendon Press, 1910.
45  Arbesmann, P. R. *Das Fasten bei den Griechen und Römern.* Giessen: Töpelmann, 1929. [Religionsgeschichtliche Versuche und Vorarbeiten, XXI, 1.]
46  Archer, John Clark. *Faiths Men Live By.* New York: Ronald, 1934.
47  _____. *Mystical Elements in Mohammed.* New Haven: Yale U.P., 1924. [Yale Oriental Series, Researches, XI, 1.]
48  Arderne, John of. *De arte phisicali et de cirurgia of Master John Arderne, Surgeon of Newark, dated 1412,* transl. by Sir D'Arcy Power. London: Bale Sons & Danielsson, 1922.
49  Aretaeus. *Aretaeus,* ed. Carolus Hude. Leipzig—Berlin: Teubner, 1923. [C.M.G., II.]
50  _____. *The Extant Works of Aretaeus, the Cappadocian,* ed. and transl. by Francis Adams. London: The Sydenham Society, 1856.

51  Aristophanes, with the English transl. of B. B. Rogers, vol. 1. Loeb, 1927.
52  Aristotle. *Minor Works*, with an English transl. by W. S. Hett. Loeb, 1936.
53  _____. *On the Soul, Parva naturalia, On Breath*, with an English transl. by
     W. S. Hett. Loeb, 1957.
54  _____. *Parva naturalia*, a revised text with introduction and commentary by
     Sir David Ross. Oxford: Clarendon, 1955.
55  _____. *Problems*, with an English transl. by W. S. Hett, 2 vols. Loeb, 1936
     and 1937.
56  _____. *The Works of Aristotle*, transl. into English under the editorship of
     W. D. Ross, vol. IX, Ethica Nicomachea by W. D. Ross, etc. Oxford U. P.,
     1925.
57  Armstrong, A. H. *The Cambridge History of Later Greek and Early Medieval
     Philosophy*. Cambridge, U.P., 1967.
58  Arnald of Villanova. *Opera omnia*. Basel, 1585.
59  D'Arnis, W. H. Maigne. *Lexicon manuale ad scriptores mediae et infimae
     latinitatis*. Paris, 1890.
60  Artemidorus Daldianus. *Artemidori Daldiani onirocriticon libri V*, ex rec. R.
     Hercheri. Leipzig, 1864.
61  Athenaeus. *The Deipnosophists*, with an English transl. by C. B. Gulick, vol.
     III. Loeb, 1929.
62  Auerbach, Erich. "Remarques sur le mot 'passion.' " *Neuphilologische
     Mitteilungen* 38 (1937): 218-24.
63  Aulus Gellius. *The Attic Nights of Aulus Gellius*, with an English transl. by
     J. C. Rolfe, vol. III. Loeb, 1928.
64  Averroës. *Colliget Averrois*. Venice, 1542.
65  _____. *Compendia librorum Aristotelis qui parva naturalia vocantur*, rec.
     A. L. Shields and H. Blumberg. Cambridge, Mass.: The Medieval Academy
     of America, 1949. [Corpus commentariorum Averrois in Aristotelem, ver-
     sionum latinorum vol. VII.]
66  Avery, Harry C. "Heracles, Philoctetes, Neoptolemus." *Hermes* 93 (1965):
     279-97.
67  Avesta. *Die Heiligen Bücher der Parsen*, übersetzt von F. Wolff. Berlin—
     Leipzig: de Gruyter, 1924.
68  Avicenna. *Avicenna's De anima (Arabic text), Being the Psychological Part of
     Kitāb al-Shifā'*, ed. by F. Rahman. London: Oxford U.P., 1959.
69  _____. *Kutubu l-qānūni fī ṭ-ṭibbi*. Rome: Typographia Medicea, 1593.
70  _____. *Liber de anima seu sextus de naturalibus IV-V*, ed. S. van Riet, intro-
     duction . . . par G. Verbeke. Leiden: Brill, 1968. [Avicenna Latinus.]
71  _____. *Libri in re medica omnes*. Venice, 1564.
72  Babbitt, Irving. *Literature and the American College*. Essays in Defense of
     the Humanities. Boston—New York: Houghton Mifflin, 1908.
73  Baglivi, Georgius. *Opera omnia medico-practica et anatomica*. Nuremberg,
     1751.
74  Baillarger. *Recherches sur les maladies mentales*, t. 1. Paris, 1890.
75  Baily, Pearce. "The problem of temporal lobe epilepsy—purpose of col-
     loquium," in Baldwin and Bailey (editors), *Temporal Lobe Epilepsy*,
     pp. 7-12.
76  Baldwin, M. and Bailey, P. [editors]. *Temporal Lobe Epilepsy: A Col-
     loquium Sponsored by the National Institute of Neurological Diseases and
     Blindness, National Institutes of Health, Bethesda, Maryland, in Coopera-
     tion with the International League Against Epilepsy*. Springfield, Ill.:
     Charles C Thomas, 1958.
77  Ballonius, Gulielmus. *Consiliorum medicinalium libri II*. Paris, 1635.

78  Barbette, Paul. *The Practice of the Most Successful Physitian Paul Barbette, . . . with the Notes and Observations of Frederick Deckers.* London, 1675.

79  Bargheer. "Fallsucht," *Handwörterbuch des Deutschen Aberglaubens,* vol. 2, cols. 1168–78. Berlin–Leipzig: de Gruyter, 1929–30.

80  Barker, Wayne. *Brain Storms: A Study of Human Spontaneity.* New York: Grove Press, 1968.

81  Barth, Michael. "De epilepsia," in: *Quaestiones cum conclusionibus ac problematis, candidatis doctoratus in arte medica numero IIII pro insignibus doctoralibus, Lipsiae in aede Paulina per Martinum a Drembach . . . consequendis, explicandae et defendendae.* Leipzig, 1571.

82  Bartholinus, Thomas. *Historiarum anatomicarum rariorum centuria I et II.* Copenhagen, 1654.

83  Barton, John K. *The Pathology and Treatment of Syphilis, Chancroid Ulcers, and Their Complications.* Dublin: Fannin and Co., 1868.

83a  Baruk, Henri. *La psychiatrie française de Pinel à nos jours.* Paris: Presses Universitaires de France, 1967.

84  Bastholm, E. *The History of Muscle Physiology.* Copenhagen: Munksgaard, 1950.

85  Bastian, H. Charleton. "Consciousness." *Journal of Mental Science* 15 (1870): 501–23.

86  Battus, Johannes. *Theses medicae de epilepsia.* Leiden, 1603.

87  Baudissin, Wolf Wilhelm, Graf. *Adonis und Esmun.* Leipzig: Hinrichs, 1911.

88  Baumann, E. D. "Die heilige Krankheit." *Janus* 29 (1925): 7–32.

89  ———. *Die heilige Ziekte.* Rotterdam: Nijgh and Van Ditmar, 1923.

90  ———. "Die Katalepsie der Antiken." *Janus* 42 (1938): 7–24.

91  Beau. "Recherches statistiques pour servir à l'histoire de l'épilepsie et de l'hystérie." *Archives générales de médecine,* 2e série 11 (1836): 328–52.

92  Beck, P. *Die Ekstase, ein Beitrag zur Psychologie und Völkerkunde.* Bad Sachsa im Harz: Haacke, 1906.

93  Beddoes, Thomas. *Hygëia, or Essays Moral and Medical, on the Causes Affecting the Personal State of Our Middling and Affluent Classes,* vol. 3. Bristol, 1803.

94  Beevor, Charles E. and Horsley, Victor. "A minute analysis (experimental) of the various movements produced by stimulating in the monkey different regions of the cortical centre for the upper limb, as defined by Professor Ferrier." *Philosophical Transactions of the Royal Society of London,* (B) for the year 1887, 178 (London 1888): 153–67; and: "A further minute analysis by electrical stimulation of the so-called motor-region of the cortex cerebri in the monkey (Macacus sinicus)," *ibid.* 179 (B) (1888): 205–56.

95  Bekker, I. *Anecdota graeca,* 3 vols. Berlin, 1814–21.

96  Bell, Charles. *The Anatomy and Philosophy of Expression as Connected with the Fine Arts.*[4] London, 1847.

97  ———. *Idea of a New Anatomy of the Brain.* London, 1811.

98  ———. *The Nervous System of the Human Body.*[3] London, 1844.

99  Bell, Richard. *Introduction to the Qur'ān.* Edinburgh: U.P., 1958.

100  Benedum, J. "Die 'balnea pensilia' des Asklepiades von Prusa." *Gesnerus* 24 (1967): 93–107.

101  Benivenius, Antonius. *De abditis nonnullis ac mirandis morborum et sanationum causis.* Florence, 1507.

102  ———. *De abditis nonnullis ac mirandis morborum et sanationum causis,* transl. by Charles Singer. Springfield, Ill.: Thomas, 1954.

103 Berendes, J. *Des Pedanios Dioskurides aus Anazarbos Arzneimittellehre in fünf Büchern.* Stuttgart: Enke, 1902.

104 Berengarius a Carpi. *Tractatus de fractura calve sive cranei a Carpo editus.* Bologna, 1518.

105 Berg, Alexander. "Die Lehre von der Faser als Form- und Funktionselement des Organismus." *Virchows Archiv* 309 (1942): 333–460.

106 Bernard of Gordon. *Omnium aegritudinum a vertice ad calcem, opus praeclariss. quod lilium medicinae appellatur.* Paris, 1542.

107 Berthelot, M. *Collection des anciens alchimistes grecs,* 2 vols. Paris, 1887–88.

108 Beverwyck, Johannes von. *Allgemeine Artzney* . . . auss der Holländischen in die Hochteutsche Sprache übersetzt. Frankfurt a. M., 1674.

109 Bey, M. L. Moharrem. "War Mohammed Epileptiker?" *Psychiatrisch-neurologische Wochenschrift* 33 (1902): 353–57, and no. 34, pp. 367–73.

110 Bezdechi, St. "Das psychopathische Substrat der 'Bacchantinnen' Euripides'." *Sudhoffs Arch.* 25 (1932): 279–306.

111 Bidez, Joseph et Cumont, Franz. *Les mages hellénisés,* 2 vols. Paris: Les Belles Lettres, 1938.

112 Billings, John S. "The surgical treatment of epilepsy." *Cincinnati Lancet & Observer* 4 (1861): 334–41.

113 Billod. "Recherches et considérations relatives à la symptomatologie de l'épilepsie." *Annales médico-psychologiques* 2 (1843): 381–423.

114 Bing, R. "Bemerkungen zur Frühgeschichte der Epilepsie." *Schweizerische medizinische Wochenschrift* 85 (1955): 97–102.

115 Bingley, Torsten. *Mental Symptoms in Temporal Lobe Epilepsy and Temporal Lobe Gliomas.* Copenhagen: Munksgaard, 1958. [Acta Psychiatrica et Neurologica, Supplementum 120, vol. 33.]

116 Binz, Carl. *Doktor Johann Weyer, ein rheinischer Arzt, der erste Bekämpfer des Hexenwahns.*[2] Berlin, 1896.

117 Black, William George. *Folk medicine; A Chapter in the History of Culture.* London, 1883. [Publications of the Folklore Society, XII.]

118 Blaiklock, E. M. "The epileptic." *Greece and Rome* 14 (1945): 48–63.

119 Blancardus, Stephanus. *Anatomia practica rationalis, sive rariorum cadaverum morbis denatorum anatomica inspectio.* Amsterdam, 1688.

120 _____. *The Physical Dictionary.*[3] London, 1697.

121 Blau, Ludwig. *Das altjüdische Zauberwesen.*[2] Berlin: Lamm, 1914.

122 Bloch, Marc. *Les rois thaumaturges.* Strasbourg, 1924. [Publications de la Faculté des Lettres de l'Université de Strasbourg, 19.]

123 Bloedner, Karl. *Petronus, Petronius, Petroncellus.* Diss. Leipzig, 1925.

124 Blum, Elisabeth. *Das staatliche und kirchliche Recht des Frankenreichs in seiner Stellung zum Dämonen-, Zauber- und Hexenwesen.* Paderborn: Schöningh, 1936. [Görres-Gesellschaft zur Pflege der Wissenschaft im katholischen Deutschland. Veröffentlichungen der Sektion für Rechts- und Staatswissenschaft, 72.]

125 Blumer, Dietrich. "Hypersexual episodes in temporal lobe epilepsy." *American Journal of Psychiatry* 126 (1970): 1099–1106.

126 _____. "The temporal lobes and paroxysmal behavior disorders." *Beiheft zur Schweizerischen Zeitschrift für Psychologie und ihre Anwendungen* 51 (1967): 273–85 (Szondiana VII).

127 Blumer, Dietrich and Walker, A. Earl. "Sexual behavior in temporal lobe epilepsy." *A.M.A. Archives of Neurology* 16 (1967): 37–43.

128 Bodin, Jean. *De la demonomanie des sorciers.* Paris, 1582.

129 Boerhaave, Abraham Kaau. *Impetum faciens dictum Hippocrati.* Leiden, 1745.

130 Boerhaave, Hermann. *Praelectiones academicae de morbis nervorum*, cur.
    Jacobus van Eems, t. II. Leiden, 1761.
131 Boguet, Henry. *An Examen of Witches*, transl. by E. Allen Ashwin, ed. by
    the Rev. Montague Summers. John Rodker, 1929.
132 Bonaparte, Marie. "L'épilepsie et le sado-masochisme dans la vie et l'oeuvre
    de Dostoïevski." *Revue Française de Psychanalyse* 26 (1962): 715–30.
133 Bonetus, Theophilus. *Medicina septentrionalis collatitia*, 2 vols. Geneva,
    1685–86.
134 _____. *Sepulchretum sive anatomia practica*, ed. J.J. Mangetus, 3 vols.
    Lyons, 1700.
135 Bootius, Arnoldus. *Observationes medicae de affectibus omissis.* Frankfurt–
    Leipzig, 1676. [Together with: Petrus Borellus, *Historiarum et observa-
    tionum medico-physicarum centuriae IV.*]
136 Borellus, Io. Alphonsus. *De motu animalium*, pars altera. Rome, 1681.
137 Borellus, Petrus. *Historiarum et observationum medico-physicarum centuriae
    IV.* Frankfurt–Leipzig, 1676.
138 Boretius, Matthias Ern. et Arnoldt, J. Godofredus. "Disput. inaugur. de
    epilepsia ex depresso cranio," in: *Disputationes ad morborum historiam et
    curationem facientes*, quas collegit, edidit et recensuit Albertus Hallerus, t.
    primus. Lausanne, 1757.
139 Bouché-Leclerq, A. *L'astrologie grecque.* Paris, 1899.
140 Bouchet et Cazauvieilh. "De l'épilepsie considérée dans ses rapports avec
    l'aliénation mentale. Recherches sur la nature et le siège de ces deux
    maladies." *Archives générales de médecine* 9 (1825): 510–42; 10 (1826):
    5–50.
141 Boudin, J. Ch. M. *Traité de géographie et de statistique médicales*, 2 vols.
    Paris, 1857.
142 Bouillaud, J. "Recherches cliniques propres à démontrer que la perte de la
    parole correspond à la lésion des lobules antérieurs du cerveau, et à con-
    firmer l'opinion de M. Gall, sur le siège de l'organe du langage articulé."
    *Archives générales de médecine* 8 (1825): 25–45.
143 Bourget, Paul. *Essais de psychologie contemporaine*, tome second, édition
    définitive augmentée d'appendices. Paris: Plon, n.d.
144 Boyer (Le Baron). *Traité des maladies chirurgicales et des operations qui leur
    conviennent*, t. 5. Paris, 1816.
145 Bräutigam, Walther. "Zur epileptischen Wesensänderung." *Psyche* 5 (1951):
    523–44.
146 Brain, Russell. "The concept of hysteria in the time of William Harvey."
    *Proceedings of the Royal Society of Medicine* (Section of the History of
    Medicine) 56 (2 April 1963): 317–24.
147 Bratz. "Das Ammonshorn bei Epileptischen, Paralytikern, Senildementen
    und anderen Hirnkranken." *Monatsschrift für Psychiatrie und Neurologie*
    47 (1920): 56–62.
148 Bravais, L. -F. *Recherches sur les symptômes et le traitement de l'épilepsie
    hémiplégique.* Paris, 1827. [Thèse de Paris No. 118.]
149 Brazier, Mary A. "The EEG in epilepsy: a historical note." *Epilepsia*, fourth
    series, vol. 1 (1959–60): 328–36.
150 Bresler, Johannes. *Die Simulation von Geistesstörung und Epilepsie.* Halle:
    Marhold, 1904.
151 Briand, Jh. et Brosson, J. -X. *Manuel complet de médecine légale*, nouv. éd.
    Paris, 1828.
152 Brierre de Boismont, A. *Des hallucinations.*[2] Paris: Baillière, 1852.

153  Bright, Richard. "Cases illustrative of the effects produced when the arteries and brain are diseased." *Guy's Hospital Reports* 1 (1836): 9-40.

154  _____. *Reports of Medical Cases*, vol. II, part II. London, 1831.

155  Briquet, P. *Traité clinique et thérapeutique de l'hystérie.* Paris, 1859.

156  Brissaud, Édouard. *Histoire des expressions populaires relatives à l'anatomie, à la physiologie et à la médecine.* Paris, 1892.

157  British Medical Association, annual meeting, Cambridge, 1880. *Journal of Mental Science* 26 (1881): 460-74.

158  Broadbent, W. H. "An attempt to remove the difficulties attending the application of Dr. Carpenter's theory of the function of the sensori-motor ganglia to the common form of hemiplegia." *British and Foreign Medico-Chirurgical Review* 37 (1866): 468-81.

159  _____. "Hughlings Jackson as pioneer in nervous physiology and pathology." *Brain* 26 (1903): 305-66.

160  Broca, Paul. "Remarques sur le siège de la faculté du langage articulé, suivies d'une observation d'aphémie (perte de la parole)." *Bulletin de la Société Anatomique*, 2e série 6 (1861): 330-57.

161  _____. *Sur la trépanation du crâne et les amulettes crâniennes à l'époque néolithique.* Paris, 1877.

162  _____. "Trépanation du crâne pratiquée avec succès dans un cas de fracture avec enfoncement." *Bulletin de la Société Impériale de Chirurgie de Paris pendant l'année 1866*, 2e série 7 (1867): 508-12.

163  Brock, Arthur J. *Greek Medicine.* New York: Dutton, 1929.

164  Brodie, Benjamin C. *Lectures Illustrative of Certain Local Nervous Affections.* London, 1837.

165  "Bromide of potassium in epilepsy." *Medical Times and Gazette* 2 (1864): 173.

166  Brothwell, Don and Sandison, A. T. [editors]. *Diseases in Antiquity.* Springfield, Illinois: Thomas, 1967.

167  Broussais, F. J. V. *De l'irritation et de la folie.* Paris, 1828.

168  Brovaert, Joannes. *Disputatio medica de morbo comitiali* [praeside Petro Pawio]. Leiden, 1610.

169  Brown, John. *The Elements of Medicine*, vol. II. London, 1788.

170  Brown-Séquard, Ed. "Experimental and clinical researches applied to physiology and pathology." *Boston Medical and Surgical Journal* 55 (1856-57): 337-42, 377-80, 421-27, 457-61; 56 (1857): 54-58, 112-15, 155-58, 174-76, 216-20, 271-78, 338-40, 433-37, 473-78.

171  _____. *Experimental Researches Applied to Physiology and Pathology.* New York, 1853.

172  _____. "Nouvelles recherches sur l'épilepsie due à certaines lésions de la moelle épinière." *Archives de physiologie normale et pathologique* 2 (1869): 211-20, 422-38, 496-503.

173  _____. "Quelques faits nouveaux relatifs à l'épilepsie qu'on observe à la suite de diverses lésions du système nerveux, chez les cobayes." *Archives de physiologie normale et pathologique* 4 (1871-72): 116-20.

174  Browne, J. Crichton. "Notes on epilepsy, and its pathological consequences." *Journal of Mental Science* 19 (1874): 19-46.

175  Browne, W. A. F. *Epileptics: Their Mental Condition.* London, 1865.

176  Bru, Paul. *Histoire de Bicêtre.* Paris, 1890.

177  Bruno, Johann. *Theses inaugurales medicae de epilepsia.* Leiden, 1612.

178  Bryan, Leon S., Jr. "Blood-letting in American medicine, 1830-1892." *Bull. Hist. Med.* 38 (1964): 516-29.

179 Bubnoff, N. and Heidenhain, R. "On excitatory and inhibitory processes within the motor centers of the brain," transl. by G. v. Bonin and W. S. McCulloch, in: *The Precentral Motor Cortex*, ed. by Paul C. Bucy, pp. 173-210. Urbana, Ill.: The University of Illinois Press, 1949.

180 _____. "Ueber Erregungs-und Hemmungsvorgänge innerhalb der motorischen Hirncentren." [*Pflügers*] *Archiv für die gesammte Physiologie* 26 (1881): 137-200.

181 Buchan, William. *Domestic Medicine*[2]. London, 1772.

182 Bucher, Heini W. *Tissot und sein Traité des nerfs.* Zurich: Juris, 1958. [Zürcher medizingeschichtliche Abh., neue Reihe, 1.]

183 Budge, E. A. Wallis. *The Book of the Saints of the Ethiopian Church*, a transl. . . . made . . . by Sir E. A. Wallis Budge, vol. III. Cambridge U.P., 1928.

184 Buhl, Frants. *Das Leben Muhammeds.*[3] Deutsch von Hans Heinrich Schaeder. Darmstadt: Wissenschaftliche Buchgesellschaft, 1961.

185 Bumke, Oswald. *Lehrbuch der Geisteskrankheiten.* Munich: Bergmann, 1924.

186 Burdach, Karl Friedrich. *Vom Baue und Leben des Gehirns*, 3. Band. Leipzig, 1826.

187 Burdett, Henry C. *Hospitals and Asylums of the World*, vol. I. London, 1891.

188 Burgener, P. *Die Einflüsse des zeitgenössichen Denkens in Morel's Begriff der 'dégénérescence.'* Zurich: Juris, 1964 (Zürcher medizingeschichtliche Abh., neue Reihe, 16).

189 Burton, Robert. *The Anatomy of Melancholy.*[8] London, 1676.

190 Busacchi, Vincenzo. "La trapanazione del cranio nei popoli preistorici (neolitici e precolombiani) e nei primitivi moderni." *Atti e memorie dell' Accademia di Storia dell'Arte Sanitaria*, serie II, anno I (1935): 64-104, 128-63.

191 Buzzard, Thomas. *Clinical Aspects of Syphilitic Nervous Affections.* Philadelphia: Lindsay and Blakiston, 1874.

192 Caelius Aurelianus. *On Acute Diseases and on Chronic Diseases*, ed. and transl. by I. E. Drabkin. Chicago: The University of Chicago Press, 1950.

193 Caesalpinus, Andreas. *Quaestionum peripateticarum lib. V . . . Daemonum investigatio peripatetica,*[2] *Quaestionum medicarum libri II, De medicament. facultatibus lib. II.* Venice, 1593.

194 Calderon-Gonzalez, Raul, Hopkins, Ian, and McLean, Jr., William T. "Tap seizures: a form of sensory precipitation epilepsy." *JAMA* 5 (1966): 521-23.

195 Callimachus. *Callimachus and Lycophron*, with an English transl. by A. W. Mair. Loeb, 1921.

196 Calmeil, L. -F. *De la folie considérée sous le point de vue pathologique, philosophique, historique et judiciaire*, 2 vols. Paris, 1845.

197 _____. *De l'épilepsie, étudiée sous le rapport de son siège et de son influence sur la production de l'aliénation mentale.* Thèse de Paris, 1824.

198 Campanella, Tommaso. *La città del sole*, ed. E. Solmi. Modena: Provincia, 1904.

199 Canguilhem, Georges. *La formation du concept de réflexe aux XVIIe et XVIIIe siècles.* Paris: Presses Universitaires de France, 1955.

200 Cannon, Walter B. *Bodily Changes in Pain, Hunger, Fear and Rage.*[2] New York: Appleton-Century, 1934.

201 Cardanus, Hieronymus. *Opera*, vols. 9 and 10. Lyons, 1663.

202 Carlyle, Thomas. *On Heroes, Hero Worship, and the Heroic in History.* Everyman's Library, [reprinted] 1959.

203 Carpenter, William B. *Principles of Human Physiology*. A new American from the last London edition, ed. F. G. Smith. Philadelphia, 1858.

204 Carr, Edward Hallett. *Dostoevsky, 1821–1881*. [Reprinted] New York: Barnes and Noble, 1963 [Unwin Books].

205 Casaubon, Meric. *A Treatise Concerning Enthusiasme, as It is an Effect of Nature: but is Mistaken by Many for either Divine Inspiration, or Diabolicall Possession.*[2] London, 1656.

206 Casper, Johann Ludwig. *A Handbook of the Practice of Forensic Medicine*, vol. IV, transl. by G. W. Balfour. London: The New Sydenham Society, 1865.

207 Cassius Felix. *De medicina*, ed. Valentin Rose. Leipzig, 1879.

208 Castiglioni, Arturo. *Incantesimo e magia.* Milan: Mondadori, 1934.

209 *Catalogus codicum astrologorum Graecorum.* Brussels, 1898 ff.

210 Caton, Richard. "The electric currents of the brain." *British Medical Journal* (28 August 1875): 278.

211 Cawthorne, Terence. "Julius Caesar and the falling sickness." *Proceedings of the Royal Society of Medicine* (Section of the History of Medicine) 51 (1958): 27–30.

212 Celsus. *De medicina*, with an English transl. by W. G. Spencer, 3 vols. Loeb, 1935–38.

213 Cerulli, Enrico. *Il "Libro della Scala" et la questione delle fonti, Arabo-Spagnole della Divina Commedia.* Vatican City: Biblioteca Apostolica Vaticana, 1949. [Studi e Testi 150.]

214 Cesbron, Henri. *Histoire critique de l'hystérie.* Paris: Asselin et Houzeau, 1909.

215 Charcot, J. -M. *Lecons du mardi à la Salpêtrière.* Paris, 1887.

216 ———. *Leçons sur les maladies du système nerveux*, recueillies et publiées par Bourneville, t. I. Paris, 1886. [Oeuvres complètes, I.]

217 Charcot, J. -M. et Pitres, A. "Contribution à l'étude des localisations dans l'écorce des hémisphères du cerveau." *Revue mensuelle de médecine et de chirurgie* 1 (1877): 1–18, 113–23, 180–95, 357–76, 437–57.

218 Cheyne, George. *The English Malady.* London, 1733.

219 Cheyne, J. "Epilepsy," in John Forbes et al. [editors], *The Cyclopaedia of Practical Medicine*, revised by Robley Dunglison, vol. 2, pp. 75–91. Philadelphia: Lea and Blanchard, 1845.

220 Cholmeley, H. P. *John of Gaddesden and the Rosa Medicinae.* Oxford: Clarendon Press, 1912.

221 Christ, Wilhelm von. *Geschichte der griechischen Literatur*, zweiter Teil, erste Hälfte.[6] Munich: C. H. Beck, 1920. [Handbuch der klassischen Altertumswissenschaft, VII, 2, 1.]

222 Cicero. *De senectute, De amicitia, De divinatione*, with an English transl. by W. A. Falconer. Loeb, 1927.

223 Clark, L. Pierce. "A study of epilepsy of Dostojewsky." *Boston Medical and Surgical Journal* 172 (1915): 46–51.

224 Clarke, Edward Goodman. *The Modern Practice of Physic.* London, 1805.

225 Clarke, Edwin. "The Doctrine of the hollow nerve in the seventeenth and eighteenth centuries," *Medicine, Science, and Culture*, eds. Lloyd G. Stevenson and Robert P. Multhauf, pp. 123–41. Baltimore: The Johns Hopkins Press, 1968.

226 Clarke, Edwin and O'Malley, C. D. *The Human Brain and Spinal Cord.* Berkeley and Los Angeles: University of California Press, 1968.

227 Clemens Alexandrinus. *Opera*, ex rec. G. Dindorfii, vol. III. Oxford, 1869.

228  Clossy, Samuel. *Observations on Some of the Diseases of the Parts of the Human Body*. London, 1763.
229  Cobb, Stanley. "Consciousness and cerebral localization." *Epilepsia*, third series, 1 (1952): 17–20.
230  Cockayne, Oswald. *Leechdoms, Wortcunning, and Starcraft of Early England*, 3 vols. London, 1864–66.
231  Collie, Sir John. *Malingering and Feigned Sickness.*[2] London: Arnold, 1917.
232  Comrie, John D. *History of Scottish Medicine*,[2] 2 vols. London: Baillière, Tindall and Cox, 1932.
233  Conringius, Hermannus. *De hermetica medicina libri duo.*[2] Helmestedt, 1669.
234  Constantinus Africanus. *Omnia opera ysaac in hoc volumine contenta: cum quibusdam aliis opusculis.* Lyons, 1515.
235  ———. *Opera*, 2 vols. Basel, 1536–39.
236  Cooper, Sir Astley. "Some experiments and observations on tying the carotid and vertebral arteries, and the pneumogastric, phrenic, and sympathetic nerves." *Guy's Hospital Reports* 1 (1836): 457–75.
237  Cordes, E. "Die Platzangst (Agoraphobie), Symptom einer Erschöpfungsparese." *Archiv für Psychiatrie und Nervenkrankheiten* 3 (1872): 521–74.
238  *Corpus glossariorum Latinorum*, ed. G. Goetz, vols. 3–5. Leipzig, 1889–94.
239  *Corpus iuris canonici*, ed. Aemilius Friedberg, 2 vols. Leipzig, 1879–81.
240  *Corpus iuris civilis*,[8] vol. I, Institutiones, rec. Paulus Krueger; Digesta, rec. Theodorus Mommsen. Berlin, 1899.
241  Corsellis, J. A. N. "The incidence of Ammon's Horn Sclerosis." *Brain* 80 (1957): 193–208.
242  Coulton, C. G. *Life in the Middle Ages*, 4 vols. in one. New York—Cambridge: Macmillan, 1933.
243  Crawfurd, Raymond. "The blessing of cramp-rings, a chapter in the history of the treatment of epilepsy." *Studies in the History and Method of Science*, ed. Charles Singer, vol. 1, pp. 165–87. Oxford: Clarendon Press, 1917.
244  Creutz, Walter. *Die Neurologie des 1.-7. Jahrhunderts N. Chr.* Leipzig: Thieme, 1934. [Sammlung psychiatrischer und neurologischer Einzeldarstellungen, VI.]
245  Critchley, Macdonald. "Hughlings Jackson, the man; and the early days of the National Hospital." *Proceedings of the Royal Society of Medicine* 53 (1960): 613–18.
246  ———. *Sir William Gowers 1845-1915*. London: Heinemann, 1949.
247  Cullen, William. *First Lines of the Practice of Physic*, vol. III. Edinburgh, 1783.
248  ———. *Nosology: or a Systematic Arrangement of Diseases, by Classes, Orders, Genera, and Species*, transl. from the Latin of William Cullen, M.D. Edinburgh—London, 1810.
249  ———. *Synopsis nosologiae methodicae.*[6] Edinburgh, 1803.
250  Cutter, Irving S. "Benjamin W. Dudley and the surgical relief of traumatic epilepsy (Landmarks in surgical progress)." *International Abstract of Surgery* 50 (1930): 189–94.
251  Dalton, John C. *A Treatise on Human Physiology.*[4] Philadelphia, 1867.
252  Daly, D. D. "Reflections on the concept of petit mal." *Epilepsia* 9 (1968): fourth series 175–78.
253  Dante. *La divina commedia di Dante Alighieri con il commento di Tommaso Casini.*[6] Florence: Sansoni, 1923.

254 ———. *The Divine Comedy of Dante Alighieri*, transl. by H. W. Longfellow. London, n.d. [Routledge's Hearth and Home Library].

255 Daquin, Joseph. *La philosophie de la folie.*[2] Chambéry, 1804.

256 Darwin, Erasmus. *Zoonomia: or the Law of Organic Life*, vol. 1. London, 1794.

257 Dawson, Warren R. *A Leechbook or Collection of Medical Recipes of the Fifteenth Century.* London: Macmillan, 1934.

258 Debus, Allen G. *The English Paracelsians.* London: Oldbourne, 1965.

259 Deichgräber, Karl. *Die griechische Empirikerschule.* Berlin: Weidmann, 1930.

260 ———. *Hippokrates über Entstehung und Aufbau des menschlichen Körpers.* Leipzig–Berlin: Teubner, 1935.

261 Delasiauve. *Traité de l'épilepsie.* Paris, 1854.

262 Delatte, A. *Les conceptions de l'enthousiasme chez les philosophes présocratiques.* Paris: Les belles lettres, 1934. [Collection d'études anciennes.]

263 ———. *Herbarius.*[2] Liége–Paris, 1938. [Bibliothèque de la Faculté de Philosophie et Lettres de l'Université de Liége, 31.]

264 Demosthenes. *Against Meidias, Androtion, Aristocrates, Timocrates, Aristogeiton*, with an English transl. by J. H. Vince. Loeb, 1935.

265 Descartes. *Oeuvres de Descartes*, publiées par C. Adam et P. Tannery, vol. IV. Paris: Cerf, 1901.

266 Detienne, Marcel. *De la pensée religieuse à la pensée philosophique: La notion de Daïmōn dans le pythagorisme ancien.* Paris: Les belles letters, 1963. [Bibliothèque de la Faculté de Philosophie et Lettres de l'Université de Liége, 165.]

267 Deutsch, Albert. *The Mentally Ill in America.* Garden City, N.Y.: Doubleday Doran, 1937.

268 *Dictionary of National Biography*, ed. L. Stephen and S. Lee. New York: Macmillan, 1908 ff.

269 *Dictionnaire encyclopédique des sciences médicales*, 2e série, t. 3, pp. 186–90 (article, *Lunatiques*). Paris, 1876.

270 Diels, Hermann. *Die Fragmente der Vorsokratiker*,[4] erster Band. Berlin: Weidmann, 1922.

271 Diepgen, Paul. "Die Dämonen- und Zauberkrankheit bei den Theologen und Medizinern im Mittelalter." *Janus* 25 (1921): 112–13.

272 ———. *Die Frauenheilkunde der alten Welt.* Munich: Bergmann, 1937. [Veit-Stoeckel, Handbuch der Gynäkologie, 12, I.]

273 ———. "Geistliche und diätetische Ratschläge für Krampfsüchtige." *Beiträge zur Inkunabelkunde*, neue Folge 2 (1938): 104–7.

274 ———. *Geschichte der Medizin.* Berlin–Leipzig: de Gruyter, vol. 1,[2] 1923; vols. 2–5, 1914–28. [Sammlung Göschen.]

275 ———. "Studien zu Arnald von Villanova IV." *Sudhoff's Arch.* 5 (1912): 88–115.

276 ———. "Die Weltanschauung Arnalds von Villanova und seine Medizin." *Scientia* 61 (1937): 38–47.

277 Dieterich, Albrecht. *Kleine Schriften.* Leipzig–Berlin: Teubner, 1911.

278 Dietz, Fridericus Reinholdus [editor]. *Apollonii Citiensis, Stephani, Palladii, Theophili, Meletii, Damascii, Joannis, aliorum scholia in Hippocratem et Galenum*, 2 vols. Königsberg, 1834.

279 Diller, Hans. *Wanderarzt und Aitiologe.* Leipzig: Dieterich, 1934. [Philologus, Supplementband 26, Heft 3.]

280 ———. "Zur Hippokratesauffassung des Galen." *Hermes* 68 (1933): 167–81.

281 Dio Cassius. *Dio's Roman History*, with an English transl. by E. Cary, vol. IV. Loeb, 1916.

282 Dioscurides, Pedanius, Anazarbeus. *De materia medica libri quinque*, ed. M. Wellman, 3 vols. Berlin: Weidmann, 1907-14.

283 Dodds, E. R. *The Greeks and the Irrational.* Berkeley—Los Angeles: University of California Press, 1951 [Sather Classical Lectures, 25].

283a _____. *Pagan and Christian in an Age of Anxiety.* Cambridge: U.P., 1965.

284 Dodonaeus, Remb. *Medicinalium observationum exempla rara.* Leiden, 1585.

285 Dölger, Franz Joseph. "Der Ausschluss der Besessenen (Epileptiker) von Oblation und Kommunion nach der Synode von Elvira." *Antike und Christentum* 4 (1934): 110-29.

286 _____. "Der Ausschluss der Besessenen von Oblation u. Kommunion nach seinen kultur- u. religionsgeschichtlichen Grundlagen untersucht." *Antike und Christentum* 4 (1934): 130-37.

287 _____. "Der Einfluss des Origenes auf die Beurteilung der Epilepsie und Mondsucht im christlichen Altertum." *Antike und Christentum* 4 (1934): 95-109.

288 _____. "Gladiatorenblut und Martyrerblut," *Vorträge der Bibliothek Warburg*, 1923-24, pp. 196-214. Leipzig—Berlin: Teubner, 1926.

289 _____. ΙΧΘΥC, 2. Band: Der heilige Fisch in den antiken Religionen und im Christentum. Münster in Westf.: Aschendorff, 1922.

290 Donatus, Marcellus. *De historia medica mirabili libri sex*, opera et studio Gregori Horsti. Frankfurt, a. M., 1613.

291 Donnadieu. "La prétendue épilepsie de Jules César." *Mémoires de la Société Nationale des Antiquaires de France* 80 (1937): 27-36.

292 Doose, H. "Aus der Geschichte der Epilepsie." *Münchener medizinische Wochenschrift* 107 (1965): 189-96.

293 Dostoievski, F. M. *Pis'ma, II, 1867-1871*, pod redaktsiei i s primechaniyami A. S. Dolinina, pp. 69-73. Moscow—Leningrad: Gosudarstvennoie izdatel'stvo, 1930 [Slavica-Reprint Nr. 11].

294 _____. *Letters of Fyodor Dostoevsky*, transl. by E. C. Mayne. New York: McGraw-Hill, 1964.

295 _____. *The Notebooks for the Idiot*, ed. by Edward Wasiolek, transl. Katherine Strelsky. Chicago—London: University of Chicago Press, 1967.

296 _____. *Sobranie sochinenii v desyati tomakh.* Moscow: Gosudarstvennoe izdatel'stvo khudozhestvennoi literatury, 1956-58. *Idiot*, t. 6, 1957; *Besy*, t. 7, 1957; *Brat'ya Karamazovy*, t. 9-10, 1958.

297 Doussin-Dubreuil, J. -L. *De l'épilepsie en général, et particulièrement de celle qui est déterminée par des causes morales.* [2] Paris, 1825.

298 Dragotti, G. "Furono epilettici Cesare e Napoleone?" *Policlinico* (sezione pratica), 65 (1958): 271-73.

299 Drelincurtius, Carolus. *Experimenta anatomica*, [2] ed. per Ernestum Gottfried Heyseum. Leiden, 1684.

300 Drossaart Lulofs, H. J. "Kanttekeningen biy Hippocrates' 'Over heilige ziekte'." *Ned. Tijdschrift voor Geneeskunde* 98 (1954): 1852-63.

301 Du Cange. *Glossarium mediae et infimae latinitatis*, editio nova. Niort, 1883-87.

302 Duffy, John. "Masturbation and clitoridectomy: a nineteenth century view." *JAMA* 186 (1963): 246-48.

303 Dunbar, H. Flanders. *Emotions and Bodily Changes.* New York: Columbia U.P., 1938.

304 Duncan, Andrew. *Medical Cases, Selected from the Records of the Public Dispensary at Edinburgh.* Edinburgh, 1778.

305 Ebbell, B. "Die ägyptischen Krankheitsnamen." *Zeitschrift für ägyptische Sprache und Altertumskunde* 62 (1926): 13-16.

306 Ebstein, Erich. "Dostojewskijs Krankheit und seine Aerzte." *Die medizinische Welt*, 1928, Nr. 43, [Reprint].

307 Ebstein, Wilhelm. *Die Medizin im Neuen Testament und im Talmud.* Stuttgart: Enke, 1903.

308 Echeverria, M. Gonzalez. "Criminal responsibility of epileptics, as illustrated by the case of David Montgomery." *American Journal of Insanity* 29 (1872-73): 341-425.

309 _____. "De la trépanation dans l'épilepsie par traumatismes du crâne." *Archives générales de médecine*, VIIe série, 2 (1878): 529-54; 652-76.

310 _____. "Marriage and hereditariness of epileptics." *Journal of Mental Science* 26 (1881): 346-69 [also in *American Journal of Insanity* 37 (1880-81): 177-216].

311 _____. *On Epilepsy: Anatomo-Pathological and Clinical Notes.* New York, 1870.

312 _____. "On epileptic insanity." *American Journal of Insanity* 30 (1873): 1-51.

313 Edelstein, Ludwig. *Ancient Medicine: Selected Papers of Ludwig Edelstein*, ed. by Owsei Temkin and C. Lilian Temkin. Baltimore: The Johns Hopkins Press, 1967.

314 _____. "Antike Diätetik." *Die Antike* 7 (1931): 255-70.

315 _____. "Hippokrates von Kos," in *Pauly-Wissowa*, Supplementband VI, 1935, cols. 1290-1345.

316 Edwards, Chilperic. *The Hammurabi Code, and the Sinaitic Legislation.*[3] London: Watts, 1921.

317 Eis, Gerhard. *Vor und nach Paracelsus*, Untersuchungen über Hohenheims Traditionsverbundenheit und Nachrichten über seine Anhänger. Stuttgart: Gustav Fischer, 1965.

318 Eitrem, S. "Lykos and Chimaireus." *Classical Review* 34 (1920): 87-89.

319 Eliade, Mircea. *Shamanism, Archaic Techniques of Ecstasy*, transl. from the French by Willard R. Trask. New York: Pantheon Books, 1964. [Bollingen Series 76.]

320 Elias, Norbert. *Über den Prozess der Zivilisation*, 2 vols. Basel: Haus zum Falken, 1937-39.

321 *Encyclopédie, ou dictionnaire raisonné des sciences, des arts et des métiers, par une société de gens de lettres*, nouvelle édition, t. 12, pp. 691-97. Geneva, 1777.

322 *Epistolographi Graeci*, rec. R. Hercher. Paris, 1873.

323 Epstein, Arthur W. and Ervin, Frank. "Psychodynamic significance of seizure content in psychomotor epilepsy." *Journal of the American Psychosomatic Society* 18 (1956): 43-55.

324 Erastus, Thomas. *Comitis Montani Vincentini novi medicorum censoris, quinque librorum de morbis nuper editorum viva anatome.* Basel, 1581.

325 Erb, Wilhelm. *Ueber die neuere Entwicklung der Nervenpathologie und ihre Bedeutung für den medicinischen Unterricht.* Leipzig, 1880.

326 Ermerins, F. Z. *Anecdota medica Graeca.* Leiden, 1840.

327 Erotianus. *Vocum Hippocraticarum conlectio*, rec. J. Klein. Leipzig, 1865.

328 Esculapius. *De morborum, infirmitatum, passionumque corporis humani origine, descriptionibus et cura.* Strasbourg: Schott, 1532 and 1544.

329  Esquirol, E. *Des maladies mentales*, 2 vols. Paris, 1838.

330  Esser, Albert. *Cäsar und die Julisch-Claudischen Kaiser im biologisch-ärztlichen Blickfeld*. Leiden: Brill, 1958 [Janus, Suppléments, 1].

331  [Ettmüller, Michael]. *Etmullerus abridg'd*. London, 1699.

332  Eugalenus, Severinus. *De morbo scorbuto liber*. The Hague, 1658.

333  Eulenburg, Albert. *Lehrbuch der Nervenkrankheiten*,[2] 2. Theil. Berlin, 1878.

334  Euripides. *Euripides*, with an English transl. by A. S. Way, vols. II and III. Loeb, 1929-30.

335  ――――. *Hippolytus*, ed. J. E. Harry. Boston―London, 1899.

336  Eustathius, Archiepiscopus Thessalonicensis. *Commentarii ad Homerii Iliadem*, 4 vols. Leipzig, 1827-30.

337  Euthymius Zigabenus. *Opera*, vol. II. Paris, 1889. [Patrologia Graeca, ed. Migne, 129.]

338  Fabricius Hildanus, Guilhelmus. *Opera observationum et curationum medico-chirurgicarum*. Frankfurt, 1646.

339  Fahd, Toufic. *La divination Arabe*. Leiden: Brill, 1966.

340  Falconer, Murray A., Serafetinides, Eustace A., and Corsellis, J. A. Nicholas. "Etiology and pathogenesis of temporal lobe epilepsy." *A.M.A. Archives of Neurology* 10 (1964): 233-48.

341  Falconer, William. *A Dissertation on the Influence of the Passions upon Disorders of the Body*. London, 1788.

342  Falloppius, Gabriel. *Opera omnia*. Frankfurt, 1600.

343  Falret, Jules. "De l'état mental des épileptiques." *Archives générales de médecine, Ve série* 16 (1860): 661-79; 17 (1861): 461-91; 18 (1861): 423-43.

344  ――――. *Études cliniques sur les maladies mentales et nerveuses*. Paris, 1890.

345  Falret, Ferrus et Renauldin [reporters.] "Mémoire sur Mahomet, considéré comme aliéné, par Jean-Jacques Beaux, docteur en médecine, -Rapport de MM. Falret, Ferrus et Renauldin." *Bulletin de l'Académie de Médecine* (Paris, 1842): 762-99.

346  Fasbender, Heinrich. *Geschichte der Geburtshülfe*. Jena: Gustav Fischer, 1906.

347  Fearing, Franklin. *Reflex Action, a Study in the History of Physiological Psychology*. Baltimore: Williams & Wilkins, 1930.

348  Feindel, William and Penfield, Wilder. "Localization of discharge in temporal lobe automatism." *A.M.A. Archives of Neurology and Psychiatry* 72 (1954): 605-30.

349  Fenner, Friedrich. *Die Krankheit im Neuen Testament*. Leipzig: Hinrichs, 1930. [Untersuchungen zum Neuen Testament, 18.]

350  Ferdinandus, Epiphanius. *Centum historiae seu observationes et casus medici*. Venice, 1621.

351  Fernelius, Joannes. *Universa medicina*. Frankfurt, a. M., 1577.

352  Ferrarius, Matthaeus. *Practica D. Magistri Joannis Matthei de gradi noviter correcta*. Venice, 1502.

353  Ferrier, David. "Experimental researches in cerebral physiology and pathology." *West Riding Lunatic Asylum Medical Reports* 3 (1873): 30-96.

354  Festus, Sextus Pompeius. *De verborum significatu*, ed. W. M. Lindsay. Leipzig: Teubner, 1933.

355  Fichtner, Horst. *Die Medizin im Avesta*. Leipzig: Pfeiffer, 1924.

356  Ficinus, Marsilius. *Theologia Platonica, De immortalitate animorum duo de viginti libris, Marsilio Ficino Florentino ... authore comprehensa*. Paris, 1559.

357 Fienus, Thomas. *Libri chirurgici duodecim, de praecipuis artis chirurgicae controversiis,*[2] Opera posthuma Hermanni Conringii cura edita. London, 1733.

358 Findeisen, Hans. *Schamanentum,* dargestellt am Beispiel der Besessenheitspriester nordeurasischer Völker. Stuttgart: Kohlhammer, 1957.

359 Fink, Arthur E. *Causes of Crime: Biological Theories in the United States.* Philadelphia: University of Pennsylvania Press, 1938.

360 Firmicius Maternus, Julius. *Matheseos libri VIII,* eds. W. Kroll et F. Skutsch. Leipzig, 1897-1913.

361 Fischer, A. "Kāhin," *The Encyclopaedia of Islām,* vol. 2, pp. 624-26. Leiden (Brill)—London (Luzac), 1927.

362 Fischer-Homberger, Esther. "Hysterie und Misogynie—ein Aspect der Hysteriegeschichte." *Gesnerus* 26 (1969): 117-27.

363 Flashar, Hellmut. *Melancholie und Melancholiker in den medizinischen Theorien der Antike.* Berlin: de Gruyter, 1966.

364 Flemming, C. F. "Ueber das Causal-Verhältniss der Selbstbefleckung zur Geistesverwirrung." *Zeitschrift für die Beurtheilung und Heilung der krankhaften Seelenzustände* 1 (1838): 205-15.

365 Flourens, P. "Recherches physiques sur les propriétés et les fonctions du système nerveux dans les animaux vertébrés." *Archives générales de médecine* 2 (1823): 321-70.

366 [Flowerden, Joseph]. *A Compendium of Physic and Surgery.* London, 1769.

367 Foderé, François-Emmanuel. *Les lois éclairées par les sciences physiques; ou traité de médecine-légale et d'hygiène publique,* t. premier. Paris, l'an septième.

368 Foerster, Richard. *Scriptores physiognomici graeci et latini,* 2 vols. Leipzig, 1893.

369 Forestus, Petrus. *Observationum et curationum medicinalium ac chirurgicarum opera omnia.* Frankfurt, 1634.

370 Foroliviensis, Jacobus. *In Hippocratis aphorismos, et Galeni super eisdem commentarios, expositio et quaestiones . . . additis Marsilii de Sancta Sophia interpretationibus in eos aphorismos, qui a Jacobo expositi non fuerant.* Venice, 1574.

371 Fossel, Victor. *Volksmedicin und medicinischer Aberglaube in Steiermark.* Graz, 1886.

372 Foster, Sir M. *Lectures on the History of Physiology during the Sixteenth, Seventeenth and Eighteenth Centuries.* Cambridge: U.P., 1901.

373 Fournier, H. *De l'onanisme.*[4] Paris, 1885.

374 Foville, A. "Épilepsie," *Dictionnaire de médecine et de chirurgie pratiques,* t. 7, pp. 412-28. Paris, 1831.

375 Fragment of Medicine, *Papyri Osloenses,* fasc. III, eds. S. Eitrem and Leiv Amundsen, pp. 26-29. Oslo, 1936.

376 Franz, Adolph. *Die kirchlichen Benediktionen im Mittelalter,* 2 vols. Freiburg im Breisgau: Herder, 1909.

377 Frazer, J. G. *The Scapegoat.* London: Macmillan, 1914. [The Golden Bough,[3] vol. 9.]

378 French, John D. and Darling, Louise. "The surgical treatment of epilepsy in 1861." *Journal of the International College of Surgeons* 34 (1960): 685-91.

379 Freud, Sigmund. "Dostoevsky and parricide (1928)," *Sigmund Freud, M.D., LL.D.: Collected Papers,* ed. by James Strachey, vol. 5, pp. 222-42. London: Hogarth Press and the Institute of Psycho-Analysis, 1950.

380  Friedlander, Walter J. "Shakespeare on epilepsy." *Boston Medical Quarterly* 14 (1963): 113-20.

381  Fritsch, G. und Hitzig, E. *Ueber die elektrische Erregbarkeit des Grosshirns.* Berlin, n.d. [reprinted from Reichert's und du Bois-Reymond's Archiv, 1870, Heft 3].

382  Fuchs, Leonhard. *De medendis singularum humani corporis partium . . . passionibus.* Basel, 1539.

383  Fuchs, Robert. "Anecdota medica Graeca." *Rheinisches Museum für Philologie*, Neue Folge, 49 (1894): 532-58; 50 (1895): 576-99.

384  ———. "Aus Themisons Werk ueber die acuten und chronischen Krankheiten." *Rheinisches Museum für Philologie*, Neue Folge, 58 (1903): 67-114.

385  Fünfgeld, E. W. " 'Morbus sacer,' ein Ueberblick vom Altertum bis zur Gegenwart." *Medizinische Welt* 5 (1966): 258-66.

386  Fulton, John F. "Clifford Allbutt's description of psychomotor seizures." *Journal of the History of Medicine and Allied Sciences* 12 (1957): 75-77.

387  ———. "History of focal epilepsy." *International Journal of Neurology* 1 (1959): 21-33.

388  Gabucinius, Hieronymus. *De comitiali morbo libri III.* Venice, 1561.

389  Galen. *Compendium Timaei Platonis*, eds. Paulus Kraus et Richardus Walzer. London: Warburg Institute, 1951. [Plato Arabus, 1.]

390  ———. *De sanitate tuenda, De alimentorum facultatibus, De bonis malisque sucis, De victu attenuante, De ptisana*, eds. K. Koch, G. Helmreich, C. Kalbfleisch, O. Hartlich. Leipzig–Berlin: Teubner, 1923. [C.M.G. V, 4, 2.]

391  ———. "Galen's 'Advice for an Epileptic Boy,' transl. by O. Temkin. *Bull. Hist. Med.* 2 (1934): 179-89.

392  ———. *In Hippocratis de natura hominis, In Hippocratis de victu acutorum, De diaeta Hippocratis in morbis acutis*, eds. J. Mewaldt, G. Helmreich, J. Westenberger—*In Hippocratis prorrheticum I, De comate secundum Hippocratem, In Hippocratis prognosticum*, eds. H. Diels, J. Mewaldt, J. Heeg. Leipzig–Berlin: Teubner, 1914-15. [C.M.G. V, 9, 1, and V, 9, 2.]

393  ———. *In Platonis Timaeum commentarii fragmenta*, coll. H. O. Schröder. Leipzig–Berlin: Teubner, 1934. [C.M.G., Supplementum I.]

394  ———. *Opera omnia*, ed. C. G. Kühn. Leipzig, 1821 ff.

395  ———. *Scripta minora*, rec. I. Marquardt, I. Mueller, G. Helmreich, vol. II. Leipzig, 1891.

396  ———. *A Translation of Galen's Hygiene (De sanitate tuenda)* by Robert Montraville Green. Springfield, Ill.: Thomas, 1951.

397  Ganschinietz. "Katochos," *Pauly-Wissowa*, vol. 10, 1917, cols. 2526-34.

398  Gardet, Louis. *L'Islam, religion et communauté*, Paris: Desclée de Brouwer, 1967. [Bibliothèque française de philosophie.]

399  Gariopontus. *Passionarius Galeni.* Lyons, 1526.

400  Garrison, Fielding H. *An Introduction to the History of Medicine.*[4] Philadelphia–London: Saunders, 1929.

401  Gastaut, Henri. "La maladie du Vincent van Gogh envisagée à la lumière des conceptions, nouvelles sur l'épilepsie psychomotrice." *Annales médico-psychologiques*, (tome premier) 114 (1956): 196-238.

402  ———. "So-called 'psychomotor' and 'temporal' epilepsy, a critical study." *Epilepsia*, third series, 2 (1953): 59-76 (discussion pp. 76-99).

403  Gastaut, Henri et al. "A proposed international classification of epileptic seizures." *Epilepsia*, fourth series, 5 (1964): 297-306.

404  Gautier, Aubin. *Histoire du somnambulisme*, 2 vols. Paris, 1842.

405 Genil-Perrin, Georges. *Histoire des origines et de l'évolution de l'idée de dégénérescence en médecine mentale.* Paris: Leclerc, 1913.

406 Georget. "Épilepsie," *Dictionnaire de médecine.* vol. 8 (Paris 1823), pp. 206-25.

407 Geraldus de Solo. *Almansoris liber nonus cum expositione Geraldi de Solo doctoris Montispessulani.* Lyons, 1504.

408 Gibbon, Edward. *The Decline and Fall of the Roman Empire,* 2 vols. [reprinted]. New York: The Modern Library, 1932.

409 Gibbs, F. A., Gibbs, E. L., and Lennox, W. G. "Cerebral dysrhythmias of epilepsy." *Archives of Neurology and Psychiatry* 39 (1938): 298-314.

410 ———. "Epilepsy: a paroxysmal cerebral dysrhythmia." *Brain* 60 (1937): 377-88.

411 ———. "The likeness of the cortical dysrhythmias of schizophrenia and psychomotor epilepsy." *American Journal of Psychiatry* 95 (1938): 255-69.

412 Gilbertus Anglicus. *Compendium medicine Gilberti anglici tam morborum universalium quam particularium nondum medicis sed et cyrurgicis utilissimum.* Lyons, 1510.

413 Glaser, G. H. "The problem of psychosis in psychomotor temporal lobe epileptics." *Epilepsia,* fourth series, 5 (1964): 271-78.

414 Glauber, John Rudolph. *The Works of the Highly Experienced and Famous Chymist John Rudolph Glauber . . .* transl. into English and published for publick good by the labour, care, and charge of Christopher Packe, philochymico-medicus. London, 1689.

415 Glisson, Franciscus. *Tractatus de ventriculo et intestinis.* London, 1677.

416 *Glossae medicinales,* ed. J. L. Heiberg. Copenhagen: Høst, 1924. [Det Kgl. Danske Videnskabernes Selskab. Historisk-filologiske Meddelelser. IX, 1.]

417 Goldziher, Ignaz. *Abh. zur arabischen Philologie,* erster Theil. Leiden, 1896.

418 Gorn, Walther. *Die historische Behandlung der Frage nach der Lokalisation der genuinen Epilepsie,* Diss. Leipzig, 1911.

419 Gorter, Joannes de. *Medicinae compendium in usum exercitationis domesticae.* Venice, 1757.

420 Gowers, W. R. *Epilepsy and Other Chronic Convulsive Diseases.* London, 1881.

421 Grabner, Elfriede (ed.). *Volksmedizin: Probleme und Forschungsgeschichte.* Darmstadt: Wissenschaftliche Buchgesellschaft, 1967 [Wege der Forschung, 63].

422 Grässe, J. G. Th. *Sagenbuch des Preussischen Staats,* 2 vols. Glogau, 1868-71.

423 Greding, Johann Ernst. *Sämmtliche medizinische Schriften,* herausgegeben von C. W. Greding, 2 vols. Greiz, 1790-91.

423a Green, John R. and Steelman, Henry F. (eds.). *Epileptic Seizures.* Baltimore: Williams and Wilkins, 1956.

424 Greenblatt, Samuel H. *John Hughlings Jackson: the Development of his Main Ideas to 1864,* M.A. essay (unpublished), The Johns Hopkins University.

425 ———. "The major influences on the early life and works of John Hughlings Jackson." *Bull. Hist. Med.* 39 (1965): 346-76.

426 Gregorius Nyssenus. *Opera,* vol. I. Paris, 1863 [Patrologia Graeca, ed. Migne, 44].

427 Gregory of Tours. *Opera,* pars I, Historia Francorum, eds. W. Arndt et Br. Krusch. Hannover, 1884. [Monumenta Germaniae historica, Scriptores rerum Merovingicarum, I, 1.]

428 ———. *Opera*, pars II, Miracula et opera minora, eds. W. Arndt et Br. Krusch. Hannover, 1885. [Monumenta Germaniae historica, Scriptores rerum Merovingicarum, I, 2.]

429 Grensemann, Hermann. *Die hippokratische Schrift "Über die heilige Krankheit."* Berlin: de Gruyter, 1968 [Ars medica, II. Abteilung, Band 1].

430 Griesinger, Wilhelm. *Gesammelte Abh.*, erster Band. Berlin, 1872.

431 ———. *Mental Pathology and Therapeutics*, transl. from the German (second edition) by C. L. Robertson and J. Rutherford. London: The New Sydenham Society, 1867.

432 ———. *Die Pathologie und Therapie der psychischen Krankheiten.* Stuttgart, 1845.

433 ———. "Ueber einige epileptoide Zustände." *Archiv für Psychiatrie und Nervenkrankheiten* 1 (1868–69): 320–33; also in Griesinger (430), pp. 163–79.

434 Grön, Fredrik. "Altnordische Heilkunde." *Janus* 12 (1907): 665–79; 13 (1908): 569–84, 631–53.

435 Grossman, L. *Dostoevski.* Moscow: Molodaya Gvardiya, 1965 [Šiznj zamechatelnykch lyudei].

436 Gruhle, H. W. et al. (ed.). *Psychiatrie der Gegenwart*: Forschung und Praxis, Band I, 1 A. Berlin–Heidelberg–New York: Springer–Verlag, 1967.

437 Gruppe, O. *Griechische Mythologie und Religionsgeschichte.* Munich: C. H. Beck, 1906. [Handbuch der klassischen Altertumswissenschaft, herausgegeben von Iwan von Müller, V, 2.]

438 Guainerius, Antonius. *Practica Antonii Guainerii papiensis doctoris preclarissimi*, Impressum opus mandato et expensis heredum quondam domini Octaviani Scoti civis Modoetiensis et Sociorum, 27. Augusti 1516.

439 Guazzo, Francesco Maria. *Compendium maleficarum*, ed. with notes by the Rev. Montague Summers . . . transl. by E. A. Ashwin. London: Rodker, 1929.

440 Guillain, Georges. *J. -M. Charcot, 1825–1893, His Life—His Work*, ed. and transl. by Pearce Bailey. New York: Hoeber, 1959.

441 ———. *J.-M. Charcot, 1825–1893: Sa vie—son oeuvre.* Paris: Masson, 1955.

442 Guintherius Andernacus, Joannes. *De medicina veteri et nova tum cognoscenda, tum faciunda*, commentarii duo. Basel, 1571.

443 Guitard, J. F. *Recherches sur les maladies héréditaires.* Paris: Richomme, an XI (1803).

444 Gundel, Wilhelm and Gundel, Hans Georg. *Astrologumena: Die astrologische Literatur in der Antike und ihre Geschichte.* Wiesbaden: Steiner, 1966. [Sudhoffs Archiv, Beihefte, 6.]

445 Gundel, Wilhelm. *Neue astrologische Texte des Hermes Trismegistos.* Munich, 1936. [Abh. d. Bayerischen Akademie d. Wissenschaften, Philosoph.– histor. Abt. Neue Folge, 12.]

446 De Haen, Antonius. *Pars quinta rationis medendi in nosocomio practico.* Vienna, 1760.

447 Haeser, Heinrich. *Lehrbuch der Geschichte der Medicin und der epidemischen Krankheiten*,[3] 3 vols. Jena: 1875 –82.

448 Hagecius ab Hagek, Thaddaeus. *Astrologica opuscula antiqua.* Prague, 1564.

449 Hall, Marshall. *On the Diseases and Derangements of the Nervous System.* London, 1841.

450 ———. "On the reflex function of the medulla oblongata and medulla spinalis." *Philosophical Transactions* (1833): 635–65.

451 Haller, Albrecht von. *A Dissertation on the Sensible and Irritable Parts of Animals*, reprint of the London translation of 1755 with introduction by O. Temkin. Baltimore: The Johns Hopkins Press, 1936.

452 _____. *Elementa physiologiae corporis humani*, t. IV. Lausanne, 1762.

453 Hammond, William A. *Clinical Lectures on Diseases of the Nervous System*, ed. by T. M. B. Cross. New York, 1874.

454 Harle, Jonathan. *An Historical Essay on the State of Physick in the Old and New Testament and the Apocryphal Interval*. London, 1729.

455 Harman, Thomas. *A Caueat or Warening for Commen Cursetors Vulgarely Called Vagabones*, ed. E. Viles and F. J. Furnivall, Early English Text Society, 1869.

456 Harnack, Adolph. *Medicinisches aus der ältesten Kirchengeschichte*. Leipzig, 1892.

457 Harrell, Jerry D. "The sickness of Philoctetes." *Transactions and Studies of the College of Physicians of Philadelphia*, fourth series, 29 (1961-62): 71-76.

458 Hartley, Sir Percival Horton-Smith and Aldridge, Harold Richard. *Johannes de Mirfeld of St. Bartholomew's, Smithfield, His Life and Works*. Cambridge U.P., 1936.

459 Hartmann, Friedrich. *Die Literatur von Früh- und Hochsalerno und der Inhalt des Breslauer Codex Salernitanus*, Diss. Leipzig, 1919.

460 Harva, Uno. *Die religiösen Vorstellungen der altaischen Völker*. Helsinki, 1938 [Folklore Fellows Communications, vol. 52, No. 125].

461 Hasse, K. E. "Die Krankheiten des Nervensystems," in: *Handbuch der speciellen Pathologie und Therapie*, . . . redigirt von R. Virchow, vierter Band, erste Abtheilung. Erlangen, 1855.

462 Hassler, R. "Funktionelle Neuroanatomie und Psychiatrie," *Psychiatrie der Gegenwart* (ed. Gruhle et al.), Band 1, 1A, pp. 152-285. Berlin—Heidelberg—New York: Springer, 1967.

463 Haupt, Mauricius. *Opuscula*, vol. III, ii. Leipzig, 1876.

464 Haustein, Hans. "Die Frühgeschichte der Syphilis 1495-1498." *Archiv für Dermatologie und Syphilis* 161 (1930): 255-388.

465 Hauthal, F. [editor]. *Acronis et Porphyrionis commentarii in Q. Horatium Flaccum*, vol. II. Berlin, 1866.

466 Haymaker, Webb [editor]. *The Founders of Neurology*. Springfield, Ill.: Thomas, 1953.

467 Head, Henry. "Hughlings Jackson on asphasia and kindred affections of speech." *Brain* 38 (1915): 1-27.

468 Heberden, William. *Commentaries on the History and Cure of Diseases*, [reprinted]. New York: Hafner, 1962.

469 Hecker, J. F. C. *Die grossen Volkskrankheiten des Mittelalters*, erweiterte Bearbeitung von A. Hirsch. Berlin, 1865.

470 Hecquet, Philippe. *Le naturalisme des convulsions dans les maladies de l'épidémie convulsionnaire*. Soleure, 1733.

471 Heers, Henricus ab. *Spadacrene, hoc est fons Spadanus . . . et observationum medicarum . . . liber unicus*. Leiden, 1645.

472 Heiberg, J. L. "Geisteskrankheiten im klassischen Altertum." *Allgemeine Zeitschrift für Psychiatrie u. psychisch-gerichtliche Medizin* 86 (1927): 1-44.

473 Heidel, William Arthur. "Hippocratea, 1," *Harvard Studies in Classical Philology*, Cambridge, Harvard U.P., 25 (1914): 139-203.

474  Heim, Ricardus. *Incantamenta magica Graeca Latina*, Diss. Bonn, 1892. [Annales philologorum, Suppl. 19.]

475  Heinrich, Fritz [ed.]. *Ein mittelenglisches Medizinbuch*. Halle, 1896.

476  Heinroth, J. C. A. *System der psychisch-gerichtlichen Medizin*. Leipzig, 1825.

477  Heister, L. *A General System of Surgery*. London, 1743.

478  Hellpach, Willy. *Die geopsychischen Erscheinungen.*[2] Leipzig: Engelmann, 1917.

479  Helmont, Joannes Baptista van. *Oriatrike or Physick Refined*, faithfully rendered into English . . . by J. Chandler, London, 1662.

480  _____. *Ortus medicinae*, editio nova. Amsterdam, 1652.

481  Henle, J. *Handbuch der rationellen Pathologie*, 2. Band, 2. Abtheilung. Braunschweig, 1853.

482  Henry, Marthe. *La Salpêtrière sous l'ancien régime*. Paris: Le François, 1922. [Les origines de l'élimination des antisociaux et de l'assistance aux aliénés chroniques.]

483  Henslow, G. *Medical Works of the Fourteenth Century*. London, 1899.

484  Héricourt, Jules. "La 'bête humaine' de M. Zola." *Revue politique et littéraire, Revue Bleue* 45 (7 June 1890): 710-18.

485  Herodotus. *Herodotus*, with an English transl. by A. D. Godley, vol. II. Loeb, 1921.

486  Herpin, Th. *Des accès incomplets d'épilepsie*. Paris, 1867.

487  _____. *Du pronostic et du traitement curatif de l'épilepsie*. Paris, 1852.

488  Herzog, Rudolf. *Die Wunderheilungen von Epidauros*. Leipzig: Dieterich, 1931. [Philologus, Supplementband 22, Heft 3.]

489  Hippocrates. *Hippocrates*, with an English transl. by W. H. S. Jones, 4 vols. (vol. 3 transl. by E. T. Withington). Loeb, 1923-31.

490  _____. Ἱπποκράτους περὶ ἱερῆς νούσου βίβλιον, rec. Fridericus Dietz. Leipzig, 1827.

491  _____. *Oeuvres complètes d'Hippocrate . . . par* É. Littré, 10 vols. Paris, 1839-61.

492  _____. *Opera*, vol. I, 1, ed. I. L. Heiberg. Leipzig–Berlin: Teubner, 1927. [C.M.G. I, 1.]

493  Hirsch, August [ed.]. *Biographisches Lexikon der hervorragenden Aerzte aller Zeiten und Völker*, 6 vols. Vienna and Leipzig, 1884-88.

494  _____. *Handbuch der historisch-geographischen Pathologie, dritte Abtheilung: Die Organkrankheiten.*[2] Stuttgart, 1886.

495  *Histoire de l'Académie Royale des Sciences*, années: 1705 [Paris, 1730]; 1706 [Paris, 1731]; 1711 [Paris, 1730]; 1734 [Paris, 1736]; 1737 [Paris, 1740]; 1757 [Paris, 1762.]

496  Hobart, William Kirk. *The Medical Language of St. Luke*. Dublin–London, 1882.

497  Höfler, M. "Altgermanische Heilkunde," in: Neuburger-Pagel, *Handbuch der Geschichte der Medizin*, erster Band. Jena: Gustav Fischer, 1902.

498  _____. *Deutsches Krankheitsnamen Buch*. Munich, 1899.

499  _____. "Die Verhüllung, ein volksmedizinischer Heilritus." *Janus* 18 (1913): 104-8.

500  _____. *Die volksmedizinische Organotherapie und ihr Verhältnis zum Kultopfer*. Stuttgart–Berlin–Leipzig, n.d.

501  Höring, C. F. F. *Über Epilepsie*, eine Inaugural–Dissertation unter dem Praesidium von Dr. W. Griesinger. [Diss. Tübingen, 1859.]

502  Hoffmann, Fr.. "Ueber die Eintheilung der Geisteskrankheiten in Siegburg." *Allgemeine Zeitschrift für Psychiatrie und psychisch-gerichtliche Medicin* 19 (1862): 367-91.

503 Hoffmann, Fridericus. *Opera omnia physico-medica*, 6 vols. Geneva, 1748-60.

504 Hoffmann, Gerda. *Beiträge zur Lehre von der durch Zauber verursachten Krankheit und ihrer Behandlung in der Medizin des Mittelalters.* Leiden: Brill, 1933.

505 Holland, Henry. *Chapters on Mental Physiology.* London, 1852.

506 Hollerius, Jacobus. . . . *Omnia opera practica. Doctissimis eiusdem scholiis et observationibus illustrata: Deinde Lud. Dureti . . . in eundem enarrationibus, annotationibus, et Antonii Valetii D. Medici exercitationibus luculentis.* Geneva, 1623.

507 _____. *Omnia opera practica.* Paris, 1664.

508 Holmes, Gordon. "The evolution of clinical medicine as illustrated by the history of epilepsy." *British Medical Journal* 2 (1946): 1-4.

509 _____. *The National Hospital Queen Square 1860-1948.* Edinburgh–London: Livingstone, 1954.

510 Holmes, Oliver Wendell. *Medical Essays 1842-1882.* Boston–New York, 1891.

511 Home, Francis. *Clinical Experiments, Histories and Dissections.* Edinburgh, 1780.

512 Horsley, Victor. "Brain-surgery." *British Medical Journal* 2 (1886): 670-75.

513 _____. "Remarks on ten consecutive cases of operations upon the brain and cranial cavity to illustrate the details and safety of the method employed." *British Medical Journal* 1 (1887): 863-65.

514 Horsley, Victor and Schäfer, Edward Albert. *A Record of Experiments upon the Functions of the Cerebral Cortex.* London, 1888 [*Philosophical Transactions*, 179 (1888), B, 1-45].

515 Horstius, Gregorius. *Opera medica quae extant omnia.* Nuremberg, 1660.

516 Hovorka, O. v., und Kronfeld, A. *Vergleichende Volksmedizin*, 2 vols. Stuttgart: Strecker und Schröder, 1908-9.

517 Howden, James C. "The religious sentiment in epileptics." *Journal of Mental Science* 18 (1873): 482-97.

518 Huette, Georges. *Histoire thérapeutique du bromure de potassium.* Paris, 1878.

519 Hunter, John. *The Works of John Hunter*, ed. J. F. Palmer, vol. I. London, 1835.

520 Hunter, Richard A. "Status epilepticus: history, incidence and problems." *Epilepsia*, 4th series, 1 (1959-60): 162-88.

521 Hunter, Richard and Macalpine, Ida. *Three Hundred Years of Psychiatry 1535-1860.* London: Oxford U.P., 1963.

522 Hyperides. *The Orations Against Athenogenes and Philippides*, ed. with a transl. by F. G. Kenyon. London, 1893.

523 Iamblichus. *De mysteriis liber*, rec. Gustavus Parthey. Berlin, 1857.

524 Ibn Abī Uṣaibi'ah. *Ibn Abi Useibia*, herausgegeben von A. Müller. Königsberg, 1884.

525 Ibn Isḥāq. *The Life of Muhammed*, a transl. of Isḥāq's *Sīrat Rasūl Allāh*, with introduction and notes by A. Guillaume. Oxford U.P., Pakistan Branch, 1967.

526 Ibn Jazla. *Tacuini aegritudinum . . . Buhahylyha Byngezla autore.* Strasbourg, 1532.

527 Ibn Khaldūn. *The Muqaddimah*, transl. from the Arabic by Franz Rosenthal, 3 vols. New York: Pantheon Books, 1958. [Bollingen Series, 43.]

528 Ibn Saad. *Biographie Muhammeds bis zur Flucht*, herausgegeben von Eugen Mittwoch. Leiden: Brill, 1905 [Ibn Saad, Biographien, herausgegeben von Eduard Sachau, 1905-28, Band 1, Theil 1].

529  Ibn Zuhr. *Theizir Abynzoar.* Venice, 1542 [with Averroës' *Colliget*].
530  Ideler, Julius Ludwig. *Physici et medici Graeci minores,* 2 vols. Berlin, 1841–42.
531  Institoris, Henricus. *Malleus maleficarum,* 2 vols. Lyons, 1596 and 1620.
532  ———. *Malleus maleficarum,* transl. with an introduction, bibliography, and notes by the Rev. Montague Summers. London: Rodker, 1928.
533  "Institutions for treatment and care of epilepsy in the different countries of the world." *Epilepsia,* 2nd series, 1 (1937–40): 105–13.
534  Irving, Washington. *Life of Mahomet.* New York: Dutton (Everyman's Library).
535  Ioannes Anglicus. *Praxis medica, rosa anglica dicta,* recens edita opera ac studio clar. V. Doct. Philippi Schopffi, Medici Physici Durlacensis, 2 vols. Augsburg, 1595.
536  Isidorus Hispalensis. *Etymologiarum sive originum, libri XX,* rec. W. M. Lindsay. Oxford U.P., 1911.
537  Isler, Hansruedi. *Thomas Willis, ein Wegbereiter der modernen Medizin 1621–1675.* Stuttgart: Wissenschaftliche Verlagsgesellschaft, 1965.
538  Iuvencus, C. Vettius Aquilinus. *Libri evangeliorum IIII,* ed. C. Marold. Leipzig, 1886.
539  Jackson, John Hughlings. "Cases of epilepsy associated with syphilis." *Medical Times and Gazette* 1 (1861): 648–52; 2: 59–60.
540  ———. "Cases of recovery from epilepsy." *Ibid.* 2 (1862): 107–9.
541  ———. "Clinical remarks on cases of temporary loss of speech and of power of expression (epileptic aphemia? aphrasia? aphasia?), and on epilepsies." *Ibid.* 1 (1866): 442–43.
542  ———. "Clinical remarks on the occasional occurrence of subjective sensations of smell in patients who are liable to epileptiform seizures, or who have symptoms of mental derangement, and in others." *Lancet* 1 (1866): 659–60.
543  ———. "Convulsions," in: *A System of Medicine,* ed. J. Russell Reynolds, vol. 2,[2] pp. 252–91. Philadelphia, 1872.
544  ———. "Convulsive spasms of the right hand and arm preceding epileptic seizures." *Medical Times and Gazette* 1 (1863): 110–11.
545  ———. "Epilepsy following some months after injury to the head." *Ibid.,* 2 (1863): 65.
546  ———. "Epileptic aphemia with epileptic seizures on the right side." *Ibid.* 2 (1864): 167.
547  ———. "Epileptic or epileptiform seizures occurring with discharge from the ear." *British Medical Journal* 1 (1869): 591.
548  ———. "Epileptiform convulsions (unilateral) after an injury to the head." *Medical Times and Gazette* 2 (1863): 65–66.
549  ———. "Epileptiform seizures—aura from the thumb—attacks of coloured vision." *Ibid.* 1 (1863): 589.
550  ———. "Loss of speech: its association with valvular disease of the heart and with hemiplegia on the right side.—Defect of smell.—Defects of speech in chorea.—Arterial lesions in epilepsy." [Reprinted in *Brain* 38 (1915): 28–42.]
551  ———. "Loss of speech, with hemiplegia on the left side—valvular diesase—epileptiform seizures affecting the side paralyzed." *Medical Times and Gazette* 2 (1864): 166–67.
552  ———. *Neurological Fragments* [with biographical memoir by James Taylor ..., and including the "Recollections" of the late Sir Jonathan Hutchinson and the late Dr. Charles Mercier]. Oxford U.P., 1925.

553 _____. "Note on lateral deviation of the eyes in hemiplegia and in certain epileptiform seizures." *Lancet* 1 (1866): 311-12.

554 _____. "Observations on defects of sight in brain disease," reprinted in *Medical Classics*. Baltimore: Williams and Wilkins, 3 (1938-39): 918-26. [Published originally in *Royal London Ophthalmic Hospital Reports* 4 (1863): 10-19.]

555 _____. "Remarks on the disorderly movements of chorea and convulsion, and on localisation." *Medical Times and Gazette* 2 (1867): 669-70.

556 _____. *Selected Writings of John Hughlings Jackson*, ed. J. Taylor, 2 vols. London: Hodder and Stoughton, 1931-32.

557 _____. "Syphilis, followed by unilateral convulsions four months afterwards—temporary hemiplegia—paralysis of the sixth nerve on the same side—recovery." *Medical Times and Gazette* 1 (1863): 111.

558 _____. "Unilateral epileptiform seizures, attended by temporary defect of sight." *Ibid.* 1 (1863): 588.

559 _____. "Unilateral epileptiform seizures beginning by a disagreeable smell." *Ibid.* 2 (1864): 168.

560 James, William. *The Varieties of Religious Experience*, [reprinted]. New York, The Modern Library.

561 Janz, Dieter. *Die Epilepsien.* Stuttgart: Thieme, 1969.

562 Jeanselme, E. "L'épilepsie sur le trône de Byzance." *Bulletin de la Société Française d'Histoire de la Médecine* 18 (1924): 225-74.

563 Jefferson, Geoffrey. *Selected Papers.* London: Pitman, 1960.

564 Joel, Franciscus. *Opera medica.* Amsterdam, 1663.

565 Jörimann, Julius. *Frühmittelalterliche Rezeptarien.* Zürich—Leipzig: Orell Füssli, 1925. [Beiträge zur Geschichte der Medizin, 1.]

566 Johnson, Robert. *Enchiridion Medicum: or a Manual of Physick.* London, 1684.

567 Jones, C. Handfield. "Clinical lecture on cases of paralysis agitans." *British Medical Journal* (March 1, 1873): 221-23, and (March 8, 1873): 248-49.

568 _____. *Studies on Functional Nervous Disorders.* London, 1870.

569 Josat. *Recherches historiques sur l'épilepsie.* Paris, 1856.

570 Jühling, Johannes. *Die Tiere in der deutschen Volksmedizin alter und neuer Zeit.* Mittweida, n.d.

571 Kanner, Leo. "The folklore and cultural history of epilepsy." *Medical Life*, new series, 37 (1930): 167-214.

572 _____. "Mistletoe, magic and medicine." *Bull. Hist. Med.* 7 (1939): 875-936.

573 _____. "The names of the falling sickness, an introduction to the study of the folklore and cultural history of epilepsy." *Human Biology* 2 (1930): 109-27.

574 Kanngiesser, Friedrich. "Notes on the pathology of the Julian Dynasty." *Glasgow Medical Journal* 77 (1912): 428-32.

575 Kaufmann, Walter A. *Nietzsche: Philosopher, Psychologist, Antichrist.* Princeton: Princeton U.P., 1950.

576 Keenan, Mary Emily. "St. Gregory of Nazianzus and early Byzantine medicine." *Bull. Hist. Med.* 9 (1941): 8-30.

577 Kehrer, Hugo. *Die heiligen drei Könige in Literatur und Kunst*, 1. Band. Leipzig: Seemann, 1908.

578 Kerler, Dietrich Heinrich. *Die Patronate der Heiligen.* Ulm: Kerler, 1905.

579 Kiesewetter, Carl. *Franz Anton Mesmer's Leben und Lehre.* Leipzig, 1893.

580 King, Lester S. *The Growth of Medical Thought.* Chicago: University of Chicago Press, 1963.

581 _____. *The Medical World of the 18th Century.* Chicago: University of Chicago Press, 1958.

582 Kinnier Wilson, J. V. "Organic diseases of ancient Mesopotamia," in Don Brothwell and A. T. Sandison (eds.) *Diseases in Antiquity*, pp. 191–208. Springfield, Ill.: Thomas, 1967.

583 _____. "Two medical texts from Nimrud." *Iraq* (1956) 18(2): 130–46 and (1957) 19(1): 40–49.

583a Kipling, Rudyard. *Rudyard Kipling's Verse*, definitive edition. Garden City, N.Y.: Doubleday and Co., 1954.

584 Kirchhoff, Th. "Geschichte der Psychiatrie," in: *Handbuch der Psychiatrie*, herausgegeben von G. Aschaffenburg, Allgemeiner Teil, 4. Abteilung. Leipzig—Vienna: Deuticke, 1912.

585 Klibansky, Raymond, Panofsky, Erwin, and Saxl, Fritz. *Saturn and Melancholy*: Studies in the History of Natural Philosophy, Religion and Art. New York: Basic Books, 1964.

586 Knapp, Ludwig. *Beiträge zur Geschichte der Eklampsie.* Berlin: Karger, 1901.

587 Kobert, Rudolf. "Zur Geschichte des Mutterkorns," *Historische Studien aus dem Pharmakologischen Institute der Kaiserlichen Universität Dorpat*, vol. I, pp. 1–47. Halle, 1889.

588 Köhm, Joseph. *Zur Auffassung und Darstellung des Wahnsinns im klassischen Altertum.* Mainz: Wilckens, 1928. [Beilage zum Jahresbericht des Hessischen Gymnasiums in Mainz, 1927–28.]

589 Kölliker, A. *Manual of Human Histology*, transl. and ed. by G. Buck, and T. Huxley, vol. 1. London: The Sydenham Society, 1853.

590 Kolle, Kurt. *Grosse Nervenärzte*, 3 vols. Stuttgart: Thieme, 1956–63.

591 Konrad von Megenberg. *Das Buch der Natur*, ed. F. Pfeiffer. Stuttgart, 1861.

592 Koty, John. *Die Behandlung der Alten und Kranken bei den Naturvölkern.* Stuttgart: Hirschfeld, 1934. [Forschungen zur Völkerpsychologie und Soziologie, 13.]

593 Kovalevskaya, S. V. *Vospominaniya detstva i avtobiographicheskie ocherki.* Akademiya Nauk, SSSR, 1945.

594 Krafft-Ebing, R. V. *Lehrbuch der Psychiatrie auf klinischer Grundlage.*[2] 2 vols. Stuttgart, 1883.

595 Krogmann, Willy. "Pro cadente morbo." *Archiv für das Studium der neureren Sprachen* 173 (1938): 1–11.

596 Kroll. Ἕρμιππος ἣ περὶ ἀστρολογίας, Pauly-Wissowa, vol. 8, 1913, cols. 854–57.

596a Kruta, Vladislav und Teich, Mikuláš. *Jan Evangelista Purkyně.* Prag: Staatsverlag für Literatur, 1962.

597 Kudlien, Fridolf. "Der Arzt des Körpers und der Arzt der Seele." *Clio Medica* 3 (1968): 1–20.

598 _____. "Early Greek primitive medicine." *Clio Medica* 3 (1968): 305–36.

599 _____. "Poseidonios und die Ärzteschule der Pneumatiker." *Hermes* 9 (1962): 419–29.

600 _____. *Untersuchungen zu Aretaios von Kappadokien.* Mainz: Akademie der Wissenschaften und der Literatur, 1964. [Abh. der Geistes- und sozialwissenschaftlichen Klasse, 1963, no. 11.]

601 Kunkle, E. Charles. "The 'Jumpers' of Maine: A reappraisal." *Archives of Internal Medicine* 119 (1967): 355–58.

602 Kussmaul, A., and Tenner, A.. *On the Nature and Origin of Epileptiform Convulsions Caused by Profuse Bleeding, and also Those of True Epilepsy*, transl. by E. Bronner. London: The New Sydenham Society, 1859.

603  Labat, René. *Traité akkadien de diagnostics et pronostics médicinaux.*
     Paris–Leiden: Académie internationale d'histoire des sciences, Brill, 1951.
604  Laehr, Heinrich. *Die Literatur der Psychiatrie, Neurologie und Psychologie
     von 1459-1799,* 3 vols. Berlin: Reimer, 1900.
605  Lallemand, F. *Recherches anatomico-pathologiques sur l'encéphale et ses
     dépendances,* vols. 1 and 2. Paris, 1824-25.
606  Lammert, G. *Volksmedizin und medizinischer Aberglaube in Bayern und den
     angrenzenden Bezirken.* Würzburg, 1869.
607  La Motte, Guillaume Mauquest de. *Traité complet de chirurgie,*[3] 2 vols. Paris,
     1771.
608  Lanata, Giuliana. *Medicina magica e religione popolare in Grecia fino all' età
     di Ippocrate.* Rome: Edizioni dell'Ateneo, 1967.
609  Lancisius, Jo. Maria. *De subitaneis mortibus libri duo.*[2] Lucca, 1707.
610  Landouzy, H. *Traité complet de l'hystérie.* Paris–London, 1846.
611  Langius, Christianus Johannes. "De morbo caduco," in: *Opera omnia medica
     theoretico-practica,* pars III, 58-68. Leipzig, 1704.
612  Langworthy, Orthello R. "Hughlings Jackson–his opinions concerning
     epilepsy." *Journal of Nervous and Mental Disease* 76 (1932): 574-85.
613  Lasègue, Ch. "Morel.–Sa vie médicale et ses oeuvres." *Archives générales de
     médecine,* 1 (6e série, tome 21) (1873): 589-600.
614  Laski, Marghanita. *Ecstasy, A Study of Some Secular and Religious Expe-
     riences.* Bloomington: Indiana U.P., 1962.
615  Lastres, Juan B. *Epilepsia y delito.* Lima (Peru), 1955.
616  Laycock, Thomas. *An Essay on Hysteria.* Philadelphia, 1840.
617  _____. *Mind and Brain,*[2] 2 vols. London, 1869.
618  _____. "On the reflex function of the brain." *British and Foreign Medical
     Review* 19 (1845): 298-311.
619  _____. *A Treatise on the Nervous Diseases of Women.* London, 1840.
620  Lea, Henry Charles. *Materials toward a History of Witchcraft,* collected by
     Henry Charles Lea, vol. III, ed. by A. C. Howland, with an introduction
     by G. L. Burr. Philadelphia: University of Pennsylvania Press, 1939.
621  Leake, John. *A Practical Essay on Diseases of the Viscera.* London, 1792.
622  Lehmann, Alfred. *Aberglaube und Zauberei,*[3] ed. D. Petersen I. Stuttgart:
     Ferdinand Enke, 1925.
623  Leibbrand, Werner and Wettley, Annemarie. *Der Wahnsinn, Geschichte der
     abendländischen Psychopathologie.* München: Alber, 1961. [Orbis
     Academicus.]
624  Lemnius, Levinus. *De occultis naturae miraculis.* Cologne, 1573.
625  _____. *The Secret Miracles of Nature.* London, 1658.
626  Lemperière, Th. "Histoire de l'évolution des idées sur la mentalité épilep-
     tique." *Histoire de la médecine,* 5(i) (1955): 69-75.
627  Lennox, William G. "Antonius Guainerius on epilepsy." *Annals of Medical
     History,* third series, 2 (1940): 482-99.
628  _____. "Bernard of Gordon on epilepsy." *Annals of Medical History,* third
     series, 3 (1941): 372-83.
629  _____. "John of Gaddesden on epilepsy." *Annals of Medical History,* third
     series, 1 (1939): 283-307.
630  _____. "Phenomena and correlates of the psychomotor triad." *Neurology* 1
     (1951): 357-71.
631  _____. *Science and Seizures.* New York–London: Harper, 1941.
632  Lennox, William Gordon with the collaboration of Margaret A. Lennox.
     *Epilepsy and Related Disorders,* 2 vols. Boston–Toronto: Little, Brown
     and Co., 1960.

633 Le Pois, Charles. *Caroli Pisonis . . . selectiorum observationum et con-siliorum . . . liber singularis*, ed. H. Boerhaave. Leiden, 1733.

634 Lesky, Erna. *Die Wiener medizinische Schule im 19. Jahrhundert.* Graz–Köln: Böhlau, 1965.

635 ———. *Die Zeugungs–und Vererbungslehren der Antike und ihr Nachwirken.* Wiesbaden: Steiner (Kommission), 1951. [Akademie der Wissenschaften und der Literatur in Mainz, Abh. der Geistes- und sozialwissenschaftlichen Klasse, 1950, Nr. 19.]

636 Lesky, E. and Waszink, J. H. "Epilepsie," *Reallexikon für Antike und Christentum*, Lieferung 38, cols. 819–31. Stuttgart: Hiersemann, 1961.

637 Lessiak, Primus. "Gicht." *Zeitschrift für deutsches Altertum* 53 (1912): 101–82.

638 Leuret. "Recherches sur l'épilepsie." *Archives générales de médecine*, 4ᵉ série, 2 (1843): 32–50.

639 Levin, Max. "Our debt to Hughlings Jackson." *JAMA* 191 (1965): 991–96.

640 Liddell and Scott. *A Greek-English Lexicon*, new edition by H. S. Jones and R. McKenzie, 2 vols. Oxford U.P., 1925–40.

641 Littré, É. *Dictionnaire de la langue française*, 6 vols. Paris, n.d.

642 Lloyd, A. C. "The later neo-Platonists," in: *The Cambridge History of Later Greek and Early Medieval Philosophy*, A. H. Armstrong (ed.), pp. 269–325. Cambridge, U.P., 1967.

643 Lombroso, Cesare. *Genio e follia in rapporto alla medicina legale, alla critica ed alla storia.*⁴ Rome–Torino–Florence, 1882.

644 ———. *L'homme criminel*, Traduit sur la IVe édition italienne par M. M. Regnier et Bournet. Paris, 1887.

645 ———. *L'homme de génie*, Traduit de la 6e édition italienne par F. Colonna d'Istria. Paris, 1889.

646 ———. *The Man of Genius.* New York, 1891.

647 ———. *L'uomo di genio in rapporte alla psichiatria, alla storia ed all-estetica*, Quinta edizione del Genio e Follia, Completamente mutata. Torino, 1888.

648 Lopez Piñero, Jose M. and García Ballester, Luis. *La obra de Andrés Alcázar sobre la trepenación.* Valencia, 1964. [Cuadernos Valencianos de historia de la medicina y de la ciencia, II, serie B.]

649 Lotze, Rudolph Hermann. *Allgemeine Pathologie und Therapie als mechanische Naturwissenschaften.*² Leipzig, 1848.

650 Lucas-Championnière. "Trépanation du crâne faite pour une fracture de la voûte sans plaie communicante; guérison complète." *Bulletins et mémoires de la Société de Chirurgie de Paris* 1 (1875): 226–31.

651 ———. *Trépanation néolithique, trépanation pré-Colombienne, trépanation des Kabyles, trépanation traditionnelle* (Les origines de la trépanation décompressive). Paris: Steinheil, 1912.

652 Lucian. *Lucian*, with an English transl. by A. M. Harmon. Loeb, 1927 ff.

653 Lucretius. *Of the Nature of Things*, a metrical transl. by W. E. Leonard. Everyman's Library, 1928.

654 Macbride, David. *A Methodical Introduction to the Theory and Practice of Physic.* London, 1772.

655 MacDonald, Carlos F. "Feigned epilepsy, case of James Clegg, alias James Lee, the 'Dummy Chucker'." *American Journal of Insanity.* 37 (1880–81): 1–22.

656 Macewen, William. "An address on the surgery of the brain and spinal cord." *British Medical Journal* 2 (1888): 302–9.

657 McKenzie, Dan. *The Infancy of Medicine.* London: Macmillan, 1927.

658  McNaughton, Francis L. "The classification  of the epilepsies." *Epilepsia*, third ser., 1 (1952): 7-16.

659  Magnan, V. "Leçons cliniques sur l'épilepsie," in: *Leçons cliniques sur les maladies mentales faites à l'asile clinique* (Sainte-Anne). Paris, 1882-91.

660  ———. "Recherches de physiologie pathologique avec l'alcool et l'essence d' absinthe.—Épilepsie." *Archives de physiologie normale et pathologique* 5 (1873): 115-42.

661  Maisonneuve, J. G. F. *Recherches et observations sur l'épilepsie, présentées à l'école de médecine de Paris.* Paris, an XII.

662  Malpighi, Marcellus. *Consultationum medicinalium centuria prima*, quam in gratiam clinicorum evulgat Hieronymus Gaspari. Padua, 1713.

663  Manetho. "Apotelesmatica," ed. A. Koechly, in: *Poetae bucolici et didactici.* Paris, 1862.

664  Mankowsky, Abraham. "Ueber Bryonia alba." *Historische Studien aus dem Pharmakologischen Institute der Kaiserlichen Universität Dorpat*, vol. II, pp. 143-80. Halle, 1890.

664a Manley, John. "On epilepsy." *Journal of Mental Science* 4 (1858): 245-48.

665  Marc. "Epilepsie simulée," *Dictionaire des sciences médicales, par une société de médecins et de chirurgiens*, t. 12, pp. 539-44. Paris, 1815.

666  Marcellus. *De medicamentis liber*, rec. M. Niedermann. Leipzig—Berlin: Teubner, 1916. [Corpus Medicorum Latinorum, V.]

667  Marchant. "Sur les vertus de la racine de la grande valeriane sauvage." *Histoire de l'Académie Royale des Sciences*, année 1706 [Paris 1731]: 333-35.

668  Marci a Kronland, Marcus. *Liturgia mentis seu disceptatio medica, philosophica et optica de natura epilepsiae illius ortu et causis.* Regensburg, 1678.

669  Margetts, Edward L. "Trepanation of the skull by the medicine men of primitive cultures, with particular reference to present-day native East African practice," in: Brothwell and Sandison (editors) *Diseases in Antiquity*, ch. 53. Springfield, Ill.: Thomas, 1967.

670  Marsan, C. Ajmone. "A newly proposed classification of epileptic seizures. Neurophysiological basis." *Epilepsia*, fourth series, 6 (1965): 275-96.

671  Martin, Alfred. "Warum galten Epilepsie und Geisteskrankheit (Frenesis) als ansteckend?" *Deutsche Zeitschrift für Nervenheilkunde* 75 (1922): 103-10.

672  Marzell. "Pfingstrose," *Handwörterbuch des deutschen Aberglaubens*, vol. 6, cols. 1698-1700. Berlin—Leipzig: de Gruyter, 1934-35.

673  Masland, Richard L. "Classification of the epilepsies." *Epilepsia*, fourth series, 1 (1959-60): 512-20.

674  Maudsley, Henry. *Responsibility in Mental Disease.* New York, 1874.

675  Mayow, John. *Medico-physical Works*, Edinburgh, 1907. [Alembic Club Reprints, 17.]

676  Mead, Richard. *De imperio solis ac lunae in corpora humana, et morbis inde oriundis.* [2] London, 1746.

677  ———. *Medica sacra.* London, 1749.

678  ———. *The Medical Works of Richard Mead.* London, 1762.

679  Mechler, Achim. "Zur Eponymik der Epilepsie." *Medizinische Welt* 10 (1963): 535-38.

680  Meier, Carl Alfred. "The dream in ancient Greece and its use in temple cures (incubation)," in: G. E. von Grunebaum and Roger Caillois [editors] *The*

*Dream and Human Society*, pp. 303-19. Berkeley and Los Angeles: University of California Press, 1966.

681 Mély, F. de. *Les lapidaires de l'antiquité et du moyen âge*, t. II. Paris, 1898.

682 Mercier, Charles Arthur. *Astrology in Medicine*. London: Macmillan, 1914. [The Fitzpatrick Lectures, 1913.]

683 Mercurialis, Hieron. *Hippocratis Coi opera quae extant*, ed. Hieron. Mercurialis. Venice, 1588.

684 ———. *Medicina practica.* Lyons, 1623.

685 Merritt, H. Houston and Putnam, Tracy, J. "Sodium diphenyl hydantoinate in the treatment of convulsive disorders." *JAMA* 111 (1938): 1068-73.

686 Mesue, Joannes. "Grabadin, idest compendii secretorum medicamentorum liber secundus," in: *Ioannis Mesuae Damasceni ... opera.* Venice, 1623.

687 Métraux, Alfred. "Le shamanisme chez les Indiens de l'Amérique du sud tropicale." *Acta Americana* (Review of the Inter-American Society of Anthropology and Geography) 2 (1944): 197-219, 320-41.

688 Meyer, Alfred and Hierons, Raymond. "On Thomas Willis's concepts of neurophysiology." *Medical History* 9 (1965): 1-15 and 142-55.

689 Meyer, Ludwig. "Aus der Krampfkranken-Abtheilung der Charité." *Annalen des Charité-Krankenhauses*, sechster Jahrgang, 2. Heft (Berlin, 1855): 1-34.

690 ———. "Einige Fälle aus der Abtheilung für Krampfkranke des Charité-Krankenhauses (Mai, Juni, Juli, 1853)." *Annalen des Charité-Krankenhauses* 4 (Berlin, 1853): 321-30.

691 ———. "Ueber Mania transitoria." *Virchows Arch.* 8 (1855): 192-210.

692 Meyerhof, Max. " 'Alī aṭ-Ṭabarī's 'Paradise of Wisdom,' one of the oldest Arabic compendiums of medicine." *Isis* 16 (1931): 6-54.

693 ———. "The 'Book of Treasure', an early Arabic treatise on medicine." *Isis* 14 (1930): 55-76.

694 ———. "Thirty-three clinical observations by Rhazes (circa 900 A.D.)." *Isis* 23 (1935): 321-72.

695 Meynert, Theodor. *Der Bau der Gross-Hirnrinde und seine örtlichen Verschiedenheiten, nebst einem pathologisch—anatomischen Corollarium.* Neuwied—Leipzig: Heuser, 1872. [Separat-Abdruck aus der Vierteljahrsschrift für Psychiatrie etc.]

696 Meynert, Theodor. *Skizzen über Umfang und wissenschaftliche Anordnung der klinischen Psychiatrie.* Vienna: Braumüller, 1876.

697 Michler, Markwart. "Die Atemtheorie in 'De morbo sacro'," in: *Current Problems in History of Medicine*, R. Blaser and H. Buess [editors], pp. 188-94. Basel—New York: Karger, 1966.

698 ———. "Die Krüppelleiden in 'De morbo sacro' und 'De articulis'." *Sudhoffs Archiv* 45 (1961): 303-28.

699 Mihles, S. *Medical Essays and Observations ... Abridg'd from the Philosophical Transactions*, vol. II. London, 1745.

700 Mildner, Th. "Die Behandlung der 'Fallenden Sucht' im 18. Jahrhundert." *Medizinische Klinik* 61 (1966): 2014-17.

701 Miller, Harold W. "The concept of the divine in De morbo sacro." *Transactions and Proceedings of the American Philological Association*, 84 (1953): 1-15.

702 Minder, Robert. *Der Hexenglaube bei den Jatrochemikern des 17. Jahrhunderts.* Zurich: Juris, 1963. [Zürcher medizingeschichtliche Abh., neue Reihe, no. 12.]

703 Mingazzini, G. "Symptomatic epilepsy in birds. An anatomico-pathological and clinical report." *Archives of Neurology and Psychiatry* 9 (1923): 576-81.
704 Minkowski, E. et Fusswerk, J. "Le problème Dostoievsky et la structure de l'épilepsie." *Annales médico-psychologiques* (2), 113 (1955): 369-409.
705 Mirfeld, John of. *Sinonima Bartholomei*, ed. J. L. G. Mowat. Oxford, 1882. [Anecdota Oxoniensia; mediaeval and modern series, vol. I, part 1.]
706 Mochulsky, Konstantin. *Dostoevsky: His Life and Work*, transl. with an introduction by Michael A. Minihan. Princeton U.P., 1967.
707 Montanus, Jo. Baptista. *Consultationum medicinalium centuria prima*, a Valentino Lublino . . . collecta. Venice, 1554.
708 Moreau, J. (de Tours). *De l'étiologie de l'épilepsie et des indications que l'étude des causes peut fournir.* Paris, 1854. [Extrait des mémoires de l'Académie Impériale de Médecine, t. XVIII, 1854.]
709 _____. *La psychologie morbide dans ses rapports avec la philosophie de l'histoire.* Paris, 1859.
710 Morel, Bénédict Augustin. "D'une forme de délire, suite d'une surexcitation nerveuse se rattachant à une variété non encore décrite d'épilepsie (Épilepsie larvée)." *Gazette hebdomadaire de médecine et de chirurgie* 7 (1860): 773-75, 819-21, 836-41.
711 _____. *Etudes cliniques. Traité théorique et pratique des maladies mentales considérées dans leur nature, leur traitement, et dans leur rapport avec la médecine légale des aliénes*, 2 vols. Nancy—Paris, 1852-53.
712 _____. *Traité des dégénérescences physiques, intellectuelles et morales de l'espèce humaine et des causes qui produisent ces variétés maladives.* Paris—London—New York, 1857.
713 _____. *Traité des maladies mentales.* Paris, 1860.
714 Morgagni, J. B. *De sedibus et causis morborum per anatomen indagatis, libri quinque,*[9] t. I. Paris, 1820.
715 Moss, Gerald C. "The mentality and personality of the Julio-Claudian emperors." *Medical History* 7 (1963): 165-75.
716 Muchnic, Helen. *Dostoevsky's English Reputation (1881-1936)*, Northampton, Mass., Smith College, 1939. [Smith College Studies in Modern Languages, 1938-39, vol. 20, 3-4.]
717 Müllener, Eduard-Rudolf. "Pierre-Charles-Alexandre Louis' (1787-1872) Genfer Schüler und die 'méthode numérique'." *Gesnerus* 24 (1967): 46-74.
718 Müller, Gottfried. *Aus mittelenglischen Medizintexten.* Leipzig: Tauchnitz, 1929. [Kölner anglistische Arbeiten, 10.]
719 Müller, Johannes. *Über die phantastischen Gesichtserscheinungen.* Eingeleitet und herausgegeben von M. Müller. Leipzig: Barth, 1927. [Klassiker der Medizin, 32.]
720 Müri, Walter. "Melancholie und schwarze Galle." *Museum Helveticum* 10 (1953): 21-38.
721 Muir, William. *The Life of Mahomet*, vol. 2. London, 1861.
722 Murphy, Edward L. "The saints of epilepsy." *Medical History* 3 (1959): 303-11.
723 Murray, James A. H. [editor]. *A new English Dictionary on Historical Principles.* Oxford, 1888 ff.
724 Muschg, Walter. *Tragische Literaturgeschichte.*[2] Bern: Francke, 1953.
725 Muskens, L. J. J. *Epilepsy.* New York: W. Wood, 1928.

726 Muth, Robert. *Träger der Lebenskraft: Ausscheidungen des Organismus im Volksglauben der Antike.* Vienna: Rohrer, 1954.

727 Myerson, Abraham. *The Inheritance of Mental Diseases.* Baltimore: Williams and Wilkins, 1925.

728 Nachmanson, Ernst. *Erotianstudien.* Uppsala—Leipzig, 1917.

729 Nasse, Fried. [editor]. "Phantasieen in einem epileptischen Anfalle." *Zeitschrift für Anthropologie* (1825): 190-91, English transl. by Owsei Temkin and C. Lilian Temkin, *Bull. Hist. Med.* 42 (1968): 566-68.

730 Neuburger, Max. *Geschichte der Medizin,* 2 vols. Stuttgart: Enke, 1906-11.

731 _____. *Die historische Entwicklung der experimentellen Gehirn- und Rückenmarksphysiologie vor Flourens.* Stuttgart, 1897.

732 Neuburger, Max, and Pagel, Julius [editors]. *Handbuch der Geschichte der Medizin,* 3 vols. Jena: Fischer, 1902-05.

733 Nicolson, Frank W. "The saliva superstition in classical literature." *Harvard Studies in Classical Philology* 8 (1897): 23-40.

734 Nietzsche, Friedrich. *Gesammelte Werke,* zehnter Band. Munich: Musarion, 1924.

735 Nioradze, Georg. *Der Schamanismus bei den sibirischen Völkern.* Stuttgart: Strecker und Schröder, 1925.

736 Nöldeke, Theodor. *Geschichte des Qorāns,*[2] ed. Friedrich Schwally, Erster Teil. Leipzig: Dieterich, 1909.

737 _____. *Das Leben Muhammed's.* Hannover, 1863.

738 Nörenberg, Heinz-Werner. *Das Göttliche und die Natur in der Schrift über die heilige Krankheit.* Bonn: Habelt, 1968.

739 Nonnus. *Dionysiaca,* rec. A. Ludwich, vol. II. Leipzig: Teubner, 1911.

740 Nothnagel, H. "Die Entstehung allgemeiner Convulsionen vom Pons und von der Medulla oblongata aus." *Virchow's Arch.* 44 (1868): 1-12.

741 _____. "Epilepsy and eclampsia," in: *Ziemssen's Cyclopaedia of the Practice of Medicine,* American edition by A. H. Buck, vol. XIV, pp. 183-311. New York, 1877.

742 _____. *Ueber den epileptischen Anfall.* Leipzig, 1872. [Sammlung klinischer Vorträge herausg. v. R. Volkmann, 39.]

743 _____. "Zur Lehre vom klonischen Krampf." *Virchows Arch.* 49 (1870): 267-90.

744 Nyffeler, Johann Rudolf. *Joseph Daquin und seine "Philosophie de la Folie,"* Diss. Zurich, 1961.

745 Nymmanus, Gregorius. *De epilepsia disputatio* [praeside Daniele Sennerto]. Wittenberg, 1618.

746 Obersteiner, H. "Ueber den Status epilepticus." *Wiener Medizinische Wochenschrift* 23 (1873): 544-47.

747 O'Brien-Moore, Ainsworth. *Madness in Ancient Literature,* Diss. Princeton, 1922. Weimar: R. Wagner Sohn, 1924.

748 O'Donoghue, Edward Geoffrey. *The Story of Bethlehem Hospital.* London—Leipzig: Unwin, 1914.

749 Oesterreich, T. K. *Possession, Demoniacal and Other,* authorized transl. by D. Ibberson. London: Kegan Paul, Trench, Trubner, 1930.

750 Ogden, Margaret Sinclair [ed.]. *The 'Liber de diversis medicinis' in the Thornton Manuscript (MS. Lincoln Cathedral A.5.2).* London: published for the Early English Text Society by Humphrey Milford, Oxford U.P., 1938.

751 Ohrt. "Fallsuchtsegen," *Handwörterbuch des deutschen Aberglaubens,* vol. 2, cols. 1178-81. Berlin—Leipzig: de Gruyter, 1929-30.

752 Onians, Richard Broxton. *The Origins of European Thought.* Cambridge, U.P., 1951.

753 Oribasius. *Collectionum medicarum reliquiae,* ed. I. Raeder. Leipzig—Berlin: Teubner, 1928 ff. [C.M.G., VI, 1.]

754 _____. *Oeuvres d'Oribase,* . . . par Bussemaker et Daremberg, 6 vols. Paris, 1851-76.

755 _____. *Synopsis ad Eustathium,* ed. I. Raeder. Leipzig—Berlin: Teubner, 1926. [C.M.G., VI, 3.]

756 Origenes. *Opera,* vol. III. Paris, 1862. [Patrologia Graeca, ed. Migne, 13.]

757 Orpheus. *Orphica et Procli hymni,* rec. E. Abel. Leipzig—Prague, 1885.

758 Pagel, Walter. "Helmont Leibniz Stahl." *Sudhoffs Arch.* 24 (1931): 19-59.

759 _____. *Jo. Bapt. van Helmont, Einführung in die philosophische Medizin des Barock.* Berlin: Julius Springer, 1930.

760 _____. "Medieval and renaissance contributions to knowledge of the brain and its functions," in: F. N. L. Poynter (ed.) *The History and Philosophy of Knowledge of the Brain and Its Functions: an Anglo-American Symposium, London, July 15th-17th, 1957,* pp. 95-114. Springfield, Ill.: Thomas, 1958.

761 _____. *Das medizinische Weltbild des Paracelsus.* Seine Zusammenhänge mit Neuplatonismus und Gnosis. Wiesbaden: Steiner, 1962. [Kosmosophie, Bd. 1.]

762 _____. *Paracelsus, an Introduction to Philosophical Medicine in the Era of the Renaissance.* Basel—New York: Karger, 1958.

763 _____. "Paracelsus' ätherähnliche Substanzen und ihre pharmakologische Auswertung an Hühnern." *Gesnerus* 21 (1964): 113-25.

764 _____. "Paracelsus: traditionalism and medieval sources," in: L. G. Stevenson and R. P. Multhauf (editors), *Medicine, Science and Culture,* pp. 51-75. Baltimore: The Johns Hopkins Press, 1968.

765 _____. Review of Gerhard Eis, Vor und nach Paracelsus. *Deutsche Literaturzeitung* 88 (1967): 160-62.

766 _____. "Religious motives in the medical biology of the 17th century." *Bull. Hist. Med.* 3 (1935): 97-128, 213-31, 265-312.

767 _____. "The 'wild spirit' (Gas) of John Baptist van Helmont (1579-1644) and Paracelsus." *Ambix* 10 (1962): 1-13.

767a _____. *William Harvey's Biological Ideas.* New York: Hafner, 1967.

768 Pagel, Walter and Winder, Marianne. "Harvey and the 'modern' concept of disease." *Bull. Hist. Med.* 42 (1968): 496-509.

769 Paracelsus. *Four Treatises of Theophrastus von Hohenheim called Paracelsus,* transl. from the original German, with introductory essays by C. L. Temkin, G. Rosen, G. Zilboorg, H. E. Sigerist. Baltimore: The Johns Hopkins Press, 1941.

770 Paracelsus. *Sämtliche Werke,* 1. Abteilung, medizinische naturwissenschaftliche und philosophische Schriften, herausgegeben von K. Sudhoff. 14 vols. Munich—Berlin: Oldenbourg, 1922-33.

771 Parchappe, Max. *Des principes à suivre dans la fondation et la construction des asiles d'aliénés.* Paris, 1853.

772 Paré, Ambroise. *Oeuvres complètes d'Ambroise Paré,* revues etc. par J. -F. Malgaigne, 3 vols. Paris, 1840-41.

773 _____. *The Workes of that Famous Chirurgion Ambrose Parey,* transl. out of Latine and compared with the French by Tho. Johnson. London, 1649.

774 Parker, Harry L. "Jacksonian convulsions: an historical note." *Journal-Lancet,* new series, 49 (1929): 107-11.

775 *Paroemiographi Graeci*, eds. E. L. a Leutsch et F. G. Schneidewin, 2 vols. Göttingen, 1839-51.

776 Patak, Martin. *Die Angst vor dem Scheintod in der 2. Hälfte des 18. Jahrhunderts.* Zurich: Juris-Verlag, 1967. [Zürcher medizingeschichtliche Abh., Neue Reihe Nr. 44.]

777 Pattie, Frank A. "Mesmer's medical dissertation and its debt to Mead's De Imperio Solis ac Lunae." *Journal of the History of Medicine and Allied Sciences* 11 (1956): 275-87.

778 Paulus of Aegina. *Paulus Aegineta*, ed. I. L. Heiberg, 2 vols. Leipzig–Berlin: Teubner, 1921-24. [C.M.G. IX, 1-2.]

779 _____. *The Seven Books of Paulus Aegineta*, transl. etc. by F. Adams, 3 vols. London: The Sydenham Society, 1844-47.

780 Paulus Alexandrinus. *Scriptoris Pauli Alexandrini*, Εἰσαγωγὴ εἰς τὴν ἀποτελεσματικήν [ed. Andreas Schato]. Wittenberg, 1586.

781 Payne, Joseph Frank. *English Medicine in the Anglo-Saxon Times.* Oxford, Clarendon Press, 1904. [The Fitz-Patrick Lectures for 1903.]

782 Penfield, Wilder and Erickson, Theodore C. *Epilepsy and Cerebral Localization.* Springfield–Baltimore: Thomas, 1941.

783 Penfield, Wilder and Jasper, Herbert. *Epilepsy and the Functional Anatomy of the Human Brain.* Boston: Little, Brown and Company, 1954.

784 Penfield, Wilder and Kristiansen, Kristian. *Epileptic Seizure Patterns.* Springfield, Ill.: Thomas, 1951.

785 Peters, U. H. "Das pseudopsychopathische Affektsyndrom der Temporallappenepileptiker." *Der Nervenarzt* 40 (1969): 75-82.

786 _____. "Sexualstörungen bei psychomotorischer Epilepsie," (paper read at the Symposium über zentralnervöse Sexualsteuerung (30. Sept. bis 2. Okt. 1969 in der Stadthalle zu Göttingen veranstaltet von der Deutschen Neurovegetativen Gesellschaft).

787 Petersen, William F. *The Patient and the Weather*, vol. II. Ann Arbor: Edwards Brothers, 1934.

788 Petrarch. *Pétrarque, Vie de César*, réproduction phototypique du manuscrit autographe manuscrit Latin 5784 de la Bibliothèque Nationale, Précédée d'une introduction par Léon Dorez. Paris: Champion, 1906.

789 Petrus de Abbano. *Tractatus de venenis.* Padua, 1473.

790 Pflüger, Eduard. *Die sensorischen Functionen des Rückenmarks der Wirbelthiere.* Berlin, 1853.

791 Philipsborn, A. " Ἱερὰ νόσος und die Spezial–Anstalt des Pantokrator–Krankenhauses." *Byzantion* 33 (1963): 223-30.

792 Philodemus. *De ira liber*, ed. C. Wilke. Leipzig: Teubner, 1914.

793 Philostratus. *Philostratos über Gymnastik*, von J. Jüthner. Leipzig–Berlin, 1909. [Sammlung wissenschaftlicher Kommentare zu griechischen und römischen Schriftstellern.]

794 Photius. *Bibliotheca*, ed. Immanuel Bekker. Berlin, 1824.

795 Phriesen, Laurentius. *Spiegel der Artzney*, Gebessert und widerumb fleissig übersehen durch Othonem Brunfels. Strasbourg, 1529.

796 Pickthall, Mohammed Marmaduke (transl.). *The Meaning of the Glorious Koran.* Mentor Books.

797 Pinel, Ph.. *Nosographie philosophique*,[5] t. 3. Paris, 1813.

798 Pitcairn, Archibald. *Elementa medicinae physico-mathematica.* The Hague, 1718.

799 Plater, Felix. *Praxeos medicae tomi tres.* Basel, 1625.

800  Platner, Ernestus. *Opuscula academica . . . post mortem auctoris edidit C. G. Neumann.* Berlin, 1824.
801  Plato. *Plato,* with an English transl., I, Euthyphro, Apology, Crito, Phaedo, Phaedrus, by H. N. Fowler. Loeb, 1960.
802  _____. *Plato,* with an English transl., VII, Timaeus, etc., by R. G. Bury. Loeb, 1929.
803  _____. *Plato,* with an English transl., IX and X, Laws, by R. G. Bury. Loeb, 1926.
804  _____. *The Republic,* transl. with introduction and notes by Francis Macdonald Cornford. New York: Oxford U.P., 1963.
805  Plautus. *Plautus,* with an English transl. by P. Nixon, vol. I. Loeb, 1921.
806  Pliny. *Naturalis historia,* rec. L. Janus. Leipzig, vol. I, 1870; vols. 2-6, 1856-65.
807  _____. *The Natural History of Pliny,* transl. etc. by J. Bostock and H. T. Riley. London, 1893-98.
808  Pliny (Pseudo). *Plinii Secundi quae fertur una cum Gargilii Martialis medicina,* ed. V. Rose. Leipzig, 1875.
809  Plutarch. *Fragmenta et spuria,* ed. Fr. Dübner. Paris, 1876.
810  _____. *The Greek Questions of Plutarch,* with a new transl. and commentary by W. R. Halliday. Oxford: Clarendon Press, 1928.
811  _____. *Moralia,* ed. Wyttenbach, editio nova, t. III. Leipzig, 1828.
812  _____. *Plutarch's Lives,* with an English transl. by B. Perrin. Loeb, 1914 ff.
813  _____. *Plutarch's Moralia,* with an English transl. by F. C. Babbitt, and others. Loeb, 1927 ff.
814  Podach, Erich F. *Friedrich Nietzsches Werke des Zusammenbruchs.* Heidelberg: Rothe, 1961.
815  Pohlenz, Max. *Hippokrates und die Begründung der wissenschaftlichen Medizin.* Berlin: de Gruyter, 1938.
816  _____. *Hippokratesstudien.* Göttingen: Vandenhoeck und Ruprecht, 1937. [Nachrichten von der Gesellschaft der Wissenschaften zu Göttingen. Philol.-hist. Klasse, Fachgruppe I, Altertumswissenschaft, N.F., Band II, Nr. 4.]
817  Politzer, Heinz. "Dostoevsky and the epilepsy of the modern world." *Ciba Symposium* 11 (1963): 106-14.
818  Pollard, John. *Seers, Shrines and Sirens.* London: Allen and Unwin, 1965.
819  Portal (Le Baron). *Observations sur la nature et le traitement de l'épilepsie.* Paris, 1827.
820  Pradel, Fritz. *Griechische und süditalienische Gebete, Beschwörungen und Rezepte des Mittelalters.* Giessen: Töpelmann, 1907. [Religionsgeschichtliche Vorarbeiten, III, 3.]
821  Premuda, Loris. *Il "Morbus Comitatialis" degli antichi e la singolare teoria etiopatogenetica de Platone ed Apuleio.* Undine, 1944.
822  Preuss, Julius. *Biblisch-talmudische Medizin.*[3] Berlin: Karger, 1923.
823  Price, George E. "Shakespeare as a neuropsychiatrist." *Annals of Medical History* 10 (1928): 159-64.
824  Prichard, J. C. *A Treatise on Diseases of the Nervous System,* Part the first. London, 1822.
825  Pritchard, James B. [editor]. *Ancient Near Eastern Texts Relating to the Old Testament.*[2] Princeton: Princeton U.P., 1955.
826  Proksch, J. K. *Die Geschichte der venerischen Krankheiten,* zweiter Theil, Neuzeit. Bonn, 1895.

827 Pruyser, Paul W. "Psychological testing in epilepsy, II. Personality." *Epilepsia*, third series, 2 (1953): 23-36.
828 Prosperus de Lambertinis. *De servorum Dei beatificatione et beatorum canonizatione*, liber tertius. Bologna, 1737.
829 Psellos, Michael. *Chronographie ou Histoire d'un siècle de Byzance* (976-1077), texte établi et traduit par Emile Renauld, 2 vols. Paris: Les Belles Lettres, 1926-28. [Collection Byzantine publiée sous le patronage de l'Association Guillaume Budé.]
830 Purcell, John. *A Treatise of Vapours or, Hysterick Fits.* London, 1702.
831 Purkyně, Jan Ev. *Opera omnia*, vols. 2 and 3. Prague, 1937-39.
832 Purpura, Dominick P. "An historical study of neurophysiologic concepts in epilepsy." *Epilepsia*, third series, 2 (1953): 115-26.
833 Quercetanus, Jos. *Tetras gravissimorum totius capitis affectuum.*[2] Marburg, 1609.
834 Rabbow, Paul. *Antike Schriften über Seelenheilung und Seelenleitung*, I. Die Therapie des Zorns. Leipzig—Berlin: Teubner, 1914.
835 Radcliffe, Charles Bland. *Lectures on Epilepsy, Pain, Paralysis and Certain Other Disorders of the Nervous System.* Philadelphia, 1866.
836 Rahman, F. *Prophecy in Islam: Philosophy and Orthodoxy.* London: Allen and Unwin, 1958.
837 Ramat, Paolo. "Gr. ἱερός, Scr. iṣíráḥ e la loro famiglia lessicale." *Die Sprache*, Zeitschrift für Sprachwissenschaft 8 (1962): 4-28.
837a Rattansi, P. M. "The Helmontian—Galenist controversy in restoration England." *Ambix* 12 (1964): 1-23.
838 Rayer, P. *Histoire de l'épidémie de suette-miliaire, qui a régné, en 1821, dans les départements de l'Oise et de Seine-Et-Oise.* Paris, 1822.
839 Renan, Ernest. *Les apôtres.*[11] Paris, 1882.
840 De Renzi, Salvatore. *Collectio Salernitana*, 5 vols. Naples, 1852-59.
841 Reynolds, J. Russell. "Epilepsy," in: *A System of Medicine*, ed. J. R. Reynolds, vol. 2, second edition, pp. 292-327. Philadelphia, 1872.
842 _____. *Epilepsy: Its Symptoms, Treatment, and Relation to Other Chronic Convulsive Diseases.* London, 1861.
843 Rhazes. *Continens.* Venice, 1509.
844 Rhodius, Joannes. *Observationum medicinalium centuriae tres.* Frankfurt, 1676. [Together with Petrus Borellus: *Historiarum et observationum medicophysicarum centuriae IV.*]
845 Ribton-Turner, C. J. *A History of Vagrants and Vagrancy and Beggars and Begging.* London, 1887.
846 Richer, Paul. *Études cliniques sur l'hystéro-épilepsie ou grande hystérie.* Paris, 1881.
847 Riese, Walther. "Changing concepts of cerebral localization." *Clio medica* 2 (1967): 189-230.
848 _____. "History and principles of classification of nervous diseases." *Bull. Hist. Med.* 18 (1945): 465-512.
849 _____. "Hughlings Jackson's doctrine of consciousness: sources, versions and elaborations." *Journal of Nervous and Mental Disease* 120 (1954): 330-37.
849a _____. "La maladie de Vincent van Gogh. Son rôle dans la vie et l'oeuvre de l'artiste." *Symposium Ciba*, 6 (no. 5) (1958): 198-205.
850 _____. "The sources of Jacksonian neurology." *Journal of Nervous and Mental Disease* 124 (1956): 125-34.
851 Riolanus, Joannes. *Opera omnia.* Paris, 1610.

852  Riolanus, Joannes, filius. *Encheiridium anatomicum et pathologicum.* Leiden, 1649.

853  Riverius, Lazarus. *The Compleat Practice of Physick*, by Nicholas Culpeper [and others]. Being Chiefly a Translation of the Works of That Learned and Renowned Doctor, Lazarus Riverius. London, 1655.

854  Rivier, André. *Recherches sur la tradition manuscrite du traité hippocratique "De morbo sacro."* Bern: Editions Francke, 1962. [Travaux publiés sous les auspices de la Société suisse des sciences morales.]

855  Robb, Preston. *Epilepsy: a Review of Basic and Clinical Research.* U.S. Department of Health, Education, and Welfare, National Institute of Neurological Diseases and Blindness, 1965 (NINDB Monograph No. 1).

856  Robinson, Nicholas. *A New System of the Spleen, Vapours, and Hypochondriack Melancholy.* London, 1729.

857  Robinson, Trevor. "On the nature of sweet oil of vitriol." *Journal of the History of Medicine and Allied Sciences* 14 (1959): 231-33.

858  Robinson, Victor. "Medico-theologic consultations in the seventeenth century" [transl. with notes from *Bulletin de la Société Française d'Histoire de la Médecine* (1932): 218-25], *Medical Life*, new series, 43 (1936): 153-61.

859  Roelans von Mecheln, Cornelis. *Liber de aegritudinibus infantium.* [Facsimile reprint in Karl Sudhoff, Erstlinge der pädiatrischen Literatur, Münchner Drucke, 1925.]

860  Röschlaub, Andreas. *Untersuchungen über Pathogenie oder Einleitung in die Heilkunde*, dritter Theil, zweite veränderte Auflage. Frankfurt am Main, 1803.

861  Rohde, Erwin. *Der griechische Roman und seine Vorläufer.*[2] Leipzig: Breitkopf und Härtel, 1900.

862  Rohde, Erwin. *Psyche.*[7-8] Tübingen: Mohr, 1921.

863  Rolleston, J. D. "The folk-lore of epilepsy." *Medical Press and Circular* 209 (1943): 154-57.

864  _____. "Jean Baptiste Bouillaud (1796-1881). A pioneer in cardiology and neurology." *Proceedings of the Royal Society of Medicine*, 24, part 2 (1931): 1253-62.

865  Romberg, Moritz Heinrich. *A Manual of the Nervous Diseases of Man*, transl. and ed. by E. H. Sieveking, vol. II. London: Sydenham Society, 1853.

866  Rondeletius, Gulielmus. *Methodus curandorum omnium morborum corporis humani.* Frankfurt, 1592.

867  Roscher, Wilhelm Heinrich. *Ausführliches Lexikon der griechischen und römischen Mythologie*, dritter Band. Leipzig, 1897-1909.

868  _____. "Nachträge zu meinem Buche 'Über Selene und Verwandtes'," in: *Jahresbericht des Königlichen Gymnasiums zu Wurzen in Sachsen für das Schuljahr 1894-1895*, pp. 1-50. Wurzen, 1895.

869  _____. *Über Selene und Verwandtes.* Leipzig, 1890. [Studien zur griechischen Mythologie und Kulturgeschichte, 4.]

870  Rose, Valentin. *Anecdota Graeca et Graecolatina*, 2. Heft. Berlin, 1870.

871  Rosen, George. "Enthusiasm, 'a dark lanthorn of the spirit'." *Bull. Hist. Med.* 42 (1968): 393-421.

872  _____. *Madness in Society, Chapters in the Historical Sociology of Mental Illness.* Chicago: The University of Chicago Press, 1968.

873  Rosenberg, Harold. " 'The Idiot': second century." *The New Yorker*, October 5, 1968, pp. 159-81.

874  Ross, W. D. *Aristotle*, [reprinted]. New York: Meridian Books, 1959.

875  Roth, Walter E. *An Inquiry into the Animism and Folklore of the Guiana Indians.* Washington: Government Printing Office, 1915. [Thirtieth Annual Report of the Bureau of American Ethnology to the Secretary of the Smithsonian Institution, 1908-09, pp. 103-386.]

876  Rowley, William. *A Treatise on Female, Nervous, Hysterical, Hypochondriacal, Bilious, Convulsive Diseases; Apoplexy and Palsey; with Thoughts on Madness, Suicide, etc.* London, 1788.

877  Rudius, Eustachius. *De humani corporis affectibus . . .* Liber primus. Venice, 1590.

878  Rüsche, Franz. *Blut, Leben und Seele.* Paderborn: Schöningh, 1930. [Studien zur Geschichte und Kultur des Altertums, fünfter Ergänzungsband.]

879  Rufus of Ephesus. *Oeuvres de Rufus d'Éphèse,* ed. Daremberg-Ruelle. Paris, 1879.

880  Rulandus, Martinus. *Curationum empiricarum et historicarum . . . centuriae.* Basel, 1580 ff.

881  Ryan, Michael. *A Manuel of Medical Jurisprudence.* London, 1831.

882  Sadger, J. *Sleep Walking and Moon Walking, a Medico-Literary Study* (transl. by L. Brink). New York—Washington: Nervous and Mental Disease Publishing Company, 1920. [Nervous and Mental Diseases Monograph Series, 31.]

883  St. Hildegard. *Causae et curae,* ed. P. Kaiser. Leipzig: Teubner, 1903.

884  _____. *Heilkunde: Das Buch von dem Grund und Wesen und der Heilung der Krankheiten.* Übersetzt und erläutert von Heinrich Schipperges. Salzburg: Müller, 1957.

885  Samt, P. "Epileptische Irreseinsformen." *Archiv für Psychiatrie und Nervenkrankheiten* 5 (1875): 393-444, and 6 (1876): 110-216.

886  Sanct a Cruz, Antonio Ponze. *Praelectiones Vallisoletanae, in librum magni Hipp. Coi de morbo sacro.* Madrid, 1631.

887  Sanctorius, Sanctorius. *De statica medicina . . .* cum commentario Martini Lister. London, 1701.

888  Sarton, George. *Introduction to the History of Science,* 3 vols. Baltimore: Williams and Wilkins, 1927-47.

889  De Saussure, R. "Jehan Taxil, auteur du premier traité sur l'épilepsie écrit en langue française." *Bulletin de la Société Française d'Histoire de la Médecine* 29 (1935): 143-55.

890  Sauvages, Franc. Boissier de. *Nosologia methodica,* castigavit emendavit auxit etc. C. F. Daniel, t. III. Leipzig, 1795.

891  Savonarola, Joannes Michael. *Practica maior.* Venice, 1547.

892  Schenckius a Grafenberg, Joannes. *Observationum medicarum rariorum, libri VII.* Lyons, 1644.

893  Schiff, J. M. *Lehrbuch der Physiologie des Menschen, I. Muskel- und Nervenphysiologie.* Lahr, 1858-59.

894  Schiller, Francis. "Stilling's nuclei—turning point in basic neurology." *Bull. Hist. Med.* 43 (1969): 67-84.

895  _____. "The vicissitudes of the basal ganglia." *Bull. Hist. Med.* 41 (1967): 515-38.

896  Schöffler, Herbert. *Beiträge zur mittelenglischen Medizinliteratur.* Halle: Niemeyer, 1919. [Sächsische Forschungsinstitute in Leipzig, III. Anglistische Abteilung, 1.]

897  Schönbach, Anton E. *Studien zur Geschichte der altdeutschen Predigt.* Zweites Stück: Zeugnisse Bertholds von Regensburg zur Volkskunde.

Vienna, 1900. [S.B. der philosophisch-historischen Classe der Kaiserlichen Akademie der Wissenschaften. 142. Band, VII, Abh.]

898 *Scholia in Apollonium Rhodium vetera*, rec. C. Wendel, Berlin: Weidmann, 1935. [Bibliothecae Graecae et Latinae auctarium Weidmannianum, IV.]

899 *Scholia in Euripidem*, ed. E. Schwartz, vol. II. Berlin, 1891.

900 *Scholia in Sophoclis tragoedias*, e cod. ms. Laurentiano descr. P. Elmsley. Leipzig, 1826.

901 Schott, Gaspar. *Physica curiosa, sive mirabilia naturae et artis.* Würzburg, 1667.

902 Schroeder van der Kolk. *On the Minute Structure and Functions of the Spinal Cord and Medulla Oblongata, and on the Proximate Cause and Rational Treatment of Epilepsy*, transl. by W. D. Moore. London: The New Sydenham Society, 1859.

903 Schüle, Heinrich. *Handbuch der Geisteskrankheiten.*[2] Leipzig, 1880.

904 Schurigius, Martinus. *Chylologia historico-medica.* Dresden, 1725.

905 Schwenn. "Selene," *Pauly-Wissowa*, Zweite Reihe, Zweiter Band, 1923, cols. 1136–44.

906 Scot, Reginald. *The Discoverie of Witchcraft*, with an Introduction by the Rev. Montague Summers. [Suffolk] : John Rodker, 1930.

907 Scribonius Largus. *Conpositiones*, ed. G. Helmreich. Leipzig, 1887.

908 Seidelius, Jacobus. *De natura et causis epilepsiae theses* [praeside D. Thoma Erasto]. Heidelberg, 1573.

909 Semelaigne, René. *Les pionniers de la psychiatrie française, avant et après Pinel*, 2 vols. Paris: Baillière, 1930–32.

910 Seneca. *Moral Essays*, with an English transl. by J. W. Basore, vol. I. Loeb, 1928.

911 ———. *Tragedies*, with an English transl. by F. J. Miller, vol. I. Loeb, 1927.

912 Senn, G. *Die Entwicklung der biologischen Forschungsmethode in der Antike und ihre grundsätzliche Förderung durch Theophrast von Eresos.* Aarau: Sauerländer, 1933. [Veröffentlichungen der Schweizerischen Gesellschaft für Geschichte der Medizin und der Naturwissenschaften, VIII.]

913 Sennert, Daniel. *Opera omnia*, 3 vols. Paris, 1641.

914 Septalius, Ludovicus. *In librum Hippocratis Coi de aeribus aquis locis commentarii V.* Cologne, 1590.

915 Serapion, Joannes. *Necessarium ac perutile opus totius medicine practice, profundissimi ac antiquissimi Arabis domini Joannis filii Serapionis... Practica etiam brevis Domini Joannis Platearij Salernitani utilissima.* Venice, 1530.

916 Serenus, Quintus. *Liber medicinalis*, ed. F. Vollmer. Leipzig–Berlin: Teubner, 1916. [Corpus Medicorum Latinorum, II, 3.]

917 Servít, Zdeněk. "In memory of Jan Marek (Joannes Marcus Marci, 1595-1667) who stood at the origin of Czech epileptology," (Proceedings of the International Symposium on Comparative and Cellular Pathophysiology of Epilepsy, Liblice near Prague, September, 1965) *Excerpta medica International Congress Series* No. 124, 4–6.

918 ———. "Joannes Marcus Marci à Cronland (Jan Marek, 1595-1667)." *Acta historiae rerum naturalium necnon technicarum.* Prague, 1967, special issue 3, pp. 27–37.

919 Severinus, Marcus Aurelius. *De efficaci medicina libri III.* Frankfurt, 1671.

920 Sextus Empiricus. *Sextus Empiricus*, with an English transl. by R. G. Bury, 4 vols. Loeb, 1933–49.

921 Shanahan, William T. "History of the development of special institutions for epileptics in the United States." *Psychiatric Quarterly* 2 (1928): 422–34.

922 Shanks, Lewis Piaget. *Flaubert's Youth 1821–1845.* Baltimore: The Johns Hopkins Press, 1927.

923 Shrady, John (ed.). *The Medical Register of New York City, Brooklyn and Vicinity for the Year Commencing June 1, 1869,* vol. 7. New York, 1869.

924 Siegel, Rudolph E. *Galen's System of Physiology and Medicine,* Basel—New York: Karger, 1968.

925 Sieveking, Edward H. "Analysis of fifty-two cases of epilepsy observed by the author." *Lancet* (1) (1857): 527–28.

926 _____. *On Epilepsy and Epileptiform Seizures.* London, 1858.

927 Sigerist, Henry E. *Studien und Texte zur frühmittelalterlichen Rezept-literatur.* Leipzig: Barth, 1923. [Studien zur Geschichte der Medizin, 13.]

928 Silvaticus, Matheus. *Pandectarum opus.* Venice, 1524.

929 Simon, John. *General Pathology, as Conducive to the Establishment of Rational Principles for the Diagnosis and Treatment of Disease.* Philadelphia, 1852.

930 Slater, Eliot, Beard, A. W., and Glithero, Eric. "The schizophrenia-like psychoses of epilepsy." *British Journal of Psychiatry* 109 (1963): 95–150.

931 Smith, Stephen. "The surgical treatment of epilepsy, with statistical tables, comprising all the recorded cases of ligature of the carotid artery: and also of trephining the cranium by American surgeons." *New York Journal of Medicine* 8 (1852): 220–42.

932 Smith, Wesley D. "So-called possession in pre-Christian Greece." *Transactions and Proceedings of the American Philological Association.* 96 (1965): 403–26.

933 Sobhy, G. [editor]. *The Book of Al Dakhîra.* Cairo: Government Press, 1928.

934 Société médico-psychologique. "De l'épilepsie larvée." *Annales médico-psychologiques,* 5e série, 9 (1873): 139–53, 155–63, 281–300, 301, 490–91, 493–530; and 10: 97–153, 154–70, 297–312, 472–73.

935 Solmsen, Friedrich. "Greek philosophy and the discovery of the nerves." *Museum Helveticum* 18 (1961): 150–67 and 169–97.

936 Sommer, Wilhelm. "Erkrankung des Ammonshorns als aetiologisches Moment der Epilepsie." *Archiv für Psychiatrie und Nervenkrankheiten* 10 (1880): 631–75.

937 Soranus. *Soranus' Gynecology,* transl. by Owsei Temkin with the assistance of Nicholson J. Eastman, Ludwig Edelstein, and Alan F. Guttmacher. Baltimore: The Johns Hopkins Press, 1956.

938 _____. *Gynaeciorum libri IV,* ed. I. Ilberg. Leipzig—Berlin: Teubner, 1927. [C.M.G., IV.]

939 Soury, Jules. *Le système nerveux central, structure et fonction. Histoire critique des théories et des doctrines.* Paris, 1899.

940 Spachius, Israel. *Nomenclator scriptorum medicorum.* Frankfurt, 1591.

941 Spencer, Herbert. *The Principles of Psychology.* London, 1855.

942 _____. *The same,* second edition, 2 vols. New York, 1873.

943 "Spicelegia epileptica" (by J. H.) *Journal of Mental Science* 4 (1858): 437–44.

944 Spigelius, Adrianus. *De humani corporis fabrica libri decem.* Venice, 1627.

945 Spitaler, A. (Review of Alfred Siggel, Die indischen Bücher aus dem Paradies der Weisheit über die Medizin des 'Alī ibn Sahl Rabban aṭ-Ṭabarī) *Orientalistische Literaturzeitung* 48 (1953): cols. 529-36.

946 Sprengel, Kurt. *Versuch einer pragmatischen Geschichte der Arzneykunde,*[3] 5 vols. Halle, 1821-28.

947 Sprenger, A. *Das Leben und die Lehre des Mohammad,*[2] 1. Band. Berlin, 1869.

948 Stahl, Georg. Ern. *Theoria medica vera,* ed. L. Choulant, 3 vols. Leipzig, 1831-33. [Scriptorum classicorum de praxi medica nonullorum opera collecta, 14-16.]

949 _____. *Über den mannigfaltigen Einfluss von Gemütsbewegungen auf den menschlichen Körper* (Halle, 1695) [and other writings], Eingeleitet, ins Deutsche übertragen und erläutert von B. J. Gottlieb. Leipzig: Barth, 1961. [Sudhoffs Klassiker der Medizin, 36.]

950 Stahl, William Harris. "Moon madness." *Annals of Medical History,* new series, 9 (1937): 248-63.

951 Stannard, Jerry. "Materia medica and philosophic theory in Aretaeus." *Sudhoffs Archiv* 48 (1964): 27-53.

952 Steckerl, Fritz. *The Fragments of Praxagoras of Cos and His School.* Leiden: Brill, 1958. [Philosophia Antiqua, 8.]

953 Steeghius, Godefridus. *Ars medica.* Frankfurt, 1606.

954 Steinmeyer, Elias von. *Die kleineren althochdeutschen Sprachdenkmäler.* Berlin: Weidmann, 1916.

955 Steinschneider, M. "Constantinus Africanus und seine arabischen Quellen." *Virchows Arch.* 37 (1866): 351-410.

956 Stephanus, Robertus. *Dictionarium, seu Latinae linguae thesaurus.* Paris, 1531.

957 Stern, Arthur. "Zum Problem der Epilepsie des Paulus." *Psychiatria et Neurologia* 133 (1957): 276-84.

958 Stevens, Harold. "Jumping Frenchmen of Maine." *Archives of Neurology* 12 (1965): 311-14.

959 Stewart, F. Campbell. *The Hospitals and Surgeons of Paris.* New York— Philadelphia, 1843.

960 Sticker, Georg. "Hiera nousos," in: *Quellen und Studien zur Geschichte der Naturwissenschaften und der Medizin,* 3 (Heft 4) (1933): 139-50.

961 Stigter, D. "Boerhaave and epilepsy." *Janus* 6 (1901): 140-45 and 187-95.

962 Stollreiter-Butzon, Leonie. "Über die Epilepsie des Fürsten Myschkin." *Psyche* 15 (1961): 517-31.

963 Stookey, Byron. "Samuel Clossy, A.B., M.D., F.R.C.P. of Ireland." *Bull. Hist. Med.* 38 (1964): 153-67.

964 Streeter, Edward C. "A note on the history of the convulsive state prior to Boerhaave," in: *Epilepsy and the Convulsive State, an Investigation of the Most Recent Advances,* part I, pp. 5-29. Baltimore: Williams and Wilkins, 1931. [Association for Research in Nervous and Mental Diseases, 7.]

965 Strömgren, Erik. "Psychiatrische Genetik," in: *Psychiatrie der Gegenwart,* ed. by Gruhle et al. (436) I, 1 A, 1-69.

966 Strümpell, Adolf. *Lehrbuch der speciellen Pathologie und Therapie der inneren Krankheiten,*[2] Zweiter Band, erster Theil. Leipzig, 1885.

967 Sudhoff, Karl. *Ärztliches aus griechischen Papyrus-Urkunden.* Leipzig: Barth, 1909. [Studien zur Geschichte der Medizin, 5-6.]

968 _____. *Beiträge zur Geschichte der Chirurgie im Mittelalter*, 2 vols. Leipzig: Barth, 1914-18. [Studien zur Geschichte der Medizin, 10-12.]

969 _____. "Die acht ansteckenden Krankheiten einer angeblichen Baseler Ratsverordnung vom Jahre 1400," [reprinted in] *Sudhoffs Arch.* 21 (1929): 219-27.

970 _____. "Epilepsie," in: *Reallexicon der Vorgeschichte*, herausgegeben von Max Ebert, vol. 3, pp. 107-9. Berlin: de Gruyter, 1925.

971 _____. "Die Krankheiten *bennu* und *sibtu* der babylonisch-assyrischen Rechtsurkunden." *Sudhoffs Arch.* 4 (1911): 353-69.

972 _____. "Ein spätmittelalterliches Epileptikerheim (Isolier- und Pflegespital für Fallsüchtige) zu Rufach im Oberelsass." *Sudhoffs Arch.* 6 (1913): 449-55.

973 _____. "Eine deutsche Besegnung der Fallsucht aus dem 14. Jahrhundert." *Sudhoffs Arch.* 12 (1920): 191-92.

974 _____. *Iatromathematiker vornehmlich im 15. und 16. Jahrhundert.* Breslau: Kern, 1902. [Abh. zur Geschichte der Medizin, II.]

975 _____. "Magische Fallsuchtmittel." *Sudhoffs Arch.* 2 (1909): 383-84.

976 Sudhoff-Pagel. *Kurzes Handbuch der Geschichte der Medizin.*[3-4] Berlin: Karger, 1922.

977 *Suetonius*, with an English transl. by J. C. Rolfe, 2 vols. Loeb, 1964-65.

978 Suidas. *Lexicon*, ed. A. Adler, pars II. Leipzig: Teubner, 1931.

979 Surgeon-General. *Index Catalogue of the Library of the Surgeon-General's Office, United States Army.* Washington: Government Printing Office, 1880 ff.

980 "Surgery." *Lancet* (2) (1886): 346-47.

981 Sutphen, Morris C. "Magic in Theokritos and Vergil." *Studies in Honor of Basil L. Gildersleeve*, pp. 315-27. Baltimore: The Johns Hopkins Press, 1902.

982 Swieten, Gerard van. *The Commentaries Upon the Aphorisms of Dr. Herman Boerhaave*, transl. into English, vol. X. London, 1754.

983 Sydenham, Thomas. *Opera omnia*, ed. G. A. Greenhill. London: Sydenham Society, 1844.

984 Sylvius, Franciscus Deleboe. *Opera medica.* Geneva, 1693.

985 Sylvius, Jacobus. *Opera medica.* Geneva, 1635.

986 Symonds, Charles. "Classification of the epilepsies with particular reference to psychomotor seizures." *A.M.A. Archives of Neurology and Psychiatry* 72 (1954): 631-37.

987 "Symposium on reflex mechanism in the genesis of epilepsy." *Epilepsia*, fourth series, 3 (1962-63): 205-468.

988 Szondi, L. *Schicksalsanalytische Therapie.* Bern—Stuttgart: Huber, 1963.

989 Taine, H. *Les origines de la France contemporaine*, IX, Le régime moderne, t. 1.[25] Paris: Hachette, 1906.

990 Tamayo, Jacobus. *Singularis curatio affectus epileptici in praegnante faemina, ex cerebri cum male affecto, et primum patiente utero, consensu.* Hispali, 1610.

991 Tambornino, Julius. *De antiquorum daemonismo.* Giessen: Töpelmann, 1909. [Religionsgeschichtliche Versuche und Vorarbeiten VII, 3.]

992 Tanquerel des Planches, L. *Lead Diseases*, with notes and additions on the use of lead pipe and its substitutes, by Samuel L. Dana. Lowell, 1848.

993 Tarver, John Charles. *Gustave Flaubert as Seen in His Works and Correspondence.* Westminster, 1895.

994 Taxil, Jean. *Traicté de l'épilepsie, maladie vulgairement appellée au pays de Provence, la gouttete aux petits enfans.* Tournon, 1602.

995 Taylor, A. E. *A Commentary on Plato's Timaeus.* Oxford: The Clarendon Press, 1928.

996 Tellenbach, Hubertus (editor). "Epileptikergestalten Dostojewskijs, ein Seminar." *Jahrbuch für Psychologie Psychotherapie und medizinische Anthropologie,* 14(1) (1966): 1–68.

997 Temkin, Owsei. "Celsus 'On Medicine' and the ancient medical sects." *Bull. Hist. Med.* 3 (1935): 249–64.

998 ———. "The classical roots of Glisson's doctrine of irritation." *Bull. Hist. Med.* 38 (1964): 297–328.

999 ———. "The doctrine of epilepsy in the Hippocratic writings." *Bull. Hist. Med.* 1 (1933): 277–322.

1000 ———. "Epilepsy in an anonymous Greek work on acute and chronic diseases." *Bull. Hist. Med.* 4 (1936): 137–44.

1001 ———. "Guillaume Ader and his contribution to biblical medicine." *Bull. Hist. Med.* 5 (1937): 247–58.

1002 ———. "A medieval translation of Rhazes' clinical observations." *Bull. Hist. Med.* 12 (1942): 102–17.

1003 ———. "Remarks on the neurology of Gall and Spurzheim," in: E. Ashworth Underwood (ed.), *Science, Medicine and History,* pp. 282–89. London–New York–Toronto: Oxford U.P., vol. 2, 1953.

1004 ———. (Review of Ebbell's translation of the papyrus Ebers.) *Isis* 28 (1938): 126–31.

1005 Terry, Gladys C. *Fever and Psychoses. A Study of the Literature and Current Opinion on the Effects of Fever on Certain Psychoses and Epilepsy.* New York: Hoeber, 1939.

1006 Theodorus Priscianus. *Euporiston libri III,* ed. V. Rose. Leipzig, 1894.

1007 Theophanes. *Chronographia,* rec. C. Boor, 2 vols. Leipzig, 1883–85.

1008 Theophanes Nonnus. *Epitome de curatione morborum,* ed. I. S. Bernard, 2 vols. Gotha-Amsterdam, 1794–95.

1009 Theophilus Protospatharius. *De corporis humani fabrica libri V,* ed. G. A. Greenhill. Oxford, 1842.

1010 Theophrastus. *The Characters of Theophrastus,* ed. and transl. by J. M. Edmonds. Loeb, 1929.

1011 ———. *Theophrasti Eresii quae supersunt omnia,* ed. J. G. Schneider, t. I. Leipzig, 1818.

1012 Thomas Aquinas. "Commentaries on Aristotle's De somno et vigilia, De somniis, and De divinatione per somnum." *Opera,* ed. Parma, vol. 20, (reprinted 1949), pp. 215–44.

1013 ———. *Exposition suivie des Quatre Évangiles,* 8 vols., ed. J. Nicolai, transl. Em. Castan. Paris, 1854–55.

1014 ———. *Summa theologica,* rec. J. -P. Migne, 4 vols. Paris, 1872–77.

1014a Thomas, Henry. "The society of chymical physitians," in E. Ashworth Underwood (ed.), *Science, Medicine, and History,* pp. 56–71. London–New York–Toronto: Oxford U.P., vol. 2, 1953.

1015 Thomas, Robert. *The Modern Practice of Physic,* the third American, from the fourth London edition. New York, 1815.

1016 Thompson, R. Campbell. "Assyrian prescriptions for diseases of the urine, etc." *Babyloniaca* 14 (1934): 57–151.

1017 ———. "Assyrian prescriptions for the 'hand of a ghost'." *Journal of the Royal Asiatic Society* (1929): 801–23.

1018 _____. "A Babylonian explanatory text." *Ibid.* (1924): 452.

1019 Thomson, J. B. "The hereditary nature of crime." *Journal of Mental Science* 15 (1870): 487-98.

1020 Thorndike, Lynn. "Henri Bate on the occult and spiritualism." *Archives internationales d'histoire des sciences* 7 (1954): 133-40.

1021 _____. *A History of Magic and Experimental Science.* Vols. I-II, New York: Macmillan, 1923; vols. III-VIII, New York: Columbia U.P., 1934-58.

1022 Tissot, Simon André. *An Essay on Onanism*, transl. by A. Hume. Dublin, 1772. [In: *Three essays . . .* by S. A. Tissot, Dublin, 1772.]

1023 _____. *L'onanisme, dissertation sur les maladies produites par la masturbation*, nouvelle édition. Lausanne, 1782.

1024 _____. *Traité de l'épilepsie, faisant le tome troisième du traité des nerfs et de leurs maladies.* Paris, 1770.

1025 Tobler-Lommatzsch. *Altfranzösisches Wörterbuch.* Berlin: Weidmann, 1925 ff.

1026 Todd, Robert Bentley. "Clinical lecture on a case of renal epilepsy, and on the treatment of epilepsy in general." *Medical Times and Gazette*, new series, 9 (1854): 129-31 and 153-56.

1027 _____. *Clinical Lectures on Paralysis, Certain Diseases of the Brain, and Other Affections of the Nervous System.*[2] London, 1856.

1028 _____. The Lumleian lectures for 1849.—"On the pathology and treatment of convulsive diseases" [Review, probably by Carpenter]. *British and Foreign Medico-Chirurgical Review* 5 (1850): 1-36.

1029 _____. "Physiology of the nervous system," in: *The Cyclopaedia of Anatomy and Physiology*, vol. III. London, 1839-47.

1030 Todd, Robert Bentley, and Bowman, William. *The Physiological Anatomy and Physiology of Man.* Philadelphia, 1857.

1031 Trillerus, D. W. *Hippocrates atheismi falso accusatus.* Rudolstadt, 1719.

1032 Trousseau, A. *Clinique médicale de l'Hôtel-Dieu de Paris*,[3] t. II. Paris, 1868.

1033 Tuke, Daniel Hack. *Chapters in the History of the Insane in the British Isles.* London, 1882.

1034 _____. *Illustrations of the Influence of the Mind upon the Body in Health and Disease.*[2] Philadelphia, 1884.

1035 Turner, William Aldren. *Epilepsy, a Study of the Idiopathic Disease.* New York: Macmillan, 1907.

1036 Ueberweg, Friedrich. *Grundriss der Geschichte der Philosophie*, fünfter Teil, Die Philosophie des Auslandes vom Beginn des 19. Jahrhunderts bis auf die Gegenwart.[12] Herausgegeben von T. K. Oesterreich. Berlin: Mittler, 1928.

1037 "Una formola magica Bizantina." *Bessarione* 2 (1897): 374-88.

1038 Untzer, Matthias. Ιερονοσολογια chymiatrica. *Hoc est epilepsiae seu morbi sacri, accuratissima, juxta Hippocratico-Galenica atque Hermetica principia, descriptio.* Halle, 1616.

1039 Valescus de Tharanta. *Philonium.* Venice, 1523.

1040 Vallerie-Radot, Pierre. "Épilepsie et génie: vingt ans de la vie de Dostoievski (1837-1857)." *La Presse médicale* 64 (1956): 2065-66.

1041 Valleriola, Franciscus. *Enarrationum medicinalium libri sex.* Lyons, 1554.

1042 _____. *Observationum medicinalium lib. VI.* Lyons, 1588.

1043 Vallette, Paul. *L'apologie d'Apulée.* Paris: Klincksieck, 1908. [Thèse de Paris.]

1044 [Van Buren.] "Trephining in epilepsy." *Medical and Surgical Reporter* 5 (1860): 338.

1045 Van der Loos, H. *The Miracles of Jesus*. Leiden: Brill, 1956. [Supplements to Novum Testamentum, 9.]

1046 Veith, Ilza. *Hysteria, the History of a Disease*. Chicago—London: University of Chicago Press, 1965.

1047 Vettius Valens. *Anthologiarum libri*, ed. G. Kroll. Berlin: Weidmann, 1908.

1048 Vicq-d'Azyr. "Recherches sur la structure du cerveau, du cervelet, de la moelle alongée, de la moelle épinière; et sur l'origine des nerfs de l'homme et des animaux." *Histoire de l'Académie Royale des Sciences, Année 1781*, pp. 495–622. Paris, 1784.

1049 Viets, Henry R. "West Riding, 1871–1876." *Bull. Hist. Med.* 6 (1938): 477–87.

1050 Voegele, George E. and Dietze, Hans J. "An historical reflection on the medico-social aspects of epilepsy." *Delaware Medical Journal* 36 (1964): 131–36.

1051 Vogel, Paul. "Joh. Purkinjes Auffassung der Epilepsie." *Der Nervenarzt* 8 (1935): 228–32.

1051a ———. "Von der Selbstwahrnehmung der Epilepsie, der Fall Dostojewski." *Ibid.* 32 (1961): 438–41.

1052 De Vogüé, E. M. *The Russian Novel*, transl. by J. L. Edmands. Boston, 1887.

1053 Voisin, Aug. "Epilepsie," in: *Nouveau dictionnaire de médecine et de chirurgie pratiques*, t. 13. Paris, 1879.

1054 Von Storch, Edna P. and Theo. J. C. "Arnold of Villanova on epilepsy." *Annals of Medical History*, new series, 10 (1938): 251–60.

1055 Von Storch, T. C. "An essay on the history of epilepsy." *Ibid.*, new series, 2 (1930): 614–50.

1056 Wächter, Theodor. *Reinheitsvorschriften im griechischen Kult.* Giessen: Töpelmann, 1910. [Religionsgeschichtliche Versuche und Vorarbeiten IX, 1.]

1057 Walker, A. Earl. "The development of the concept of cerebral localization in the nineteenth century." *Bull. Hist. Med.* 31 (1957): 99–121.

1058 ———(ed.). *A History of Neurological Surgery*. Baltimore: Williams and Wilkins, 1951.

1059 ———. "A prospectus," in: Jasper, Herbert H.; Ward, Arthur A.; Pope, Alfred (editors), *Basic Mechanisms of the Epilepsies*, pp. 807–14. Boston: Little, Brown and Co., 1969.

1060 Walker, Nigel. *Crime and Insanity in England*, vol. 1. Edinburgh: U.P., 1968.

1061 Walshe, F. M. R. "The brain-stem conceived as the 'highest level' of function in the nervous system; with particular reference to the 'automatic apparatus' of Carpenter (1850) and to the 'centrencephalic integrating system' of Penfield." *Brain* 80 (1957): 510–39.

1062 ———. "Contributions of John Hughlings Jackson to neurology." *A.M.A. Archives of Neurology* 5 (1961): 119–31.

1063 ———. "Thoughts upon the equation of mind with brain." *Brain*, 76(1) (1953): 1–18.

1064 Waltershausen, Bodo Sartorius, Freiherr von. *Paracelsus am Eingang der deutschen Bildungsgeschichte*. Leipzig: Meiner, 1936. [Forschungen zur Geschichte der Philosophie und der Pädagogik, 16.]

1065 Walzer, Richard. *Greek into Arabic*. Cambridge: Harvard U.P., 1962.

1066 Watson, Gilbert. *Theriac and Mithridatium*. London: Wellcome Historical Medical Library, 1966.

1067 Watson, Thomas. *Lectures on the Principles and Practice of Physic*. Philadelphia, 1844.

1068  Watt, W. Montgomery. *Muhammad at Mecca*. Oxford: Clarendon, 1953.
1069  Wavell, Stewart; Butt, Audrey; and Epton, Nina. *Trances*. New York: Dutton, 1967.
1070  Weidlich, Theodor. *Die Sympathie in der antiken Litteratur*. Stuttgart, 1894. [Programm des Karls-Gymnasiums in Stuttgart z. Schlusse des Schuljahrs 1893-1894.]
1071  Weil, Gustav. *Mohammed der Prophet, sein Leben und seine Lehre*. Stuttgart, 1843.
1072  Weinreich, Otto. *Menekrates Zeus und Salmoneus*, Religionsgeschichtliche Studien zur Psychopathologie des Gottmenschentums in Antike und Neuzeit. Stuttgart: Kohlhammer, 1933. [Tübinger Beiträge zur Altertumswissenschaft, XVIII.]
1073  Weizsäcker, Viktor von. "Epileptische Erkrankungen, Organneurosen des Nervensystems und allgemeine Neurosenlehre," in: *J. von Mehring's Lehrbuch der inneren Medizin*,[16] herausgegeben von L. Krehl, 2. Band pp. 354-92. Jena: Fischer, 1929.
1074  Wellek, René (editor). *Dostoevsky, a Collection of Critical Essays*. Englewood Cliffs: Prentice-Hall, 1962.
1075  Wellhausen, J. *Reste arabischen Heidentums*.[2] Berlin, 1897.
1076  Wellmann, Max. "Erasistratos," *Pauly-Wissowa*, vol. 6 (1909): cols. 333-50.
1077  _____. *Die Fragmente der sikelischen Ärzte*. Berlin: Weidmann, 1901. [Fragmentsammlung der griechischen Ärzte, 1.]
1078  _____. *Hippokrates-Glossare*. Berlin: Springer, 1931. [Quellen und Studien zur Geschichte der Naturwissenschaften und der Medizin, 2.]
1079  _____. *Die pneumatische Schule bis auf Archigenes in ihrer Entwickelung dargestellt*. Berlin, 1895. [Philologische Untersuchungen, 14.]
1080  _____. "Die Schrift περὶ ἱρῆς νούσου des Corpus Hippocraticum." *Sudhoffs Arch.* 22 (1929): 290-312.
1081  _____. "Zu Herodots Schrift Περὶ τῶν ὀξέων καὶ χρονίων νοσημάτων." *Hermes* 48 (1913): 141-43.
1082  Wenger, O. "Geschichte der Epilepsie, ein Rückblick auf vier Jahrtausende." *Monatsschrift für Psychiatrie und Neurologie* 106 (1942): 163-216.
1083  Wenkebach, E. *Beiträge zur Textgeschichte der Epidemienkommentare Galens*, II. Teil. Berlin, 1928. [Abh. d. Preussischen Akademie d. Wissenschaften, Jahrg. 1928, Phil.-Hist. Klasse, Nr. 9.]
1084  Wepfer, Joh. Jacob. *Cicutae aquaticae historia et noxae*. Basel, 1679.
1085  _____. *Observationes medico-practicae de affectibus capitis internis et externis*.[2] Zurich, 1745.
1086  West, C. "Clitoridectomy." *British Medical Journal* (2) (1866): 585.
1087  West, W. J. "On a peculiar form of infantile convulsions." *Lancet* (1) (1841): 724-25.
1088  Westermann, W. L. "Sklaverei," *Pauly-Wissowa*, Supplementband VI (1935): cols. 894-1068.
1089  Westphal, C. "Die Agoraphobie, eine neuropathische Erscheinung." *Archiv für Psychiatrie und Nervenkrankheiten* 3 (1872): 138-61.
1090  _____. "Einige Beobachtungen über die epileptiformen und apoplectiformen Anfälle der paralytischen Geisteskranken mit Rücksicht auf die Körperwärme." *Ibid.* 1 (1868-69): 337-86.
1091  _____. "Tracheotomie bei Epilepsie." *Annalen des Charité-Krankenhauses*, neunter Band, 1. Heft, pp. 7-24. Berlin, 1860.
1092  Wettley, Annemarie. "Entartung und Erbsünde: Der Einfluss des medizinischen Entartungsbegriffs auf den literarischen Naturalismus." *Hochland* 51 (1959): 348-58.

1093 _____. "Hysterie, ärztliche Einbildung oder Wirklichkeit?" *Münchener medizinische Wochenschrift* 101 (1959): 193-96.

1094 Weyer, Johann. *De praestigiis daemonum, et incantationibus ac veneficiis libri sex.* Basel, 1583.

1095 _____. *Histoires, disputes et discours des illusions et impostures des diables*, 2 vols. Paris, 1885.

1096 Whiting, B. J. "A dramatic clyster." *Bull. Hist. Med.* 16 (1944): 511-13.

1097 Whytt, Robert. *The Works of Robert Whytt.* Edinburgh, 1768.

1098 Van der Wiel, C. Stalpartius. *Observationum rariorum . . . centuria prior.* Leiden, 1687.

1099 Wilamowitz-Moellendorff, Ulrich von. *Euripides Herakles*,[2] 2 vols. Berlin: Weidmann, 1895.

1100 _____. *Der Glaube der Hellenen*, I. Berlin: Weidmann, 1931.

1101 _____. *Griechisches Lesebuch*, I. Text, zweiter Halbband.[6] Berlin: Weidmann, 1926.

1102 _____. *Isyllos von Epidauros.* Berlin, 1886. [Philologische Untersuchungen, 9.]

1103 Wilks, Samuel. "Bromide and iodide of potassium in epilepsy. Cases and clinical remarks by Dr. Wilks." *Medical Times and Gazette* 2 (1861): 635-36.

1104 _____. *Lectures on Diseases of the Nervous System.*[2] Philadelphia, 1883.

1105 _____. "Observations on the pathology of some of the diseases of the nervous system." *Guy's Hospital Reports*, third series, 12 (1866): 152-244.

1106 Williams, Dennis. "Epilepsy." *Royal Institute of Public Health and Hygiene Journal* 30 (1967): 38-41.

1107 Willis, Thomas. *Dr. Willis' Practice of Physick, Being the Whole Works of That . . . Physician.* London, 1684.

1108 _____. *Opera omnia.* Amsterdam, 1682.

1109 Wittich, J. *Libellus de infantilium aegritudinum medicatione, Das ist: Artzneybüchlein wie man den armen Kinderlein für allerhand Leibs gebrechen vom Haupt an biss auff die Fussohle helffen und rathen soll.* Leipzig, 1607.

1110 Wood, George B. *A Treatise on the Practice of Medicine*,[2] vol. II. Philadelphia, 1849.

1111 Wülfing-v. Martitz, Peter. " Ἱερός bei Homer und in der älteren griechischen Literatur." *Glotta* 38 (1960): 272-307; 39 (1961): 24-43.

1112 Yarmolinsky, Avrahm. *Dostoevsky.* New York: Harcourt, Brace, 1934.

1113 Young, Robert M. "The functions of the brain: Gall to Ferrier (1808-1886)." *Isis* 59 (1968): 251-68.

1114 _____. *Mind, Brain and Adaptation in the Nineteenth Century.* Oxford: Clarendon Press, 1970.

1115 Zacchias, Paulus. *Quaestionum medico-legalium tomi tres*, editio nova . . . cura J. D. Horstii. Frankfurt, 1666.

1116 Zacutus Lusitanus. *Historiarum medicarum libri sex*,[2] t. I. Amsterdam, 1637.

1117 Zilboorg, Gregory, and Henry, George, W. *A History of Medical Psychology.* New York: Norton, 1941.

1118 Zimmermann, J. G. *Dissertatio physiologica de irritabilitate.* Göttingen, 1751.

1119 Zola, Emile. "La bête humaine," in: *Les Rougon-Macquart*, vol. IV, études, notes et variantes par Henri Mitterand. Paris: Bibliothèque de la Pléiade, 1966.

1120 Zweig, Stefan. *Drei Meister, Balzac, Dickens, Dostojewski.* Leipzig: Insel, 1922.

# Index of
# Personal Names

Abt, Adam, 12, 13, 48
Abulqasim, 102, 106, 107, 140, 159, 185, 233, 235
Açaravius. *See* Abulqasim
Ackerknecht, Erwin H., viii, 144, 238, 257, 317, 365, 373
Adam, 113, 175–76
Adamantius, 39
Adams, Francis, 7, 9, 32, 36, 39, 42, 43, 44, 65, 69, 76, 89, 155, 348
Adie, W. J., 250
Aelianus, Claudius, 25
Aetius of Amida, 43, 64, 77, 80
Agatharchides, 155
Agilon, Walter, 105, 107, 127, 140
Agricola, Georg, 164, 181
Agricola, Johann, 8
Agrippa of Nettesheim, 160–61
Ahrens, Karl, 152
'Ā'isha, 152
Ajax, 161
Alajouanine, T., 373, 376, 377, 393
Albers, 321
Alberti, Michael, 133, 168
Albertus Magnus, 131, 194
Albich, Siegmund, 116
Albright, W. F., xi
Alcmaeon, 5, 54
Aldrovandi, Ulysses, 178–80
Alexander, *the Great*, 380
Alexander of Aphrodisias, 26
Alexander of Tralles, 13, 22, 25, 26, 39, 64, 77
Alexida, 14
Al-Fārābī, 148
Alī Ibn Abbās, 102, 122, 125, 127, 131
Alī b. Rabban al-Ṭabarī, 151
Allbutt, T. Clifford, 370
Alsarius a Cruce Genuense, Vincentius, 138–39, 248
Althaus, Julius, 298
Amacher, M. Peter, 328
Amphiaraus, 14
Anderson, James, 345
Andrae, Tor, 151
Andrée, 225
Anonymus Christianus, 95
Anonymus Parisinus, 5, 36, 40, 41, 42, 45, 46, 74

Anstie, Francis E., 343
Antheia, 165
Antyllus, 26
Apollo, 15, 18
Apollodorus, 21
Apollonius, 10
Apollonius Rhodius, 19
Appian, 162
Apuleius, 6, 7, 8, 9, 21, 35, 44, 48, 49, 59–60, 85, 144, 155
Arago, 264, 265
Arbesmann, P. R., 11
Archelaus, 12, 13, 14
Archer, John Clark, 152, 153
Arderne, John of, 111, 112
Ares, 15
Aretaeus, 7, 9, 20, 28, 32, 36, 38–39, 40–41, 42, 43, 44, 45, 50, 59, 60, 65, 68–69, 76, 77, 78, 89, 155, 218, 305, 317
Aristophanes, 19
Aristotle, 12, 21, 22, 34, 44, 45, 52, 55, 59, 60, 87, 90, 116, 121, 127, 128, 138, 150, 154, 155, 156, 157, 158, 161, 167
Arnald of Villanova, 104, 122, 123, 124, 164, 165, 171, 233, 297
Artemidorus Daldianus, 11
Artemis, 6, 16, 18
Artemon, 23
Artephius, 179
Asclepiades, 36, 57, 67
Asclepius, 14, 18, 47
Ashwin, E. A., 139, 142
Athenaeus, 17
Audi, Barbara, viii
Auerbach, Erich, 98
Augustinus, 85, 158, 160
Aulus Gellius. *See* Gellius, Aulus
Aussoleil, *Dr.*, 359
Averroës, 128–30, 160
Avicenna, 102, 115, 122, 125, 126, 127, 128, 142, 156, 187, 189

Baal, 89, 149
Babbitt, Irving, 378
Bacchus, 16
Bacon, *Dr.*, 231–32

445

# Index to Subjects

THE JOHNS HOPKINS PRESS

Composed in Baskerville text with Univers display
by Jones Composition Company

Printed on 60-lb. Sebago, MF, Regular
by Universal Lithographers, Inc.

Bound in Joanna Kennett, #39450
by L. H. Jenkins, Inc.